McGraw-Hill's **RadReviewEasy**
Internet Subscription Access Number

McGraw-Hill
LANGE Q&A

- Better than a CD, the electronic tests that you depend on to prepare for the ARRT exam are now online. Access is included with this book, nothing more to buy.
- Now you can use either Mac or PC!
- With in-depth test results, you can hone in on subject weaknesses!
- Practice in an online setting that simulates the ARRT exam interface!
- Compare your scores to other test takers!

SCRATCH OFF*
your registation code.

*NOTE: This book cannot be returned once label is scratched off.

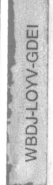

WBDJ-LOYV-GDEI

To Access **RadReviewEasy:**

1 Open a web browser and go to http://register.radrevieweasy.com

2 Enter your unique registration code in the space provided. You must enter the entire code as it appears in the scratch off box when you register. This code can be used only once.

3 After you have entered your registration code, click on the "Register" button to continue the registration process.

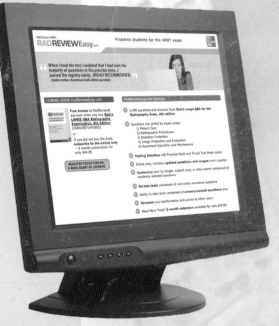

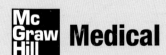

P/N 0-07-146325-9 of set 0-07-144166-2,
and set 0-07-110296-5
Lange Q&A for the Radiography Examination • SAIA

SIXTH EDITION

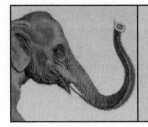

LANGE Q&A™

RADIOGRAPHY EXAMINATION

(handwritten notes)
1800 656 2575
ADHD
free Road map
to success
www.FreetriplescoresS.com
Credit report
Revlon age define makeup

D.A. Saia, MA, RT(R) (M)
Director, Radiography Program
Stamford Hospital
Stamford, Connecticut

McGraw-Hill
Medical Publishing Division

New York   Chicago   San Francisco   Lisbon   London
Madrid   Mexico City   New Delhi
San Juan   Seoul   Singapore   Sydney   Toronto

Lange Q&A™ for the Radiography Examination, Sixth Edition

2 3 4 5 6 7 8 9 0 QPD/QPD 0 9 8 7 6

Book ISBN 0-07-146324-0; Internet Access Code Card ISBN 0-07-146325-9; Set ISBN 0-07-144166-2

Notice

Medicine is an ever-changing science. As new research and clinical experience broaden our knowledge, changes in treatment and drug therapy are required. The authors and the publisher of this work have checked with sources believed to be reliable in their efforts to provide information that is complete and generally in accord with the standards accepted at the time of publication. However, in view of the possibility of human error or changes in medical sciences, neither the authors nor the publisher nor any other party who has been involved in the preparation or publication of this work warrants that the information contained herein is in every respect accurate or complete, and they disclaim all responsibility for any errors or omissions or for the results obtained from use of the information contained in this work. Readers are encouraged to confirm the information contained herein with other sources. For example and in particular, readers are advised to check the product information sheet included in the package of each drug they plan to administer to be certain that the information contained in this work is accurate and that changes have not been made in the recommended dose or in the contraindications for administration. This recommendation is of particular importance in connection with new or infrequently used drugs.

This book was set in Palatino by Techbooks.
The editors were Michael Brown and Christie Naglieri.
The production supervisor was Sherri Souffrance.
Project management was provided by Techbooks.
The cover designer was Aimee Nordin.
Quebecor World Dubuque was the printer and binder.

This book is printed on acid-free paper.

Library of Congress Cataloging-in-Publication Data

Saia, D. A. (Dorothy A.)
  Lange Q & A for the radiography examination / Dorothy A. Saia.—6th ed.
    p. ; cm. — (Appleton & Lange reviews)
  Rev. ed. of: Appleton & Lange review for the radiography exam. 5th ed. 2003.
  Includes bibliographical references and index.
  ISBN 0-07-144166-2 (softcover)
 1. Radiography, Medical—Examinations, questions, etc.
  [DNLM: 1. Radiography—Examination Questions. 2. Technology, Radiologic—Examination Questions. WN 18.2 S132L 2005] I. Title: Q & A for the radiography examination. II. Saia, D. A. (Dorothy A.). Appleton & Lange review for the radiography exam. III. Title. IV. Appleton & Lange's review series.
  RC78.15.S25 2003
  616.07′572′076—dc22

                                                                        2005050504

Please tell the author and publisher what you think of this book by sending your comments to radtech@mcgraw-hill.com. Please put the author and title of this book in the subject line.

International Edition Book ISBN 0-07-110516-6; Internet Access Code Card ISBN 0-07-146325-9; Set ISBN 0-07-110296-5 Copyright © 2006. Exclusive rights by The McGraw-Hill Companies, Inc. for manufacture and export. This book may not be re-exported from the country to which it is consigned by McGraw-Hill. The International Edition is not available in North America.

Contents

With love to Tony

Reviewers

Jacqueline M. Kralik, BAS, RT(R)(CT)(MR)
Radiography Program Director
Pima Medical Institute
Seattle, Washington

Wanda E. Wesolowski, RT, MAEd
Professor/Diagnostic Medical Imaging Program
Community College of Philadelphia
Philadelphia, Pennsylvania

To the Student

Your feedback on the previous five editions of this book has been encouraging; I appreciate all the comments and suggestions I have received. I hope that all who use this book, educators and students alike, will continue to provide me with their input in order that this book may continue to meet their needs. I invite and encourage you to contact me at dsaia@stamhealth.org with comments, questions, and suggestions for future editions. This sixth edition contains new and revised material to reflect changes to the ARRT Content Specifications implemented January 2005. It includes questions on Digital/Electronic Imaging including computed and direct digital radiography. Also included is processing of electronic images including their acquisition, manipulation, and exposure indication.

New to this edition is our *RadReviewEasy.com* website. I am very excited about this additional tool. RadReviewEasy.com is a powerful website that includes all the questions and answers from this book *and more!* New questions and answers will be added regularly.

RadReviewEasy.com lets you:

- customize your review by length
- customize your review by exam subject area
- customize your review by specific subcategory
- take simulated certification exams
- compare your score to other students using the site

The website affords the student an opportunity to practice CBT prior to taking the computerized ARRT examination. This edition also addresses the ARRT's most recent revision of the *Conventions Specific to the Radiography Examination.*

I am sure you realize that a review book is not intended to be a "quick fix" preparation for the certification examination administered by the ARRT. It takes at least two years of didactic instruction and testing, and hours of clinical practice, to prepare oneself as an entry-level radiographer. During about the last four months of radiography education, the Registry ("R-word") becomes a new and more horrific reality. Confident, competent, even cavalier students suddenly become sober when the "R-word" is mentioned. They begin to question all they ever felt confident about. If you use this book the way it is designed to be used, and perhaps in conjunction with its companion book, *Radiography PREP (Program Review and Examination Preparation),* you should be able to set aside any fears you may have.

I believe that proper use of the materials presented here and online will help you overcome your anxieties. First, read the introductory section carefully. It presents proven, sensible suggestions to help improve test-taking performance. It elaborates on simple processes to help selection of the correct answer, and several methods and strategies that may be employed while taking "the" test. Probably the most important key to reducing apprehension is to reduce the unknowns to the fewest number. You will also find an introduction to CBT with a description of what to expect, and helpful hints to enhance preparation and reduce anxiety. Secondly, the format and content of the book and its new companion website RadReviewEasy.com have been specially designed in many ways to provide focus and direction for your review, and thus to help you do your very best on your certification examination. The ARRT has no secrets and springs no surprises on you. Just as your instructors have made known what is expected of you during your education, the ARRT has made known the content, question format, and terminology used on the certification examination. Each educational program receives the ARRT newsletter, *Educator Update,* and each program director receives the *ARRT Educator's Handbook.* The newsletter is published regularly by the ARRT and functions to keep educators and students current on the activities and policies of the ARRT. The *Educator's Handbook* is also published by the ARRT and serves as a source for general information, policies and procedures, and reprints of a number of documents, including *Content Specifications for the Examination in Radiography, Conventions Specific to the Radiography Examination,* and *Standard Terminology for Positioning and Protection.* These documents are revised periodically and advise educators of terminology, categories, content, and approximate weight of content areas on the ARRT examination. Although the *Content Specifications* by no means serves as a comprehensive radiography curriculum, it does serve as a suitable guide for examination review and preparation. It makes sense to design a review book in which the content, question format, and terminology is similar to that which students can expect to find on their certification examination.

The number of questions found in each chapter is proportional to the number found in that category on the ARRT examination. The questions are designed to test your problem-solving skills and your ability to integrate facts that fit the situation.

Most important and practical, I believe, are the detailed explanations found at the end of each chapter. By themselves, the explanations are good reviews of essential material; they provide a "mini-lecture" for each question. Use them to confirm your correct answers and to better understand your weaker areas. You will see that most explanations will tell you not only why the correct answer is correct, but also why the other answer choices (distractors) are incorrect.

Once you have finished reviewing the first five chapters, set aside special time for the practice tests in Chapters 6 and 7. Try to simulate the actual examination environment as much as possible. Choose a quiet place free from distractions and interruptions, gather the necessary materials, and arrange to be uninterrupted for up to three hours.

In summary, use this book as recommended to help ease your precertification exam jitters. Excessive anxiety can impair clear thinking and lower your score. Avoiding excessive stress can improve your concentration and information retrieval process. Remember, you have been well prepared by your program director and instructors, and you have studied and worked hard for at least two years. So follow the advice found in the Introduction: prepare yourself sensibly, and keep a positive attitude. I wish you good luck and much happiness in your radiography career!

D.A. Saia

Acknowledgments

I would like to recognize and express my sincere appreciation to those who again have been so helpful and supportive during the preparation of this sixth edition.

The assistance offered by Courtney Kraemer and Tom Belmont of Fuji Medical Systems USA is greatly appreciated. A very special note of thanks goes to George Spahn, also of Fuji Medical Systems USA, for returning calls, patiently answering questions, and sharing his immense expertise. His participation in this sixth edition of the book (as in the first edition) is greatly appreciated.

Many of the images are reproduced through the courtesy of Stamford Hospital, Department of Radiology. Many of the images in Chapter 4, Image Production and Evaluation, have been reproduced courtesy of the American College of Radiology.

Thank you to Mr. Joel R. Schenck, Marketing Product Manager of RMI, for permission to reproduce the mammographic phantom image found in Chapter 4. I wish to express appreciation again to the Dunlee Corporation, and their Marketing Manager, Mr. Roger Flees, for his assistance in granting permission to reproduce various tube rating charts. I am grateful to the professional staff of McGraw-Hill, with special notes of appreciation to Michael Brown, Christie Naglieri, Karen Edmonson, and Jack Farrell and to my terrific Project Manager, Seema Koul, for their support and assistance. Everyone at McGraw-Hill has been helpful in the development of this project; it is always a pleasure to work with their creative and skilled staff.

I greatly appreciate the suggestions and expertise shared with me by the professionals who reviewed this project. Jacqueline M. Kralik, BAS, RT(R)(CT)(MR) and Wanda E. Wesolowski, RT, MAEd were thorough and timely, and a pleasure to work with.

Special and fond recognition goes to my coworker Olive Peart, MS, RT(R)(M) for her generous support day-to-day and through the preparation of this project.

Appreciative and affectionate acknowledgment is sent to my students, particularly my class of 2006: Richard, Nickol, Micheal, LeeAnn, Minh, Al, Beth, Ron, and Deog—and all students—past, present, and those still to come. Their questions, enthusiasm, and desire to learn make my job a most pleasant task and served as the original stimulation for the preparation of this text.

I would like to accord special acknowledgment to two of my graduates Daniel DiPaola, RT(R) and Racheal Bennette, RT(R), as well as Jeff Lesnikoski, RT(R) for their willingness to help with the development and proofing of our new companion website, saiaradreview.com.

Finally and most especially, a loving message of appreciation goes to my husband Tony. His love, understanding, and encouragement are invaluable and deeply appreciated throughout the preparation of this edition.

Introduction

Completion of the American Registry of Radiologic Technologists (ARRT) radiography certification examination is often a high point in the career of a radiologic professional. Certification indicates that the individual has acquired a recognized level of knowledge and expertise and is qualified to deliver ionizing radiation in the performance of medical diagnostic testing. On what does success or failure depend?

Relax! It isn't as bad as it seems! As the student radiographer nears graduation, there is, understandably, an anxiety that begins to grow. It is a time when you wonder if you are smart enough and if you are skillful enough. Although there will always be room for growth, these concerns arise from the realization that an important landmark has been reached. Formal education will soon be at an end—no more written examinations, no more competencies to complete. You will be on your own, proclaimed competent. How will you perform on the certification examination? How will you perform in the clinical arena? These are indeed sobering thoughts.

I believe that proper use of the materials presented here will help you overcome your anxieties. You will find several easy and effective suggestions for intelligent preparation and test taking. The suggestions are proven, sensible recommendations to help improve test-taking performance. Special focus has been placed on suggestions for the ARRT computer-based testing (CBT) system. They elaborate on simple processes to help in selection of the correct answer, and several methods and strategies that may be employed while taking your certification examination. Probably the most important key to reducing apprehension is to reduce the unknowns to the fewest number.

You will find the format and content of this review book is very helpful and is specially designed to provide focus and direction for your review, thus helping you do your very best on the certification examination. The ARRT has no secrets and springs no suprises on you. Just as your instructors have made known what is expected of you during your education, the ARRT has made known the content, question format, and terminology used on the certification examination. The following are some tried-and-true tips and strategies for test taking in general, and specifics to help you through CBT. The later sections on Preparing for Success in CBT, Test-Taking Strategies, and Practice Tests will be particularly useful.

HOW THIS BOOK IS ORGANIZED

There are three primary sections in this book: a topic-by-topic review with 1,000 exam-type questions and paragraph-length explanations; two 200-question practice tests, also with paragraph-length explanations; and this Introduction, which includes information necessary to help you get the most out of the book and to do your best on the CBT system.

This is a current book of practice questions that are designed to mimic actual test questions. Additionally, the new companion website saiaradreview. com. has these and additional questions and answers for further practice in simulated certification conditions.

In summary, this book will provide you, the student, with a review that will better enable you to simulate and prepare for the certification exam by providing an excellent and comprehensive review of radiography.

ABOUT THE EXAMINATION

ARRT examinations are administered via computer. Candidates are presented with multiple-choice questions on a computer screen and directed to select an answer using either the keyboard or a mouse. The process allows candidates to review or change any answers to any questions prior to submitting the completed examination for scoring.

A tutorial is offered at the beginning of each examination that allows the candidate to answer several practice questions. This ensures that the candidate is thoroughly familiar with the process.

Radiography	200	20	220	3.5

The national certification examination for radiography is a standardized test administered by the American Registry of Radiologic Technologists and includes 220 multiple-choice questions; 200 questions are scored, 20 questions are unidentified pilot questions. The time allotted for the test is 3 ½ hours; passing score is 75 percent.

Beginning January 2000, the ARRT discontinued paper and pencil testing and began to use computer-based testing (CBT) for the administration of its radiography examinations. Pearson VUE testing centers will administer the ARRT exam. There is postmarking deadline for ARRT applications for CBT. Applicants may apply for the examination prior to graduation, but will schedule their examination date within an assigned 90-day window that starts at graduation. To gain admittance to the test center, the candidate must show two current identifications; at least one must show a photo, and both must show signatures. Positive identification will include fingerprinting at the test site. A four-function non-programmable calculator will be given to the examinee upon request. A tutorial of practice questions is offered at the start of the examination. This helps the candidate become familiar with the testing process. Test questions are administered in random order; that is, they are not grouped together by subject (and that is the way the two practice tests in this book are designed). Multiple-choice questions are presented with on the computer screen and the candidate is directed to select the best answer—the mouse or keyboard may be used. The candidate is permitted to review or change answers to questions before indicating that he/she is finished with the examination.

You will find much more information on CBT as you read through this Introduction and, in particular, in the section entitled *TEST-TAKING STRATEGIES.*

STRATEGIES FOR STUDYING AND TEST TAKING

The purpose of a test strategy is to make the most of your knowledge, although no strategy, however elaborate, can help you if you don't know your subject.

A good test strategy can do the following:

(1) prevent you from making mistakes
(2) help you to use your time efficiently
(3) improve your odds of getting the right answer.

The single most important trait of a good test strategy is *simplicity.* There are two ways to make and keep a procedure simple. The first way is to design it to be simple. The second is to practice the procedure as it is designed. The second part is up to you. If you use the following test strategies (particularly the elimination strategy) while using this review book, the strategies will become second nature to you, and you can then concentrate all your attention on passing your certification exam.

PREPARING FOR THE EXAM

Designing a Study Schedule
It is important to establish a routine study schedule. This schedule should allow you to study at a time when you are at your optimum. Some students are more alert in the morning for this kind of work, while others have better success in the afternoon. It would not be a good plan to try and study late at night after a full day unless this is an optimum time for you.

There are several advantages to designing a schedule. The first is that it forces you to face the reality of your study load. Many students underplay the amount of time it will take to complete a thorough study, and this can adversely affect performance. If you write out a schedule that includes both your daily responsibilities and the time you need to study, you will have a sense of the pace needed to complete your review.

The second advantage to designing a schedule is that it will allow you to increase your concentration because the schedule defines the allotted amount of time for each topic you need to cover. Otherwise, a lot of time can be wasted in determining what to study during each session.

Setting up a Study Plan

After completing the best of radiography programs, even the best of students will have gaps in his or her knowledge, subjects that were somehow missed or forgotten, or that will not come to mind when needed. These gaps in your knowledge are often small; but since one piece of information often builds upon other pieces, a small gap in your knowledge can sometimes lead to a large drop in your test score. The best way to get around this problem is to use a well-defined study plan. Listed below are two alternative plans for you to consider. The first is *diagnosis and remediation*, and the second is "*SQ3R.*"

Diagnosis and Remediation

This is a two-step approach: *diagnosis* (finding out what you do not know), and *remediation* (learning the material).

Diagnosis. Many students graduate from their programs without a good idea of what they do or do not know. Fortunately, this book has been designed to make diagnosis simple. By following the steps listed below, you will know what you need to learn before you take the certifying examination.

Step 1. Begin with Chapter 1, Patient Care, or any of the other first five chapters. Go through the questions in one sitting, making the experience as similar to the actual exam as possible. Remember to practice test strategies while answering the questions. This will produce a more valid diagnosis.

While taking the test, you should note or highlight words and phrases from the questions that you do not understand. After you have finished the questions (but before you have graded your work) make a list of the terms you noted and the numbers of the questions that contained them.

Step 2. Analyze your results. Read the answers and make a list of the questions you missed. Compare this list with the subspecialty list at the end of the chapter. This will tell you if you are weak in a particular area. Once you have defined an area of weakness, pay special attention to the explanations provided. If the answer is still unclear, use the exact page references to your textbook for further study.

Anytime you go through your work, picking out and correcting your mistakes, you will gain a greater understanding of your strengths and weaknesses. However, by approaching the analysis systematically, the improvement can be dramatic. Concentrate on your areas of weakness, but be sure to read all the explanations at least once. This will allow you to compare your reasoning on right and wrong answers and to check for the possibility that you put down the right answer for the wrong reason.

Step 3. Repeat the process. The purpose of this study plan is to get important information into your long-term memory. The best way to ensure this is to begin your study plan early enough to allow yourself time to repeat your chapter study one more time before the examination. Keep and compare your results from each review and focus on any weaknesses still apparent from the comparison.

Remediation

Step 1. Read and cross-read. Starting with the subspecialty that you missed most often, make a reading list. For those areas in which you missed three or four questions, a single reference will probably be enough, but if you missed more than four, you should cross-read to cover the same information in more than one text. (You might also want to review these topics in your old class notes.)

When you study from texts, use the index and the table of contents to find the section you need. If you are using more than one text, compare and look for common ideas. Sometimes, writing a summary of your reading helps to clarify the information. This technique has been proven to improve retention and understanding, but it can be time consuming.

Step 2. Once you have finished your reading, go back to the questions that you missed. If they still aren't clear, consult an expert. Most students are reluctant to approach an instructor with a question that doesn't relate directly to a class. However, most instructors are glad to answer questions that will improve the chances for their students to obtain a high passing score on the certification examination. Instructors appreciate questions that are specific, well thought out, and which show that the student has done some independent work.

SQ3R

The second method for study is best suited for reviewing your textbooks for further study once you have identified a weakness. It is called the SQ3R and is presented by Frances P. Robinson in his book *Effective Study*. It makes study reading more efficient and long-term remembering more probable. *SQ3R* stands for *Survey, Question, Read, Recite,* and *Review*. The steps are as follows:

Survey. First, skim through an entire chapter.

1. Think about the title of the chapter. What do you already know about the subject? Write ideas in the margins. Read the conclusion. What better way is there to discover the main ideas of a chapter?
2. Read the headings. These are the main topics that have been developed by the author.
3. Read the captions under the diagrams, charts, and graphs.

Allow approximately 10 to 12 minutes for the survey step. Surveying will help increase your focus and interest in the material.

Question. Write out two or three questions relating to each heading. These should be questions that you believe will be answered within each section. Use the "who, what, when, where, why, and how" application when generating these questions.

Read. Now read the first section. Keep in mind the questions you have created and read, with a purpose, as quickly as possible.

Recite. At the end of the section, look away from the book for a few seconds. Recite and think about what you've just learned. It is best to recite aloud because hearing the information will help increase your memorization.

Review. Reviewing is a key step if you want to retain the material you've read. Reviewing as you study results in less time needed for test preparation.

Learning to utilize the SQ3R method is a skill that takes practice. Often, students feel that it takes too long and is too complicated, but its use results in an increase in comprehension, interest, and memorization. The SQ3R method allows you to study at the same time that you are doing your course reading.

Summary

Everyone does not have the same learning style, and, as a result, effective study techniques are not the same for everyone. It is important to choose the method that is best for you, and this will take some experimentation. For instance, some students become frustrated when they cannot comprehend the textbook material while reading when seated at a desk. Sometimes, just getting up and pacing while memorizing can facilitate the learning process if you are having trouble at your desk. Other students learn faster with audio aids. If these are available to you and you are having trouble with learning just from your books, it may be worth the experiment to see if hearing the material will enhance your learning.

Study Groups

While preparing for an examination, properly organizing or attending a study group can be extremely helpful. However, a study group needs to be very focused with a specific agenda for each session. Otherwise, it can be a time waster. Listed below are some important points to keep in mind when organizing and conducting a study group:

1. Limit the group size to four or five people.
2. Select classmates who share your academic goals.
3. Meet the first time to discuss the meeting times, meeting place, and group goals.
4. Select a group leader and time keeper. The group should meet for 2 to 3 hours for each session to ensure a thorough review.
5. Establish an agenda for each meeting that specifies the topics of discussion. This will save time and lend focus to the group. It ensures that the group reviews all pertinent topics by slotting time for all areas.
6. Establish group norms that define how the group will act. This would include things such as getting there on time, being prepared, and ending on time. It is important to emphasize that all members must do their fair share of the work for the group to gain the maximum benefit.

Study groups are used to review and compare both lecture and reading notes, to review textbook information together, and to review examination topics. Group sessions are a good time to review the question types used on the certification examination, to discuss test-taking strategies, to help each other design study plans, and to drill or review together all material expected to be on the examination.

The support of a study group is extremely helpful in building self-confidence and in overall preparation for examinations. They are not intended to replace individual study time, but serve as a supplement. If properly utilized, study groups are an enormous asset for test preparation. Finally, when working within a group, many students are more likely to exert their best effort because they are accountable to the other members of the group.

Practice Tests

The practice tests (Chapter 6 and 7) can be used in one of the following two ways: (1) as a way of determining strengths and weaknesses before you go through the review book, or (2) as a final preparation for the test after you have done your chapter- by-chapter review.

The practice tests have been designed in an effort to duplicate the experience of taking the certification examination. CBT administers test questions in *random order,* questions are not ordered according to topic. Therefore, the practice test questions in this book are in randomized sequence—just as you will find questions presented on the ARRT CBT. Taking the practice tests, and using the companion website, will make the process more familiar, so you won't be as nervous when you face the real test. The practice test will help you to determine whether or not you are answering the questions quickly enough, and whether your score is high enough to pass. In summary, the practice tests simply give you a chance to practice. Using these materials, and the new companion website, will give you the opportunity to practice for the ARRT CBT examination.

TEST-TAKING STRATEGIES

Time Management

Keeping track of your time and progress is harder than it might first appear. Most of us have been surprised while taking a test by how little time was left. This experience is even more upsetting in the middle of a certification exam. Knowing when there is a problem and knowing what to do about it are the objectives of time management.

Even with your eye on the clock, calculating the time you have left is not always easy. On the radiography examination, you have 3 ½ hours to finish 220 questions. That gives you about 57 seconds (0.9 minute) per question. In other words, you have to answer approximately 66 questions per hour.

Another way to look at this is by breaking the time into two blocks. If, when you are halfway through the allotted examination time, you have finished a minimum of 110 questions, you are working on time. However, there is one additional complication. Not all questions require equal time to work. It is quite possible to run across a string of difficult questions early in the test and fall behind, then make up the time with easy questions later in the test. For this reason, being a few questions short at the halfway mark is not a cause for concern. However, if you have finished significantly less than 110 questions after 90 minutes, you may be starting to fall behind.

If you do fall behind, what can you do to catch up? Sometimes, simply seeing that you are behind and trying to work faster will be enough to motivate you to catch up. If not, you have other options. Try to read through the questions and answers faster. If you have checked only one answer as likely to be right, put that choice down immediately; do not reconsider your answer. Always mark your best choice and move forward.

As a rule of thumb, if a fact question (one requiring you to recall a fact) takes more than a minute or two, select your best answer, "mark" the question (CBT has a "mark" button you can click), and go on. You may not skip a question; you must indicate an answer but you may mark the question and return to it later for further consideration. For a calculation problem (one requiring you to calculate some quantity), give yourself an extra minute or two. The CBT examination will indicate the number question you are currently answering, compared to the total number of questions (eg, number 62 of 220). The computer counts down from your allotted time, and the computer screen will indicate the amount of time you have remaining.

Elimination: Finding the Correct Answer

Good test performance is sometimes determined by the ability to recognize the incorrect answers as well as the correct ones. *Eliminating incorrect answers* (termed *distractors*) not only improves your score, it actually makes the test a more accurate measure of your knowledge.

Eliminating a distractor reduces the possible wrong choices. If your knowledge allows you to eliminate two incorrect responses, your odds of a correct response would be increased from one out of four to one out of two. If you can eliminate three distractors, you would have a 100 percent probability of getting the right answer. Every distractor you eliminate increases your odds of picking the right answer.

Multiple choice questions usually have one distractor that is obviously wrong, one distractor that is closer to the correct response, and one distractor that is very close to the correct answer. If you know the subject, you can eliminate the distractors that are most incorrect and improve your chances. If you prepare thoroughly, you will be able to eliminate the others. The more you know, the better you will do.

Many books on test taking suggest complicated systems to eliminate bad answers and rank good ones, but in order to use elimination effectively, you need a procedure that is both quick and simple. For the ARRT CBT exam, you must select an answer in order for the next question to be displayed. If you are unsure of your selection, or just want to come back later to review it, you are able to *mark* the question. All the questions you have marked in this manner will be displayed one by one after you have completed all 220 questions. There is an optional tutorial that you may take prior to starting the exam. Taking the tutorial is a good way to become more familiar with navigating through the exam with greater ease and assurance.

Changing Answers

Everyone has had the experience of trying to remember the answer to a question without success and then *finding that piece of information further along in the test.* A problem that you stare at for an hour without progress might seem simple if you go on to other problems and come back to it later. Very often, another question will jog your memory; this technique can work for you during the CBT exam.

If you are unsure of the correct way to answer a question:

1. If one of the answers seems better than the rest, put it down and mark the question for future reference. Come back and check the question at the end if you have time.
2. If you can eliminate two of the possible answers, make an educated guess between the two remaining possibilities. Then, mark the question for future reference.
3. Ask yourself, "Will more time really help me answer this question?" If your answer is no, do the best you can with what you know, using the process of elimination and making an educated guess. Again, mark the question for future reference so you can reread it if there is time at the end.

Guessing

You've probably been given a great deal of information and advice about guessing on tests. Most of what you've been told may be confusing or contradictory. It may make the problem easier to think in terms of rolling a die. Imagine a game in which you get a point every time the number 1, for example, comes up. How could you improve your score in this game? One way would be to roll the die as many times as you could. Another way would be to reduce the number of sides on the die so the "right" side would be more likely to come up; this way is called *the process of elimination,* and it plays a good part in test taking when you are unsure of the correct response.

Although we do *not* suggest guessing as an effective method of test taking, we do recognize that there will be times when it can be effective for you. Keep in mind the following things if you need to use this method:

1. The process of elimination will help you significantly in determining the right answer. Use this technique to narrow down the possible choices.
2. *Mark* the question so that, if you have time, you can come back to it. It is possible that the correct response may reveal itself through a question further ahead on the test.
3. Remember that guessing really doesn't work as an effective strategy by itself. You will need to study hard and use guessing in conjunction with other methods for it to be effective.

PRACTICE TESTS

Taking the Practice Test

In order to use the practice test to determine how long the test will take you to complete or how high you will score, you must take it under conditions matching, as closely as possible, the actual test conditions. If you try to eat supper while taking the test, take a 5 hour break in the middle of the test, or stop after every question to look up the answer, you will not get a clear picture of your current standing or potential to pass the exam. Following are some suggestions on how you can get the most out of the practice test:

1. Keep your schedule completely free. Find a time and a place that will guarantee that you

will not be disturbed for the duration of the test. Most libraries work well for this purpose, as do unoccupied classrooms if you can get access to them. If you have to take the test at home, make sure that you won't be bothered by friends or family.

Minimize your distractions, don't take phone calls, and don't try to watch TV or concentrate on anything else other than the test.

2. Start at a predetermined time. You may choose to take the practice test at the same time of day your test will be given at the testing center.

3. Bring everything you will need to take the test. The CBT test center will supply you with scrap paper and a simple nonprogrammable calculator. You must remember to *request* a calculator from the testing center personnel during your check-in at the center.

4. Approach the practice tests with the same strategies and attitudes that you plan on using with the actual examination. (Rereading the section on test strategies would be a good idea.)

5. Note time-consuming questions. While taking the test, mark the questions that take longer than 2 or 3 minutes. Don't spend too much time on any one question.

6. Note how far you get. You should be able to finish the whole practice test in the allotted time, but if you do run out of time, draw a line across the test book to show how far you got and then finish the rest of the test.

Checking Your Results

You should be able to finish all of the questions with enough time left over to go back and check your answers on those problems you marked as difficult. Your score should be at least 160 correct answers (80 percent). If you fail at either of these two goals, you need to go over the test carefully and try to analyze your problem.

Two questions you can address while analyzing a problem are "Was there a common factor in the questions that gave me trouble?" and "What were the subspecialties of the questions that I missed?" If you keep missing the same type of question, the problem could be easy to fix. Try going back and reworking the section of the book that corresponds to that topic.

Review your test-taking techniques. Did you spend too much time on a few questions? Did you spend too much time rereading answers that you had already eliminated as potential answers? If the answer to either of these questions is *yes*, you might want to review the earlier section on test strategies.

TEST STRATEGY CHECKLIST

1. CROSS AND CHECK
   Cross out bad answers and put checks next to good answers.
2. DO 50 EVERY 45
   Try to do at least 50 problems every 45 minutes.
3. MARK UNCERTAIN ANSWERS
   Mark questions you guessed on so you can come back and double-check them.

PREPARING FOR SUCCESS IN CBT

Reducing the unknown to a minimum is one of the best ways to prepare for success in any endeavor. This will be discussed later in the stress reduction section. Before proceeding to methods for improving your test performance, the following is a review of CBT facts that will help you better understand what to expect:

- You have the option to review a tutorial before starting your test, and it is a good idea to do that.
- Your responses can be given by using either the mouse or particular keystrokes that the tutorial will explain.
- The screen will show your name and the examination you are taking (eg, radiography, advanced mammography, etc.).
- The computer screen will let you know what question you are currently working on, out of the total number of questions (eg, number 62 of 220).
- The computer counts down your allotted time, and the computer screen will indicate the amount of time you have remaining.
- One question at a time will appear on the computer screen.
- You will indicate your answer (A, B, C, or D) by clicking on a little circle in front of the corresponding letter.
- The bar along the bottom of the screen will probably have 4 or 5 buttons on which you may click.
- A click on the "Previous" button brings you back to the last question you answered.
- A click on the "Next" button advances you to the question that follows.

- A click on the "Mark" button will signal that you want to look at that question again after you have completed answering all 200 questions.
- You may change your answer while you are working on any one question, or when you return to the question later.
- You must indicate an answer to a question before you can advance to the next question.
- When your "marked" questions are returned to you for review, you may change the answer or leave it as it is. You will then click "unmark" to indicate that you are satisfied with your answer and do not need to see that question again.
- Once you have reviewed and unmarked all your marked questions, the screen will tell you that all your questions have been answered and give you the opportunity to return to review any and/or all questions.
- A "Comment" button appears with each question and allows you to communicate a comment to the ARRT about that particular question. Your comments will be welcome and can be useful and constructive, but any comment should be concise because you will be using your running time.

OPTIMIZING YOUR RESULTS

When you take the radiography examination, two factors determine your score:

- your knowledge of the subject
- your performance on the exam

Of the two, knowledge is the key element needed for success. *Performance is harder to guarantee.* For some people, it seems to come naturally. These people apply test-taking strategies almost unconsciously, concentrating all their attention on the test. For the rest of the population (which includes most people), standardized tests are some of the most stressful and unpleasant experiences that they will ever have to face.

Fortunately, it is possible to significantly improve your performance on tests, even if you've been taking tests all of your life with no apparent improvement. By mastering the following three areas, you can have better results and greatly reduce the trauma of test taking:

1. Know your test strategies.
2. Learn to manage your stress.
3. Avoid surprises on the day of the test.

The important points for each of these areas are explained in detail in the following sections and are summarized in checklists included at the end of each part of the Introduction. These checklists are designed so that you can read them on the day of the test to reassure yourself that you haven't forgotten anything.

Test-Taking Strategies
The strategies recommended earlier serve two purposes: (1) to give you a simple, systematic way of eliminating bad choices and improving your odds of getting a correct response; and (2) to help you manage your time most efficiently during the test.

Managing Stress
Over the past 20 or so years, educators have become increasingly concerned about the problems of test anxiety and excessive stress that prevent students from doing their best on examinations. In the following sections, you will learn some basics about the nature of stress, the difference between good stress and bad stress, and some management techniques. All of the items listed will be helpful in reducing test anxiety, but the most important point for you to remember is that you are well prepared for the test you are about to take and the odds of your doing well are very good.

Where You Stand
The best way to reduce test anxiety is to address the following points:

1. know the subject
2. master a test-taking routine
3. avoid surprises
4. understand the role of stress in test taking
5. practice relaxation techniques

The Stress Curve
Recently, stress has received national attention. Magazines discuss it, doctors warn against it, commercials promise to reduce it, and seminars claim to eliminate it. Stress is often treated as a psychological cancer. There is, however, another aspect of stress that receives less attention. In demanding situations requiring optimal performance, moderate stress is not only natural, it is actually helpful. The relationship between stress and performance is called the stress curve; the most important aspect of the curve is the location of the maxima. The maxima is the

point of optimal performance, which occurs somewhere between too much stress and no stress at all.

There are plenty of familiar examples of stress improving performance. Athletes often set personal records during pressure situations such as playoff games or international events. Actors give their best performances and musicians play or sing best before an audience. You can probably think of personal examples as well. Most of us have surprised ourselves at one time or another by doing better than we expected under pressure.

How to Recognize Good Stress

If everyone dealt with stress equally well and experienced the same level of stress in the same situation, setting up guidelines for optimal stress levels would be easy. Unfortunately, everyone handles stress differently, and determining what level of stress is best must be judged on an individual basis. Given the importance of the radiography exam and the amount of time you have spent preparing for it, there is little chance of your stress level being too low when you sit for the test.

How do you know if you have too much stress? Feeling nervous does not indicate excessive stress. You are just as likely to feel nervous when you are at your optimal stress level. Stress is excessive when it interferes with the test-taking process. If you have trouble reading the questions, if you lose your place because you're worrying about the test, or if you're too distracted to follow the test strategies you've been practicing, you are experiencing test anxiety.

Relaxation Techniques

Whether or not you anticipate problems with stress, it is a good idea to take a couple of minutes to relax before the test. Stretch your muscles; take deep, slow breaths; and try to think about something unrelated to the test. If, during the test, you have trouble working effectively because of stress, stop, close your eyes, and count to five while taking some deep, slow breaths. Remind yourself that you are extremely well prepared for this test. Not many people realize that breathing and anxiety are related, or that a deep-breathing relaxation exercise can be helpful in reducing anxiety.

When you feel anxious, you tend to tighten your chest muscles. This results in breathing changes, with movement predominantly in your upper chest rather than your lower abdomen. Breathing this way often leads to undesirable conditions:

1. A reduction of oxygen in your blood, which can affect the way you think and lead to anxiety or fatigue.
2. Too much oxygen in your blood, resulting in an uncomfortable condition called *hyperventilation*.

It is important, therefore, to learn how to control your breathing, which, in turn, will result in relaxation. When attempting the following breathing exercise, don't try too hard to relax—it can work against you. Instead, try to be as peaceful as possible.

First, take a deep, full breath and exhale fully and completely. Next, inhale again, mentally counting from 1 to 4 while breathing in. Hold this breath in while again counting from 1 to 4. Then, begin fully exhaling, while slowly counting from 1 to 8. Repeat this sequence four times. If you run out of breath before reaching number 8, take deeper breaths and exhale more slowly. If you can learn this technique ahead of time, you can use it while in the exam room without anyone else knowing.

If the stress continues, try to think less about what you are doing. After practicing on 1200 questions, you have developed a kind of "automatic pilot," which will allow you to answer questions almost by reflex. Of course, this isn't the best way to take the test, but if you are faced with serious stress problems, it is an option.

Avoiding Surprises
The Week Before the Test

You have spent the past 2 to 4 years studying radiography, and the past 2 to 4 months reviewing for this examination. You probably know a great deal more than you think you do. Your top priority now should be getting yourself up to your best testing performance. If you follow these suggestions, you should have a good start.

Take Care of Yourself. When you take the test, you want to be as healthy and well rested as possible. The time it takes to get enough sleep, take a walk, or prepare a balanced meal is better spent than hours of last-minute cramming.

Reread This Introduction. This may be unnecessary advice, but it is worth mentioning. Pay close attention to the figures and checklists.

Gather Your Supplies. You want to be sure to get everything you need, but, almost as importantly, you want everything organized so you can avoid extra effort and worry. You might want to bring a sweater or light jacket. This may seem like a strange item, particularly if your test is taken in the summer, but an uncomfortably cold room is extremely distracting, and many public buildings have a wide variation in temperature from room to room. A sweater or windbreaker is a quick, easy solution. Avoid bringing a large purse or other large bundle. Lockers are available for stowing your personal items not allowed in the CBT room, but they are fairly small lockers and will not accommodate a very large purse or other large package.

Scout the Location. It is a very good idea to visit the location of the exam if possible. Getting lost on the morning of a test will add unwanted stress. Keep in mind the following questions: (1) What is the best route to the exam? (2) Where is the parking? (3) Where are the doors to the building? If possible, go into the building and look around.

Treat Yourself. Go out and do something special. See a movie. Eat out. Go for a drive. Just let yourself unwind.

The Day of the Test

There are few things more irritating then being told not to worry when you feel like worrying, but not worrying is the best thing to do. To help you avoid worrying, two checklists have been included, one physical checklist (things you need to bring) and one mental checklist (things you need to remember). Check off each item and put it out of your mind. Knowing you have both mentally and physically prepared will help you to relax before the exam.

You should plan to arrive a few minutes early. Many test centers require you to be there 30 minutes ahead of the scheduled test time.

You will probably want to eat a light meal before taking the test. Digestion tends to slow down when a person is under stress, so a large meal is, in most cases, a bad idea. You will also want to avoid excessive stimulants (and caffeine is definitely considered a stimulant).

This brings up another point. Though you want to be well rested and alert, you should be careful not to disrupt your normal routine any more than necessary. Getting extra rest, eating light, and avoiding stimulants are relative suggestions—relative to your habits and lifestyle. Don't make drastic changes on the day of the test. Get an extra half hour or hour of sleep. Eat a lighter meal than you usually would. If you drink coffee, drink a little less than normal.

When you get to the testing center, take a few minutes to relax. Walk around. Stretch your muscles. Remind yourself that you've put a great deal of work into doing well on this test and that work is the main factor for determining success.

PHYSICAL CHECKLIST(What to Bring)

1. Your admission ticket
2. Two current ID's
3. Sweater or windbreaker

MENTAL CHECKLIST

1. Remind yourself that you are well prepared.
2. Take the computer tutorial.
3. Use your test-taking strategies.
4. Focus on the test, not on the surroundings.
5. After you have finished, use the same strategies to go over any questions you marked for review.

REFERENCES

Benson H, Klipper M. *The Relaxation Response.* New York: Avon Books; 1990.

Bosworth S, Brisk M. *Learning Skills for the Science Student.* Florida: H&H Publishing Company; 1986.

Bragstad B, Stumpf S. *A Guidebook for Teaching: Study Skills and Motivation.* Boston: Allyn and Bacon; 1982.

Coffman S. *How to Survive at College.* Indiana: College Town Press; 1988.

Hamachek A. *Coping in College: A Guide for Aca-demic Success.* Boston: Allyn and Bacon; 1994.

Krantz H, Kemmelman J. *Keys to Reading and Study Skills.* New York: Holt, Rinehart & Winston; 1985.

Nieves L. *Coping in College.* Princeton, NJ: Educational Testing Service; 1984.

Palav S. *Learning Strategies for Allied Health Students.* Philadelphia: W. B. Saunders; 1995.

Robinson F. *Effective Study.* New York: Harper and Row; 1970.

Saia DA. *Radiography Program Review Exam Preparation,* 3rd ed. NY: McGraw-Hill; 2003.

Vitale B, Nugent P. *Test Success: Test-Taking Techniques for the Health Care Student.* Philadelphia: F. A. Davis; 1996.

Master Bibliography

Here is a list of reference books pertaining to the Answers and Explanations sections found at the end of each chapter in this book.

On the last line of each answer/explanation, there appears the last name of the author or editor of one of the publications listed here, along with a number or numbers indicating the correct page or range of pages where information relating to the correct answer may be found. For example, *(Bushong, p 45)* refers to page 45 of Bushong's *Radiologic Science for Technologists.*

Adler AM, Carlton RR. *Introduction to Radiography and Patient Care* (3rd ed). Philadelphia: W. B. Sanders, 2003.

Ballinger PW, Frank ED. *Merrill's Atlas of Radiographic Positions and Radiologic Procedures*, Vols 1, 2, and 3 (10th ed). St. Louis, MO: Mosby, 2004.

Bontrager KL. *Textbook of Radiographic Positioning and Related Anatomy* (5th ed). St. Louis, MO: Mosby, 2001.

Bushong SC. *Radiologic Science for Technologists* (8th ed). St. Louis, MO: Mosby, 2004.

Carlton RR, Adler AM. *Principles of Radiographic Imaging* (3rd ed). Albany, NY: Delmar, 2001.

Dowd SB, Tilson ER. *Practical Radiation Protection and Applied Radiobiology* (2nd ed). WB Saunders, 1999.

Ehrlich RA, McCloskey ED. *Patient Care in Radiography* (6th ed). St. Louis, MO: Mosby, 2004.

Fauber TL. *Radiographic Imaging and Exposure* (1st ed). Mosby, 2000.

Fosbinder RA, Kelsey CA. *Essentials of Radiologic Science* (1st ed). McGraw-Hill, 2002.

Gurley LT, Callaway WJ. *Introduction to Radiologic Technology* (5th ed). St. Louis, MO: Mosby, 2002.

Laudicina P. *Applied Pathology for Radiographers.* Philadelphia: W. B. Saunders, 1989.

Mill WR. *The relation of bodily habitus to visceral form, tonus, and motility.* Am J. Roentgengr 1917;4:155–169.

McKinney WEJ. *Radiographic Processing and Quality Control.* Philadelphia: Lippincott, 1988.

NCRP Report no 116: *Recommendations on Limits for Exposure to Ionizing Radiation.* NCRP, 1987.

Peart O. *A&L Mammography Review* (1st ed). McGraw-Hill, 2002.

Saia DA. *Radiography PREP* (3rd ed). McGraw-Hill 2003, 1997.

Seeram, E. *Rad Techs Guide to Equipment Operation and Maintenance.* Blackwell Science, Inc, 2001.

Selman J. *The Fundamentals of X-ray and Radium Physics* (9th ed). Springfield, IL: Charles C Thomas, 2000.

Shephard, CT. *Radiographic Image Production and Manipulation* (1st ed). McGraw-Hill, 2003.

Statkiewicz-Sherer, MA.. *Radiation Protection for Student Radiographers* (4th ed). St. Louis, MO: Mosby, 2002.

Taber's Cyclopedic Medical Dictionary (20th ed). Thomas CL, ed. Philadelphia: F. A. Davis, 2005.

Thompson, Hattaway, Hall, et al. *Principles of Imaging Science and Protection* (1st ed). Philadelphia: WB Saunders Co, 1994.

Torres LS, Linn-Watson Norcutt TA, Dutton AG. *Basic Medical Techniques and Patient Care in Imaging Technology* (6th ed). Philadelphia: Lippincott, 2003.

Tortora GJ, Derrickson B. *Principles of Anatomy and Physiology* (11th ed). John Wiley & Sons, Inc, 2006.

Travis EL. *Primer of Medical Radiobiology* (2nd ed). Chicago: Year Book, 1989.

Wolbarst, AB. *Physics of Radiology* (1st ed). Stamford, CT: Appleton & Lange, 1993.

CHAPTER 1

Patient Care
Questions

DIRECTIONS (Questions 1 through 130): Each of the numbered items or incomplete statements in this section is followed by answers or by completions of the statement. Select the *one* lettered answer or completion that is *best* in each case.

1. Which of the following blood pressure measurements might indicate shock?

    (A) Systolic pressure lower than 60 mm Hg
    (B) Systolic pressure higher than 140 mm Hg
    (C) Diastolic pressure higher than 140 mm Hg
    (D) Diastolic pressure lower than 90 mm Hg

2. Sterile technique is required when contrast agents are administered

    (A) rectally.
    (B) orally.
    (C) intrathecally.
    (D) through a nasogastric tube.

3. For medicolegal reasons, radiographic images are required to include all the following information, *except*

    (A) the patient's name and/or identification number.
    (B) the patient's birth date.
    (C) a right- or left-side marker.
    (D) the date of the examination.

4. A radiographer who discloses confidential information to unauthorized individuals could be found guilty of

    (A) invasion of privacy.
    (B) slander.
    (C) libel.
    (D) defamation.

5. A diabetic patient who has prepared for a fasting radiographic examination is susceptible to a hypoglycemic reaction. This is characterized by

    1. shaking and nervousness.
    2. cold, clammy skin.
    3. cyanosis.

    (A) 1 only
    (B) 2 only
    (C) 1 and 2 only
    (D) 1, 2, and 3

6. Which of the following instructions should be given to the patient following a barium sulfate contrast examination?

    1. Increase fluid and fiber intake for several days.
    2. Changes in stool color will occur until all barium has been evacuated.
    3. Contact a physician if no bowel movement occurs in 24 hours.

    (A) 1 only
    (B) 2 only
    (C) 1 and 3 only
    (D) 1, 2, and 3

7. *Logrolling* is a method of moving patients with suspected

   (A) head injury.
   (B) spinal injury.
   (C) bowel obstruction.
   (D) extremity fracture.

8. A patient is usually required to drink a barium sulfate suspension in order to demonstrate which of the following structures?

   1. Pylorus
   2. Sigmoid
   3. Ilium

   (A) 1 only
   (B) 1 and 3 only
   (C) 2 and 3 only
   (D) 3 only

9. The normal average rate of respiration for a healthy adult patient is

   (A) 5 to 7 breaths/min.
   (B) 8 to 12 breaths/min.
   (C) 12 to 20 breaths/min.
   (D) 20 to 30 breaths/min.

10. Examples of COPD include

   1. bronchitis.
   2. pulmonary emphysema.
   3. asthma.

   (A) 1 only
   (B) 1 and 2 only
   (C) 2 and 3 only
   (D) 1, 2, and 3

11. Administration of contrast agents for radiographic purposes is usually performed by which of the following parenteral routes?

   (A) Subcutaneous
   (B) Intravenous
   (C) Intramuscular
   (D) Intradermal

12. A patient developed hives several minutes after injection of an iodinated contrast agent. What type of drug should be readily available?

   (A) Analgesic
   (B) Antihistamine
   (C) Anti-inflammatory
   (D) Antibiotic

13. Which of the following sites are commonly used for an intravenous injection?

   1. Antecubital vein
   2. Basilic vein
   3. Popliteal vein

   (A) 1 and 2 only
   (B) 1 and 3 only
   (C) 2 and 3 only
   (D) 1, 2, and 3

14. The mechanical device used to correct an ineffectual cardiac rhythm is a

   (A) defibrillator.
   (B) cardiac monitor.
   (C) crash cart.
   (D) resuscitation bag.

15. You have encountered a person who is apparently unconscious. Although you open his airway, there is no rise and fall of the chest, and you can hear no breath sounds. You should

   (A) begin mouth-to-mouth rescue breathing, giving two full breaths.
   (B) proceed with the Heimlich maneuver.
   (C) begin external chest compressions at a rate of 80 to 100/min.
   (D) begin external chest compressions at a rate of at least 100/min.

16. In classifying intravenous (IV) contrast agents, the total number of dissolved particles in solution per kilogram of water defines

   (A) osmolality.
   (B) toxicity.
   (C) viscosity.
   (D) miscibility.

17. Which of the following procedures requires that the patient be placed in the lithotomy position?

(A) Myelography
(B) Venography
(C) T-tube cholangiography
(D) Hysterosalpingography

18. A nosocomial infection is a (n)

(A) infection acquired from frequent hand-shaking.
(B) upper respiratory tract infection.
(C) infection acquired in a hospital.
(D) type of rhinitis.

19. The legal doctrine *res ipsa locquitur* means which of the following?

(A) Let the master answer.
(B) The thing speaks for itself.
(C) A thing or matter settled by justice.
(D) A matter settled by precedent.

20. The usual patient preparation for an upper gastrointestinal (GI) examination is

(A) NPO 8 hours before the examination.
(B) light breakfast only on the morning of the examination.
(C) clear fluids only on the morning of the examination.
(D) 2-ounce castor oil and enemas until clear.

21. Conditions in which there is a lack of normal bone calcification include

1. rickets.
2. osteomalacia.
3. osteoarthritis.

(A) 1 only
(B) 1 and 2 only
(C) 2 and 3 only
(D) 1, 2, and 3

22. Abnormal accumulation of air in pulmonary tissues, resulting in overdistention of the alveolar spaces, is

(A) emphysema.
(B) empyema.
(C) pneumothorax.
(D) pneumoconiosis.

23. Anaphylactic shock manifests early symptoms that include

1. dysphagia.
2. itching of palms and soles.
3. constriction of the throat.

(A) 1 only
(B) 2 only
(C) 2 and 3 only
(D) 1, 2, and 3

24. *Anaphylaxis* is the term used to describe

(A) an inflammatory reaction.
(B) bronchial asthma.
(C) acute chest pain.
(D) allergic shock.

25. Of the four stages of infection, which is the stage during which the infection is *most* communicable?

(A) Latent period
(B) Incubation period
(C) Disease phase
(D) Convalescent phase

26. When performing cardiopulmonary resuscitation (CPR) on an infant, it is required that the number of compressions per minute, compared to that for an adult,

(A) remain the same.
(B) double.
(C) decrease.
(D) increase.

27. All of the following statements regarding hand washing and skin care are correct *except*

    (A) hands should be washed after each patient examination.
    (B) faucets should be opened and closed with paper towels.
    (C) hands should be smooth and free from chapping.
    (D) any cracks or abrasions should be left uncovered to facilitate healing.

28. A patient whose systolic blood pressure is less than 90 mm Hg is usually considered

    (A) hypertensive.
    (B) hypotensive.
    (C) average/normal.
    (D) baseline.

29. When a patient arrives in the radiology department with a urinary Foley catheter bag, it is important to

    (A) place the drainage bag above the level of the bladder.
    (B) place the drainage bag at the same level as the bladder.
    (C) place the drainage bag below the level of the bladder.
    (D) clamp the Foley catheter.

30. Instruments required to assess vital signs include

    1. a thermometer.
    2. a tongue blade.
    3. a watch with a second hand.

    (A) 1 only
    (B) 1 and 2 only
    (C) 1 and 3 only
    (D) 1, 2, and 3

31. Lyme disease is caused by bacteria carried by deer ticks. The tick bite may cause fever, fatigue, and other associated symptoms. This is an example of transmission of an infection by

    (A) droplet contact.
    (B) a vehicle.
    (C) the airborne route.
    (D) a vector.

32. Possible side effects of an iodinated contrast medium that is administered intravenously include all of the following *except*

    (A) a warm feeling.
    (B) altered taste.
    (C) nausea.
    (D) hypotension.

33. Blood pressure may be expressed as 120/95. What does 95 represent?

    1. The phase of relaxation of the cardiac muscle tissue
    2. The phase of contraction of the cardiac muscle tissue
    3. A higher-than-average diastolic pressure

    (A) 1 only
    (B) 2 only
    (C) 1 and 3 only
    (D) 2 and 3 only

34. All drug packages must provide certain information required by the U.S. Food and Drug Administration. Some of the information that must be provided includes

    1. the generic name.
    2. contraindications.
    3. the usual dose.

    (A) 1 only
    (B) 1 and 2 only
    (C) 1 and 3 only
    (D) 1, 2, and 3

35. Forms of intentional misconduct include

1. slander.
2. invasion of privacy.
3. negligence.

(A) 1 only
(B) 2 only
(C) 1 and 2 only
(D) 1, 2, and 3

36. When a patient with an arm injury needs help in undressing, the radiographer should

(A) remove clothing from the injured arm first.
(B) remove clothing from the uninjured arm first.
(C) always remove clothing from the left arm first.
(D) always cut clothing away from the injured extremity.

37. Which of the following conditions describes a patient who is unable to breathe easily while in the recumbent position?

(A) Dyspnea
(B) Apnea
(C) Orthopnea
(D) Oligopnea

38. You and a fellow radiographer have received an unconscious patient from a motor vehicle accident. As you perform the examination, it is important that you

1. refer to the patient by name.
2. make only those statements that you would make with a conscious patient.
3. reassure the patient about what you are doing.

(A) 1 only
(B) 1 and 2 only
(C) 2 and 3 only
(D) 1, 2, and 3

39. A diuretic is used to

(A) induce vomiting.
(B) stimulate defecation.
(C) promote elimination of urine.
(D) inhibit coughing.

40. When radiographing the elderly, it is helpful to

1. move quickly.
2. address them by their full name.
3. give straightforward instructions.

(A) 1 only
(B) 1 and 2 only
(C) 2 and 3 only
(D) 1, 2, and 3

41. The complete killing of all microorganisms is termed

(A) surgical asepsis.
(B) medical asepsis.
(C) sterilization.
(D) disinfection.

42. Involuntary patient motion can be caused by

1. posttraumatic shock.
2. medication.
3. low room temperature.

(A) 1 only
(B) 1 and 2 only
(C) 1 and 3 only
(D) 1, 2, and 3

43. When caring for a patient with an IV, the radiographer should keep the medication

(A) 18 to 20 inches above the level of the vein.
(B) 18 to 20 inches below the level of the vein.
(C) 28 to 30 inches above the level of the vein.
(D) 28 to 30 inches below the level of the vein.

44. Which of the following may be used to effectively reduce the viscosity of contrast media?

    (A) Warming
    (B) Refrigeration
    (C) Storage at normal room temperature
    (D) Storage in a cool, dry place

45. The type of shock associated with pooling of blood in the peripheral vessels is classified as

    (A) neurogenic.
    (B) cardiogenic.
    (C) hypovolemic.
    (D) septic.

46. Which of the following must be included in the patient's medical record or chart?

    1. Diagnostic and therapeutic orders
    2. Medical history
    3. Informed consent

    (A) 1 and 2 only
    (B) 1 and 3 only
    (C) 2 and 3 only
    (D) 1, 2, and 3

47. What type of precautions prevents the spread of infectious agents in aerosol form?

    (A) Strict isolation
    (B) Protective isolation
    (C) Airborne precautions
    (D) Contact precautions

48. Which of the following conditions must be met in order for patient consent to be valid?

    1. The patient must sign the consent form before receiving sedation.
    2. The physician named on the consent form must perform the procedure.
    3. All the blanks on the consent form must be filled in before the patient signs the form.

    (A) 1 and 2 only
    (B) 1 and 3 only
    (C) 2 and 3 only
    (D) 1, 2, and 3

49. The Heimlich maneuver is used if a patient is

    (A) in cardiac arrest.
    (B) choking.
    (C) having a seizure.
    (D) suffering from hiccups.

50. Which of the following is a violation of correct sterile techniques?

    (A) Gowns are considered sterile in the front down to the waist, including the arms.
    (B) Sterile gloves must be kept above the waist level.
    (C) Persons in sterile dress should pass each other face to face.
    (D) A sterile field should not be left unattended.

51. Which of the following legal phrases defines a circumstance in which both the health-care provider's and the patient's actions contributed to an injurious outcome?

    (A) Intentional misconduct
    (B) Contributory negligence
    (C) Gross negligence
    (D) None of the above

52. If extravasation occurs during an IV injection of contrast media, correct treatment includes which of the following?

    1. Remove the needle and locate a sturdier vein immediately.
    2. Apply pressure to the vein until bleeding stops.
    3. Apply warm, moist heat.

    (A) 1 only
    (B) 1 and 2 only
    (C) 2 and 3 only
    (D) 1, 2, and 3

53. Which of the following diastolic pressure readings might indicate hypertension?

    (A) 40 mm Hg
    (B) 60 mm Hg
    (C) 80 mm Hg
    (D) 100 mm Hg

54. To reduce the back strain associated with transferring patients from stretcher to x-ray table, the radiographer should

(A) pull the patient.
(B) push the patient.
(C) hold the patient away from his or her body and lift.
(D) bend at the waist and pull.

55. A small bottle containing a single dose of medication is termed

(A) an ampule.
(B) a vial.
(C) a bolus.
(D) a carafe.

56. If an emergency trauma patient experiences hemorrhaging from a leg injury, the radiographer should

1. apply pressure to the bleeding site.
2. call the emergency department for assistance.
3. apply a pressure bandage and complete the examination.

(A) 1 and 2 only
(B) 1 and 3 only
(C) 2 and 3 only
(D) 1, 2, and 3

57. Ingestion of a gas-producing powder or crystals is usually preliminary to which of the following examinations?

1. Double-contrast GI
2. Oral cholecystogram
3. IV urogram

(A) 1 only
(B) 2 only
(C) 1 and 2 only
(D) 2 and 3 only

58. Which ethical principle is related to the theory that patients have the right to decide what will or will not be done to them?

(A) Autonomy
(B) Beneficence
(C) Fidelity
(D) Veracity

59. When disposing of contaminated needles, they are placed in a special container using what procedure?

(A) Recap the needle, remove the syringe, and dispose of the needle.
(B) Do not recap the needle, remove the syringe, and dispose of the needle.
(C) Recap the needle and dispose of the entire syringe.
(D) Do not recap the needle and dispose of the entire syringe.

60. You receive a patient who is complaining of pain in the area of the left fourth and fifth metatarsals; however, the requisition asks for a left ankle examination. What should you do?

(A) Perform a left foot examination.
(B) Perform a left ankle examination.
(C) Perform both a left foot and a left ankle examination.
(D) Check with the referring physician.

61. You receive an ambulatory patient for a GI series. As the patient is seated on the x-ray table, he feels faint. You should

1. lay the patient down on the x-ray table.
2. elevate the patient's legs or place the table slightly Trendelenburg.
3. leave quickly and call for help.

(A) 1 only
(B) 1 and 2 only
(C) 1 and 3 only
(D) 1, 2, and 3

62. Which of the following examinations require(s) restriction of the patient's diet?

    1. GI series
    2. Abdominal survey
    3. Pyelogram

    (A) 1 only
    (B) 1 and 2 only
    (C) 1 and 3 only
    (D) 2 and 3 only

63. The radiographer must perform which of the following procedures prior to entering a contact isolation room with a mobile x-ray unit?

    1. Put on gown and gloves only.
    2. Put on gown, gloves, mask, and cap.
    3. Clean the mobile x-ray unit.

    (A) 1 only
    (B) 2 only
    (C) 1 and 3 only
    (D) 2 and 3 only

64. Examples of nasogastric tubes include

    1. Swan–Ganz.
    2. Salem-sump.
    3. Levin.

    (A) 1 and 2 only
    (B) 1 and 3 only
    (C) 2 and 3 only
    (D) 1, 2, and 3

65. Rapid onset of severe respiratory or cardiovascular symptoms after ingestion or injection of a drug, vaccine, contrast agent, or food, or after an insect bite, best describes

    (A) asthma.
    (B) anaphylaxis.
    (C) myocardial infarction.
    (D) rhinitis.

66. The *most* effective method of sterilization is

    (A) dry heat.
    (B) moist heat.
    (C) pasteurization.
    (D) freezing.

67. The condition in which pulmonary alveoli lose their elasticity and become permanently inflated, causing the patient to consciously exhale, is

    (A) bronchial asthma.
    (B) bronchitis.
    (C) emphysema.
    (D) tuberculosis.

68. Chest drainage systems should always be kept

    1. below the level of the patient's chest.
    2. above the patient's chest.
    3. at the level of the patient's diaphragm.

    A. 1 only
    B. 1 and 2 only
    C. 2 and 3 only
    D. 1, 2, and 3

69. Which of the following patient rights is violated by discussing privileged patient information with an individual who is not involved with the patient's care?

    1. The right to considerate and respectful care
    2. The right to privacy
    3. The right to continuity of care

    (A) 1 only
    (B) 2 only
    (C) 1 and 3 only
    (D) 2 and 3 only

70. Nitroglycerin is used

    (A) to relieve pain from angina pectoris.
    (B) to prevent a heart attack.
    (C) as a vasoconstrictor.
    (D) to increase blood pressure.

71. In which of the following situations should a radiographer wear protective eye gear (goggles)?

    1. When performing an upper GI radiography examination
    2. When assisting the radiologist during an angiogram
    3. When assisting the radiologist in a biopsy/aspiration procedure

    (A) 1 and 2 only
    (B) 1 and 3 only
    (C) 2 and 3 only
    (D) 1, 2, and 3

72. In reviewing a patient's blood chemistry, which of the following blood urea nitrogen (BUN) ranges is considered normal?

    (A) 0.6 to 1.5 mg/100 mL
    (B) 4.5 to 6 mg/100 mL
    (C) 8 to 25 mg/100 mL
    (D) Up to 50 mg/100 mL

73. A quantity of medication introduced intravenously over a period of time is termed

    (A) an IV push.
    (B) an infusion.
    (C) a bolus.
    (D) hypodermic.

74. A patient who is *diaphoretic* has

    (A) pale, cool, clammy skin.
    (B) hot, dry skin.
    (C) dilated pupils.
    (D) warm, moist skin.

75. In what order should the following examinations be performed?

    1. Upper GI
    2. IV urogram
    3. Barium enema

    (A) 3, 1, 2
    (B) 1, 3, 2
    (C) 2, 1, 3
    (D) 2, 3, 1

76. An MRI procedure is contraindicated for a patient who has

    (A) herniated disc.
    (B) aneurysm clips.
    (C) dental fillings.
    (D) subdural bleeding.

77. An inanimate object that has been in contact with an infectious microorganism is termed a

    (A) vector.
    (B) fomite.
    (C) host.
    (D) reservoir.

78. The advantages of using nonionic, water-soluble contrast media include

    1. cost-containment benefits.
    2. low toxicity.
    3. fewer adverse reactions.

    (A) 1 only
    (B) 1 and 2 only
    (C) 2 and 3 only
    (D) 1, 2, and 3

79. A vasodilator would *most* likely be used for

    (A) angina.
    (B) cardiac arrest.
    (C) bradycardia.
    (D) antihistamine.

80. Which of the following statements are true regarding a two-member team performing mobile radiography on a patient with MRSA precautions?

    1. One radiographer remains "clean"—that is, he or she has no physical contact with the patient.
    2. The radiographer who positions the mobile unit also makes the exposure.
    3. The radiographer who positions the cassette also retrieves the cassette and removes it from its plastic protective cover.

    (A) 1 and 2 only
    (B) 1 and 3 only
    (C) 2 and 3 only
    (D) 1, 2, and 3

81. Symptoms associated with a respiratory reaction to contrast media include

    1. sneezing.
    2. dyspnea.
    3. asthma attack.

    (A) 1 and 2 only
    (B) 1 and 3 only
    (C) 2 and 3 only
    (D) 1, 2, and 3

82. While in your care for a radiologic procedure, a patient asks to see his chart. Which of the following is the appropriate response?

    (A) Inform the patient that the chart is for health-care providers to view, not for the patient.
    (B) Inform the patient that you do not know where the chart is.
    (C) Inform the patient that he has the right to see his chart, but that he should request to view it with his physician, so that it is properly interpreted.
    (D) Give the patient the chart and leave him alone for a few minutes to review it.

83. Skin discoloration due to cyanosis may be observed in the

    1. gums.
    2. nailbeds.
    3. cornea.

    (A) 1 only
    (B) 1 and 2 only
    (C) 3 only
    (D) 1, 2, and 3

84. With a patient suffering abdominal pain, it is frequently helpful to

    1. elevate the head slightly with a pillow.
    2. perform the examination in the Trendelenburg position.
    3. place a support under the knees.

    (A) 1 and 2 only
    (B) 1 and 3 only
    (C) 2 and 3 only
    (D) 1, 2, and 3

85. While performing mobile radiography on a patient, you note that the requisition is for a chest image to check placement of a Swan–Ganz catheter. A Swan–Ganz catheter is a (n)

    (A) pacemaker.
    (B) chest tube.
    (C) IV catheter.
    (D) urinary catheter.

86. The medical term for *nosebleed* is

    (A) vertigo.
    (B) epistaxis.
    (C) urticaria.
    (D) aura.

87. Blood pressure is measured in units of

    (A) mm Hg.
    (B) beats per minute.
    (C) °F.
    (D) liters per minute.

88. Which of the following radiographic procedures requires an intrathecal injection?

    (A) IV pyelogram
    (B) Myelogram
    (C) Lymphangiogram
    (D) Computed tomography (CT)

89. According to the CDC (Centers for Disease Control and Prevention), all of the following precaution guidelines are true, *except*

    (A) Airborne precautions require that the patient wear a mask.
    (B) Masks are indicated when caring for patients on MRSA precautions.
    (C) Patients under MRSA precautions require a negative-pressure room.
    (D) Gloves are indicated when caring for a patient on droplet precautions.

90. The medical term for *congenital clubfoot* is

    (A) coxa plana.
    (B) osteochondritis.
    (C) talipes.
    (D) muscular dystrophy.

91. The pain experienced by an individual whose coronary arteries are not conveying sufficient blood to the heart is called

    (A) tachycardia.
    (B) bradycardia.
    (C) angina pectoris.
    (D) syncope.

92. Hypochlorite bleach (Clorox) and Lysol are examples of

    (A) antiseptics.
    (B) bacteriostatics.
    (C) antifungal agents.
    (D) disinfectants.

93. The condition that allows blood to shunt between the right and left ventricles is called

    (A) patent ductus arteriosus.
    (B) coarctation of the aorta.
    (C) atrial septal defect.
    (D) ventricular septal defect.

94. When radiographing young children, it is helpful to

    1. let them bring a toy.
    2. tell them it will not hurt.
    3. be cheerful and unhurried.

    (A) 1 only
    (B) 1 and 3 only
    (C) 2 and 3 only
    (D) 1, 2, and 3

95. A drug's chemical name is called its

    (A) generic name.
    (B) trade name.
    (C) brand name.
    (D) proprietary name.

96. The act of inspiration will cause elevation of the

    1. sternum.
    2. ribs.
    3. diaphragm.

    (A) 1 only
    (B) 1 and 2 only
    (C) 2 and 3 only
    (D) 1, 2, and 3

97. A radiologic technologist can be found guilty of a *tort* in which of the following situations?

    1. Failure to shield a patient of childbearing age from unnecessary radiation
    2. Performing an examination on a patient who has refused the examination
    3. Discussing a patient's condition with a third party

    (A) 1 only
    (B) 1 and 2 only
    (C) 2 and 3 only
    (D) 1, 2, and 3

98. Guidelines for cleaning contaminated objects or surfaces include the following:

    1. Clean from the least contaminated to the most contaminated area.
    2. Clean in a circular motion, starting from the center and working outward.
    3. Clean from the top down.

    (A) 1 only
    (B) 1 and 2 only
    (C) 1 and 3 only
    (D) 1, 2, and 3

99. If the radiographer performed a lumbar spine examination on a patient who was supposed to have an elbow examination, which of the following charges may be brought against the radiographer?

    (A) Assault
    (B) Battery
    (C) False imprisonment
    (D) Defamation

100. Physical changes characteristic of gerontologic patients usually include

    1. loss of bone calcium.
    2. loss of hearing.
    3. loss of mental alertness.

    (A) 1 only
    (B) 1 and 2 only
    (C) 1 and 3 only
    (D) 1, 2, and 3

101. Which statement(s) would be true regarding tracheostomy patients?

    1. Tracheostomy patients have difficulty speaking.
    2. A routine chest x-ray requires the tracheostomy tubing to be rotated out of view.
    3. Audible rattling sounds indicate a need for suction.

    (A) 1 only
    (B) 1 and 2 only
    (C) 1 and 3 only
    (D) 1, 2, and 3

102. An esophagogram might be requested for patients with which of the following esophageal disorders/symptoms?

    1. Varices
    2. Achalasia
    3. Dysphasia

    (A) 1 only
    (B) 1 and 2 only
    (C) 1 and 3 only
    (D) 1, 2, and 3

103. Medication can be administered by which of the following routes?

    1. Orally
    2. Intravenously
    3. Intramuscularly

    (A) 1 and 2 only
    (B) 1 and 3 only
    (C) 2 and 3 only
    (D) 1, 2, and 3

104. Protective or "reverse" isolation is required in which of the following conditions?

    1. Tuberculosis
    2. Burns
    3. Leukemia

    (A) 1 only
    (B) 1 and 2 only
    (C) 2 and 3 only
    (D) 1, 2, and 3

105. When a GI series has been requested on a patient with a suspected perforated ulcer, the type of contrast medium that should be used is

    (A) thin barium sulfate suspension.
    (B) thick barium sulfate suspension.
    (C) water-soluble iodinated media.
    (D) oil-based iodinated media.

106. Which of the following statements are true regarding the proper care of a patient with a tracheostomy?

1. Employ sterile technique if you must touch a tracheostomy for any reason.
2. Before you suction a tracheostomy, the patient should be well aerated.
3. Never suction for longer than 15 seconds, permitting the patient to rest in between.

(A) 1 and 2 only
(B) 1 and 3 only
(C) 2 and 3 only
(D) 1, 2, and 3

107. A patient experiencing an episode of syncope should be placed in which of the following positions?

(A) Dorsal recumbent with head elevated
(B) Dorsal recumbent with feet elevated
(C) Lateral recumbent
(D) Seated with feet supported

108. The diameter of a needle is termed its

(A) bevel.
(B) gauge.
(C) hub.
(D) length.

109. A patient in a recumbent position with the head lower than the feet is said to be in which of the following positions?

(A) Trendelenburg
(B) Fowler's
(C) Sims'
(D) Stenver's

110. Which of the following drugs is considered a bronchodilator?

(A) Epinephrine
(B) Lidocaine
(C) Nitroglycerin
(D) Verapamil

111. Which of the following is a vasopressor and may be used for an anaphylactic reaction or cardiac arrest?

(A) Nitroglycerin
(B) Epinephrine
(C) Hydrocortisone
(D) Digitoxin

112. Chemical substances that are used to kill pathogenic bacteria are called

1. antiseptics.
2. germicides.
3. disinfectants.

(A) 1 only
(B) 1 and 2 only
(C) 2 and 3 only
(D) 1, 2, and 3

113. All of the following rules regarding proper hand washing technique are correct *except*

(A) keep hands and forearms lower than elbows.
(B) use paper towels to turn water on.
(C) avoid using hand lotions whenever possible.
(D) carefully wash all surfaces and between fingers.

114. Where is the "sterile corridor" located?

(A) Just outside the surgical suite
(B) Immediately inside each operating room door
(C) Between the draped patient and the instrument table
(D) At the foot end of the draped patient

115. The medical abbreviation meaning "three times a day" is

(A) tid.
(B) qid.
(C) qh.
(D) pc.

116. During a grand mal seizure, the patient should be

(A) protected from injury.
(B) placed in a semiupright position to prevent aspiration of vomitus.
(C) allowed to thrash freely.
(D) given a sedative to reduce jerky body movements and reduce the possibility of injury.

117. A patient suffering from orthopnea would experience the *least* discomfort in which body position?

(A) Fowler's
(B) Trendelenburg
(C) Recumbent
(D) Erect

118. In which of the following conditions is a double-contrast barium enema (BE) essential for demonstration of the condition?

1. Polyps
2. Colitis
3. Diverticulosis

(A) 1 only
(B) 1 and 2 only
(C) 1 and 3 only
(D) 1, 2, and 3

119. When a radiographer is obtaining a patient history, both subjective and objective data should be obtained. An example of *subjective* data is that

(A) the patient appears to have a productive cough.
(B) the patient has a blood pressure of 130/95.
(C) the patient states that he experiences extreme pain in the upright position.
(D) the patient has a palpable mass in the right upper quadrant of the left breast.

120. Symptoms of impending diabetic coma include

1. increased urination.
2. sweet-smelling breath.
3. extreme thirst.

(A) 1 and 2 only
(B) 1 and 3 only
(C) 2 and 3 only
(D) 1, 2, and 3

121. The condition of slow heart rate, below 60 beats/min, is termed

(A) hyperthermia.
(B) hypotension.
(C) hypoxia.
(D) bradycardia.

122. Which of the following is (are) symptom(s) of shock?

1. Pallor and weakness
2. Increased pulse
3. Fever

(A) 1 only
(B) 1 and 2 only
(C) 1 and 3 only
(D) 1, 2, and 3

123. Increased pain threshold, breakdown of skin, and atrophy of fat pads and sweat glands are all important considerations when working with which group of patients?

(A) Infants
(B) Children
(C) Adolescents
(D) Geriatric patients

124. The medical abbreviation meaning "every hour" is

(A) tid.
(B) qid.
(C) qh.
(D) pc.

125. Radiographs are the property of the

    (A) radiologist.
    (B) patient.
    (C) health-care institution.
    (D) referring physician.

126. When reviewing patient blood chemistry levels, what is considered the normal creatinine range?

    (A) 0.6 to 1.5 mg/100 mL
    (B) 4.5 to 6 mg/100 mL
    (C) 8 to 25 mg/100 mL   *BUN*
    (D) Up to 50 mg/100 mL

127. Which of the following medical equipment is used to determine blood pressure?

    1. Pulse oximeter
    2. Stethoscope
    3. Sphygmomanometer

    (A) 1 and 2 only
    (B) 1 and 3 only
    (C) 2 and 3 only
    (D) 1, 2, and 3

128. Diseases whose mode of transmission is through the air include

    1. tuberculosis.
    2. mumps.
    3. rubella.

    (A) 1 only
    (B) 1 and 2 only
    (C) 1 and 3 only
    (D) 1, 2, and 3

129. All of the following statements regarding oxygen delivery are true, *except*

    (A) oxygen is classified as a drug and must be prescribed by a physician.
    (B) rate of delivery and mode of delivery must be part of a physician order for oxygen.
    (C) oxygen may be ordered continuously or as needed by the patient.
    (D) none of the above; they are all true.

130. Which of the following imaging procedures do *not* require the use of ionizing radiation to produce an image?

    1. Ultrasound
    2. Computed axial tomography
    3. MRI

    (A) 1 and 2 only
    (B) 1 and 3 only
    (C) 2 and 3 only
    (D) 1, 2, and 3

Answers and Explanations

1. **(A)** *Shock* is indicated by extremely low blood pressure, that is, a systolic blood pressure reading *lower than 60 mmHg* (below 90 mmHg is considered low blood pressure). Normal blood pressure is 110 to 140 mmHg systolic and 60 to 80 mmHg diastolic. High blood pressure is indicated by systolic pressure higher than 140 mmHg and diastolic pressure higher than 90 mmHg. *(Torres et al, p 163)*

2. **(C)** *Sterile technique* is required for the administration of contrast media by the IV and intrathecal (intraspinal) methods. Sterile technique is also required for injection of contrast media during arthrography. *Aseptic technique* is used for administration of contrast media by means of the oral and rectal routes, as well as through the nasogastric tube. *(Torres et al, p 270)*

3. **(B)** Every radiographic image *must* include (1) the patient's name or ID number; (2) the side marker, right or left; (3) the date of the examination; and (4) the identity of the institution or office. Additional information *may* be included: the patient's birth date or age, name of the attending physician, and the time of day. When multiple examinations (eg, chest examinations or small bowel images) of a patient are made on the same day, it becomes crucial that the time the radiographs were taken be included on the image. This allows the physician to track the patient's progress. *(Ballinger & Frank, vol 1, pp 22–23)*

4. **(A)** A radiographer who discloses confidential information to unauthorized individuals may be found guilty of *invasion of privacy*. If the disclosure is in some way detrimental or otherwise harmful to the patient, the radiographer may also be accused of *defamation*. Spoken defamation is *slander;* written defamation is *libel. (Saia, p 8)*

5. **(C)** Hypoglycemic reactions can be very severe and should be treated with an immediate dose of sugar (e.g., in juice). Early symptoms of an insulin reaction are shaking, nervousness, dizziness, cold and clammy skin, blurred vision, and slurred speech. Convulsions and coma may result if the patient is not treated. *Cyanosis* is the lack of oxygenated blood, which is a symptom of shock. *(Torres et al, p 169)*

6. **(D)** Physicians often prescribe a mild laxative to aid in the elimination of barium sulfate. If a laxative is not given, the patient should be instructed to increase dietary fluid and fiber and to monitor bowel movements (the patient should have at least one within 24 hours). Patients should also be aware of the white appearance of their stool that will be present until all barium is expelled. *(Torres et al, p 222)*

7. **(B)** Patients arriving from the emergency department (ED) with suspected *spinal injury* should not be moved. AP and horizontal lateral projections of the suspected area should be evaluated and a decision made about the

advisability of further images. For a lateral projection, the patient should be moved along one plane, that is, rolled like a log. It is imperative that twisting motions be avoided. *(Torres et al, p 87)*

8. **(A)** Oral administration of barium sulfate is used to demonstrate the upper digestive system—the esophagus, fundus, body, and pylorus of the stomach—and barium progression through the small bowel. The small bowel includes the duodenum, jejunum and ileum (ilium is part of the pelvis). The large bowel, including the sigmoid colon, is usually demonstrated via *rectal* administration of barium. *(Gurley & Callaway, pp 125–126)*

9. **(C)** The normal average rate of respiration for a healthy adult patient is between 12 and 20 breaths/min. For children, the rate is higher, averaging between 20 and 30 breaths/min. In addition to monitoring the respiratory rate, it is also important to monitor the depth (shallow or labored) and pattern (regularity) of respiration. A respiratory rate greater than 20 breaths/min in an adult would be considered *tachypnea*. *(Adler & Carlton, p 163)*

10. **(D)** COPD is the abbreviation for chronic obstructive pulmonary disease; it refers to a group of disorders, including bronchitis, emphysema, asthma, and bronchiectasis. COPD is irreversible and decreases the ability of the lungs to perform their ventilation functions. There is often less than half the normal expected maximal breathing capacity. *(Taber's, p 416)*

11. **(B)** A parental route of drug administration is one that bypasses the digestive system. In radiography, the IV method is most commonly used to administer contrast agents. The four parenteral routes require different needle placements: under the skin *(subcutaneous)*, through the skin and into the muscle *(intramuscular)*, between the layers of the skin *(intradermal)*, and into the vein *(intravenous)*. *(Adler & Carlton, p 267)*

12. **(B)** When a contrast medium is injected, histamines are produced to protect the body from the foreign substance. An *antihistamine* (such as diphenhydramine [Benadryl]) blocks the action of the histamine and reduces the body's inflammatory response to the contrast medium. An *analgesic* (such as aspirin) relieves pain. An *anti-inflammatory* drug (such as ibuprofen) suppresses the inflammation of tissue. *Antibiotics* (such as penicillin) help fight bacterial infections. *(Torres et al, p 166)*

13. **(A)** Either the *antecubital vein* or the *basilic vein*, both found in the elbow region, may be used for an IV injection. Other veins in the area include the cephalic and accessory veins. The *popliteal* vein, found in the area of the knee, is not commonly used for an IV injection. *(Adler & Carlton, p 275)*

14. **(A)** The mechanical device used to correct an ineffectual cardiac ventricular rhythm is a *defibrillator*. The two paddles attached to the unit are placed on a patient's chest and used to introduce an electric current in an effort to correct the dysrhythmia. *Automatic implantable cardioverter defibrillators* (AICDs) are fairly new devices that are implanted in the body and which deliver a small shock to the heart if a life-threatening dysrhythmia occurs. A *cardiac monitor* is used to display, and sometime record, electrocardiogram (ECG) readings and some pressure readings. The *crash cart* is a supply cart with various medications and equipment necessary for treating a patient who is suffering from a myocardial infarction or some other serious medical emergency. It is periodically checked and restocked. A *resuscitation bag* is used for ventilation, as during cardiopulmonary resuscitation. *(Torres et al, pp 173–175)*

15. **(A)** The victim's airway should first be opened. This is accomplished by tilting back the head and lifting the chin. However, if the victim may have suffered a spinal cord injury, the spine should not be moved and the airway should be opened using the jaw-thrust method. The rescuer next listens to breathing sounds and watches for the rise and fall of the chest to indicate breathing. If there is no breathing, the rescuer pinches the victim's

nose and delivers two full breaths via mouth-to-mouth rescue breathing. If rise and fall of the chest is still not present, the Heimlich maneuver is instituted. If ventilation does not take place during the two full breaths, the victim's circulation is checked next (using the carotid artery). If there is no pulse, external chest compressions are begun at a rate of 80 to 100/min for adults and at least 100/min for infants. (*Torres et al, p 172*)

16. **(A)** In classifying contrast agents, the total number of dissolved particles in solution per kilogram of water defines the *osmolality* of the contrast agent. The *toxicity* defines how noxious or harmful a contrast agent is. Contrast agents with low osmolality have been found to cause less tissue toxicity than the ionic IV contrast agents. The *viscosity* defines the thickness or concentration of the contrast agent. The viscosity of a contrast agent can affect the injection rate. A thicker, or more viscous, contrast agent will be more difficult to inject (more pressure is needed to push the contrast agent through the syringe and needle or the angiocatheter). The *miscibility* of a contrast agent refers to its ability to mix with body fluids, such as blood. Miscibility is an important consideration in preventing thrombus formation. It is generally preferable to use a contrast agent with low osmolality and low toxicity because such an agent is safer for the patient and less likely to cause any untoward reactions. When ionic and nonionic contrast agents are compared, a nonionic contrast agent has a lower osmolality. To further understand osmolality, remember that whenever IV contrast media are introduced, there is a notable shift in fluid and ions. This shift is caused by an inflow of water from interstitial regions into the vascular compartment, which increases the blood volume and cardiac output. Consequently, there will be an increase in systemic arterial pressure and peripheral vascular resistance with peripheral *vasodilation*. Additionally, the pulmonary pressure and heart rate increase. When the effects of osmolality on the patient are understood, it becomes clear that an elderly patient or one with cardiac disease or impaired circulation would greatly benefit from the use of an agent with lower osmolality. (*Adler & Carlton, p 289*)

17. **(D)** The *lithotomy* position is generally employed for hysterosalpingography. The lithotomy position requires that the patient lie on the back with buttocks at the edge of the table. The hips are flexed, the knees are flexed and resting on leg supports, and the feet rest in stirrups. (*Adler & Carlton, p 202*)

18. **(C)** *Nosocomial* diseases are those acquired in hospitals, especially by patients whose resistance to infection has been diminished by their illness. Cleanliness is essential to decrease the number of nosocomial infections. The x-ray table must be cleaned and the pillowcase changed between patients. The most common nosocomial infection is the *urinary tract infection* (UTI). (*Gurley & Callaway, pp 178–179*)

19. **(B)** The legal doctrine *res ipsa locquitur* relates to a thing or matter that speaks for itself. For instance, if a patient went into the hospital to have a kidney stone removed and ended up with an appendectomy, that speaks for itself, and negligence can be proven. *Respondeat superior* is the phase meaning "let the master answer" or "the one ruling is responsible." If a radiographer was negligent, there may be an attempt to prove that the radiologist was responsible, because the radiologist oversees the radiographer. *Res judicata* means a thing or matter *settled by justice*. *Stare decisis* refers to a matter *settled by precedent*. (*Gurley & Callaway, p 194*)

20. **(A)** To obtain a diagnostic examination of the stomach, it must first be empty. The usual preparation is NPO (nothing by mouth) after midnight (approximately 8 hours before the examination). Any material in the stomach can simulate the appearance of disease. (*Torres et al, p 233*)

21. **(B)** *Rickets* and *osteomalacia* are disorders in which there is softening of bone. Rickets results from a deficiency of vitamin D and usually is found affecting the growing bones of young children. The body's weight on the soft bones of the legs results in bowed and misshapen legs. Osteomalacia is an adult condition in which new bone fails to calcify. It is a painful condition and can result in easily fractured bones, especially in the lower extremities.

Osteoarthritis is often seen in the elderly and is characterized by degeneration of articular cartilage in adjacent bones. The resulting rubbing of bone against bone results in pain and deterioration. *(Tortora & Derrickson, p 190)*

22. **(A)** Overdistention of the alveoli with air is *emphysema*. The condition is often a result of many years of smoking and is characterized by *dyspnea*, especially when recumbent. *Empyema* is pus in the thoracic cavity; *pneumothorax* is air or gas in the pleural cavity. *Pneumoconiosis* is a condition of the lungs characterized by particulate matter having been deposited in lung tissue; it sometimes results in emphysema. *(Bontrager, pp 69, 80)*

23. **(D)** Adverse reactions to the intravascular administration of iodinated contrast are not uncommon, and although the risk of a life-threatening reaction is relatively low, the radiographer must be alert to recognize the situation and deal with it effectively should a serious reaction occur. A minor reaction is characterized by flushed appearance and nausea, and occasionally by vomiting and a few hives. *Early* symptoms of a possible anaphylactic reaction include constriction of the throat, possibly because of laryngeal edema, dysphagia (difficulty swallowing), and itching of the palms and soles. The radiographer must maintain the patient's airway, summon the radiologist, and call a "code." *(Adler & Carlton, p 240)*

24. **(D)** A severe allergic reaction affecting several tissue functions is referred to as *anaphylaxis* or anaphylactic shock. It is characterized by *dyspnea* (difficulty breathing) caused by rapid swelling of the respiratory tract and a sharp drop in blood pressure. Individuals who are sensitive to bee stings and certain medications, including iodinated contrast agents, are candidates for this reaction. *(Adler & Carlton, p 240)*

25. **(C)** Of the four stages of infection, the stage during which the infection is most communicable is the *disease phase*. In the initial phase, the *latent period*, the infection is introduced and lies dormant. As soon as the microbes begin to shed, the infection becomes communicable. The microbes reproduce (during the

incubation period), and during the actual disease period signs and symptoms of the infection may begin. The infection is most active and communicable at this point. As the patient fights off the infection, and the symptoms regress, the *convalescent (recovery) phase* occurs. *(Torres et al, p 56)*

26. **(D)** The heart rate of an infant is much faster than that of an adult; therefore, the number of compressions per minute is also greater. Infant CPR requires 5 compressions to 1 breath. There should be at least 100 compressions per minute. *(Adler & Carlton, p 244)*

27. **(D)** In the practice of aseptic technique, *hand washing* is the most important precaution. The radiographer's hands should be thoroughly washed with warm, soapy running water after each patient examination. To avoid contamination of, or contamination by, the faucets, they should be opened and closed using paper towels. Care should be taken to avoid chapped hands by the use of hand cream. Skin function is a major factor in protecting bodies from the invasion of bacteria and infection. Any cuts, abrasions, or other breaks in the continuity of this protective barrier should be protected from bacterial invasion with a bandage. *(Torres et al, pp 61–62)*

28. **(B)** *Systolic* blood pressure describes the pressure during *contraction* of the heart. It is expressed as the top number when recording blood pressure. *Diastolic* blood pressure is the reading during *relaxation* of the heart and is placed on the bottom when recording blood pressure. A patient is considered *hypertensive* when systolic pressure is consistently above 140 mm Hg, and *hypotensive* when the systolic pressure is lower than 90 mm Hg. *(Adler & Carlton, p 160)*

29. **(C)** When caring for a patient with an indwelling Foley catheter, place the drainage bag and tubing *below the level of the bladder* to maintain the gravity flow of urine. Placement of the tubing or bag above or level with the bladder will allow backflow of urine into the bladder. This reflux of urine can increase the chance of UTI. *(Adler & Carlton, pp 216, 217)*

30. (C) The four *vital signs* are *temperature, pulse, respiration,* and *blood pressure.* Because radiographers may be required to take vital signs in an emergency, they should practice these skills. A *thermometer* is required to measure the patient's temperature. A *watch with a second hand* is required to measure the patient's pulse and respiration. To measure blood pressure, a *blood pressure cuff, sphygmomanometer,* and *stethoscope* are required. This is the skill that the radiographer should practice most frequently, as it is the one most likely to be needed in an emergency situation. A *tongue blade* is used to depress the tongue for inspection of the throat and is not used in vital sign assessment. *(Torres et al, p 139)*

31. (D) Lyme disease is a condition that results from the transmission of an infection by a *vector* (in this case, a deer tick). Vectors are insects and animals carrying disease. *Droplet contact* involves contact with secretions (from the nose, mouth, or eye) that travel via a sneeze or cough. The *airborne route* involves evaporated droplets in the air that transfer disease. A *vehicle* can transmit infection via contaminated water, food, blood, or drugs. *(Adler & Carlton, p 190)*

32. (D) Nonionic, low-osmolality iodinated contrast agents are associated with far fewer side effects and reactions than ionic, higher osmolality contrast agents. A *side effect* is an effect that is unintended but possibly expected and fundamentally *not harmful.* An *adverse reaction* is a *harmful* unintended effect. Possible *side effects* of iodinated contrast agents include a warm, flushed feeling, a metallic taste in the mouth, nausea, headache, and pain at the injection site. *Adverse reactions* include itching, anxiety, rash or hives, vomiting, sneezing, dyspnea, and hypotension. *(Adler & Carlton, p 240)*

33. (C) The normal blood pressure range for men and women is 110 to 140 mm Hg *systolic* reading (top number) and 60 to 80 mm Hg *diastolic* reading (bottom number). Systolic pressure is the contraction phase of the left ventricle, and diastolic pressure is the relaxation phase in the heart cycle. *(Torres et al, pp 148–149)*

34. (D) The U.S. Food and Drug Administration mandates that certain information be included in every drug package. Some of the information that drug companies are required to provide is *trade* and *generic* names, *indications* and *contraindications, usual dose, chemical composition* and *strength,* and any reported *side effects.* *(Adler & Carlton, pp 252–253)*

35. (C) Verbal defamation of another, or *slander,* is a type of intentional misconduct. *Invasion of privacy* (i.e., public discussion of privileged and confidential information) is intentional misconduct. However, if a radiographer leaves a weak patient standing alone to check images or get supplies, and that patient falls and sustains an injury, that would be considered unintentional misconduct or *negligence.* *(Saia, p 8)*

36. (B) When assisting the patient in changing, first remove clothing from the unaffected side. If this is done, removing clothing from the affected side will require less movement and effort. The patient's clothing should be cut away only as a last resort in cases of extreme emergency and with the patient's consent. *(Torres et al, p 96)*

37. (C) A patient with *orthopnea* is unable to breathe while lying down. When the body is recumbent, the diaphragm and abdominal viscera move to a more superior position. It is therefore more difficult to breathe deeply. Patients with orthopnea must be examined in an erect or semierect position. *Dyspnea* refers to difficulty breathing in any body position. *Apnea* describes cessation of breathing for short intervals. *Oligopnea* is infrequent breathing—as slow as 6 to 10 respirations per minute. *(Ehrlich, McCloskey, & Daly, p 127)*

38. (D) An unconscious patient is frequently able to hear and understand all that is going on, even though he or she is unable to respond. Therefore, while performing the examination, the radiographer should always refer to the patient by name and take care to continually explain what is being done and reassure the patient. *(Adler & Carlton, p 117)*

39. (C) *Diuretics* are used to promote urine elimination in individuals whose tissues are retaining excessive fluid. *Emetics* induce vomiting, and *cathartics* stimulate defecation. *Antitussives* are used to inhibit coughing. *(Torres et al, p 283)*

40. **(C)** Elderly patients dislike being pushed or hurried along. They appreciate the radiographer who is caring enough to take the extra few minutes necessary to comfort them. Some elderly patients are easily confused, and it is best to address them by their full name and keep instructions simple and direct. The elderly require the same respectful, dignified care as all other patients. *(Adler & Carlton, pp 120–121)*

41. **(C)** The complete killing of all microorganisms is termed *sterilization*. *Surgical asepsis* refers to the technique used to prevent contamination when performing procedures. *Medical asepsis* refers to practices that reduce the spread of microbes, and therefore the chance of spreading disease or infection. Hand washing is an example of medical asepsis. It reduces the spread of infection, but does not eliminate all microorganisms. *Disinfection* involves the use of chemicals to either inactivate or inhibit the growth of microbes. *(Adler & Carlton, p 184)*

42. **(D)** The radiographer must be aware that the patient's condition has a significant impact on motion control. The patient may wish to be very cooperative, but conditions beyond his or her control may exist. Patients often exhibit uncontrolled motion following a *traumatic injury*. *Medication* can worsen the condition. Traumatized patients are often more sensitive and likely to feel *chilled*. *Peristalsis* is another type of involuntary motion. *(Adler & Carlton, pp 146–147)*

43. **(A)** It is generally recommended that the IV bottle/bag be kept 18 to 20 inches above the level of the vein. If the container is too high, the pressure of the IV fluid can cause it to pass through the vein into surrounding tissues, causing a painful and potentially harmful condition. If the IV container is too low, blood may return through the needle into the tubing, form a clot, and obstruct the flow of IV fluid. *(Torres et al, p 323)*

44. **(A)** Iodinated contrast material can become somewhat *viscous* (thick and sticky) at normal room temperatures. This makes injection much more difficult. Warming the contrast medium to body temperature serves to reduce viscosity. This may be achieved by placing the vial in warm water or putting it into a special warming oven. *(Adler & Carlton, p 291)*

45. **(A)** The type of shock associated with the pooling of blood in the peripheral vessels is classified as *neurogenic shock*. This occurs in cases of trauma to the central nervous system that results in decreased arterial resistance and pooling of blood in peripheral vessels. *Cardiogenic shock* is related to cardiac failure and results from interference with heart function. It can occur in cases of cardiac tamponade, pulmonary embolus, or myocardial infarction. *Hypovolemic shock* is related to loss of large amounts of blood, either from internal bleeding or from hemorrhage associated with trauma. *Septic shock*, along with *anaphylactic shock*, is generally classified as *vasogenic shock*. *(Adler & Carlton, p 240)*

46. **(D)** The Joint Commission on the Accreditation of Healthcare Organizations *(JCAHO)* is the organization that accredits health-care organizations in the United States. The JCAHO sets forth certain standards for medical records. In keeping with these standards, all diagnostic and therapeutic orders must appear on the patient's medical record or chart. Additionally, patient identification information, medical history, consent forms, and any diagnostic and therapeutic reports should also be part of the patient's permanent record. The patient's chart is a means of communication between various health-care providers. *(Torres et al, p 19)*

47. **(C)** Category-specific isolations have been replaced by *transmission-based precautions: airborne, droplet,* and *contact*. Under these guidelines, some conditions or diseases can fall into more than one category. *Airborne precautions* are employed with patients suspected or known to be infected with the *tubercle bacillus (TB)*, *chickenpox (varicella)*, or *measles (rubeola)*. Airborne precautions *require that the patient wear a mask* to avoid the spread of bronchial secretions or other pathogens during coughing.

If the patient is unable or unwilling to wear a mask, the radiographer must wear one. The radiographer should wear gloves, but a gown is required only if flagrant contamination is likely. Patients under *airborne precautions* require a *private, specially ventilated (negative-pressure) room*. A private room is also indicated for all patients on *droplet precautions*, that is, with diseases transmitted via *large droplets* expelled from the patient while speaking, sneezing, or coughing. The pathogenic droplets can infect others when they come in contact with mouth or nasal mucosa or conjunctiva. *Rubella* ("German measles"), *mumps*, and *influenza* are among the diseases spread by droplet contact; *a private room is required* for the patient, and health-care practitioners should use *gown and gloves*. Any diseases spread by direct or close *contact*, such as *MRSA, conjunctivitis,* and *hepatitis A*, require *contact precautions. Contact precautions* require a *private patient room* and the use of *gloves, mask, and gown* for anyone coming in direct contact with the infected individual or his or her environment. *(Adler & Carlton, p 196)*

48. **(D)** All of the statements in the question are true and necessary in order for patient consent to be valid. The patient must sign the consent form before receiving sedation. The physician named on the consent form must perform the procedure; no other physician should perform it. Also, the consent form should be complete prior to being signed; there should be no blank spaces on the consent form when the patient signs it. In the case of a minor, a parent or guardian is required to sign the form. If a patient is not competent, then the legally appointed guardian should sign the consent. Remember that obtaining consent is the physician's responsibility, and so the explanation of the procedural risks should be performed by the physician, not by the radiographer. *(Ehrlich, McCloskey, & Daly, pp 54–56)*

49. **(B)** The Heimlich maneuver is used when a person is choking. If you suspect that an individual is choking, be certain that the airway is indeed obstructed before attempting the Heimlich maneuver. A person with a completely obstructed airway will not be able to speak or cough. If the person cannot speak or cough, then the airway is obstructed, and the Heimlich maneuver should be performed. The proper method is to stand behind the choking victim with one hand in a fist, thumb side in, midway between the navel and the xiphoid tip. Place the other hand over the closed fist with the palm open and apply pressure in and up. Repeat the thrust several times, until the object is dislodged. For an infant, the procedure is modified. Four back blows are given, midway between the scapulae, using the heel of the hand. If the object is not dislodged, the baby is turned over (being very careful to support the baby's head and spine), and four chests thrusts are performed just below the nipple line, using several fingers. *(Adler & Carlton, p 241)*

50. **(C)** Persons in sterile dress should not pass each other face to face. Rather, they should pass each other *back to back*, to avoid contaminating each other. Gowns are considered sterile in the front down to the waist, including the arms. Sterile gloves must be kept above the waist level. If the hands are accidentally lowered or placed behind the back, they are no longer sterile. A sterile field should not be left unattended. Sterile fields should be set up immediately prior to a procedure, and should be covered with a sterile drape if a few moments are to elapse before the procedure can begin. A sterile field should be constantly monitored to be certain that it has not been contaminated. *(Adler & Carlton, p 213)*

51. **(B)** A circumstance in which both the health-care provider's and the patient's actions contribute to an injurious outcome is termed *contributory negligence*. An example would be a patient who fails to follow the physician's orders or show up for follow-up care, and then sues when the condition causes permanent damage. Another example would be a patient who deliberately gives false information about the ingestion of drugs, leading to adverse effects from medications administered. Most states do not completely dismiss injury if there has been negligence on the part of the health-care institution, even if the patient's actions contributed substantially to the

injury. Rather, comparative negligence is applied, with the percentage of the injury due to the patient's actions is compared with the total amount of injury. A jury may decide that a doctor was negligent in his or her actions, but because the patient lied about using an illegal street drug that contributed to the injurious outcome, the patient is 80% responsible for his or her condition. The party suing may be awarded $100,000 for injuries, but would actually receive only $20,000. *Gross negligence* occurs when there is willful or deliberate neglect of the patient. Assault, battery, invasion of privacy, false imprisonment, and defamation of character all fall under the category of *intentional misconduct*. (*Ehrlich, McCloskey, & Daly, p 57*)

52. **(C)** *Extravasation* of contrast media into surrounding tissue is potentially very painful. If it does occur, the needle should be removed and the extravasation cared for immediately (before looking for another vein). *Pressure* should be applied to the vein until bleeding stops. Application of *warm, moist heat* to the affected area helps relieve pain. (*Adler & Carlton, p 275*)

53. **(D)** The *diastolic* number is the bottom number in a blood pressure reading. The normal range for diastolic pressure is considered to be 60 to 80 mm Hg. A diastolic pressure reading of 110 mm Hg might indicate hypertension. A diastolic pressure of 50 mm Hg might indicate shock. The *systolic* number is the top number in a blood pressure reading. The normal systolic pressure range is 110 to 140 mm Hg. (*Torres et al, p 148*)

54. **(A)** When transferring patients from stretcher to x-ray table, there are several rules that will reduce back strain. Pull, do not push, the patient; pushing increases friction and makes the transfer more difficult. Do not bend at the waist and pull; use your biceps for pulling the patient. Draw the patient as close to you as possible and then lift if necessary. (*Torres et al, p 82*)

55. **(A)** Injectable medications are available in two different kinds of containers. An *ampule* is a small container that usually holds a single dose of medication. A *vial* is a larger container that holds several doses of the medication. The term *bolus* is used to describe an amount of fluid to be injected. A *carafe* is a narrow-mouthed container; it is not likely to be used for medical purposes. (*Adler & Carlton, p 269*)

56. **(A)** It is unlikely that the radiographer will be faced with a wound hemorrhage, because bleeding from wounds is controlled before the patient is seen for x-ray examination. However, if a patient does experience hemorrhaging from a wound, you should apply pressure to the bleeding site and call for assistance. Delay can lead to serious blood loss. (*Adler & Carlton, p 248*)

57. **(A)** A *double-contrast GI* examination requires that the patient ingest gas-producing powder, crystals, pills, or beverage followed by a small amount of high-density barium. The patient may then be asked to roll in the recumbent position in order to coat the gastric mucosa, while the carbon dioxide expands. This procedure provides optimal visualization of the gastric walls. An *oral cholecystogram* can be performed approximately 3 hours after ingestion of special ipodate calcium granules. An intravenous urogram (IVU) requires an IV injection of iodinated contrast medium. (*Ballinger & Frank, vol 2, p 99*)

58. **(A)** *Autonomy* is the ethical principle that is related to the theory that patients have the right to decide what will or will not be done to them. *Beneficence* is related to the idea of doing good and being kind. *Fidelity* is faithfulness and loyalty. *Veracity* is not only telling the truth, but also not practicing deception. (*Adler & Carlton, p 308*)

59. **(D)** Most needle sticks occur during attempts to recap a needle. Proper disposal of contaminated needles and syringes is becoming more vital as HIV, AIDS, and HBV reach epidemic proportions. To prevent the spread of any possible infection, handle contaminated materials as little as possible. Therefore, do not attempt to recap a needle; instead, dispose of the entire syringe with the needle attached in the special container that is available. (*Torres et al, p 309*)

60. (D) Although it is never the responsibility of the radiographer to diagnose a patient, it is the responsibility of every radiographer to be alert. The patient should not be subjected to unnecessary radiation from an unwanted examination. Rather, it is the radiographer's responsibility to check with the referring physician and report the patient's complaint. *(Ehrlich & McCloskey, p 14)*

61. (B) A patient who has been NPO since midnight or who is anxious, frightened, or in pain may suffer an episode of syncope (fainting) on exertion. The patient should be helped to a recumbent position with feet elevated, to increase blood flow to the head. A patient who feels faint should never be left alone. *(Adler & Carlton, pp 247–248)*

62. (C) A patient who is having a *GI series* is required to be NPO for at least 8 hours prior to the examination; food or drink in the stomach can simulate disease. A patient who is scheduled for a *pyelogram* must have the preceding meal withheld to avoid the possibility of aspirating vomitus in case of an allergic reaction. An *abdominal survey* does not require the use of contrast media, and no patient preparation is necessary. *(Torres et al, p 234)*

63. (B) When performing bedside radiography in a contact isolation room, the radiographer should wear a gown, gloves, mask, and cap. The cassettes are prepared for the examination by placing a pillowcase over them to protect them from contamination. Whenever possible, one person should manipulate the mobile unit and remain "clean" whereas the other handles the patient. The mobile unit should be cleaned with a disinfectant upon exiting the patient's room, not prior to entering. *(Torres et al, p 69)*

64. (C) The Levin and Salem-sump tubes are nasogastric (NG) tubes used for gastric decompression. The *Salem-sump* tube is radiopaque and has a double lumen. One lumen is for gastric air compression, and the other is for removal of fluids. The *Levin* tube is a single-lumen tube that is used to prevent accumulation of intestinal liquids and gas during and following intestinal surgery. The *Swan–Ganz*

IV catheter is advanced to the pulmonary artery and used to measure various heart pressures. *(Adler & Carlton, p 223)*

65. (B) *Anaphylaxis* is an acute reaction characterized by the sudden onset of urticaria, respiratory distress, vascular collapse, or systemic shock, sometimes leading to death. It is caused by ingestion or injection of a sensitizing agent such as a drug, vaccine, contrast agent, or food, or by an insect bite. *Asthma* and *rhinitis* are examples of allergic reactions. Myocardial infarction (MI) is caused by partial or complete occlusion of a coronary artery. *(Torres et al, p 165)*

66. (B) The most effective method of sterilization is moist heat, using steam under pressure. This is known as autoclaving. Sterilization with dry heat requires higher temperatures for longer periods of time than sterilization with moist heat. Pasteurization is moderate heating with rapid cooling; it is frequently used in the commercial preparation of milk and alcoholic beverages such as wine and beer. It is not a form of sterilization. Freezing can also kill some microbes, but it is not a form of sterilization. *(Torres et al, pp 116–117)*

67. (C) *Emphysema* is a progressive disorder caused by long-term irritation of the bronchial passages, such as by air pollution or cigarette smoking. Emphysema patients are unable to exhale normally because of the loss of elasticity of alveolar walls. If emphysema patients receive oxygen, it is usually administered at a very slow flow rate, because their respirations are controlled by the level of carbon dioxide in the blood. *(Bontrager, pp 69, 80)*

68. (A) The chest drainage system unit should always be kept below the level of the patient's chest. Chest tubes are used to remove air, blood, or fluid from the pleural cavity. By draining fluid from the pleural cavity, a collapsed lung, or *atelectasis*, may be relieved. By relieving the pressure from air in the pleural cavity, a *pneumothorax* may be reduced. Radiographers must take care that the tubes of the chest drainage unit do not kink and do not get caught on IV poles or radiographic equipment. It is imperative that the unit remain below the level of the chest. The chest drainage system has several components. One component is a chamber that collects the draining fluid. Another component is the suction control chamber. A third component is the water seal chamber, which prevents air from the atmosphere from entering the system. The last component is the water seal venting chamber, which allows air to leave the system, thus preventing pressure buildup. In order for the unit to work properly, it must remain below the level of the chest. (*Adler & Carlton, pp 174–175*)

69. **(B)** The patient's right to privacy refers to his or her modesty and dignity being respected. It also refers to the professional health-care worker's obligation to respect the confidentiality of privileged information. Communication of privileged information to anyone but health-care workers involved with the patient's care is inexcusable. (*Gurley & Callaway, p 187*)

70. **(A)** Angina pectoris is a crushing chest pain caused by a circulatory disturbance of the coronary arteries. Nitroglycerin is used to dilate blood vessels (vasodilation) and decrease blood pressure in the treatment of pain from angina pectoris. Nitroglycerin is usually given sublingually, and thus is absorbed directly into the bloodstream. (*Torres et al, p 280*)

71. **(C)** It is recommended that a radiographer wear protective eye gear (goggles) during any procedure in which there might be splattering of blood or body fluids. This includes both angiography and biopsy/aspiration procedures. This would not be expected during a routine upper gastrointestinal examination. (*Torres et al, p 64*)

72. **(C)** The BUN level indicates the quantity of *nitrogen in the blood in the form of urea*. The normal concentration is 8 to 25 mg/100 mL. *BUN and creatinine* blood chemistry levels should be checked prior to beginning an intravenous pyelogram (IVP). An increase in the BUN level often indicates decreased renal function. Increased BUN and/or creatinine levels may forecast an increased possibility of contrast media–induced renal effects and poor visualization of the renal collecting systems.

The normal creatinine range is 0.6 to 1.5 mg/mL. (*Ballinger & Frank, vol 2, p 176*)

73. **(B)** Quantities of medication can be dispensed intravenously over a period of time via an *IV infusion*. A special infusion pump may be used to precisely regulate the quantity received by the patient. An *IV push* refers to a rapid injection; the term *bolus* refers to the quantity of material being injected. The term *hypodermic* refers to administration of medication by any route other than orally. (*Adler & Carlton, p 276*)

74. **(A)** Observation is an important part of the evaluation of acutely ill patients. The patient who is *diaphoretic* is "in a cold sweat," with pale, cool, moist skin. *Hot, dry skin* accompanies fever. *Warm, moist skin* may be a result of anxiety or simply of being in a warm room. The pupils *dilate* in dimly illuminated places in order to allow more light into the eyes. (*Torres et al, p 160*)

75. **(D)** When scheduling patient examinations, it is important to avoid the possibility of residual contrast medium covering areas that will be of interest on later examinations. The IV urogram (also referred to as intravenous Pyelogram/IVP) should be scheduled first because the contrast medium used is excreted rapidly. The barium enema should be scheduled next. Finally, the upper GI is scheduled. There should not be enough barium remaining from the previous BE to interfere with the examination of the stomach or duodenum, although a preliminary scout image should be taken in each case. (*Torres et al, p 234*)

76. **(B)** The presence of aneurysm clips is contraindication for MRI; even slight shift can cause damage. MRI can be performed for herniated disc and subdural bleeding. Dental fillings do not contraindicate MRI. (*Torres et al, p 363*)

77. **(B)** A *fomite* is an inanimate object that has been in contact with an infectious microorganism. A *reservoir* is a site where an infectious organism can remain alive and from which transmission can occur. Although an inanimate object can be a reservoir for infection, living

objects (such as humans) can also be reservoirs. For infection to spread, there must be a *host* environment. Although an inanimate object may serve as a temporary host where microbes can grow, microbes flourish on and in the human host, where there are plenty of body fluids and tissues to nourish and feed the microbes. A *vector* is an animal host of an infectious organism that transmits the infection via bite or sting. (*Torres et al, p 54*)

78. **(C)** The relatively low-osmolality and non-ionic, water-soluble contrast media available to radiology departments have outstanding advantages, especially for patients with a history of allergic reaction. They were originally used for intrathecal injections (myelography), but they were quickly accepted for intravascular injections as well. *Side effects and allergic reactions are less likely and less severe with these media.* Their one very significant disadvantage is their high cost compared to ionic contrast media. (*Adler & Carlton, p 328*)

79. **(A)** Anginal pain, caused by constriction of blood vessels, may be relieved with the administration of a *vasodilator* such as nitroglycerin. *Bradycardia* (abnormally slow heartbeat) and *cardiac arrest* are treated with *vasoconstrictors* such as dopamine or epinephrine to increase blood pressure. *Antihistamines* such as diphenhydramine (Benadryl) are used to treat allergic reactions and anaphylactic shock. (*Adler & Carlton, p 265*)

80. **(A)** When a two-member team of radiographers is performing mobile radiography on a patient with contact precautions, such as an MRSA (methicillin-resistant *Staphyloccus aureus*) patient, one radiographer remains "clean"—that is, he or she has no physical contact with the patient. The clean radiographer will position the mobile unit and make the exposure. The other member of the team will position the cassette and retrieve the cassette. As the two radiographers fold down the cassette's protective plastic cover, the clean radiographer will remove the cassette from the plastic. Both radiographers should be protected with gowns, gloves, and masks if the patient is on contact precautions. Additionally,

after the examination is completed, the mobile unit should be cleaned with a disinfectant. Conditions requiring the use of contact precautions also include hepatitis A and varicella. (*Adler & Carlton, p 196*)

81. **(D)** All of these symptoms are related to a respiratory reaction. There may also be hoarseness, wheezing, or cyanosis. The patient who has received contrast media should be watched closely. If any symptoms arise, the radiologist should be notified immediately. (*Adler & Carlton, p 293*)

82. **(C)** If a patient in your care asks to see his or her chart, the appropriate response is to refer the patient to his or her physician. A patient *does* have the right to review his or her own medical record; however, the patient should do so in the presence of the physician so that the patient does not misinterpret the information and so that the physician can address concerns or answer questions. It is not appropriate to hand over the chart to a patient, nor is it appropriate to deceive the patient into believing that the chart is not available for viewing or that the patient has no right to review the chart. (*Adler & Carlton, p 317*)

83. **(B)** *Cyanosis* is a condition resulting from a deficiency of oxygen circulating in the blood. It is characterized by bluish discoloration of the gums, nailbeds, and earlobes, and around the mouth. Cyanosis may be accompanied by labored breathing or other types of respiratory distress. (*Torres et al, p 147*)

84. **(B)** Strain on the abdominal muscles may be minimized by placing a pillow under the patient's head and a support under the patient's knees. The pillow also relieves neck strain, reduces the chance of aspiration in the nauseated patient, and allows the patient to observe his or her surroundings. The Trendelenburg position causes the diaphragm to assume a higher position and can cause a patient to become short of breath. (*Ehrlich, McCloskey, & Daly, pp 93–94*)

85. **(C)** A *Swan–Ganz catheter* is a specific type of IV catheter used to measure the pumping ability of the heart, to obtain pressure readings,

and to introduce medications and IV fluids. A *pacemaker* is a device that is inserted under the patient's skin to regulate heart rate. Pacemakers may be permanent or temporary. *Chest tubes* are used to remove fluid or air from the pleural cavity. Any of these items may be identified on a chest radiograph, provided the cassette is properly positioned and the correct exposure factors are employed. If the physician is interested in assessing the proper placement of a Swan–Ganz catheter, the lungs may have to be slightly overexposed in order to clearly delineate the proper placement of the tip of the Swan–Ganz catheter, which will overlap the denser cardiac silhouette. A *urinary catheter* will not appear on a chest radiograph. *(Adler & Carlton, p 177)*

86. **(B)** The medical term for nosebleed is *epistaxis*. *Vertigo* refers to a feeling of "whirling" or a sensation that the room is spinning. Some possible causes of vertigo include inner ear infection and acoustic neuroma. *Urticaria* is a vascular reaction resulting in dilated capillaries and edema and causing the patient to break out in hives. An *aura* may be classified as either a feeling or a sensory response (such as flashing lights, tasting metal, smelling coffee) that precedes an episode such as a seizure or a migraine headache. *(Adler & Carlton, p 247)*

87. **(A)** Blood pressure is measured in *millimeters of mercury, or mmHg*. Heart rate, or pulse, is measured in units of *beats per minute*. Temperature is measured in *degrees Fahrenheit, or °F*. Oxygen delivery is measured in units of *liters per minute, or L/min*. Table 1–1 outlines the normal ranges for vital signs in healthy adults. *(Torres et al, p 147)*

TABLE 1–1. NORMAL RANGES FOR VITAL SIGNS IN ADULTS

Blood pressure	110–140 mmHg/60–80 mmHg
Pulse rate	60–100 beats/min
Temperature	97.7–99.5°F
Respiration rate	12–20 breaths/min

88. **(B)** A *myelogram*, or radiographic examination of the spinal canal, requires an intrathecal (intraspinal) injection. Intrathecal administration of contrast medium is usually at the level

of L2/3 or L3/4. An *intravenous pyelogram* is performed with an injection of contrast medium into the venous system. A *lymphangiogram* requires that contrast medium be delivered into the lymphatic vessels. A *CT scan* may or may not require the use of an IV injection. *(Torres et al, p 369)*

89. **(C)** Category-specific isolations have been replaced by *transmission-based precautions: airborne, droplet,* and *contact.* Under these guidelines, some conditions or diseases can fall into more than one category. *Airborne precautions* are employed with patients suspected or known to be infected with the *tubercle bacillus (TB), chickenpox (varicella),* or *measles (rubeola).* Airborne precautions *require that the patient wear a mask* to avoid the spread of bronchial secretions or other pathogens during coughing. If the patient is unable or unwilling to wear a mask, the radiographer must wear one. The radiographer should wear gloves, but a gown is required only if flagrant contamination is likely. Patients under *airborne precautions* require a *private, specially ventilated (negative-pressure) room.* A private room is also indicated for all patients on *droplet precautions,* that is, with diseases transmitted via *large droplets* expelled from the patient while speaking, sneezing, or coughing. The pathogenic droplets can infect others when they come in contact with mouth or nasal mucosa or conjunctiva. *Rubella* ("German measles"), *mumps,* and *influenza* are among the diseases spread by droplet contact; *a private room is required* for the patient, and health-care practitioners should use *gown and gloves.* Any diseases spread by direct or close *contact,* such as *MRSA,* conjunctivitis, and *hepatitis A,* require *contact precautions.* Contact precautions require a *private patient room* and the use of *gloves, mask, and gown* for anyone coming in direct contact with the infected individual or his or her environment. *(Adler & Carlton, p 196)*

90. **(C)** *Talipes* is the term used to describe congenital clubfoot. There are several types of talipes, generally characterized by a deformed talus and a shortened Achilles tendon, giving the foot a *clubfoot* appearance. *Osteochondritis* (Osgood–Schlatter disease) is a painful incomplete

separation of the tibial tuberosity from the tibial shaft. It is often seen in active adolescent boys. *Coxa plana* (Legg–Calvé–Perthes disease) is ischemic necrosis leading to flattening of the femoral head. *Muscular dystrophy* is a congenital disorder characterized by wasting of skeletal muscles. *(Ballinger & Frank, vol 1, p 259)*

91. **(C)** An individual whose coronary arteries are not carrying enough blood to the heart muscle (myocardium), as a result of partial or complete blockage of a cardiac vessel, experiences crushing pain in the chest, frequently radiating to the left jaw and arm. This is termed *angina pectoris*. It may be relieved by the drug nitroglycerin, which dilates the coronary arteries, thus facilitating circulation. *Tachycardia* refers to rapid heart rate, and *bradycardia* to slow heart rate. *Syncope* is fainting. *(Adler & Carlton, p 292)*

92. **(D)** Hypochlorite bleach (Clorox) and Lysol are examples of *disinfectants*. Disinfectants are used in radiology departments to clean equipment and to remove microorganisms from areas such as radiographic tables. *Antiseptics* are also used to stop the growth of microorganisms, but they are often applied to the skin, not to radiographic equipment. *Antifungal* medications can be administered systemically or topically to treat or prevent fungal infections. *Antibacterial* medications (bacteriostatics) can also be administered systemically or externally. Tetracycline is a systemic antibacterial medication. *(Torres et al, p 116)*

93. **(D)** *Ventricular septal defect* is a congenital heart condition characterized by a hole in the interventricular septum, which allows oxygenated and unoxygenated blood to mix. Some interventricular septal defects are small and close spontaneously; others require surgery. *Coarctation of the aorta* is a narrowing or constriction of the aorta. *Atrial septal defect* is a small hole (the remnant of the fetal foramen ovale) in the interatrial septum. It usually closes spontaneously in the first months of life; if it persists or is unusually large, surgical repair is necessary. The ductus arteriosus is a short fetal blood vessel connecting the aorta and pulmonary artery that usually closes within 10 to 15 hours after birth. A *patent ductus*

arteriosus is one that persists and requires surgical closure. *(Taber's, p 2323)*

94. **(B)** Children are often fearful of leaving familiar surroundings, and being able to take along a familiar toy is helpful. A calm and cheerful radiographer can be reassuring to the anxious child. Honesty is essential, and false reassurances, such as telling the child it will not hurt, not only do more harm than good, but also focus the child's attention on pain. *(Torres et al, p 201)*

95. **(A)** A drug's *generic name* identifies its chemical family. A particular generic drug can be manufactured by several different companies and given different *trade names* (*brand* or *proprietary names*). For example, the drug with the chemical/generic name acetaminophen is known by the trade or brand name Tylenol. Drugs can be classified by either their generic name or their trade name. *(Torres et al, p 262)*

96. **(B)** The diaphragm is the major muscle of respiration. Upon inspiration/inhalation, the diaphragm and abdominal viscera are depressed, enabling the filling and expansion of the lungs, accompanied by upward movement of the sternum and ribs. During expiration/exhalation, air leaves the lungs and they deflate, while the diaphragm relaxes and moves to a more superior position along with the abdominal viscera. As the diaphragm relaxes and moves up, the sternum and ribs move inferiorly. *(Ballinger & Frank, vol 1, pp 509–510)*

97. **(D)** A *tort* is an *intentional* or *unintentional* act that involves personal injury or damage to a patient. Allowing a patient to be exposed to unnecessary radiation, either by neglecting to shield the patient or by performing an unwanted examination, would be considered a tort, and the radiographer would be legally accountable. Discussing a patient's condition with a third party would undoubtedly be considered a serious intentional tort. *(Torres et al, p 15)*

98. **(C)** Because hospitals are the refuge of the sick, they can also be places of disease transmission unless proper infection control guidelines are followed. When cleaning contaminated objects

or surfaces such as the radiographic table, it is important to *clean from the least contaminated to the most contaminated area* and *from the top down*. Soiled gowns and linens should be folded from the outside in and properly disposed of. When the patient's skin is being prepared for surgery, it is often cleaned in circular motion, starting from the center and working outward; however, this motion is not used for objects or surfaces. *(Torres et al, p 66)*

99. **(B)** A radiographer who performs the wrong examination on a patient may be charged with battery. *Battery* refers to the unlawful laying of hands on a patient. The radiographer could also be charged with battery if a patient was moved about roughly or touched in a manner that is inappropriate or without the patient's consent. *Assault* is the *threat* of touching or laying hands on someone. If a patient feels threatened by a practitioner, either because of the tone or pitch of the practitioner's voice or because the practitioner uses words that are threatening, the practitioner can be accused of assault. *False imprisonment* may be considered if a patient is ignored after stating that she no longer wishes to continue with the procedure, or if restraining devices are improperly used or used without a physician's order. The accusation of *defamation* can be upheld when patient confidentiality is not respected, and as a result the patient suffers embarrassment or mockery. *(Adler & Carlton, p 329)*

100. **(A)** *Gerontology*, or geriatrics, is the study of the elderly. While bone demineralization and loss of muscle mass occur to a greater or lesser degree in most elderly individuals, the radiographer must not assume that all gerontologic patients are hard of hearing, clumsy, or not mentally alert. Today many elderly people remain very active, staying mentally and physically agile well into their so-called golden years. The radiographer must keep this in mind as he or she provides age-specific care to the gerontologic patient. *(Torres et al, p 211)*

101. **(C)** The tracheostomy patient will have difficulty speaking as a result of the redirection of the air past the vocal cords. Gurgling or rattling sounds coming from the trachea indicate an ex-

cess accumulation of secretions, requiring suction with sterile catheters. Any rotation or movement of the tracheostomy tube may cause the tube to become dislodged, and an obstructed airway could result. *(Torres et al, p 239)*

102. **(B)** Dilated twisted veins, or *varices*, of the esophagus are frequently associated with obstructive liver disease or cirrhosis of the liver. These esophageal veins enlarge and can rupture, causing serious hemorrhage. *Achalasia* is dilation of the esophagus as a result of the cardiac sphincter's failure to relax and allow food to pass into the stomach. *Dysphasia* is a speech impairment resulting from a brain lesion; it is unrelated to the esophagus. *Dysphagia* refers to difficulty swallowing and is the most common esophageal complaint. *Hiatal hernia* is another common esophageal problem; it is characterized by protrusion of a portion of the stomach through the cardiac sphincter. It is a common condition, and many individuals with the condition are asymptomatic. Each of these conditions of the esophagus may be evaluated with an esophagogram. Positions usually include the posteroanterior, right anterior oblique, and right lateral. *(Linn-Watson, pp 102, 107)*

103. **(D)** Medications are commonly administered *orally* (by mouth). They may also be administered directly into a vein (*intravenously*), into a muscle (*intramuscularly*), or under the skin (*subcutaneously*). *(Torres et al, p 269)*

104. **(C)** Protective or "reverse" isolation is used to keep the susceptible patient from becoming infected. Patients who have suffered burns have lost a very important means of protection, their skin, and therefore have increased susceptibility to bacterial invasion. Patients whose immune systems are depressed have lost the ability to combat infection, and hence are more susceptible to infection. Active tuberculosis requires airborne precautions, not protective isolation. *(Torres et al, p 69)*

105. **(C)** Whenever a perforation of the GI tract is suspected, a water-soluble contrast agent (such as Gastrografin or oral Hypaque) should be used because it is easily absorbed from within

the peritoneal cavity. Leakage of barium sulfate into the peritoneal cavity can have serious consequences. Water-soluble contrast agents may also be used in place of barium sulfate when the possibility of barium impaction exists. Oil-based contrast agents are rarely used today. (*Ballinger & Frank, vol 2, p 94*)

106. **(D)** All of the statements in the question are true regarding the proper care of a patient with a tracheostomy. If a tracheostomy needs to be touched for any reason, sterile technique should be employed to avoid the possibility of infection. Patients with tracheostomies require frequent suction. This is usually not performed by the technologist, but radiographers may be called upon to assist with suctioning, especially for patients who must be in the radiology department for lengthy procedures. Patients who are to be suctioned should be aerated beforehand (i.e., oxygen should be administered prior to suctioning). It is also important that patients be permitted to rest during suctioning. Never suction for longer than 15 s; check breath sounds with a stethoscope to ensure that the airway is clear. It is the radiographer's responsibility to check the work area and ensure that the suction is working and that ample ancillary supplies (suction kit, catheters, tubing) are available. (*Adler & Carlton, p 214*)

107. **(B)** Syncope, or fainting, is the result of a drop in blood pressure caused by insufficient blood (oxygen) flow to the brain. The patient should be helped into a dorsal recumbent position with feet elevated to facilitate blood flow to the brain. (*Ehrlich et al, p 239*)

108. **(B)** The diameter of a needle is the needle's *gauge*. The higher the gauge number, the smaller the diameter and the thinner the needle. For example, a very tiny-gauge needle (25 gauge) may be used on a pediatric patient for an IV injection, whereas a large-gauge needle (16 gauge) may be used for donating blood. The *hub* of a needle is the portion of the needle that attaches to a syringe. The *length* of the needle varies depending on its use. A longer needle is needed for intramuscular injections, whereas a shorter needle is used for subcutaneous injection. The *bevel* of the needle is the slanted tip

of the needle. For IV injections, the bevel should always face up. (*Adler & Carlton, p 267*)

109. **(A)** The patient is said to be in the *Trendelenburg* position when the head is positioned lower than the feet. This position is helpful in several radiographic procedures, such as separating redundant bowel loops and demonstration of hiatal hernias. It is also used in treating shock. In *Fowler's* position, the head is higher than the feet. The *Sims'* position is the left posterior oblique (LPO) position with the right leg flexed up for insertion of the enema tip. *Stenver's* is a radiographic position for mastoids. (*Taber's, p 2234*)

110. **(A)** *Epinephrine* (Adrenalin) is a bronchodilator. Bronchodilators may be administered in a spray mister, such as for asthma, or by injection to relieve severe bronchospasm. *Lidocaine* (Xylocaine) is an antiarrhythmic used to prevent or treat cardiac arrhythmias (dysrhythmia). *Nitroglycerin* and *verapamil* are vasodilators. Vasodilators permit increased blood flow by relaxing the walls of the blood vessels. (*Adler & Carlton, p 265*)

111. **(B)** *Epinephrine* (Adrenalin) is the vasopressor used to treat an anaphylactic reaction or cardiac arrest. *Nitroglycerin* is a vasodilator. *Hydrocortisone* is a steroid that may be used to treat bronchial asthma, allergic reactions, and inflammatory reactions. *Digitoxin* is used to treat cardiac fibrillation. (*Adler & Carlton, p 265*)

112. **(C)** Some chemical agents used in health-care facilities function to kill pathogenic microorganisms, while others function to inhibit the growth/spread of pathogenic microorganisms. *Germicides* and *disinfectants* are used to kill pathogenic microorganisms, whereas *antiseptics* (like alcohol) are used to stop their growth/spread. *Sterilization* is another associated term; it refers to the killing of all microorganisms and their spores. (*Ballinger & Frank, vol 1, p 15*)

113. **(C)** Frequent and correct hand washing is an essential part of medical asepsis; it is the best method for avoiding the spread of microorganisms. If the faucet cannot be operated with

the knee or a foot pedal, it should be opened and closed using paper towels. Care should be taken to wash all surfaces of the hand and between the fingers thoroughly. The hands and forearms should always be kept below the elbows. Hand lotions should be used frequently to keep hands from chapping. Unbroken skin prevents the entry of microorganisms; dry, cracked skin breaks down that defense and permits the entry of microorganisms. *(Ehrlich et al, pp 153–155)*

114. **(C)** When radiographs in the surgical suite are required, the radiographer is responsible for ensuring that surgical asepsis is maintained. This requires proper dress, cleanliness of equipment, and restricted access to certain areas. An example of a restricted area is the "sterile corridor," which is located between the draped patient and the instrument table and is occupied only by the surgeon and the instrument nurse. *(Adler & Carlton, p 220)*

115. **(A)** Three times a day is indicated by the abbreviation *tid*. The abbreviation *qid* means four times a day. Every hour is represented by *qh*, and *pc* means after meals. *(Adler & Carlton, p 278)*

116. **(A)** When a patient is experiencing a seizure, he or she should be *protected* from striking any hard surfaces or falling. The patient exhibits uncontrollable body movements. Any attempt to place the patient in a semierect position or to administer a sedative would prove futile. Following the seizure, it is important to place the patient on his or her side to prevent aspiration of any vomitus or oral secretions. *(Adler & Carlton, p 248)*

117. **(D)** *Orthopnea* is a respiratory condition in which the patient has difficulty breathing *(dyspnea)* in any position other than erect. The patient is usually comfortable in the erect, standing, or seated position. The *Trendelenburg* position places the patient's head lower than the rest of the body. *Fowler's position* is a semierect position, and the *recumbent* position is lying down. *(Taber, p 1535)*

118. **(B)** Double-contrast studies of the large bowel are particularly useful for demonstration of

the *bowel wall*, and anything projecting from it, as in diverticulosis. *Polyps* are projections of the bowel wall mucous membrane into the bowel lumen. *Colitis* is inflammation of the large bowel, often associated with ulcerations of the mucosal wall. A single-contrast study would most likely obliterate these mucosal conditions, but coating of the bowel mucosa with barium and subsequent filling the bowel with air (double contrast) provides optimal delineation. *(Ballinger & Frank, vol 2, p 128)*

119. **(C)** Obtaining a complete and accurate history from the patient for the radiologist is an important aspect of a radiographer's job. Both subjective and objective data should be collected. *Objective* data include signs and symptoms that can be observed, such as a cough, a lump, or elevated blood pressure. *Subjective* data relate to what the patient feels, and to what extent. A patient may experience pain, but is it mild or severe? Is it localized or general? Does the pain increase or decrease under different circumstances? A radiographer should explore this with a patient and document the information on the requisition for the radiologist. *(Adler & Carlton, p 126)*

120. **(D)** When a diabetic patient misses an insulin injection, the body loses its ability to metabolize glucose, and ketoacidosis can occur. If this is not quickly corrected, the patient may become comatose. Symptoms of impending coma include increased urination, sweet (fruity) breath, and extreme thirst. Other symptoms are weakness and nausea. *(Torres et al, p 170)*

121. **(D)** The condition in which a patient's heart rate slows to below 60 beats/min is *bradycardia*. *Hyperthermia* is the condition in which the patient's temperature is well above the normal average range (97.7 to 99.5°F). *Hypotension* occurs if the blood pressure drops below the normal ranges (110 to 140/60 to 90 mmHg). *Hypoxia* is a condition in which there is decreased oxygen supply to body tissues. *(Adler & Carlton, p 160)*

122. **(B)** A patient who is going into shock may exhibit *pallor and weakness*, a significant *drop in blood pressure*, and an *increased pulse*. The

patient may also experience *apprehension and restlessness* and may have *cool, clammy skin*. A radiographer recognizing these symptoms should call them to the physician's attention immediately. Fever is not associated with shock. *(Torres et al, p 163)*

123. **(D)** Increased pain threshold, breakdown of skin, and atrophy of fat pads and sweat glands are all important considerations when working with *geriatric patients*. Many changes occur as our bodies age. Although muscle is replaced with fat, the amount of subcutaneous fat is decreased, and the skin atrophies. Therefore, the geriatric patient requires *extra-gentle treatment*. A mattress pad should always be placed on the radiographic table to help prevent *skin injury* or abrasions. If tape is required, paper tape should be used instead of adhesive. Geriatric patients are also more sensitive to *hypothermia* because of breakdown of the sweat glands and should always be kept covered, both to preserve modesty and for extra warmth. *Loss of sensation* in the skin increases pain tolerance, and so the geriatric patient may not be aware of excessive stress on bony prominences like the elbow, wrist, coccyx, and ankles. *(Dowd & Wilson, vol 2, p 1026)*

124. **(C)** The abbreviation for every hour is *qh*. The abbreviation *tid* means three times a day, and *qid* means four times a day. After meals is abbreviated *pc*. *(Adler & Carlton, p 278)*

125. **(C)** Radiographs are the *property of the health-care institution* and are a part of every patient's permanent medical record. They are often retained on file for about 7 years or, in the case of pediatric patients, until the patient reaches maturity. They are not the personal property of either the radiologist or the referring physician. If a patient changes doctors or needs a second opinion, copies can be requested. The patient may also borrow the originals, which must be returned, or he or she may pay for copies. *(Adler & Carlton, p 317)*

126. **(A)** *Creatinine* is a normal alkaline constituent of urine and blood, but increased quantities of creatinine are present in advanced stages of renal disease. Creatinine and *BUN* blood chemistry levels should be checked prior to beginning an IV pyelogram. Increased levels may forecast an increased possibility of contrast-media induced renal effects and poor visualization of the renal collecting systems. The normal creatinine range is 0.6 to 1.5 mg/100 mL. The normal BUN range is 8 to 25 mg/100 mL. *(Ballinger & Frank, vol 2, p 126)*

127. **(C)** A *stethoscope* and a *sphygmomanometer* are used together to measure blood pressure. The first sound heard is the systolic pressure, and the normal range is 110 to 140 mmHg. When the sound is no longer heard, the diastolic pressure is recorded. The normal diastolic range is 60 to 90 mmHg. Elevated blood pressure is called *hypertension. Hypotension*, or low blood pressure, is not of concern unless it is caused by injury or disease; in that case, it can result in shock. A *pulse oximeter* is used to measure a patient's pulse rate and oxygen saturation level. *(Adler & Carlton, p 166)*

128. **(D)** Diseases that are transmitted through the air include TB, rubella ("German measles"), mumps, and influenza. Airborne precautions *require the patient to wear a mask* to avoid the spread of acid-fast bacilli (in the bronchial secretions of TB patients) or other pathogens during coughing. If the patient is unable or unwilling to wear a mask, the radiographer must wear one. The radiographer should wear gloves, but a gown is required only if flagrant contamination is likely. Patients infected with diseases calling for *airborne precautions* require a *private, specially ventilated (negative-pressure)* room. A private room is also indicated for all patients on *droplet precautions*, that is, with diseases that are transmitted via large droplets expelled from the patient while speaking, sneezing, or coughing. The pathogenic droplets can infect others when they come in contact with the mouth or nasal mucosa or conjunctiva. *Rubella* ("German measles"), *mumps*, and *influenza* are among the diseases spread by droplet contact; *a private room is required* for the patient, and health-care practitioners must use *gown and gloves. (Adler & Carlton, p 196)*

129. **(D)** None of the statements in the question is false; all are true. Oxygen is classified as a

drug and must be prescribed by a physician. The rate and mode of delivery of oxygen must be specified in the physician's orders. It can be ordered to be delivered continuously or as needed. *(Adler & Carlton, p 168)*

130. **(B)** Both ultrasound and magnetic resonance imaging do not require the use of ionizing radiation to produce an image. Computed axial tomography does require ionizing radiation to produce an image. Ultrasound requires the use of high-frequency sound waves to produce images of soft tissue structures and certain blood vessels within the body. Magnetic resonance imaging relies on the use of a very powerful magnet and specially designed coils that are sensitive to radio-wave signals to produce the image. *(Torres et al, p 362)*

Subspecialty List

1. Physical assistance and transfer
2. Infection control
3. Ethical and legal aspects
4. Ethical and legal aspects
5. Medical emergencies
6. Interpersonal communication
7. Physical assistance and transfer
8. Contrast media
9. Physical assistance and transfer
10. Medical emergencies
11. Contrast media
12. Contrast media
13. Contrast media
14. Medical emergencies
15. Medical emergencies
16. Contrast media
17. Contrast media
18. Infection control
19. Ethical and legal aspects
20. Contrast media
21. Physical assistance and transfer
22. Medical emergencies
23. Medical emergencies
24. Medical emergencies
25. Infection control
26. Medical emergencies
27. Infection control
28. Physical assistance and transfer
29. Physical assistance and transfer
30. Physical assistance and transfer
31. Infection control
32. Contrast media
33. Physical assistance and transfer
34. Patient monitoring
35. Patient monitoring
36. Physical assistance and transfer
37. Medical emergencies
38. Medical emergencies
39. Physical assistance and transfer
40. Physical assistance and transfer
41. Infection control
42. Physical assistance and transfer
43. Contrast media
44. Contrast media
45. Medical emergencies
46. Ethical and legal aspects
47. Infection control
48. Ethical and legal aspects
49. Medical emergencies
50. Infection control
51. Ethical and legal aspects
52. Contrast media
53. Physical assistance and transfer
54. Physical assistance and transfer
55. Contrast media
56. Medical emergencies
57. Contrast media
58. Ethical and legal aspects
59. Infection control
60. Ethical and legal aspects
61. Medical emergencies
62. Contrast media
63. Infection control
64. Contrast media

65. Medical emergencies
66. Infection control
67. Medical emergencies
68. Physical assistance and transfer
69. Ethical and legal aspects
70. Medical emergencies
71. Infection control
72. Physical assistance and transfer
73. Contrast media
74. Interpersonal communication
75. Contrast media
76. Interpersonal communication
77. Infection control
78. Contrast media
79. Medical emergencies
80. Infection control
81. Contrast media
82. Interpersonal communication
83. Medical emergencies
84. Physical assistance and transfer
85. Physical assistance and transfer
86. Medical emergencies
87. Physical assistance and transfer
88. Contrast media
89. Infection control
90. Physical assistance and transfer
91. Medical emergencies
92. Infection control
93. Medical emergencies
94. Interpersonal communication
95. Contrast media
96. Physical assistance and transfer
97. Ethical and legal aspects

98. Infection control
99. Ethical and legal aspects
100. Interpersonal communication
101. Medical emergencies
102. Contrast media
103. Contrast media
104. Infection control
105. Contrast media
106. Medical emergencies
107. Medical emergencies
108. Contrast media
109. Physical assistance and transfer
110. Medical emergencies
111. Medical emergencies
112. Infection control
113. Infection control
114. Infection control
115. Interpersonal communication
116. Medical emergencies
117. Medical emergencies
118. Contrast media
119. Interpersonal communication
120. Interpersonal communication
121. Interpersonal communication
122. Physical assistance and transfer
123. Interpersonal communication
124. Interpersonal communication
125. Ethical and legal aspects
126. Physical assistance and transfer
127. Physical assistance and transfer
128. Infection control
129. Physical assistance and transfer
130. Interpersonal communication

CHAPTER 2

Radiographic Procedures
Questions

DIRECTIONS (Questions 1 through 300): Each of the numbered items or incomplete statements in this section is followed by answers or by completions of the statement. Select the *one* lettered answer or completion that is *best* in each case.

1. Which of the following statements is (are) correct regarding the parietoacanthial projection (Waters' method) of the skull?

   1. The head is rested on the extended chin.
   2. The orbitomeatal line (OML) is perpendicular to the (IR).
   3. The maxillary antra should be projected above the petrosa.

   (A) 1 only
   (B) 1 and 2 only
   (C) 1 and 3 only
   (D) 1, 2, and 3

2. Skeletal conditions characterized by faulty bone calcification include

   1. osteoarthritis.
   2. osteomalacia.
   3. rickets.

   (A) 1 only
   (B) 1 and 2 only
   (C) 2 and 3 only
   (D) 1, 2, and 3

3. Which of the positions illustrated in Figure 2–1 would best demonstrate the cervical pedicles?

   1. A
   2. B
   3. C

   (A) 1 only
   (B) 2 only
   (C) 1 and 3 only
   (D) 2 and 3 only

4. In which of the following positions/projections will the talocalcaneal joint be visualized?

   (A) Dorsoplantar projection of the foot
   (B) Plantodorsal projection of the os calcis
   (C) Medial oblique position of the foot
   (D) Lateral foot

5. When comparing the male and female bony pelves, it is noted that the

   1. male pelvis is deeper.
   2. female pubic arch is greater than 90°.
   3. female greater sciatic notch is wider.

   A. 1 only
   B. 1 and 2 only
   C. 2 and 3 only
   D. 1, 2, and 3

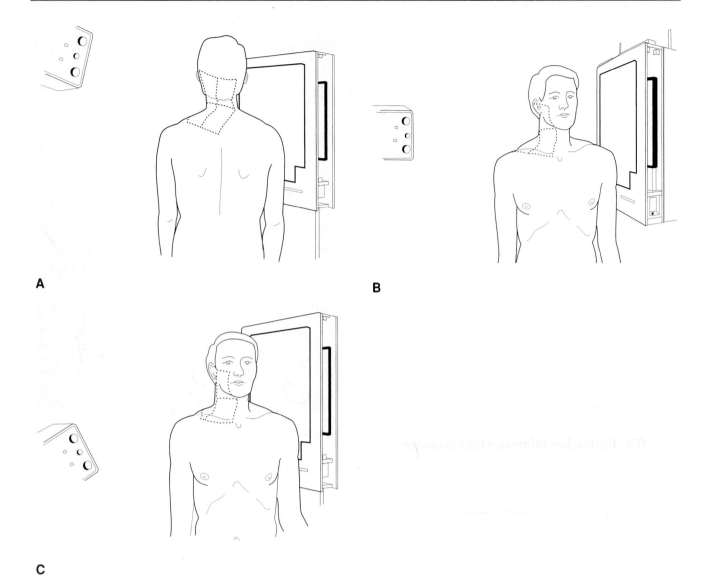

A

B

C

Figure 2–1.

6. Angulation of the central ray may be required

   1. to avoid superimposition of overlying structures.
   2. to avoid foreshortening or self-superimposition.
   3. to project through certain articulations.

   (A) 1 only
   (B) 2 only
   (C) 1 and 3 only
   (D) 1, 2, and 3

7. With the patient and the x-ray tube positioned as illustrated in Figure 2–2, which of the following will be visulaized?

   1. Intercondyloid fossa
   2. Patellofemoral articulation
   3. Tangential patella

   (A) 1 only
   (B) 1 and 2 only
   (C) 2 and 3 only
   (D) 1, 2, and 3

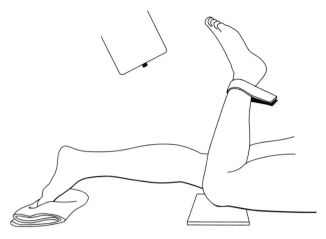

Figure 2–2.

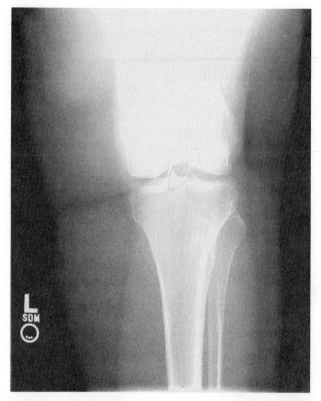

Figure 2–3. Courtesy of Stamford Hospital, Department of Radiology.

8. All of the following statements regarding respiratory structures are true *except*

   (A) the right lung has two lobes.
   (B) the uppermost portion of the lung is the apex.
   (C) each lung is enclosed in pleura.
   (D) the trachea bifurcates into mainstem bronchi.

9. All of the following statements regarding an exact PA projection of the skull, with the central ray perpendicular to the IR, are true *except*

   (A) The orbitomeatal line is perpendicular to the IR.
   (B) The petrous pyramids fill the orbits.
   (C) The midsagittal plane (MSP) is parallel to the IR.
   (D) The central ray exits at the nasion.

10. Which of the following statements regarding the radiograph in Figure 2–3 is (are) true?

   1. The tibial eminences are well visualized.
   2. The intercondyloid fossa is demonstrated between the femoral condyles.
   3. The femorotibial articulation is well demonstrated.

   (A) 1 only
   (B) 1 and 2 only
   (C) 1 and 3 only
   (D) 2 and 3 only

11. Ingestion of barium sulfate is contraindicated in which of the following situations?

   1. Suspected perforation of a hollow viscus
   2. Suspected large-bowel obstruction
   3. Presurgical patients

   (A) 1 only
   (B) 1 and 3 only
   (C) 2 and 3 only
   (D) 1, 2, and 3

12. "Flattening" of the hemidiaphragms is characteristic of which of the following conditions?

   (A) Pneumothorax
   (B) Emphysema
   (C) Pleural effusion
   (D) Pneumonia

13. Which of the following structures is (are) located in the right lower quadrant (RLQ)?

    1. Gallbladder
    2. Hepatic flexure
    3. Cecum

    (A) 1 only
    (B) 1 and 2 only
    (C) 3 only
    (D) 1, 2, and 3

14. The number 1 in the radiograph in Figure 2–4 represents which of the following renal structures?

    (A) Vesicoureteral junction
    (B) Renal pelvis
    (C) Minor calyx
    (D) Major calyx

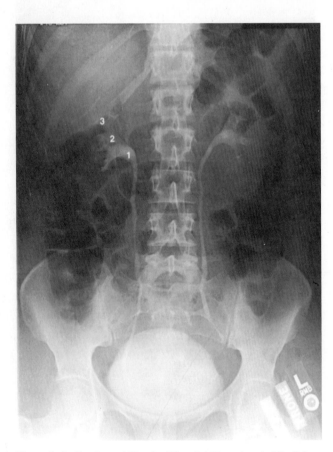

Figure 2–4. Courtesy of Stamford Hospital, Department of Radiology.

15. During an upper gastrointestinal (GI) examination, the AP recumbent projection of a stomach of average shape will usually demonstrate

    1. anterior and posterior aspects of the stomach.
    2. barium-filled fundus.
    3. double-contrast body and antral portions.

    (A) 1 only
    (B) 1 and 2 only
    (C) 2 and 3 only
    (D) 1, 2, and 3

16. The ridge that marks the bifurcation of the trachea into the right and left primary bronchi is the

    (A) root.
    (B) hilus.
    (C) carina.
    (D) epiglottis.

17. Which projection of the foot will best demonstrate the longitudinal arch?

    (A) Mediolateral
    (B) Lateromedial
    (C) Lateral weight-bearing
    (D) 30° medial oblique

18. Cells concerned with the formation and repair of bone are

    (A) osteoblasts.
    (B) osteoclasts.
    (C) osteomas.
    (D) osteons.

19. The axiolateral, or horizontal beam, projection of the hip requires the cassette to be placed

1. in contact with the lateral surface of the body.
2. in a vertical position and exactly perpendicular to the long axis of the femoral neck.
3. with top edge slightly above the iliac crest.

(A) 1 only
(B) 1 and 2 only
(C) 1 and 3 only
(D) 1, 2, and 3

20. In the AP axial projection (Towne method) of the skull, with the central ray directed 30° caudad to the OML and passing midway between the external auditory meati, which of the following is best demonstrated?

(A) Occipital bone
(B) Frontal bone
(C) Facial bones
(D) Basal foramina

21. The *best* way to control voluntary motion is

(A) immobilization of the part.
(B) careful explanation of the procedure.
(C) short exposure time.
(D) physical restraint.

22. Figure 2–5 was made in which of the following positions?

(A) AP
(B) Medial oblique
(C) Lateral oblique
(D) Partial flexion

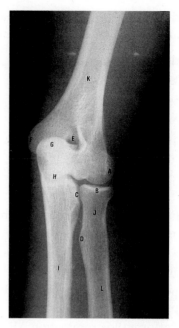

Figure 2–5. Reproduced with permission from Saia DA. *Radiography: Program Review and Examination Preparation*, 2nd ed. Stamford, CT: Appleton & Lange, 1999.

23. What are the positions most commonly employed for a radiographic examination of the sternum?

1. Lateral
2. RAO
3. LAO

(A) 1 and 2 only
(B) 1 and 3 only
(C) 2 and 3 only
(D) 1, 2, and 3

24. Which of the following are demonstrated in the oblique position of the cervical spine?

1. Intervertebral foramina   OBL
2. Apophyseal joints
3. Intervertebral joints   LAT.

(A) 1 only
(B) 1 and 2 only
(C) 2 and 3 only
(D) 1, 2, and 3

25. Aspirated foreign bodies in older children and adults are *most* likely to lodge in the

    (A) right main bronchus.
    (B) left main bronchus.
    (C) esophagus.
    (D) proximal stomach.

26. How should a chest examination to rule out air–fluid levels be obtained on a patient having traumatic injuries?

    A. Perform the examination in the Trendelenburg position.
    B. Erect inspiration and expiration images should be obtained.
    C. Include a dorsal decubitus lateral chest projection
    D. Perform the examination AP supine at 44" SID.

27. What should you do if you discover while taking the patient history that a patient scheduled for an intravenous urogram (IVU) takes Glucophage (metformin hydrochloride) daily?

    1. Proceed with the examination.
    2. Reschedule the examination until the patient has been off Glucophage for 48 hours.
    3. Instruct the patient to withhold the Glucophage for 48 hours after the examination.

    (A) 1 only
    (B) 1 and 2 only
    (C) 1 and 3 only
    (D) 1, 2, and 3

28. Which of the following methods was used to obtain the image seen in Figure 2–6?

    (A) PA, chin extended, OML forming 37° to IR
    (B) PA, OML, and CR perpendicular to IR
    (C) PA, OML perpendicular to IR, CR 25° caudad
    (D) PA, OML perpendicular to IR, CR 25° cephalad

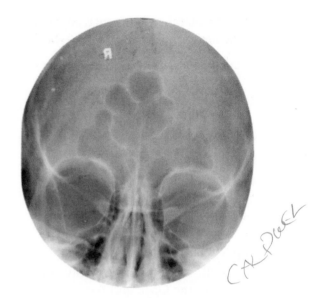

Figure 2–6. Courtesy of Stamford Hospital, Department of Radiology.

29. Which of the following statements regarding the radiograph in Figure 2–6 is (are) true?

    1. The position is used to demonstrate the frontal and ethmoidal sinuses.
    2. The sphenoidal sinuses are seen near the medial aspect of the orbits.
    3. The chin should be elevated more to bring the petrous ridges below the maxillary sinuses.

    (A) 1 only
    (B) 1 and 2 only
    (C) 1 and 3 only
    (D) 1, 2, and 3

30. Which of the following positions is obtained with the patient lying prone recumbent on the radiographic table, and the central ray directed horizontally to the iliac crest?

    (A) Ventral decubitus position
    (B) Dorsal decubitus position
    (C) Left lateral decubitus position
    (D) Right lateral decubitus position

31. All the following positions may be used to demonstrate the sternoclavicular articulations *except*

(A) weight bearing.
(B) RAO.
(C) LAO.
(D) PA.

32. Which of the following is a radiologic procedure that functions to dilate a stenotic vessel?

(A) Percutaneous nephrolithotomy
(B) Percutaneous angioplasty
(C) Renal arteriography
(D) Surgical nephrostomy

33. When examining a patient whose elbow is in partial flexion, how should an AP projection be obtained?

1. With humerus parallel to IR, central ray perpendicular
2. With forearm parallel to IR, central ray perpendicular
3. Through the partially flexed elbow, resting on the olecranon process, central ray perpendicular

(A) 1 only
(B) 1 and 2 only
(C) 2 and 3 only
(D) 1, 2, and 3

34. Which of the following positions is required to demonstrate small amounts of fluid in the pleural cavity?

(A) Lateral decubitus, affected side up
(B) Lateral decubitus, affected side down
(C) AP Trendelenburg
(D) AP supine

35. Place the following anatomic structures in order from anterior to posterior:

1. Trachea
2. Apex of heart
3. Esophagus

(A) Trachea, esophagus, apex of heart
(B) Esophagus, trachea, apex of heart
(C) Apex of heart, trachea, esophagus
(D) Apex of heart, esophagus, trachea

36. Which of the following projections will *best* demonstrate the carpal scaphoid?

(A) Lateral wrist
(B) Ulnar flexion/deviation
(C) Radial flexion/deviation
(D) Carpal tunnel

37. In which of the following positions was the radiograph in Figure 2–7 made?

(A) AP with perpendicular plantar surface
(B) 45° lateral oblique
(C) 20° medial oblique
(D) 45° medial oblique

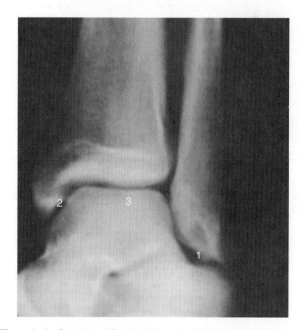

Figure 2–7. Courtesy of Stamford Hospital, Department of Radiology.

38. Which of the following anatomic structures is indicated by the number 3 in Figure 2–7?

   (A) Talus
   (B) Medial malleolus
   (C) Lateral malleolus
   (D) Lateral tibial condyle

39. Which of the following is (are) well demonstrated in the lumbar spine pictured in Figure 2–8?

   1. Intervertebral joints
   2. Pedicles
   3. Apophyseal joints *→) Oblique*

   (A) 1 only
   (B) 1 and 2 only
   (C) 1 and 3 only
   (D) 1, 2, and 3

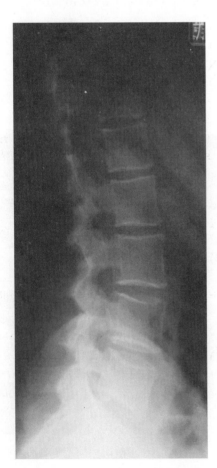

Figure 2–8. Courtesy of Stamford Hospital, Department of Radiology.

40. To better demonstrate the mandibular rami in the PA position, the

   (A) skull is obliqued toward the affected side.
   (B) skull is obliqued away from the affected side.
   (C) central ray is angled cephalad.
   (D) central ray is angled caudad.

41. Which of the following projections can be used to supplement the traditional "open-mouth" projection, when the upper portion of the odontoid process cannot be well demonstrated?

   (A) AP or PA through the foramen magnum
   (B) AP oblique with R and L head rotation
   (C) horizontal beam lateral
   (D) AP axial

42. The left sacroiliac joint is positioned perpendicular to the IR when the patient is positioned in a

   (A) left lateral position.
   (B) 25° to 30° LAO position. *→ RPO*
   (C) 25° to 30° LPO position.
   (D) 30° to 40° LPO position.

43. A lateral projection of the hand in extension is often recommended to evaluate

   1. a fracture.
   2. a foreign body.
   3. soft tissue.

   (A) 1 only
   (B) 2 only
   (C) 2 and 3 only
   (D) 1 and 3 only

44. The radiograph seen in Figure 2–9 best demonstrates the

   1. ascending colon.
   2. descending colon.
   3. right colic flexure.

   (A) 2 only
   (B) 3 only
   (C) 1 and 3 only
   (D) 2 and 3 only

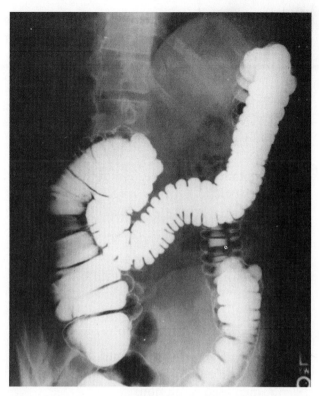

Figure 2–9. Courtesy of Stamford Hospital, Department of Radiology.

45. In which of the following positions was the radiograph in Figure 2–9 taken?

    (A) RAO
    (B) LAO
    (C) AP axial
    (D) Right lateral decubitus

46. Which of the following statements is (are) true regarding lower-extremity venography?

    1. The patient is often examined in the semi-erect position.
    2. Contrast medium is injected through a vein in the foot.
    3. Imaging begins at the hip and proceeds inferiorly.

    (A) 1 only
    (B) 1 and 2 only
    (C) 1 and 3 only
    (D) 1, 2, and 3

47. Which of the following projections or positions will best demonstrate subacromial or subcoracoid dislocation?

    (A) Tangential
    (B) AP axial
    (C) Transthoracic lateral
    (D) PA oblique scapular Y

48. Which of the following will best demonstrate the size and shape of the liver and kidneys?

    (A) Lateral abdomen
    (B) AP abdomen
    (C) Dorsal decubitus abdomen
    (D) Ventral decubitus abdomen

49. Which of the following positions will demonstrate the right axillary ribs?

    1. RAO
    2. LAO
    3. RPO

    (A) 1 only
    (B) 1 and 2 only
    (C) 2 and 3 only
    (D) 1, 2, and 3

50. In which projection of the foot are the sinus tarsi, cuboid, and tuberosity of the fifth metatarsal best demonstrated?

    (A) Lateral oblique foot
    (B) Medial oblique foot
    (C) Lateral foot
    (D) Weight-bearing foot

51. The manubrial notch is at approximately the same level as the

    (A) fifth thoracic vertebra. *sternal angle*
    (B) T2–3 interspace.
    (C) T4–5 interspace.
    (D) costal margin.   *L 3*

52. What is the position of the gallbladder in an asthenic patient?

    (A) Superior and medial
    (B) Superior and lateral
    (C) Inferior and medial
    (D) Inferior and lateral

53. To demonstrate esophageal varices, the patient must be examined in

    (A) the recumbent position.
    (B) the erect position.
    (C) the anatomic position.
    (D) Fowler's position.

54. Which of the following criteria are used to evaluate a PA projection of the chest?

    1. Ten posterior ribs should be visualized.
    2. Sternoclavicular joints should be symmetrical.
    3. The scapulae should be lateral to the lung fields.

    (A) 1 and 2 only
    (B) 1 and 3 only
    (C) 2 and 3 only
    (D) 1, 2, and 3

55. Which of the following is (are) valid criteria for a lateral projection of the forearm?

    1. The radius and ulna should be superimposed proximally and distally.
    2. The coronoid process and radial head should be superimposed.
    3. The radial tuberosity should face anteriorly.

    (A) 1 only
    (B) 1 and 2 only
    (C) 2 and 3 only
    (D) 1, 2, and 3

56. All of the following bones are associated with condyles *except* the

    (A) femur.
    (B) tibia.
    (C) fibula.
    (D) mandible.

57. Which of the following projections of the ankle would best demonstrate the distal tibiofibular joint?

    (A) Medial oblique 15° to 20°
    (B) Lateral oblique 15° to 20°
    (C) Medial oblique 45°
    (D) Lateral oblique 45°

58. To obtain an AP projection of the right ilium, the patient's

    (A) left side is elevated 40°.
    (B) right side is elevated 40°.
    (C) left side is elevated 15°.
    (D) right side is elevated 15°.

59. The advantages of digital subtraction angiography over film angiography include

    1. greater sensitivity to contrast medium.
    2. immediately available images.
    3. increased resolution.

    (A) 1 only
    (B) 1 and 2 only
    (C) 2 and 3 only
    (D) 1, 2, and 3

60. The usual patient preparation for an upper GI series is

    (A) clear fluids 8 hours prior to examination.
    (B) npo after midnight.
    (C) enemas until clear before examination.
    (D) light breakfast the day of the examination.

61. Which projection(s) of the abdomen would be used to demonstrate pneumoperitoneum?

    1. Right lateral decubitus
    2. Left lateral decubitus
    3. Upright

    (A) 2 only
    (B) 1 and 3 only
    (C) 2 and 3 only
    (D) 1, 2, and 3

62. Which of the following structures should be visualized through the foramen magnum in the AP axial projection (Grashey method) of the skull for occipital bone?

1. Posterior clinoid processes
2. Dorsum sella
3. Posterior arch of C1

(A) 1 only
(B) 2 only
(C) 1 and 2 only
(D) 2 and 3 only

63. Which of the following criteria is (are) required for visualization of the greater tubercle in profile?

1. Epicondyles parallel to the IR
2. Arm in external rotation
3. Humerus in AP position

(A) 1 only
(B) 1 and 3 only
(C) 2 and 3 only
(D) 1, 2, and 3

64. What instructions might a patient be given following an upper GI examination?

1. Drink plenty of fluids.
2. Take a mild laxative.
3. Increase dietary fiber.

(A) 1 only
(B) 1 and 2 only
(C) 2 and 3 only
(D) 1, 2, and 3

65. Which of the following tube angle and direction combinations is correct for an axial projection of the clavicle, with the patient in the PA position?

(A) 5° to 15° caudad
(B) 5° to 15° cephalad
(C) 15° to 30° cephalad
(D) 15° to 30° caudad

66. Which of the following should be performed to rule out subluxation or fracture of the cervical spine?

(A) Oblique cervical spine, seated
(B) AP cervical spine, recumbent
(C) Horizontal beam lateral
(D) Laterals in flexion and extension

67. What portion of the humerus articulates with the ulna to help form the elbow joint?

(A) Semilunar/trochlear notch
(B) Radial head
(C) Capitulum
(D) Trochlea

68. The true lateral position of the skull uses which of the following principles?

1. Interpupillary line perpendicular to the IR
2. MSP perpendicular to the IR
3. Infraorbitomeatal line (IOML) parallel to the transverse axis of the IR

(A) 1 only
(B) 1 and 2 only
(C) 1 and 3 only
(D) 1, 2, and 3

69. During myelography, contrast medium is introduced into the

(A) subdural space.
(B) subarachnoid space.
(C) epidural space.
(D) epidermal space.

70. An axiolateral inferosuperior projection of the femoral neck is particularly useful

1. when the axiolateral is contraindicated.
2. for patients with bilateral hip fractures.
3. for patients with limited movement of the unaffected leg.

(A) 1 only
(B) 1 and 2 only
(C) 1 and 3 only
(D) 1, 2, and 3

71. Which of the following statements is (are) true regarding the radiograph in Figure 2–10?

1. The patient is placed in an RAO position.
2. The midcoronal plane is about 60° to the IR.
3. The acromion process is free of superimposition.

(A) 1 only
(B) 1 and 2 only
(C) 2 and 3 only
(D) 1, 2, and 3

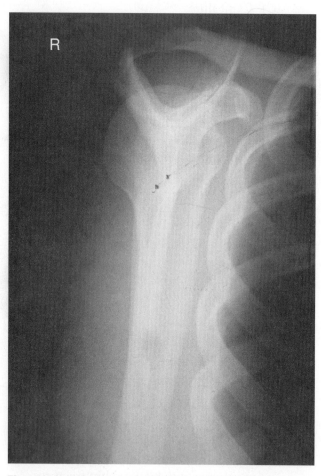

Figure 2–10. Courtesy of Stamford Hospital, Department of Radiology.

72. Examples of synovial pivot articulations include the

1. atlantoaxial joint.
2. radioulnar joint.
3. temporomandibular joint.

(A) 1 only
(B) 1 and 2 only
(C) 2 and 3 only
(D) 1, 2, and 3 only

73. The pars interarticularis is represented by what part of the "scotty dog" seen in a correctly positioned oblique lumbar spine?

(A) Eye — Pedicle
(B) Front foot Inferior articular proces
(C) Body — Lamina
(D) Neck Pars interarticulares

74. Which of the following will separate the radial head, neck, and tuberosity from superimposition on the ulna?

(A) AP
(B) Lateral
(C) Medial oblique
(D) Lateral oblique

75. In which of the following positions can the sesamoid bones of the foot be demonstrated free of superimposition with the metatarsals or phalanges?

(A) dorsoplantar metatarsals/toes
(B) tangential metatarsals/toes
(C) 30° medial oblique foot
(D) 30° lateral oblique foot

76. Tangential axial projections of the patella can be obtained in which of the following positions?

1. supine flexion 45° (Merchant)
2. prone flexion 90° (Settegast)
3. prone flexion 55° (Hughston)

(A) 1 only
(B) 1 and 2 only
(C) 2 and 3 only
(D) 1, 2, and 3 only

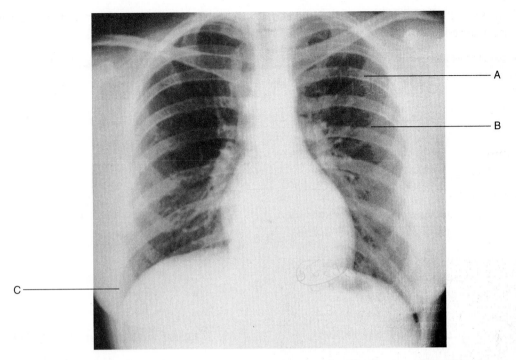

Figure 2–11. From the American College of Radiology Learning File. Courtesy of the ACR.

77. With the patient in the PA position and the OML and central ray perpendicular to the IR, the resulting radiograph will demonstrate the petrous pyramids

  (A) below the orbits.
  (B) in the lower one third of the orbits.
  (C) completely within the orbits.
  (D) above the orbits.

78. Which of the following are part of the bony thorax?

  1. 12 thoracic vertebrae
  2. Scapulae
  3. 24 ribs

  (A) 1 only
  (B) 1 and 2 only
  (C) 1 and 3 only
  (D) 1, 2, and 3

79. During atrial systole, blood flows into the right ventricle by way of what valve?

  (A) Pulmonary semilunar
  (B) Aortic
  (C) Mitral
  (D) Tricuspid

80. The PA chest radiograph seen in Figure 2–11 demonstrates

  1. rotation.
  2. scapulae removed from lung fields.
  3. adequate inspiration.

  (A) 1 only
  (B) 1 and 3 only
  (C) 2 and 3 only
  (D) 1, 2, and 3

81. The letter *B* in Figure 2–11 indicates

  (A) a left anterior rib.
  (B) a right posterior rib.
  (C) a left posterior rib.
  (D) a right anterior rib.

82. With the patient seated at the end of the x-ray table, elbow flexed 80°, CR directed 45° laterally *from the shoulder to the elbow joint*, which of the following structures will be demonstrated best?

  (A) radial head
  (B) ulnar head
  (C) coronoid process
  (D) olecranon process

83. The following procedure can be employed to better demonstrate the carpal scaphoid:

    1. elevate hand and wrist 20°.
    2. place wrist in ulnar deviation.
    3. angle CR 20° distally (toward fingers).

    (A) 1 only
    (B) 1 and 2 only
    (C) 1 and 3 only
    (D) 1, 2, and 3

84. Which of the following are demonstrated in the lateral projection of the thoracic spine?

    1. Intervertebral spaces
    2. Apophyseal joints   70° Oblique
    3. Intervertebral foramina

    (A) 1 only
    (B) 2 only
    (C) 1 and 3 only
    (D) 1, 2, and 3

85. What structure can be located midway between the anterior superior iliac spine (ASIS) and pubic symphysis?

    (A) dome of the acetabulum
    (B) femoral neck
    (C) greater trochanter
    (D) iliac crest

86. The structure labeled 3 in Figure 2–12 is the

    (A) maxillary sinus. → 4
    (B) sphenoidal sinus.
    (C) ethmoidal sinus. → 2
    (D) frontal sinus. → 1

87. Which of the following would *best* evaluate the structure labeled 4 in Figure 2–12?

    (A) PA axial projection (Caldwell method)
    (B) Parietoacanthial projection (Waters' method)
    (C) Lateral projection
    (D) Submentovertical projection

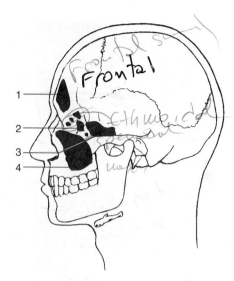

Figure 2–12.

88. During chest radiography, the act of inspiration

    1. elevates the diaphragm.
    2. raises the ribs.
    3. depresses the abdominal viscera.

    (A) 1 only
    (B) 1 and 2 only
    (C) 2 and 3 only
    (D) 1, 2, and 3

89. The radiograph shown in Figure 2–13 demonstrates the articulation between the

    1. talus and the calcaneus.
    2. calcaneus and the cuboid.
    3. talus and the navicular.

    (A) 1 only
    (B) 1 and 2 only
    (C) 2 and 3 only
    (D) 1, 2, and 3

90. What should be done to better demonstrate the mandibular rami seen in PA projection in Figure 2–14?

    (A) use a perpendicular CR
    (B) angle the CR cephalad 20°–25°
    (C) angle the CR caudad
    (D) oblique the head 15° medial

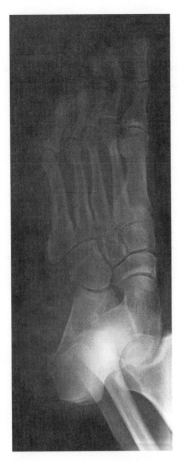

Figure 2–13. Courtesy of Stamford Hospital, Department of Radiology.

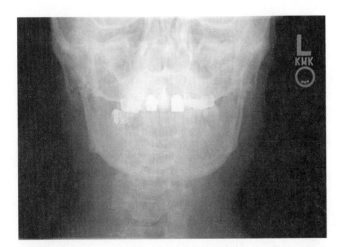

Figure 2–14. Courtesy of Stamford Hospital, Department of Radiology.

91. What process is best seen using a perpendicular CR with the elbow in acute flexion and with the posterior aspect of the humerus adjacent to the image receptor?

   (A) Coracoid
   (B) Coronoid
   (C) Olecranon
   (D) Glenoid

92. The patient's chin should be elevated during chest radiography to

   (A) permit the diaphragm to move to its lowest position.
   (B) avoid superimposition on the apices.
   (C) assist in maintaining an upright position.
   (D) keep the MSP parallel.

93. The primary center of ossification in long bones is the _____

   (A) diaphysis.
   (B) epiphysis.
   (C) metaphysis.
   (D) apophysis.

94. To make the patient as comfortable as possible during a single-contrast barium enema (BE), the radiographer should

   1. instruct the patient to relax the abdominal muscles to prevent intra-abdominal pressure.
   2. instruct the patient to concentrate on breathing deeply to reduce colonic spasm.
   3. prepare a warm barium suspension (98 to 105°F) to aid in retention. *temperature should be below body >> 85° or cold 41°*

   (A) 2 only
   (B) 1 and 2 only
   (C) 2 and 3 only
   (D) 1, 2, and 3

95. The pedicle is represented by what part of the "scotty dog" seen in a correctly positioned oblique lumbar spine?

   (A) Eye
   (B) Front foot
   (C) Body
   (D) Neck

96. The position shown in Figure 2–15 is known as

   (A) ventral decubitus.

   (B) dorsal decubitus.

   (C) left lateral decubitus.

   (D) right lateral decubitus.

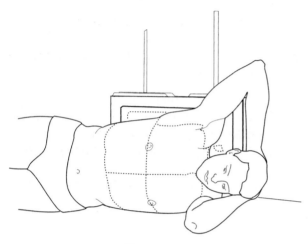

Figure 2–15.

97. Which of the following projections will best demonstrate the tarsal navicular free of superimposition?

   (A) AP oblique, medial rotation

   (B) AP oblique, lateral rotation

   (C) Mediolateral

   (D) Lateral weight bearing

98. At what level do the carotid arteries bifurcate?

   (A) Foramen magnum

   (B) Trachea

   (C) Pharynx

   (D) C4

99. During a double-contrast BE, which of the following positions would afford the *best* double-contrast visualization of both colic flexures?

   (A) LAO and RPO

   (B) Lateral

   (C) Left lateral decubitus

   (D) AP or PA erect

100. What is the structure indicated by the number 6 in Figure 2–16?

   (A) Common hepatic duct

   (B) Common bile duct

   (C) Cystic duct

   (D) Pancreatic duct

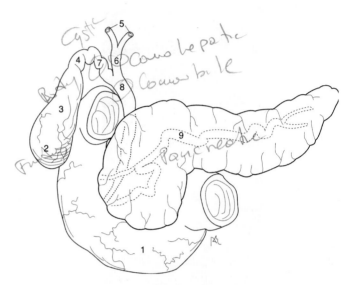

Figure 2–16.

101. What is the structure indicated by the number 7 in Figure 2–16?

   (A) Common hepatic duct

   (B) Common bile duct

   (C) Cystic duct

   (D) Pancreatic duct

102. To evaluate the interphalangeal joints in the oblique and lateral positions, the fingers

   (A) rest on the cassette for immobilization.

   (B) must be supported parallel to the IR.

   (C) are radiographed in natural flexion.

   (D) are radiographed in palmar flexion.

103. Which of the following examinations involves the introduction of a radiopaque contrast medium through a uterine cannula?

   (A) Retrograde pyelogram

   (B) Voiding cystourethrogram

   (C) Hysterosalpingogram

   (D) Myelogram

104. All of the following statements regarding large-bowel radiography are true *except*

(A) the large bowel must be completely empty prior to examination.

(B) Retained fecal material can simulate pathology.

(C) Single-contrast studies help to demonstrate polyps.

(D) Double-contrast studies help to demonstrate intraluminal lesions.

105. In the lateral projection of the knee, the

1. femoral condyles are superimposed.
2. patellofemoral joint is visualized.
3. knee is flexed about 20° to 30°.

(A) 1 only

(B) 2 only

(C) 1 and 3 only

(D) 1, 2, and 3

106. To demonstrate the pulmonary apices with the patient in the AP position, the

(A) central ray is directed 15° to 20° cephalad.

(B) central ray is directed 15° to 20° caudad.

(C) exposure is made on full exhalation.

(D) patient's shoulders are rolled forward.

107. All of the following statements regarding the inferosuperior axial (nontrauma, Lawrence method) projection of the shoulder are true, *except*

(A) the coracoid process and lesser tubercle are seen in profile.

(B) the arm is abducted about 90° from the body.

(C) the arm should be in internal rotation.

(D) the CR is directed medially 25° to 30° through the axilla.

108. Double-contrast examinations of the stomach or large bowel are performed to better visualize the

(A) position of the organ.

(B) size and shape of the organ.

(C) diverticula.

(D) gastric or bowel mucosa.

109. The sternoclavicular joints are best demonstrated with the patient PA and

(A) in a slight oblique position, affected side adjacent to the image receptor.

(B) in a slight oblique position, affected side away from the image receptor.

(C) erect and weight bearing.

(D) erect, with and without weights.

110. Which of the following statements is/are true regarding the position illustrated in Figure 2–17?

1. The left (elevated) kidney is parallel to the IR. —) 30° oblique
2. The right (adjacent to the table) kidney is parallel to the IR.
3. The degree of obliquity should be about 45°

(A) 1 only

(B) 1 and 2 only

(C) 2 and 3 only

(D) 1, 2, and 3

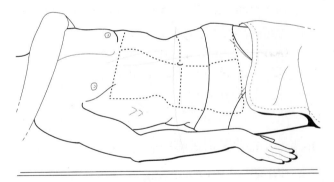

Figure 2–17.

111. For which of the following conditions is operative cholangiography a useful tool?

1. Biliary tract calculi
2. Patency of the biliary ducts
3. Function of the sphincter of Oddi

(A) 1 only

(B) 2 only

(C) 2 and 3 only

(D) 1, 2, and 3

112. With the patient positioned as illustrated in Figure 2–18, which of the following structures is best demonstrated?

    (A) Patella
    (B) Patellofemoral articulation
    (C) Intercondyloid fossa
    (D) Tibial tuberosity

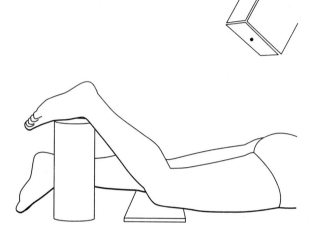

Figure 2–18.

113. Which of the following structures is illustrated by the number 2 in Figure 2–19?

    (A) Maxillary sinus 4
    (B) Coronoid process 3   [1])
    (C) Zygomatic arch   Mandibulary
    (D) Coracoid process   angle

114. Which of the following articulations may be described as diarthrotic?

    1. Knee
    2. Intervertebral joints
    3. Temporomandibular joint (TMJ)

    (A) 1 only
    (B) 2 only
    (C) 1 and 3 only
    (D) 1, 2, and 3

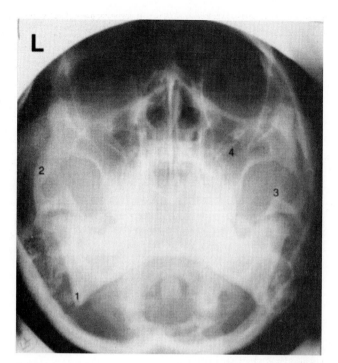

Figure 2–19. Courtesy of Stamford Hospital, Department of Radiology.

115. A patient is usually required to drink barium sulfate suspension to demonstrate which of the following structures?

    1. Esophagus
    2. Pylorus
    3. Ilium

    (A) 1 only
    (B) 1 and 2 only
    (C) 2 and 3 only
    (D) 1, 2, and 3

116. What should be done to better demonstrate the coracoid process seen in Figure 2–20?

    (A) Use a perpendicular CR
    (B) Angle the CR about 30°cephalad
    (C) Angle the CR about 30°caudad
    (D) Angle the MSP 15° toward the affected side

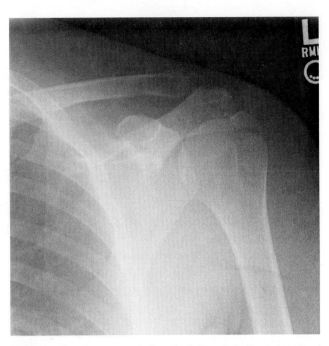

Figure 2–20. Courtesy of Stamford Hospital, Department of Radiology.

117. Which of the positions illustrated in Figure 2–21 will *best* demonstrate the lumbar intervertebral foramina?

    (A) Number 1
    (B) Number 2
    (C) Number 3
    (D) Number 4

118. Which of the positions illustrated in Figure 2–21 will *best* demonstrate the lumbar apophyseal joints closest to the IR?

    (A) Number 1
    (B) Number 2
    (C) Number 3
    (D) Number 4

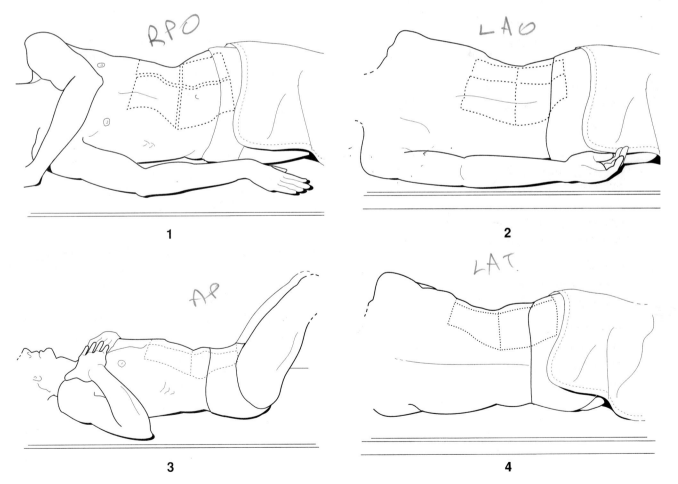

Figure 2–21.

119. The apophyseal articulations of the thoracic spine are demonstrated with the

    (A) coronal plane 45° to the IR.
    (B) midsagittal plane 45° to the IR.
    (C) coronal plane 70° to the IR.
    (D) midsagittal plane 70° to the IR.

120. Which of the following may be used to evaluate the glenohumeral joint?

    1. Scapular Y projection
    2. Inferosuperior axial
    3. Transthoracic lateral

    (A) 1 only
    (B) 1 and 2 only
    (C) 2 and 3 only
    (D) 1, 2, and 3

121. During lower-limb venography, tourniquets are applied above the knee and ankle to

    1. suppress filling of the superficial veins.
    2. coerce filling of the deep veins.
    3. fill the anterior tibial vein.

    (A) 1 and 2 only
    (B) 1 and 3 only
    (C) 2 and 3 only
    (D) 1, 2, and 3

122. Which of the following women is likely to have the most homogeneous, glandular breast tissue?

    (A) A postpubertal adolescent
    (B) A 20-year-old with one previous pregnancy
    (C) A menopausal woman
    (D) A postmenopausal 65-year-old

123. Which of the following positions/projections of the skull will result in the most shape distortion?

    (A) 0° PA
    (B) 23° Caldwell
    (C) 37° Towne/Grashey
    (D) 25° Haas

124. Which of the following examinations require(s) special identification markers in addition to the usual patient name and number, date, and side marker?

    1. IVU
    2. Tomography
    3. Abdominal survey

    (A) 1 only
    (B) 1 and 2 only
    (C) 2 and 3 only
    (D) 1, 2, and 3

125. Which of the following is *most* likely to be the correct routine for a radiographic examination of the forearm?

    (A) PA and medial oblique
    (B) AP and lateral oblique
    (C) PA and lateral
    (D) AP and lateral

126. The body habitus characterized by a long and narrow thoracic cavity and low, midline stomach and gallbladder is the

    (A) asthenic.
    (B) hyposthenic.
    (C) sthenic.
    (D) hypersthenic.

127. Which of the following fracture classifications describes a small bony fragment pulled from a bony process?

    (A) Avulsion fracture
    (B) Torus fracture
    (C) Comminuted fracture
    (D) Compound fracture

128. Which of the following is proximal to the carpal bones?

    (A) Distal interphalangeal joints
    (B) Proximal interphalangeal joints
    (C) Metacarpals
    (D) Radial styloid process

129. The scapular Y projection of the shoulder demonstrates

 1. an oblique projection of the shoulder.
 2. anterior or posterior dislocation.
 3. a lateral projection of the shoulder.

 (A) 1 only
 (B) 1 and 2 only
 (C) 1 and 3 only
 (D) 2 and 3 only

130. Which of the following projection(s) require(s) that the shoulder be placed in internal rotation?

 1. AP humerus
 2. Lateral forearm
 3. Lateral humerus

 (A) 1 only
 (B) 1 and 2 only
 (C) 3 only
 (D) 1, 2, and 3

131. The fifth metacarpal is located on which aspect of the hand?

 (A) Medial
 (B) Lateral
 (C) Ulnar
 (D) Volar

132. With the patient's head in a PA position and the central ray directed 20° cephalad, which part of the mandible will be best visualized?

 (A) Symphysis
 (B) Rami
 (C) Body
 (D) Angle

133. During intravenous (IV) urography, the prone position is generally recommended to demonstrate

 1. the filling of ureters.
 2. the renal pelvis.
 3. the superior calyces.

 (A) 1 only
 (B) 1 and 2 only
 (C) 1 and 3 only
 (D) 1, 2, and 3

134. The plane that passes vertically through the body, dividing it into anterior and posterior halves, is termed the

 (A) median sagittal plane.
 (B) midcoronal plane.
 (C) sagittal plane.
 (D) transverse plane.

135. To demonstrate a profile view of the glenoid fossa, the patient is AP recumbent and obliqued 45°

 (A) toward the affected side.
 (B) away from the affected side.
 (C) with the arm at the side in the anatomic position.
 (D) with the arm in external rotation.

136. Which of the following is (are) accurate criticism(s) of the open-mouth projection of C1–2 seen in Figure 2–22?

 1. The MSP is not centered and perpendicular to the midline of the table.
 2. The neck should be flexed more.
 3. The neck should be extended more.

 (A) 1 only
 (B) 1 and 2 only
 (C) 3 only
 (D) 1 and 3 only

137. Myelography is a diagnostic examination used to demonstrate

 1. extrinsic spinal cord compression resulting from disk herniation.
 2. posttraumatic swelling of the spinal cord.
 3. internal disk lesions.

 (A) 1 only
 (B) 2 only
 (C) 1 and 2 only
 (D) 1 and 3 only

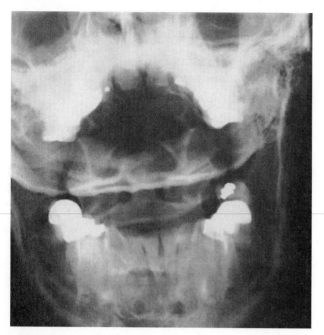

Figure 2–22. Courtesy of Stamford Hospital, Department of Radiology.

138. Which of the following techniques would provide a PA projection of the gastroduodenal surfaces of the barium-filled, high and transverse stomach?

    (A) Place the patient in a 35° to 40° RAO position.
    (B) Place the patient in a lateral position.
    (C) Angle the central ray 35° to 45° cephalad.
    (D) Angle the central ray 35° to 45° caudad.

139. Which of the following is recommended to better demonstrate the tarsometatarsal joints in the dorsoplantar projection of the foot?

    (A) Invert the foot
    (B) Evert the foot
    (C) Angle the central ray 10° posteriorly
    (D) Angle the central ray 10° anteriorly

140. The tissue that occupies the central cavity within the shaft of a long bone in an adult is

    (A) red marrow.
    (B) yellow marrow.
    (C) cortical tissue.
    (D) cancellous tissue.

141. Which of the following positions will provide an AP projection of the L5–S1 interspace?

    (A) Patient AP with 30° to 35° angle cephalad
    (B) Patient AP with 30° to 35° angle caudad
    (C) Patient AP with 0° angle
    (D) Patient lateral, coned to L5

142. Which of the following bony landmarks is in the same transverse plane as the symphysis pubis?

    (A) Ischial tuberosity
    (B) Prominence of the greater trochanter
    (C) Anterior superior iliac spine
    (D) Anterior inferior iliac spine

143. Patients are instructed to remove all jewelry, hair clips, metal prostheses, coins, and credit cards before entering the room for an examination in

    (A) sonography.
    (B) computed tomography (CT).
    (C) magnetic resonance imaging (MRI).
    (D) nuclear medicine.

144. Movement of a part toward the midline of the body is termed

    (A) eversion.
    (B) inversion.
    (C) abduction.
    (D) adduction.

145. In which of the following positions was the radiograph in Figure 2–23 probably made?

    (A) AP recumbent
    (B) PA recumbent
    (C) PA upright
    (D) AP Trendelenburg

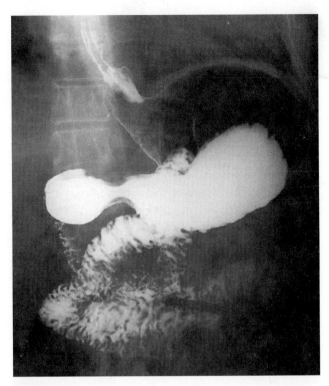

Figure 2–23. Courtesy of Stamford Hospital, Department of Radiology.

146. Which of the following vertebral groups form(s) lordotic curve(s)?

    1. Cervical
    2. Thoracic
    3. Lumbar

    (A) 1 only
    (B) 2 only
    (C) 1 and 2 only
    (D) 1 and 3 only

147. Which of the following is (are) required for a lateral projection of the skull?

    1. The IOML is parallel to the IR.
    2. The MSP is perpendicular to the IR.
    3. The CR enters 2 inches superior to the external auditory meatus (EAM).

    (A) 1 only
    (B) 1 and 3 only
    (C) 2 and 3 only
    (D) 1, 2, and 3

148. With which of the following does the trapezium articulate?

    (A) Fifth metacarpal
    (B) First metacarpal
    (C) Distal radius
    (D) Distal ulna

149. Which of the following positions will *most* effectively move the gallbladder away from the vertebrae in the asthenic patient?

    (A) LAO
    (B) RAO
    (C) LPO
    (D) Erect

150. The ileocecal valve is normally located in which of the following body regions?

    (A) Right iliac
    (B) Left iliac
    (C) Right lumbar
    (D) Hypogastric

151. Which of the following is (are) true regarding radiographic examination of the acromioclavicular joints?

    1. The procedure is performed in the erect position.
    2. Use of weights can improve demonstration of the joints.
    3. The procedure should be avoided if dislocation or separation is suspected.

    (A) 1 only
    (B) 1 and 2 only
    (C) 1 and 3 only
    (D) 2 and 3 only

152. Which of the following projections of the abdomen may be used to demonstrate air or fluid levels?

1. Dorsal decubitus
2. Lateral decubitus
3. AP Trendelenburg

(A) 1 only
(B) 1 and 2 only
(C) 1 and 3 only
(D) 1, 2, and 3

153. Which of the following articulations participate(s) in formation of the ankle mortise?

1. Talotibial
2. Talocalcaneal
3. Talofibular

(A) 1 only
(B) 1 and 3 only
(C) 2 and 3 only
(D) 3 only

154. Which of the following skull positions will demonstrate the cranial base, sphenoidal sinuses, atlas, and odontoid process?

(A) AP axial
(B) Lateral
(C) Parietoacanthial
(D) Submentovertical (SMV)

155. Which of the following statements is (are) true with respect to the radiograph in Figure 2–24?

1. The coracoid process is seen partially superimposed on the third rib.
2. This projection is performed to evaluate the acromioclavicular articulation.
3. This projection is performed to evaluate possible shoulder dislocation.

(A) 1 only
(B) 1 and 2 only
(C) 1 and 3 only
(D) 2 and 3 only

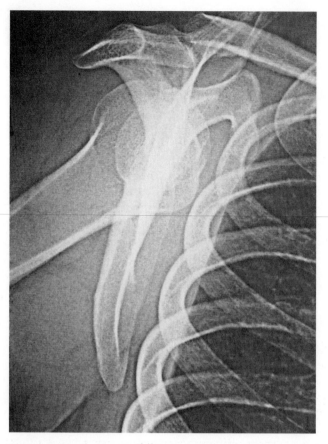

Figure 2–24. Courtesy of Stamford Hospital, Department of Radiology.

156. Which of the following is (are) located on the posterior aspect of the femur?

1. Intercondyloid fossa
2. Intertrochanteric crest
3. Intertubercular groove

(A) 1 only
(B) 1 and 2 only
(C) 1 and 3 only
(D) 2 and 3 only

157. An intrathecal injection is associated with which of the following examinations?

(A) IVU
(B) Retrograde pyelogram
(C) Myelogram
(D) Arthrogram

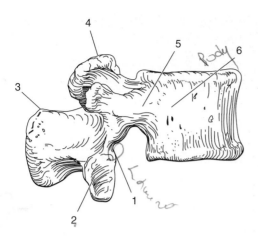

Figure 2–25.

158. In Figure 2–25, which of the following is represented by the number 5?

(A) Pedicle
(B) Transverse process
(C) Spinous process
(D) Superior articular process

159. Which of the following statements is (are) correct with respect to evaluation criteria for a PA projection of the chest for lungs?

1. The sternoclavicular joints should be symmetrical.
2. The sternum is seen lateral without rotation.
3. Ten anterior ribs are demonstrated above the diaphragm.

(A) 1 only
(B) 1 and 2 only
(C) 1 and 3 only
(D) 1, 2, and 3

160. The coronoid process should be visualized in profile in which of the following positions?

(A) Scapular Y
(B) AP scapula
(C) Medial oblique elbow
(D) Lateral oblique elbow

161. In the lateral projection of the ankle, the

1. talotibial joint is visualized.
2. talofibular joint is visualized.
3. tibia and fibula are superimposed.

(A) 1 only
(B) 1 and 2 only
(C) 1 and 3 only
(D) 1, 2, and 3

162. The position illustrated in the radiograph in Figure 2–26 may be obtained with the patient

1. supine and the central ray angled 30° caudad.
2. supine and the central ray angled 30° cephalad.
3. prone and the central ray angled 30° cephalad.

(A) 1 only
(B) 2 only
(C) 1 and 3 only
(D) 2 and 3 only

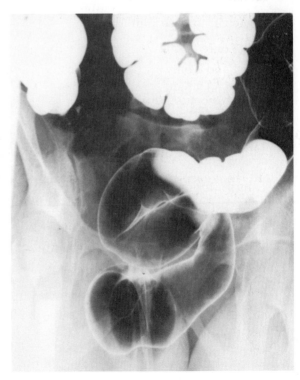

Figure 2–26. Courtesy of Stamford Hospital, Department of Radiology.

163. All of the following positions are likely to be employed for both single-contrast and double-contrast examinations of the large bowel *except*

(A) lateral rectum.
(B) AP axial rectosigmoid.
(C) right and left lateral decubitus abdomen.
(D) RAO and LAO abdomen.

164. Which of the following positions is essential in radiography of the paranasal sinuses?

(A) Erect
(B) Recumbent
(C) Oblique
(D) Trendelenburg

165. Which of the following can be used to demonstrate the intercondyloid fossa?

1. Patient PA, knee flexed 40°, central ray directed caudad 40° to the popliteal fossa
2. Patient AP, cassette under flexed knee, central ray directed cephalad to knee, perpendicular to tibia
3. Patient PA, patella parallel to IR, heel rotated 5° to 10° lateral, central ray perpendicular to knee joint

(A) 1 only
(B) 1 and 2 only
(C) 2 and 3 only
(D) 1, 2, and 3

166. The scapula pictured in Figure 2–27 demonstrates

1. its posterior aspect.
2. its costal surface.
3. its sternal articular surface.

(A) 1 only
(B) 1 and 2 only
(C) 1 and 3 only
(D) 1, 2, and 3

167. In Figure 2–27, which of the following is represented by the number 3?

(A) Acromion process
(B) Scapular spine
(C) Coracoid process
(D) Acromioclavicular joint

168. In Figure 2–27, which of the following is represented by the number 12?

(A) Vertebral border
(B) Axillary border
(C) Inferior angle
(D) Superior angle

169. AP stress studies of the ankle may be performed

1. to demonstrate fractures of the distal tibia and fibula.
2. following inversion or eversion injuries.
3. to demonstrate a ligament tear.

(A) 1 only
(B) 1 and 2 only
(C) 2 and 3 only
(D) 1, 2, and 3

170. When evaluating a PA axial projection of the skull with a 15° caudal angle, the radiographer should see

1. petrous pyramids in the lower third of the orbits.
2. equal distance from the lateral border of the skull to the lateral rim of the orbit bilaterally.
3. symmetrical petrous pyramids.

(A) 1 and 2 only
(B) 1 and 3 only
(C) 2 and 3 only
(D) 1, 2, and 3

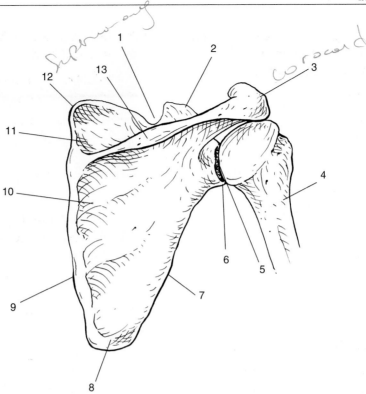

Figure 2–27. Reproduced with permission from Saia DA. *Radiography: Program Review and Examination Preparation*, 2nd ed. Stamford, CT: Appleton & Lange, 1999.

171. In the lateral projection of the knee, the central ray is angled 5° cephalad to prevent superimposition of which of the following structures on the joint space?

   (A) Lateral femoral condyle
   (B) Medial femoral condyle
   (C) Patella
   (D) Tibial eminence

172. The uppermost portion of the iliac crest is at approximately the same level as the

   (A) costal margin.
   (B) umbilicus.
   (C) xiphoid tip.
   (D) fourth lumbar vertebra.

173. Which of the following structures is (are) located in the left upper quadrant (LUQ)?

   1. Stomach
   2. Spleen
   3. Cecum

   (A) 1 only
   (B) 2 only
   (C) 1 and 2 only
   (D) 1, 2, and 3

174. In the posterior oblique position of the cervical spine, the intervertebral foramina that are best seen are those

   (A) nearest the IR.
   (B) furthest from the IR.
   (C) seen medially.
   (D) seen inferiorly.

175. Which of the following positions demonstrates all the paranasal sinuses?

(A) Parietoacanthial

(B) PA axial

(C) Lateral

(D) True PA

176. In the lateral projection of the scapula, the

1. vertebral and axillary borders are superimposed.
2. acromion and coracoid processes are superimposed.
3. patient may be examined in the erect position.

(A) 1 only

(B) 1 and 2 only

(C) 1 and 3 only

(D) 1, 2, and 3

177. Which of the following statements is/are true regarding Figure 2–28?

1. The radiograph was made in the LAO position.
2. The central ray should enter more inferiorly.
3. The sternum is projected onto the left side of the thorax.

(A) 1 only

(B) 2 only

(C) 2 and 3 only

(D) 1, 2, and 3

178. To better visualize the knee joint space in the radiograph in Figure 2–29, the radiographer should

(A) flex the knee more acutely.

(B) flex the knee less acutely.

(C) angle the CR 5° to 7° cephalad.

(D) angle the CR 5° to 7° caudad.

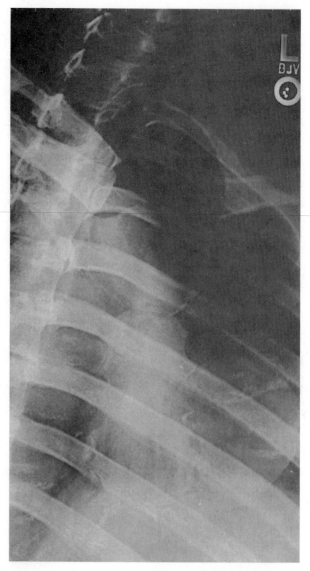

Figure 2–28. Courtesy of Stamford Hospital, Department of Radiology.

179. Which of the following is (are) demonstrated in the AP projection of the cervical spine?

1. Intervertebral disk spaces
2. C3–7 cervical bodies
3. Apophyseal joints

(A) 1 only

(B) 1 and 2 only

(C) 2 and 3 only

(D) 1, 2, and 3

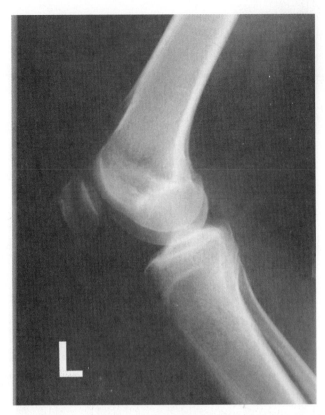

Figure 2–29. Courtesy of Stamford Hospital, Department of Radiology.

180. That ossified portion of a long bone where cartilage has been replaced by bone is known as the

(A) diaphysis.

(B) epiphysis.

(C) metaphysis.

(D) apophysis.

181. Which of the following statements is (are) true regarding the PA axial projection of the paranasal sinuses?

1. The central ray is directed caudally to the OML.
2. The petrous pyramids are projected into the lower third of the orbits.
3. The frontal sinuses are visualized.

(A) 1 only

(B) 1 and 2 only

(C) 1 and 3 only

(D) 1, 2, and 3

182. Tracheotomy and intubation are effective techniques used to restore breathing when there is (are)

(A) respiratory pathway obstruction above the larynx.

(B) crushed tracheal rings due to trauma.

(C) respiratory pathway closure due to inflammation and swelling.

(D) all of the above.

183. To demonstrate the first two cervical vertebrae in the AP projection, the patient is positioned so that

(A) the glabellomeatal line is vertical.

(B) the acanthiomeatal line is vertical.

(C) a line between the mentum and the mastoid tip is vertical.

(D) a line between the maxillary occlusal plane and the mastoid tip is vertical.

184. Which of the following is recommended to demonstrate small amounts of air within the peritoneal cavity?

(A) Lateral decubitus, affected side up

(B) Lateral decubitus, affected side down

(C) AP Trendelenburg

(D) AP supine

185. For the average patient, the central ray for a lateral projection of a barium-filled stomach should enter

(A) midway between the midcoronal line and the anterior abdominal surface.

(B) midway between the vertebral column and the lateral border of the abdomen.

(C) at the midcoronal line at the level of the iliac crest.

(D) perpendicular to the level of L2.

186. Which of the following is an important consideration to avoid excessive metacarpophalangeal joint overlap in the oblique projection of the hand?

(A) Oblique the hand no more than 45°.
(B) Use a support sponge for the phalanges.
(C) Clench the fist to bring the carpals closer to the IR.
(D) Utilize ulnar flexion.

187. Involuntary motion can be caused by

1. peristalsis.
2. severe pain.
3. heart muscle contraction.

(A) 1 only
(B) 2 only
(C) 1 and 2 only
(D) 1, 2, and 3

188. Which of the following positions is used to demonstrate vertical patellar fractures and the patellofemoral articulation?

(A) AP knee
(B) Lateral knee
(C) Tangential patella
(D) "Tunnel" view

189. In what position was the radiograph in Figure 2–30 made?

(A) Flexion
(B) Extension
(C) Left bending
(D) Right bending

190. The structure labeled 1 in Figure 2–30 is the

(A) intervertebral disk space.
(B) apophyseal joint.
(C) intervertebral foramen.
(D) spinous process.

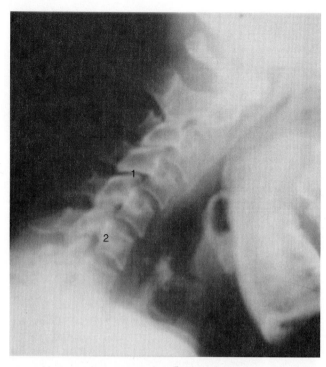

Figure 2–30. Courtesy of Stamford Hospital, Department of Radiology.

191. When the erect position is requested as part of an IVU, it is used to demonstrate

(A) the adrenal glands.
(B) the renal surfaces.
(C) kidney mobility.
(D) the bladder neck.

192. AP erect left and right bending images of the thoracic and lumbar vertebrae, to include 1 inch of the iliac crest, are performed to demonstrate

(A) spondylolisthesis.
(B) subluxation.
(C) scoliosis.
(D) arthritis.

193. In which of the following projections is the talofibular joint *best* demonstrated?

(A) AP
(B) Lateral oblique
(C) Medial oblique
(D) Lateral

194. Free air in the abdominal cavity is best demonstrated in which of the following positions?

    A. AP projection, left lateral decubitus position
    B. AP projection, right lateral decubitus position
    C. PA recumbent position
    D. AP recumbent position

195. Which of the following sequences correctly describes the path of blood flow as it leaves the left ventricle?

    (A) Arteries, arterioles, capillaries, venules, veins
    (B) Arterioles, arteries, capillaries, veins, venules
    (C) Veins, venules, capillaries, arteries, arterioles
    (D) Venules, veins, capillaries, arterioles, arteries

196. Which of the following projections of the elbow should demonstrate the coronoid process free of superimposition and the olecranon process within the olecranon fossa?

    (A) AP
    (B) Lateral
    (C) Medial oblique
    (D) Lateral oblique

197. Which of the following will *best* demonstrate acromioclavicular separation?

    (A) AP recumbent, affected shoulder
    (B) AP recumbent, both shoulders
    (C) AP erect, affected shoulder
    (D) AP erect, both shoulders

198. Which of the following statements regarding myelography is (are) correct?

    1. Spinal puncture may be performed in the prone or flexed lateral position.
    2. Contrast medium distribution is regulated through x-ray tube angulation.
    3. The patient's neck must be in extension during Trendelenburg positions.

    (A) 1 only
    (B) 1 and 2 only
    (C) 1 and 3 only
    (D) 1, 2, and 3

199. The term that refers to parts closer to the source or beginning is

    (A) cephalad.
    (B) caudad.
    (C) proximal.
    (D) medial.

200. With the patient PA, MSP centered to the grid, the OML forming a 37° angle with the IR, and the central ray perpendicular and exiting the acanthion, which of the following is *best* demonstrated?

    (A) Occipital bone
    (B) Frontal bone
    (C) Facial bones
    (D) Basal foramina

201. The inhalation of liquid or solid particles into the nose, throat, or lungs is referred to as

    (A) asphyxia
    (B) aspiration
    (C) atelectasis
    (D) asystole

202. Endoscopic retrograde cholangiopancreatography (ERCP) usually involves

1. cannulation of the hepatopancreatic ampulla.
2. introduction of contrast medium into the common bile duct.
3. introduction of barium directly into the duodenum.

(A) 1 only
(B) 1 and 2 only
(C) 1 and 3 only
(D) 1, 2, and 3

203. Which of the following is (are) associated with a Colles' fracture?

1. Transverse fracture of the radial head
2. Chip fracture of the ulnar styloid
3. Posterior or backward displacement

(A) 1 only
(B) 1 and 3 only
(C) 2 and 3 only
(D) 1, 2, and 3

204. To *best* visualize the lower ribs, the exposure should be made

(A) on normal inspiration.
(B) on inspiration, second breath.
(C) on expiration.
(D) during shallow breathing.

205. Which of the following statements regarding the male pelvis is (are) true?

1. The angle formed by the pubic arch is less than that of the female.
2. The pelvic outlet is wider than that of the female.
3. The ischial tuberosities are further apart.

(A) 1 only
(B) 1 and 2 only
(C) 2 and 3 only
(D) 1, 2, and 3

206. Which of the following interventional procedures can be used to increase the diameter of a stenosed vessel?

1. Percutaneous transluminal angioplasty (PTA)
2. Stent placement
3. Peripherally inserted central catheter (PICC line)

(A) 1 only
(B) 1 and 2 only
(C) 1 and 3 only
(D) 1, 2, and 3

207. Important considerations for radiographic examinations of traumatic injuries to the upper extremity include

1. the joint closest to the injured site should be supported during movement of the limb
2. both joints must be included in long bone studies
3. two views, at 90° to each other, are required

A. 1 only
B. 1 and 2 only
C. 2 and 3 only
D. 1, 2, and 3

208. Fluoroscopic imaging of the ileocecal valve is generally part of a(n)

(A) esophagram.
(B) upper GI series.
(C) small-bowel series.
(D) ERCP.

209. The contraction and expansion of arterial walls in accordance with forceful contraction and relaxation of the heart is called

(A) hypertension.
(B) elasticity.
(C) pulse.
(D) pressure.

210. The AP Trendelenburg position is often used during an upper GI examination to demonstrate

    (A) the duodenal loop.
    (B) filling of the duodenal bulb.
    (C) hiatal hernia.
    (D) hypertrophic pyloric stenosis.

211. Which of the following would be the best choice for a right-shoulder examination to rule out fracture?

    (A) Internal and external rotation
    (B) AP and tangential
    (C) AP and AP axial
    (D) AP and scapular Y

212. Which of the following positions would best demonstrate the proximal tibiofibular articulation?

    (A) AP
    (B) 90° mediolateral
    (C) 45° internal rotation
    (D) 45° external rotation

213. Which of the following bones participate in the formation of the acetabulum?

    1. Ilium
    2. Ischium
    3. Pubis

    (A) 1 and 2 only
    (B) 1 and 3 only
    (C) 2 and 3 only
    (D) 1, 2, and 3

214. Which of the following radiologic procedures requires that a contrast medium be injected into the renal pelvis via a catheter placed within the ureter?

    (A) Nephrotomography
    (B) Retrograde urography
    (C) Cystourethrography
    (D) IV urography

215. The AP projection of the sacrum requires that the central ray be directed

    1. 15° cephalad.
    2. to the pubic symphysis.
    3. at the level of the lesser trochanter.

    (A) 1 only
    (B) 2 only
    (C) 1 and 2 only
    (D) 1 and 3 only

216. Which of the following would best demonstrate arthritic changes in the knees?

    (A) AP recumbent
    (B) Lateral recumbent
    (C) AP erect
    (D) Medial oblique

217. Which of the following positions will demonstrate the lumbosacral apophyseal articulation?

    (A) AP
    (B) Lateral
    (C) 30° RPO
    (D) 45° LPO

218. Which of the following statements is (are) true regarding the images seen in Figure 2–31?

    1. Image A is positioned in internal rotation.
    2. Image B is positioned in internal rotation.
    3. The greater tubercle is better demonstrated in image A.

    (A) 1 only
    (B) 2 only
    (C) 1 and 3 only
    (D) 2 and 3 only

219. When the patient is recumbent and the central ray is directed horizontally, the patient is said to be in the

    (A) Trendelenburg position.
    (B) Fowler's position.
    (C) decubitus position.
    (D) Sims' position.

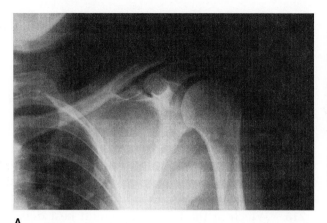

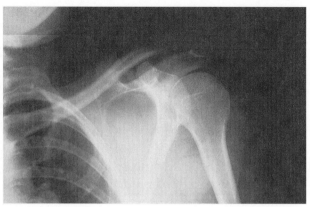

A

B

Figure 2–31. Courtesy of Stamford Hospital, Department of Radiology.

220. Which of the following radiologic examinations can demonstrate ureteral reflux?

(A) IV urogram
(B) Retrograde pyelogram
(C) Voiding cystourethrogram
(D) Nephrotomogram

221. The AP axial projection, or "frog leg" position, of the femoral neck places the patient in a supine position with the affected thigh

(A) adducted 25° from the horizontal.
(B) abducted 25° from the vertical.
(C) adducted 40° from the horizontal.
(D) abducted 40° from the vertical.

222. Which of the following precaution(s) should be observed when radiographing a patient who has sustained a traumatic injury to the hip?

1. When a fracture is suspected, manipulation of the affected extremity should be performed by a physician.
2. The AP axiolateral projection should be avoided.
3. To evaluate the entire region, the pelvis is typically included in the initial examination.

(A) 1 only
(B) 1 and 3 only
(C) 2 and 3 only
(D) 1, 2, and 3

223. Which of the following are characteristics of the hypersthenic body type?

1. Short, wide, transverse heart
2. High and peripheral large bowel
3. Diaphragm positioned low

(A) 1 and 2 only
(B) 1 and 3 only
(C) 2 and 3 only
(D) 1, 2, and 3

224. Prior to the start of an IV urogram, which of the following procedures should be carried out?

1. Have patient empty the bladder.
2. Review the patient's allergy history.
3. Check the patient's creatinine level.

(A) 1 only
(B) 2 only
(C) 1 and 2 only
(D) 1, 2, and 3

225. To demonstrate the entire circumference of the radial head, exposure(s) must be made with the

1. epicondyles perpendicular to the cassette.
2. hand pronated and supinated as much as possible.
3. hand lateral and in internal rotation.

(A) 1 only
(B) 1 and 2 only
(C) 1 and 3 only
(D) 1, 2, and 3

226. The radiograph pictured in Figure 2–32 may be used to evaluate

1. polypoid lesions.
2. the lateral wall of the descending colon.
3. the posterior wall of the rectum.

(A) 1 only
(B) 1 and 2 only
(C) 2 and 3 only
(D) 1, 2, and 3

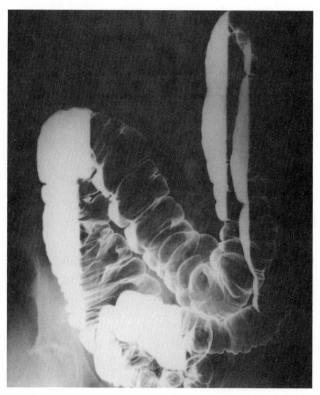

Figure 2–32. Courtesy of Stamford Hospital, Department of Radiology.

227. In myelography, the contrast medium is generally injected into the

(A) cisterna magna.
(B) individual intervertebral disks.
(C) subarachnoid space between the first and second lumbar vertebrae.
(D) subarachnoid space between the third and fourth lumbar vertebrae.

228. Which of the following conditions is often the result of ureteral obstruction or stricture?

(A) Pyelonephrosis
(B) Nephroptosis
(C) Hydronephrosis
(D) Cystourethritis

229. Which of the following is (are) effective in reducing breast exposure during scoliosis examinations?

1. Use of a high-speed imaging system
2. Use of breast shields
3. Use of compensating filtration

(A) 1 only
(B) 1 and 2 only
(C) 2 and 3 only
(D) 1, 2, and 3

230. Which type of articulation is evaluated in arthrography?

(A) Synarthrodial
(B) Diarthrodial
(C) Amphiarthrodial
(D) Cartilaginous

231. The laryngeal prominence is formed by the

A. thyroid gland.
B. thyroid cartilage.
C. vocal cords.
D. pharynx.

232. In the AP projection of the ankle, the

1. plantar surface of the foot is vertical.
2. fibula projects more distally than the tibia.
3. calcaneus is well visualized.

(A) 1 only
(B) 1 and 2 only
(C) 2 and 3 only
(D) 1, 2, and 3

233. During studies of the soft tissue of the neck, the exposure can be made

    1. during phonation before/after opacification.
    2. during Valsalva maneuver.
    3. at the height of swallowing motion with opacification.

    A. 1 only
    B. 1 and 2 only
    C. 2 and 3 only
    D. 1, 2, and 3

234. When modifying the PA axial projection of the skull to demonstrate superior orbital fissures, the central ray is directed

    (A) 20° to 25° caudad.
    (B) 20° to 25° cephalad.
    (C) 30° to 35° caudad.
    (D) 30° to 35° cephalad.

235. Deoxygenated blood from the head and thorax is returned to the heart by the

    (A) pulmonary artery.
    (B) pulmonary veins.
    (C) superior vena cava.
    (D) thoracic aorta.

236. A flat and upright abdomen is requested on an acutely ill patient, to demonstrate the presence of air–fluid levels. Because of the patient's condition, the x-ray table can be tilted upright only 70° (rather than the desired 90°). How should the central ray be directed?

    (A) Perpendicular to the IR
    (B) Parallel to the floor
    (C) 20° caudad
    (D) 20° cephalad

237. Standard radiographic protocols may be reduced to include two views, at right angles to each other, in which of the following situations?

    (A) Barium examinations
    (B) Spine radiography
    (C) Skull radiography
    (D) Emergency and trauma radiography

238. Which of the following is a condition in which an occluded blood vessel stops blood flow to a portion of the lungs?

    (A) Pneumothorax
    (B) Atelectasis
    (C) Pulmonary embolism
    (D) Hypoxia

239. Following the ingestion of a fatty meal, what hormone is secreted by the duodenal mucosa to stimulate contraction of the gallbladder?

    (A) Insulin
    (B) Cholecystokinin
    (C) Adrenocorticotropic hormone
    (D) Gastrin

240. Which of the following projections is most likely to demonstrate the carpal pisiform free of superimposition?

    (A) Radial flexion/deviation
    (B) Ulnar flexion/deviation
    (C) AP (medial) oblique
    (D) AP (lateral) oblique

241. The stomach of an asthenic patient is *most* likely to be located

    (A) high, transverse, and lateral.
    (B) low, transverse, and lateral.
    (C) high, vertical, and toward the midline.
    (D) low, vertical, and toward the midline.

242. With which of the following is zonography associated?

    1. Thick tomographic cuts
    2. Long exposure amplitude
    3. Less blurring than with pluridirectional tomography because a narrow exposure angle is used

    (A) 1 only
    (B) 2 only
    (C) 1 and 3 only
    (D) 2 and 3 only

243. Which of the following are components of a trimalleolar fracture?

1. Fractured lateral malleolus
2. Fractured medial malleolus
3. Fractured posterior tibia

(A) 1 only
(B) 1 and 3 only
(C) 2 and 3 only
(D) 1, 2, and 3

244. The functions of which body system include mineral homeostasis, protection, and triglyceride storage?

A. endocrine
B. integumentary
C. skeletal
D. muscular

245. The four major arteries supplying the brain include the

1. brachiocephalic artery.
2. common carotid arteries.
3. vertebral arteries.

(A) 1 and 2 only
(B) 1 and 3 only
(C) 2 and 3 only
(D) 1, 2, and 3

246. Which of the following articulates with the base of the first metatarsal?

(A) First cuneiform
(B) Third cuneiform
(C) Navicular
(D) Cuboid

247. Which of the following is a major cause of bowel obstruction in children?

(A) Appendicitis
(B) Intussusception
(C) Regional enteritis
(D) Ulcerative colitis

248. Which of the following are well demonstrated in the lumbar spine pictured in Figure 2–33?

1. Apophyseal articulations
2. Intervertebral foramina
3. Inferior articular processes

(A) 1 only
(B) 1 and 2 only
(C) 1 and 3 only
(D) 1, 2, and 3

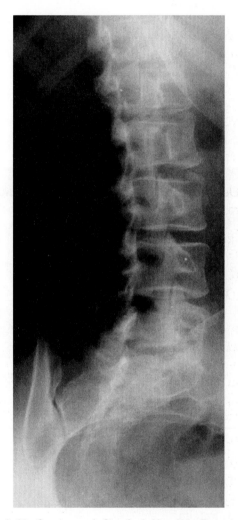

Figure 2–33. Courtesy of Stamford Hospital, Department of Radiology.

249. Which of the following is (are) recommended when positioning the patient for a lateral projection of the chest?

1. The patient should be examined upright.
2. The shoulders should be depressed.
3. The shoulders should be rolled forward.

(A) 1 only
(B) 1 and 2 only
(C) 1 and 3 only
(D) 1, 2, and 3

250. Which of the following is represented by the number 3 in Figure 2–34?

(A) Inferior vena cava
(B) Aorta
(C) Gallbladder
(D) Psoas muscle

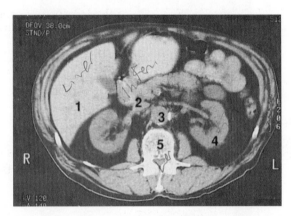

Figure 2–34. Courtesy of Stamford Hospital, Department of Radiology.

251. Which of the following bones participates in the formation of the knee joint?

1. Femur
2. Tibia
3. Patella

(A) 1 and 2 only
(B) 1 and 3 only
(C) 2 and 3 only
(D) 1, 2, and 3

252. All of the following are palpable bony landmarks used in radiography of the pelvis *except* the

(A) femoral neck.
(B) pubic symphysis.
(C) greater trochanter.
(D) iliac crest.

253. Lateral deviation of the nasal septum may be *best* demonstrated in the

(A) lateral projection.
(B) PA axial (Caldwell method) projection.
(C) parietoacanthial (Waters' method) projection.
(D) AP axial (Grashey/Towne method) projection.

254. Which of the following is/are proximal to the tibial plateau?

1. Femoral condyles
2. Tibial condyles
3. Tibial tuberosity

(A) 1 only
(B) 1 and 2 only
(C) 2 and 3 only
(D) 1, 2, and 3

255. All of the following may be determined by oral cholecystography *except*

(A) liver function.
(B) ability of the gallbladder to concentrate bile.
(C) emptying power of the gallbladder.
(D) pancreatic function.

256. The medial oblique projection of the elbow demonstrates the

1. olecranon process within the olecranon fossa.
2. radial head free of superimposition.
3. coronoid process free of superimposition.

(A) 1 only
(B) 2 only
(C) 1 and 3 only
(D) 1, 2, and 3

257. In the posterior oblique position of the cervical spine, the central ray should be directed

(A) parallel to C4.
(B) perpendicular to C4.
(C) 15° cephalad to C4.
(D) 15° caudad to C4.

258. Which of the following is a functional study used to demonstrate the degree of AP motion present in the cervical spine?

(A) Open-mouth projection
(B) Moving mandible AP
(C) Flexion and extension laterals
(D) Right and left bending AP

259. If the patient's zygomatic arch has been traumatically depressed or the patient has flat cheekbones, the arch may be demonstrated by modifying the SMV projection and rotating the patient's head

(A) 15° toward the side being examined.
(B) 15° away from the side being examined.
(C) 30° toward the side being examined.
(D) 30° away from the side being examined.

260. Which of the following barium-filled anatomic structures is *best* demonstrated in the LAO position?

(A) Hepatic flexure
(B) Splenic flexure
(C) Sigmoid colon
(D) Ileocecal valve

261. Which of the localization lines seen in Figure 2–35 is used for the SMV (Schüller method) projection of the skull?

(A) Line 1
(B) Line 2
(C) Line 3
(D) Line 4

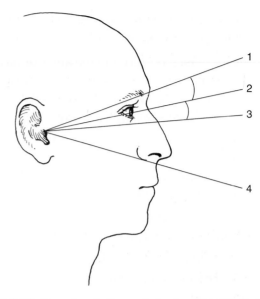

Figure 2–35. Reproduced with permission from Saia DA. *Radiography: Program Review and Examination Preparation,* 2nd ed. Stamford, CT: Appleton & Lange, 1999.

262. In Figure 2–35, which of the localization lines is used for the lateral projection of the skull?

(A) Line 1
(B) Line 2
(C) Line 3
(D) Line 4

263. Radiographic measurement of long bones of an upper or lower extremity requires the following accessories:

1. Bell-Thompson scale
2. Cannula
3. Speculum

(A) 1 only
(B) 1 and 2 only
(C) 1 and 3 only
(D) 1, 2, and 3

264. What is the name of the condition that results in the forward slipping of one vertebra on the one below it?

(A) Spondylitis
(B) Spondylolysis
(C) Spondylolisthesis
(D) Spondylosis

265. In a lateral projection of the nasal bones, the central ray is directed

    (A) 1/2 inch posterior to the anterior nasal spine.
    (B) 3/4 inch posterior to the glabella.
    (C) 3/4 inch distal to the nasion.
    (D) 1/2 inch anterior to the EAM.

266. Posterior displacement of a tibial fracture would be *best* demonstrated in the

    (A) AP projection.
    (B) lateral projection.
    (C) medial oblique projection.
    (D) lateral oblique projection.

267. Which of the following positions would *best* demonstrate the left apophyseal articulations of the lumbar vertebrae?

    (A) LPO
    (B) RPO
    (C) Left lateral
    (D) PA

268. Blowout fractures of the orbit are *best* demonstrated using the

    (A) lateral projection of the facial bones.
    (B) parietoacanthial projection (Waters' method).
    (C) posteroanterior projection with a 15° caudal angle.
    (D) Sweet's localization method.

269. Inspiration and expiration projections of the chest may be performed to demonstrate

    1. pneumothorax.
    2. foreign body.
    3. atelectasis.

    (A) 1 only
    (B) 1 and 2 only
    (C) 1 and 3 only
    (D) 1, 2, and 3

270. Shoulder arthrography may be performed to evaluate

    (A) humeral dislocation.
    (B) complete or incomplete rotator cuff tears.
    (C) osteoarthritis.
    (D) acromioclavicular joint separation.

271. What angle is formed by the median sagittal plane and the IR in the parietoorbital projection (Rhese method) of the optic canal?

    (A) 90°
    (B) 37°
    (C) 53°
    (D) 45°

272. The most significant risk factor for breast cancer is:

    (A) age.
    (B) gender.
    (C) family history.
    (D) personal history.

273. Which of the following is located at the level of the interspace between the fourth and fifth thoracic vertebrae?

    (A) Manubrium   T2–T3
    (B) Jugular notch opposite T2–T3
    (C) Sternal angle T4–T5
    (D) Xiphoid process T-10

274. For the AP projection of the scapula, the

    1. patient's arm is abducted at right angles to the body.
    2. patient's elbow is flexed with the hand supinated.
    3. exposure is made during quiet breathing.

    (A) 1 and 2 only
    (B) 1 and 3 only
    (C) 3 only
    (D) 1, 2, and 3

275. The short, thick processes that project posteriorly from the vertebral body are the

(A) transverse processes.
(B) vertebral arches.
(C) laminae.
(D) pedicles.

276. All of the following are mediastinal structures *except* the

(A) esophagus.
(B) thymus.
(C) heart.
(D) terminal bronchiole.

277. Which of the following sinus groups is demonstrated with the patient positioned as for a parietoacanthial projection (Waters' method) and the central ray directed through the patient's open mouth?

(A) Frontal
(B) Ethmoidal
(C) Maxillary
(D) Sphenoidal

278. To better demonstrate the ribs below the diaphragm,

1. suspend respiration at the end of full exhalation.
2. suspend respiration at the end of deep inhalation.
3. perform the examination in the recumbent position.

(A) 1 only
(B) 2 only
(C) 1 and 3 only
(D) 2 and 3 only

279. To obtain an exact axial projection of the clavicle, place the patient

(A) supine and angle the central ray 30° caudally.
(B) prone and angle the central ray 30° cephalad.
(C) supine and angle the central ray 15° cephalad.
(D) in a lordotic position and direct the central ray at right angles to the coronal plane of the clavicle.

280. Which of the following projections of the calcaneus is obtained with the leg extended, the plantar surface of the foot vertical and perpendicular to the IR, and the central ray directed 40° caudad?

(A) Axial plantodorsal projection
(B) Axial dorsoplantar projection
(C) Lateral projection
(D) Weight-bearing lateral projection

281. During GI radiography, the position of the stomach may vary depending on

1. respiratory phase.
2. body habitus.
3. patient position.

(A) 1 and 2 only
(B) 1 and 3 only
(C) 2 and 3 only
(D) 1, 2, and 3

282. With a patient in the PA position and the OML perpendicular to the table, a 15° to 20° caudal angulation would place the petrous ridges in the lower third of the orbit. To achieve the same result in a baby or a small child, it is necessary for the radiographer to modify the angulation to

(A) 10° to 15° caudal.
(B) 25° to 30° caudal.
(C) 15° to 20° cephalic.
(D) 3° to 5° caudal.

283. The patient positioned for an T-tube cholangiography is in a

(A) 15° to 20° LPO.
(B) 15° to 20° RPO.
(C) 45° LPO.
(D) 45° RPO.

284. The structures forming the brain stem include

1. pons.
2. medulla oblongata.
3. midbrain.

(A) 1 and 2 only
(B) 1 and 3 only
(C) 2 and 3 only
(D) 1, 2, and 3

285. Knee arthrography may be performed to demonstrate a

1. torn meniscus.
2. Baker's cyst.
3. torn rotator cuff.

(A) 1 and 2 only
(B) 1 and 3 only
(C) 2 and 3 only
(D) 1, 2, and 3

286. In which of the following tangential axial projections of the patella is complete relaxation of the quadriceps femoris required for an accurate diagnosis?

1. Supine flexion 45° (Merchant)
2. Prone flexion 90° (Settegast)
3. Prone flexion 55° (Hughston)

(A) 1 only
(B) 1 and 2 only
(C) 2 and 3 only
(D) 1, 2, and 3 only

287. In the lateral projection of the foot, the

1. plantar surface should be perpendicular to the IR.
2. metatarsals are superimposed.
3. talofibular joint should be visualized.

(A) 1 only
(B) 1 and 2 only
(C) 2 and 3 only
(D) 1, 2, and 3

288. Hysterosalpingography may be performed for demonstration of

1. uterine tubal patency.
2. mass lesions in the uterine cavity.
3. uterine position.

(A) 1 and 2 only
(B) 1 and 3 only
(C) 2 and 3 only
(D) 1, 2, and 3

289. Which of the following equipment is necessary for ERCP?

1. A fluoroscopic unit with imaging device and tilt table capabilities
2. A fiberoptic endoscope
3. Polyethylene catheters

(A) 1 and 2 only
(B) 1 and 3 only
(C) 2 and 3 only
(D) 1, 2, and 3

290. All of the following statements regarding pediatric positioning are true, *except*

(A) for radiography of the kidneys, the central ray should be directed midway between the diaphragm and the symphysis pubis.
(B) if a pediatric patient is in respiratory distress, a chest radiograph should be obtained in the AP projection rather than in the standard PA projection.
(C) chest radiography on a neonate should be performed in the supine position.
(D) radiography of pediatric patients with a myelomeningocele defect should be performed in the supine position.

291. Operative cholangiography may be performed to

1. visualize biliary stones or a neoplasm.
2. determine function of the hepatopancreatic ampulla.
3. examine the patency of the biliary tract.

(A) 1 and 2 only
(B) 1 and 3 only
(C) 2 and 3 only
(D) 1, 2, and 3

292. With the patient seated at the end of the x-ray table, elbow flexed 90°, CR directed 45° *toward the shoulder to the elbow joint*, which of the following structures will be demonstrated best?

(A) Radial head
(B) Ulnar head
(C) Coronoid process
(D) Olecranon process

293. Which of the following articulate(s) with the bases of the metatarsals?

1. The heads of the first row of phalanges
2. The cuboid
3. The cuneiforms

(A) 1 only
(B) 1 and 2 only
(C) 2 and 3 only
(D) 1, 2, and 3

294. Arthrography requires the use of

1. general anesthesia.
2. sterile technique.
3. fluoroscopy.

(A) 1 and 2 only
(B) 1 and 3 only
(C) 2 and 3 only
(D) 1, 2, and 3

295. The contrast media of choice for use in myelography are

(A) ionic non–water-soluble.
(B) ionic water-soluble.
(C) nonionic water-soluble.
(D) gas.

296. Which of the following procedures will *best* demonstrate the cephalic, basilic, and subclavian veins?

(A) Aortofemoral arteriogram
(B) Upper-limb venogram
(C) Lower-limb venogram
(D) Renal venogram

297. Which of the following devices should *not* be removed before positioning for a radiograph?

1. A ring when performing hand radiography
2. An antishock garment
3. A pneumatic splint

(A) 1 and 2
(B) 1 and 3
(C) 2 and 3
(D) 1, 2, and 3

298. Which of the following is demonstrated in a 25° RPO position with the central ray entering 1 inch medial to the elevated ASIS?

(A) Left sacroiliac joint
(B) Right sacroiliac joint
(C) Left ilium
(D) Right ilium

299. Which of the following are appropriate techniques for imaging a patient with a possible traumatic spine injury?

1. Instruct the patient to turn slowly and stop if anything hurts.
2. Maneuver the x-ray tube head instead of moving the patient.
3. Call for help and use the log-rolling method to turn the patient.

(A) 1 and 2 only
(B) 1 and 3 only
(C) 2 and 3 only
(D) 1, 2, and 3

300. In which type of fracture are the splintered ends of bone forced through the skin?

(A) Closed
(B) Compound
(C) Compression
(D) Depressed

Answers and Explanations

1. **(C)** The parietoacanthial projection (Waters' position) of the skull is valuable for the demonstration of facial bones or maxillary sinuses. The head is rested on the extended chin so that the OML forms a 37° angle with the IR. This projects the petrous pyramids below the floor of the maxillary sinuses and provides an oblique frontal view of the facial bones. *(Ballinger & Frank, vol 2, pp 316–317)*

2. **(C)** *Rickets* and *osteomalacia* are skeletal disorders characterised by abnormal calcification processes. In osteomalacia, bones become soft and are easily misshapen. Rickets affects the growing bones of children and is also characterized by soft, mishapend bones—as a result of calcium salts not being deposited in bone matrix. *Osteoarthritis* is a degeneration of articular cartilage; when these surfaces then attempt to articulate and move, bone friction and pain occur. *(Tortora & Derrickson, pp 189–190)*

3. **(C)** Three positions of the cervical spine are illustrated. Figure B shows the *left lateral position*. Lateral projections of the cervical spine are done to demonstrate the intervertebral disk spaces, apophyseal joints, and spinous processes. Apophyseal joints are formed by adjacent superior and inferior articular processes and their facets. Spinous processes are formed by the union of the laminae. Figure A is an *RAO* with caudal angulation; Figure C is an *LPO* with cephalad angulation. *Anterior oblique* positions (LAO, RAO) of the cervical spine demonstrate the intervertebral *foramina* *closer* to the IR, while *posterior oblique* positions (LPO, RPO) demonstrate the intervertebral *foramina farther* from the IR. Intervertebral foramina are formed by the vertebral notches of the *pedicles*. *(Ballinger & Frank, pp 400–403)*

4. **(B)** The talocalcaneal, or subtalar, joint is a three-faceted articulation formed by the talus and the os calcis (calcaneus). The plantodorsal and dorsoplantar projections of the os calcis should exhibit sufficient density to visualize the talocalcaneal joint (Fig. 2–36). This is the only "routine" projection that will demonstrate the talocalcaneal joint. If evaluation of the talocalcaneal joint is desired, special views

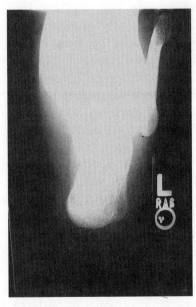

Figure 2–36. Courtesy of Stamford Hospital, Department of Radiology.

(such as the Broden and Isherwood methods) are required. *(Ballinger & Frank, vol 1, p 215)*

5. **(D)** The male and female bony pelves have several differing characteristics. A overview of comparisons is listed below.

Male pelvis
• Heavy and thick general structure
• Greater, or false, pelvis is deep
• Pelvis brim, or inlet, is small and heart-shaped
• Acetabulum is large and faces laterally
• Pubic angle is less than 90°
• Ilium is more vertical

Female pelvis
• Light and thin general structure
• Greater, or false, pelvis is shallow
• Pelvis brim, or inlet, is large and oval
• Acetabulum is small and faces anteriorly
• Pubic angle is more than 90°
• Ilium is more horizontal

(Tortora & Derrickson, p 244)

6. **(D)** If structures are overlying or underlying the area to be demonstrated (eg, the medial femoral condyle obscuring the joint space in the lateral knee projection), central ray angulation is employed (eg, 5° cephalad angulation to see the joint space in the lateral knee). If structures would be foreshortened or self-superimposed (eg, the scaphoid in a PA wrist), central ray angulation may be employed to place the structure more closely parallel with the IR. Another example is the oblique cervical spine, where cephalad or caudad angulation is required to "open" the intervertebral foramina. *(Ballinger & Frank, vol 1, p 17)*

7. **(C)** The relationship between the thigh, lower leg, patella, and central ray should be noted. The central ray is directed *parallel to the plane of the patella,* thereby providing a *tangential* projection of the patella (patella in profile) and an unobstructed view of the *patellofemoral articulation* (Fig. 2–37). A "tunnel view" is required to demonstrate the intercondyloid fossa and the articulating surfaces of the tibia and femur. *(Ballinger & Frank, vol 1, p 311)*

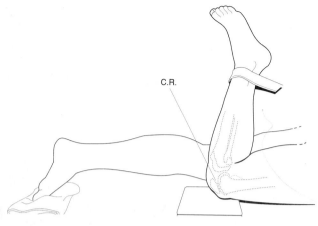

C.R.

Figure 2–37.

8. **(A)** The trachea (windpipe) bifurcates into left and right *mainstem bronchi,* each entering its respective lung hilum. The *left* bronchus divides into *two* portions, one for each lobe of the left lung. The *right* bronchus divides into *three* portions, one for each lobe of the right lung (Fig. 2–38). The lungs are conical in shape, consisting of upper pointed portions, termed the *apices* (plural of apex), and broad lower portions (or *bases*). The lungs are enclosed in a double-walled serous membrane called the *pleura. (Bontrager, pp 69–70)*

9. **(C)** In the exact PA projection of the skull with the perpendicular central ray exiting the nasion, the petrous pyramids should *fill* the orbits (Fig. 2–39). As the central ray is angled caudally, the petrous pyramids are projected lower in the orbits. At about 25° to 30° caudad they are projected *below* the orbits. The orbitomeatal line must be *perpendicular* to the IR or the petrous pyramids will not be projected into the expected location. The MSP must be *perpendicular* to the IR or the skull will be rotated. With the MSP *parallel* to the IR, a lateral skull projection is obtained. *(Ballinger & Frank, vol 2, p 242)*

10. **(C)** The pictured radiograph is an AP projection of the knee with the knee extended. The tibial *intercondylar eminences* are well demonstrated on the tibial plateau, and the *femorotibial joint* is well visualized. The intercondyloid fossa is not demonstrated here. A "tunnel" view of the knee is required to demonstrate the intercondyloid fossa. *(Ballinger & Frank, vol 1, p 290)*

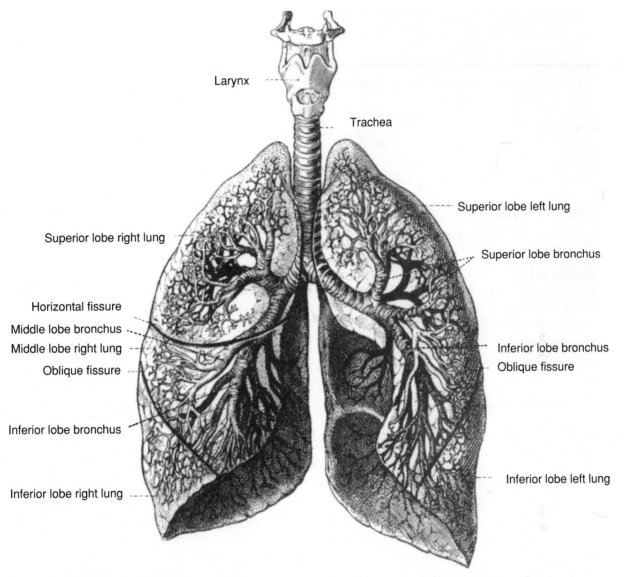

Larynx

Trachea

Superior lobe left lung

Superior lobe right lung

Superior lobe bronchus

Horizontal fissure
Middle lobe bronchus
Middle lobe right lung
Oblique fissure

Inferior lobe bronchus
Oblique fissure

Inferior lobe bronchus

Inferior lobe left lung

Inferior lobe right lung

Figure 2–38. Reproduced with permission from Montgomery RL. *Appleton & Lange's Review of Anatomy for the USMLE Step I*. East Norwalk, CT: Appleton & Lange, 1995.

11. **(D)** Barium sulfate suspension is the usual contrast medium of choice for investigation of the alimentary tract. There are, however, a few exceptions. Whenever there is the possibility of escape of contrast medium into the peritoneal cavity, barium sulfate is contraindicated and a water-soluble iodinated medium is recommended, as it is easily aspirated before surgery. Rupture of a hollow viscus (eg, perforated ulcer) and patients who are scheduled for surgery are two examples. Patients with suspected large-bowel obstruction should also ingest only water-soluble iodinated media. *(Ballinger & Frank, vol 2, p 94)*

12. **(B)** Chest radiographs demonstrating *emphysema* will show the characteristic irreversible trapping of air that gradually increases and overexpands the lungs. This produces the characteristic "flattening" of the hemidiaphragms and widening of the intercostal spaces. The increased air content of the lungs requires a compensating decrease in technical factors. *Pneumonia* is inflammation of the lungs, usually caused by bacteria, virus, or chemical irritant. *Pneumothorax* is a collection of air or gas in the pleural cavity (outside the lungs), with an accompanying collapse of the lung. *Pleural effusion* is excessive fluid between

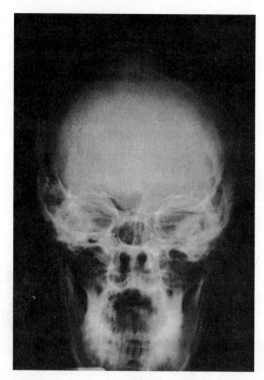

Figure 2–39. Courtesy of Stamford Hospital, Department of Radiology.

the parietal and visceral layers of pleura (*Bontrager, p 80*)

13. **(C)** The *gallbladder* is located on the posterior surface of the liver in the right upper quadrant (RUQ). The *hepatic flexure*, so named because of its close proximity to the liver, is also in the RUQ. The vermiform appendix projects from the first portion of the large bowel, the *cecum*, located in the right lower quadrant (RLQ). (*Bontrager, p 104*)

14. **(B)** The pictured radiograph is one of a series of IVU (IU) images. It was done prone at 20 minutes after injection of the contrast medium. The urinary collecting system is well demonstrated. The *renal pelvis* (number 1) is the proximal expanded end of the ureter lying within the renal sinus. The *minor calyces* (number 3) receive urine from the collecting tubules of the renal pyramids and convey it to the *major calyces* (number 2), which empty into the renal pelvis. Urine is carried down the ureters by peristaltic waves. The *vesicoureteral junction* (number 4) is located at the distal end of the ureter, where it unites with the urinary bladder. (*Bontrager, pp 543–544*)

15. **(C)** With the body in the AP recumbent position, *barium* flows easily into the *fundus* of the stomach, displacing the stomach somewhat superiorly. The fundus, then, is filled with barium, while the *air* that had been in the fundus is displaced into the *gastric body, pylorus,* and *duodenum,* illustrating them in double-contrast fashion. Air-contrast delineation of these structures allows us to see through the stomach to the retrogastric areas and structures. *Anterior and posterior aspects* of the stomach are visualized in the *lateral* position; medial and lateral aspects of the stomach are visualized in the AP projection. (*Ballinger & Frank, vol 2, p 110*)

16. **(C)** The *carina* is an internal ridge located at the bifurcation of the trachea into right and left primary, or mainstem, bronchi. The *epiglottis* is a flap of elastic cartilage that functions to prevent fluids and solids from entering the respiratory tract during swallowing. The *root* of the lung attaches the lung, via dense connective tissue, to the mediastinum. The root of the left lung is at the level of T6, and the root of the right is at T5. The *hilus* (hilum) is the slitlike opening on the medial aspect of the lung through which arteries, veins, lymphatics, and so forth, enter and exit. (*Bontrager, p 68*)

17. **(C)** The bones of the foot are arranged to form a number of longitudinal and transverse arches. The longitudinal arch facilitates walking and is evaluated radiographically in lateral weight-bearing (erect) projections. Recumbent laterals would not demonstrate any structural change that occurs when the individual is erect. (*Ballinger & Frank, vol 1, p 256*)

18. **(A)** *Osteoblasts* are cells of mesodermal origin that are concerned with formation and repair of bone. *Osteoclasts* are cells concerned with the breakdown and resorption of old or dead bone. An *osteoma* is a benign bony tumor. An *osteon* is the microscopic unit of compact bone, consisting of a haversian canal and its surrounding lamellae. (*Bontrager, p 745*)

19. **(C)** The cassette for a cross-table lateral projection of the hip is placed in a *vertical* position. The top edge of the cassette should be placed directly above the iliac crest and adjacent to

the *lateral surface* of the affected hip. The cassette is positioned *parallel* to the femoral neck; the central ray is *perpendicular* to the femoral neck and cassette. (*Ballinger, vol 2, p 290*)

20. **(A)** The AP axial position projects the anterior structures (frontal and facial bones) downward, thus permitting visualization of the *occipital bone* without superimposition (Grashey/Towne method). The dorsum sella and posterior clinoid processes of the sphenoid bone should be visualized within the foramen magnum. This projection may also be obtained by angling the central ray 30° caudad to the OML (Fig. 2–40). The *frontal bone* is best shown with the patient PA and a perpendicular central ray. The parietoacanthial projection is the single best position for *facial bones. Basal foramina* are well demonstrated in the submentovertical projection. (*Ballinger & Frank, vol 2, p 270*)

21. **(B)** Patients who are able to cooperate are usually able to control *voluntary* motion if they are provided with an adequate explanation of

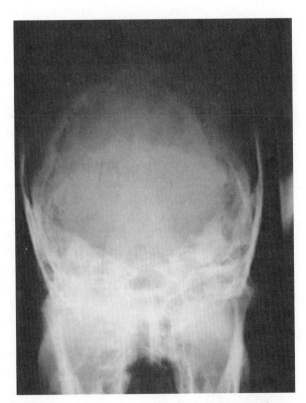

Figure 2–40. Courtesy of Stamford Hospital, Department of Radiology.

the procedure. Once patients understand what is needed, most will cooperate to the best of their ability (by suspending respiration and holding still for the exposure). Certain body functions and responses, such as heart action, peristalsis, pain, and muscle spasm, cause *involuntary* motion that is uncontrollable by the patient. The best and only way to control involuntary motion is by always selecting the shortest possible exposure time. Involuntary motion may also be minimized by careful explanation, immobilization, and (as a last resort and only in certain cases) restraint. (*Ballinger & Frank, vol 1, pp 12–13*)

22. **(C)** The radiograph is a *lateral oblique* (external rotation) projection of the elbow, *removing the proximal radius from superimposition with the ulna* and demonstrating its articulation with the ulna at the radial notch, that is, the proximal radioulnar articulation. An *AP* projection of the elbow would demonstrate partial overlap of the proximal radius and ulna. A *medial oblique* would demonstrate complete overlap of the proximal radius and ulna; this position is used to demonstrate the coronoid process in profile and the olecranon process within the olecranon fossa. (*Ballinger & Frank, vol 1, p 135*)

23. **(A)** Because the sternum and vertebrae would be superimposed in a direct PA or AP projection, a slight oblique (just enough to separate the sternum from superimposition on the vertebrae) is used instead of a direct frontal projection. In the RAO position, the heart superimposes a homogeneous density over the sternum, thereby providing clearer radiographic visualization of its bony structure. If the *LAO* position were used to project the sternum to the *right* of the thoracic vertebrae, the posterior ribs and pulmonary markings would cast confusing shadows over the sternum because of their differing densities. The *lateral* projection requires that the shoulders be rolled back sufficiently to project the sternum completely anterior to the ribs. Prominent pulmonary vascular markings can be obliterated using a "breathing technique," that is, using an exposure time long enough (with appropriately low milliamperage) to equal at least a few respirations. (*Ballinger & Frank, vol 1, pp 476–477*)

24. **(A)** *Intervertebral joints* are well visualized in the lateral projection of all the vertebral groups. Cervical articular facets (forming *apophyseal joints*) are 90° to the midsagittal plane and are therefore well demonstrated in the *lateral* projection. The cervical *intervertebral foramina* lie 45° to the midsagittal plane (and 15° to 20° to a transverse plane) and are therefore demonstrated in the *oblique* position. *(Bontrager, p 294)*

25. **(A)** Because the *right* main bronchus is *wider and more vertical,* aspirated foreign bodies are more likely to enter it than the left main bronchus, which is narrower and angles more sharply from the trachea. An aspirated foreign body does not enter the esophagus or the stomach, as they are not respiratory structures, but rather digestive structures. *(Tortora & Derrickson, p 857)*

26. **(C)** One of the most important principles in chest radiography is that it be performed, whenever possible, in the erect position. It is in this position that the diaphragm can descend to its lowest position during inspiration, and any air–fluid levels can be detected. However, patients having traumatic injuries must frequently be examined in the supine position. An AP supine chest is performed first. If the examination is also being performed to rule out air–fluid levels, this can be determined by performing the *lateral projection in the dorsal decubitus position.* The patient is lying supine, and a *horizontal* ("cross-table") x-ray beam is used. *(Ballinger & Frank, Vol 2, p 16)*

27. **(C)** *Glucophage (metformin hydrochloride)* is used as an adjunct to appropriate diet to lower blood glucose level in patients who have type 2 diabetes and whose hyperglycemia is not being managed satisfactorily with diet alone. Patients on Glucophage who are having intravascular iodinated contrast studies can develop an acute alteration of renal function or acute acidosis. If you discover while taking patient history that your IVU patient takes Glucophage daily, you should still *continue* with the examination. In these patients, however, Glucophage should be *discontinued for 48 hours* subsequent to the procedure and continued again only after renal function

has been reevaluated and found to be normal. *(PDR, 55th ed, 2001)*

28. **(C)** The illustrated radiograph is a PA axial projection (Caldwell method) of the frontal and anterior ethmoidal sinuses. The frontal sinuses are seen centrally in the vertical plate of the frontal bone behind the glabella and extending laterally over the superciliary arches. The ethmoidal sinuses are seen adjacent and inferior to the medial aspect of the orbits. The patient is positioned with the *OML perpendicular to the IR* and the *CR* angled about 25° *caudally.* This angle projects the petrous pyramids at the lower rim of the orbits; superior orbital fissures are well demonstrated in this position. A caudal angle of 15° to 20° would project the petrous pyramids in the lower third of the orbits. In the PA position with chin extended (choice A) and OML 37° to the table (parietoacanthial projection, Waters' method), the petrous pyramids are projected below the maxillary sinuses. With the patient PA and the CR angled 25° cephalad (Haas method), the occipital bone and sella turcica are demonstrated. *(Ballinger & Frank, vol 2, pp 366–367)*

29. **(A)** The illustrated radiograph is a PA axial projection (Caldwell method) of the *frontal and anterior ethmoidal* sinuses. The frontal sinuses are seen centrally in the vertical plate of the frontal bone behind the glabella and extending laterally over the superciliary arches. The ethmoidal sinuses are seen adjacent and inferior to the medial aspect of the orbits. The patient is positioned with the OML perpendicular to the IR; the central ray should be angled 15° caudally to place the petrous pyramids in the lower third of the orbits (a little too much caudal angle was used here; the petrosae are projected to the inferior rim of the orbits). Projecting the petrous pyramids below the orbits is the objective of the parietocanthial projection (Waters' method). *(Ballinger & Frank, vol 2, pp 366–367)*

30. **(A)** A decubitus projection is obtained using a horizontal x-ray beam. The type of decubitus projection is dependent on the patient's recumbent position. When the patient is lying *AP recumbent,* the patient is said to be in the dorsal decubitus position. When the patient is

lying *prone*, he or she is in the ventral decubitus position. If the patient is lying in the *left or right lateral recumbent* position with the x-ray beam directed horizontally, the patient is said to be in the left or right lateral decubitus position, respectively. *(Bontrager, p 20)*

31. **(A)** Sternoclavicular articulations may be examined with the patient PA, either bilaterally with the patient's head resting on the chin or unilaterally with the patient's head turned toward the side being examined. The sternoclavicular articulations may also be examined in the oblique position, with either the patient rotated slightly or the central ray angled slightly medialward. Weight-bearing positions are frequently used for evaluation of acromioclavicular joints. *(Ballinger & Frank, vol 1, p 485)*

32. **(B)** Plaque deposited on arterial walls in cases of atherosclerosis causes arterial stenosis. *Percutaneous transluminal angioplasty* (PTA) is a procedure that uses a balloon catheter to permanently increase the size of the arterial lumen, thus reopening the vessel and restoring blood flow. A *percutaneous nephrolithotomy* is a procedure performed to remove a renal calculus from a kidney or proximal ureter. *Renal arteriography* is the radiologic investigation of the renal arteries. *Nephrostomy* is the surgical formation of an artificial opening into the kidney. *(Ballinger & Frank, vol 2, p 561)*

33. **(B)** When a patient's elbow needs to be examined in partial flexion, the lateral projection offers little difficulty, but the AP projection requires special attention. If the AP is made with a perpendicular central ray and the olecranon process resting on the tabletop, the articulating surfaces are obscured. With the elbow in partial flexion, *two exposures are necessary*. One is made with the forearm parallel to the IR (humerus elevated), which demonstrates the proximal forearm. The other is made with the humerus parallel to the IR (forearm elevated), which demonstrates the distal humerus. In both cases, the central ray is perpendicular if the degree of flexion is not too great, or angled slightly into the joint space with greater degrees of flexion. *(Ballinger & Frank, vol 1, pp 106–107)*

34. **(B)** Air or fluid levels will be clearly delineated only if the central ray is directed parallel to them. Therefore, to demonstrate air or fluid levels, the erect or decubitus position should be used. Small amounts of *fluid* within the pleural space are best demonstrated in the lateral decubitus position, *affected side down*. Small amounts of air within the pleural space are best demonstrated in the lateral decubitus position, *affected side up*. *(Ballinger & Frank, vol 1, p 476)*

35. **(C)** The relationship of these three structures can be appreciated in a lateral projection of the chest. The *heart* is seen in the anterior half of the thoracic cavity, with its apex extending inferior and anterior. The air-filled *trachea* can be seen in about the center of the chest, and the air-filled *esophagus* just posterior to the trachea (Fig. 2–41). *(Ballinger & Frank, vol 1, p 458)*

36. **(B)** The carpal scaphoid is somewhat curved and consequently foreshortened radiographically in the PA position. To better separate it

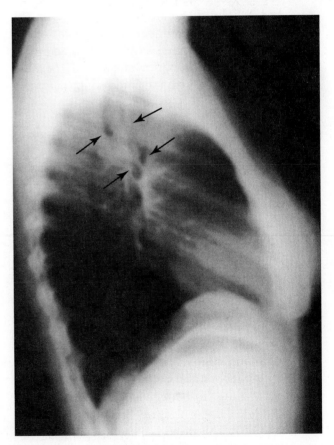

Figure 2–41. From the American College of Radiology Learning Files. Courtesy of the ACR.

from the adjacent carpals, the ulnar flexion (ulnar deviation) maneuver is frequently employed. In addition to correcting foreshortening of the scaphoid, ulnar flexion/deviation opens the interspaces between adjacent lateral carpals. Radial flexion/deviation is used to better demonstrate *medial* carpals. (*Ballinger & Frank, vol 1, p 118*)

37. **(D)** The fact that the distal tibiofibular articulation is visualized is evidence that this is a 45° medial (internal) oblique. A 15° to 20° oblique is performed for the ankle mortise (joint) and would demonstrate some superimposition of the distal tibia and fibula. In the AP ankle, there is some superimposition of the fibula over the tibia and talus, thereby obscuring the medial aspect of the ankle mortise. (*Ballinger & Frank, vol 1, p 279*)

38. **(A)** The ankle mortise is formed by the distal tibia and fibula and the talus. The distal tibia (the medial and larger bone) forms a club-shaped projection, the *medial malleolus* (number 2). The distal fibula's projection is the *lateral malleolus* (number 1). The distal articular surfaces of both the tibia and fibula articulate with the superior surface of the *talus* (number 3) to form the ankle joint. (*Bontrager, p 201*)

39. **(B)** A *lateral* projection of the lumbar spine is illustrated. The *intervertebral joints* (disk spaces) are well demonstrated. Because the *intervertebral foramina*, which are formed by the *pedicles*, are 90° to the MSP, they are also well demonstrated in the lateral projection. The *articular facets*, forming the apophyseal joints, lie 30° to 50° to the MSP and therefore are visualized in the *oblique* position. (*Ballinger & Frank, vol 1, pp 230–231*)

40. **(C)** The straight PA (0°) projection effectively demonstrates the mandibular body, but the rami and condyles are superimposed on the occipital bone and petrous portion of the temporal bone. To better visualize the rami and condyles, the central ray is directed cephalad 20° to 30°. This projects the temporal and occipital bones above the area of interest. (*Ballinger & Frank, vol 2, p 341*)

41. **(A)** A diagnostic image of C1–2 depends on adjusting the flexion of the neck *so that the maxillary occlusal plane and the base of the skull are superimposed.* Accurate adjustment of these structures will usually allow good visualization of the odontoid process and the atlantoaxial articulation. Should patient anatomy occasionally prevent the usual visualization, the odontoid process can be visualized through the foramen magnum, either AP or PA. In the AP position (Fuchs method), or the PA position (Judd method), the patient's chin is extended to be in line vertically with the mastoid tip (similar to a Water's or reverse Water's position). The CR is directed to the midline and perpendicularly at the level of the mastoid tip. The resulting image demonstrates the odontoid process through the foramen magnum. These positions should not be attempted if the patient has suspected, new, or healing fracture, or destructive disease. (*Ballinger & Frank, vol 1, pp 413, 416*)

42. **(B)** Sacroiliac joints lie obliquely within the pelvis and open anteriorly at an angle of 25° to 30° to the midsagittal plane. A 25° to 30° oblique position places the joints perpendicular to the IR. The left sacroiliac joint may be demonstrated in the LAO and RPO positions with little magnification variation. (*Ballinger & Frank, vol 1, p 327*)

43. **(C)** The lateral hand in extension, with appropriate technique adjustment, is recommended to evaluate foreign body location in soft tissue. A small lead marker is frequently taped to the spot thought to be the point of entry. The physician then uses this external marker and the radiograph to determine the exact foreign body location. Extension of the hand in the presence of a fracture would cause additional and unnecessary pain, and possibly additional injury. (*Ballinger & Frank, vol 1, p 79*)

44–45. **(44, C; 45, A)** The pictured radiograph is an oblique position of the large bowel, illustrating an "open" view of the hepatic/right colic flexure and ascending colon, with the splenic/left colic flexure superimposed on the descending colon. Therefore, the radiograph must have been made in either an *RAO* (if the patient was prone) or an *LPO* (if the patient was supine) position. The LAO and RPO positions are used to demonstrate the splenic flexure and descending colon free of self-superimposition. AP or PA axial is generally used to visualize the rectosigmoid colon. (*Ballinger & Frank, vol 2, p 146*)

46. **(B)** To increase the concentration of contrast media in the deep veins of the leg, a Fowler's position is used with the x-ray table angled at least 45°. Tourniquets can also be used to force the contrast into the deep veins of the leg, especially when the patient is examined in the recumbent position. Contrast medium is injected through a superficial vein in the foot. Imaging may be performed with or without fluoroscopy, and may include AP, lateral, and 30° obliques of the lower leg in internal rotation. Imaging begins at the ankle and proceeds superiorly, usually including the inferior vena cava. (*Ballinger & Frank, vol 2, p 542*)

47. **(D)** The "scapular Y" refers to the characteristic Y formed by the humerus, acromion, and coracoid processes. The patient is positioned in a PA oblique position—an RAO or LAO, depending on which is the affected side. The midcoronal plane is adjusted approximately 60° to the IR, and the affected arm remains relaxed at the patient's side. The scapular Y position is employed *to demonstrate anterior (subcoracoid) or posterior (subacromial) humeral dislocation*. The humerus is normally superimposed on the scapula in this position; any deviation from this may indicate dislocation. (*Ballinger & Frank, vol 1, pp 179–181*)

48. **(B)** The AP projection provides a general survey of the abdomen, showing the size and shape of the liver, spleen, and kidneys. When performed erect, it should demonstrate both hemidiaphragms. The lateral projection is sometimes requested and is useful for evaluating the prevertebral space occupied by the aorta. Ventral and dorsal decubitus positions provide a lateral view of the abdomen that is useful for demonstration of air–fluid levels. (*Ballinger & Frank, vol 1, p 38*)

49. **(C)** The axillary portion of the ribs is best demonstrated in a 45° oblique position. The axillary ribs are demonstrated in the AP oblique projection with the affected side *adjacent to* the IR, and in the PA oblique projection with the affected side *away from* the IR. Therefore, the right axillary ribs would be demonstrated in the RPO (AP oblique with affected side *adjacent to* the IR) and LAO (PA oblique with affected side *away from* the IR) positions. (*Ballinger & Frank, vol 1, pp 428–431*)

50. **(B)** To best demonstrate *most* of the tarsals and intertarsal spaces (including the cuboid, sinus tarsi, and tuberosity of the fifth metatarsal), a *medial oblique* is required (plantar surface and IR form a 30° angle). The *lateral oblique* demonstrates the interspaces between the first and second metatarsals and between the first and second cuneiforms. *Weight-bearing lateral* feet are used to demonstrate the longitudinal arches. (*Ballinger & Frank, vol 1, p 261*)

51. **(B)** Surface landmarks, prominences, and depressions are very useful to the radiographer in locating anatomic structures that are not visible externally. The fifth thoracic vertebra is at approximately the same level as the sternal angle. The T2–3 interspace is about at the same level as the manubrial (suprasternal) notch. The costal margin is about the same level as L3. (*Saia, p 74*)

52. **(C)** The position, shape, and motility of various organs can differ greatly from one body habitus to another. The *hypersthenic* individual is large and heavy; the lungs and heart are high, the stomach is high and transverse, the gallbladder is high and lateral, and the colon is high and peripheral. In contrast, the other habitus extreme is the *asthenic* individual. This patient is slender and light, and has a long and narrow thorax, a low and long stomach, a low and medial gallbladder, and a low medial and redundant colon. The radiographer must consider these characteristic differences when radiographing individuals of various body types. (*Ballinger & Frank, vol 1, p 72*)

53. **(A)** Esophageal varices are tortuous dilatations of the esophageal veins. They are much less pronounced in the erect position and must always be examined with the patient recumbent.

The recumbent position affords more complete filling of the veins, as blood flows against gravity. *(Ballinger & Frank, vol 2, p 88)*

54. (D) To evaluate sufficient inspiration and lung expansion, 10 posterior ribs should be visualized. The sternoclavicular joints should be symmetrical; any loss of symmetry indicates rotation. To visualize maximum lung area, the shoulders are rolled forward to move the scapulae laterally from the lung fields. *(Ballinger & Frank, vol 1, p 527)*

55. (C) To accurately position a lateral forearm, the elbow must form a 90° angle with the humeral epicondyles superimposed. The radius and ulna are superimposed only *distally.* Proximally, the coronoid process and radial head are superimposed, and the radial head faces anteriorly. Failure of the elbow to form a 90° angle or the hand to be lateral results in a less than satisfactory lateral projection of the forearm. *(Saia, p 95)*

56. (C) The distal *femur* is associated with two large condyles; the deep depression separating them is the intercondyloid fossa (Fig. 2–42). The proximal *tibia* has two condyles; their superior surfaces are smooth, forming the tibial plateau. The *mandible* has a condyle that articulates with the mandibular fossa of the temporal bone, forming the temporomandibular joint. The *fibula* has a proximal styloid process and a distal malleolus, but no condyle. *(Tortora & Derrickson, p 249)*

57. (C) To best demonstrate the distal tibiofibular articulation, a *45° medial oblique* projection of

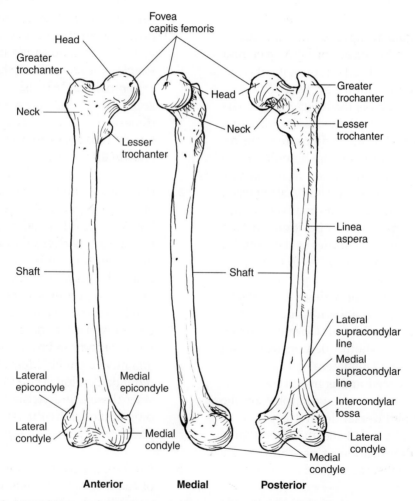

Figure 2–42. Reproduced with permission from Saia DA. *Radiography: Program Review and Examination Preparation*, 2nd ed. Stamford, CT: Appleton & Lange, 1999.

the ankle is required. The *15° medial oblique* is used to demonstrate the ankle mortise (joint). Although the joint is well demonstrated in the 15° medial oblique, there is some superimposition of the distal tibia and fibula, and greater obliquity is required to separate the bones. *(Ballinger & Frank, vol 1, pp 279–280)*

58. **(A)** When the pelvis is observed in the anatomic position, the ilia are seen to oblique forward, giving the pelvis a "basin-like" appearance. To view the *right* iliac bone, the radiographer must place it parallel to the IR by elevating the left side about 40° (RPO). The *left* iliac bone is radiographed in the 40° LPO oblique position. *(Ballinger & Frank, vol 1, p 308)*

59. **(B)** Superimposition of bony details frequently makes angiographic demonstration of blood vessels less than optimal. The method used to remove these superimposed bony details is called *subtraction. Digital subtraction angiography (DSA)* accomplishes this through a computer. The advantages of DSA over film angiography include greater sensitivity to contrast medium, immediate availability of images, and lower total cost. Although DSA applications are increasing, film angiography may be preferred in cases in which resolution is critical. *(Ballinger & Frank, vol 3, p 178)*

60. **(B)** The upper GI tract must be empty for best x-ray evaluation. Any food or liquid that mixes with the barium sulfate suspension can simulate pathology. Preparation therefore is to withhold food and fluids for 8 to 9 hours before the examination, typically after midnight, as fasting examinations are usually performed first thing in the morning. Enemas until clear prior to the examination is a part of the typical preparation for barium enema/air contrast. *(Bontrager, p 466)*

61. **(C)** An *erect* abdomen or *left lateral decubitus* should be performed for demonstration of air–fluid levels in the abdomen. The *right lateral decubitus* position is used to demonstrate the layering of gallstones. It will not show free air within the peritoneum because of the overlying gastric bubble on the elevated left side of the body. *(Bontrager, pp 107, 111)*

62. **(C)** The AP axial projection (Grashey method) of the skull requires that the central ray be angled 30° caudad if the OML is perpendicular to the image receptor (37° caudad if the IOML is perpendicular to the image receptor). The frontal and facial bones are projected down and away from superimposition on the occipital bone. If positioning is accurate, the *dorsum sella* and *posterior clinoid processes* will be demonstrated within the foramen magnum. If the central ray is angled excessively, the *posterior aspect of the arch of C1* will appear in the foramen magnum. *(Ballinger & Frank, vol 2, p 246)*

63. **(D)** The greater and lesser tubercles are prominences on the proximal humerus separated by the intertubercular (bicipital) groove. The AP projection of the humerus/shoulder places the *epicondyles parallel to the IR* and the shoulder in *external rotation*, and demonstrates the *greater tubercle in profile*. The lateral projection of the humerus places the shoulder in extreme internal rotation with the epicondyles perpendicular to the IR and demonstrates the lesser tubercle in profile. *(Ballinger & Frank, vol 1, pp 161–162)*

64. **(D)** Barium can dry and harden in the large bowel, causing symptoms ranging from mild constipation to bowel obstruction. It is therefore essential that the radiographer provide clear instructions, especially to outpatients, for follow-up care, along with the rationale for this care. To avoid the possibility of fecal impaction, patients should drink plenty of fluids for the next few days, increase their dietary fiber, and take a mild laxative such as milk of magnesia. *(Torres et al, p 233)*

65. **(D)** When the clavicle is examined in the PA recumbent position, the central ray must be directed 15° to 30° caudad to project most of the clavicle's length above the ribs. The direction of the central ray is reversed when examining the patient in the AP position. *(Bontrager, p 188)*

66. **(C)** When a cervical spine is requested to rule out subluxation or fracture, the patient will arrive in the radiology area on a stretcher. The patient should *not* be moved before a subluxation

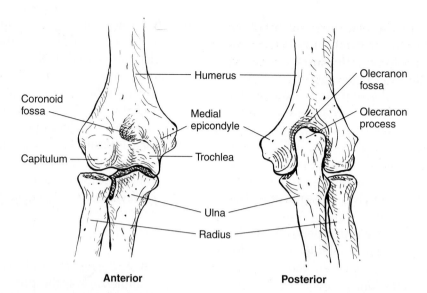

Figure 2–43. Reproduced with permission from Lindner HH. *Clinical Anatomy.* East Norwalk, CT: Appleton & Lange, 1989.

is ruled out. Any movement of the head and neck could cause serious damage to the spinal cord. A horizontal beam lateral is performed and evaluated. The physician will then decide what further images are required. *(Ballinger & Frank, vol 1, p 350)*

67. (D) The distal humerus articulates with the proximal radius and ulna to form the elbow joint. Specifically, the *semilunar/trochlear notch* of the proximal ulna articulates with the *trochlea* of the distal medial humerus. The *capitulum* is lateral to the trochlea and articulates with the *radial head* (Fig. 2–43). *(Ballinger & Frank, vol 1, p 90)*

68. (C) A lateral projection is generally included in a routine skull series. The patient is placed in a PA oblique position. The *MSP* is positioned parallel to the IR, and the *IOML* is adjusted so as to be parallel to the long axis of the cassette. The *interpupillary line* must be perpendicular to the IR. In a routine lateral projection of the skull, the central ray should enter approximately 2 inches superior to the EAM. *(Ballinger & Frank, vol 2, p 326)*

69. (B) The CNS (brain and spinal cord) is located within three protective membranes, the *meninges.* The inner membrane is the *pia mater,* the middle membrane is the *arachnoid,* and the outer membrane is the *dura mater.* The *sub-*

arachnoid space is located between the pia and arachnoid mater and contains cerebrospinal fluid (CSF). During myelography, the needle is introduced into the subarachnoid space (L3-4 or L4-5), a small amount of CSF is removed, and the contrast medium is introduced (Fig. 2–44). The *subdural space* is located between the arachnoid and dura mater. The *epidural space* is located between the two layers of the dura mater. *(Saia, pp 197–198)*

70. (D) Typically, traumatic injury to the hip requires a cross-table (axiolateral) lateral projection. Occasionally, this projection may be contraindicated, for example, a patient with suspected bilateral hip fractures, or one who

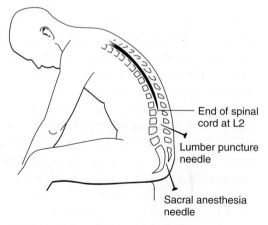

Figure 2–44. Reproduced with permission from deGroot, Correlative Neuroanatomy, 21st ed. Norwalk, CT: Appleton & Lange, 1991.

is unable to move the *un*affected hip out of the way as required by the axiolateral. In these instances, the axiolateral inferosuperior trauma projection (Clements–Nakayama method)can be employed. The patients is recumbent, lateral surface of affected side close to table/stretcher edge. The CR is directed almost horizontally to the affected femoral neck (inferosuperior), with a 15° posterior angulation. Correct placement and angulation of the grid cassette is essential to avoid grid cutoff. *(Ballinger & Frank, vol 1, p 372)*

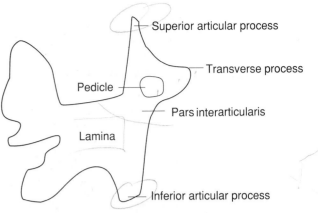

Figure 2–45.

71. **(D)** A right "scapular Y" is illustrated; this refers to the characteristic Y formed by the humerus, acromion, and coracoid. The patient is positioned in a PA oblique position—in this case, an RAO to demonstrate the right side. The midcoronal plane is adjusted to approximately 60° to the IR, and the affected arm is left relaxed at the patient's side. The scapular Y position is employed *to demonstrate anterior or posterior humeral dislocation*. The humerus is normally superimposed on the scapula in this position; any deviation from this may indicate dislocation. *(Ballinger & Frank, vol 1, pp 179–181)*

72. **(B)** Synovial pivot joints are diarthrotic, that is, freely movable. Pivot joints permit rotation motion. Examples include the proximal radioulnar joint that permits supination and pronation of the hand. The atlantoaxial joint is the articulation between C1 and C2 and permits rotation of the head. The temporomandibular joint is diarthrotic, having both hinge and plamar movements. *(Tortora & Derrickson, p 269)*

73. **(D)** The *45° oblique position* of the lumbar spine is generally performed for demonstration of the *apophyseal joints*. In a correctly positioned oblique lumbar spine, "scotty dog" images are demonstrated (Figs. 2–45 and 2–46). The scotty's ear corresponds to the superior articular process, his nose to the transverse process, his eye to the pedicle, his neck to the pars interarticularis, his body to the lamina, and his front foot to the inferior articular process. *(Saia, p 131)*

74. **(D)** In the *AP* projection of the elbow, the proximal radius and ulna are partially super-

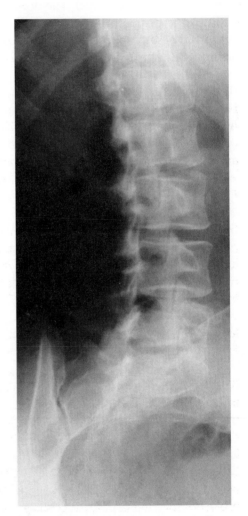

Figure 2–46. Courtesy of Stamford Hospital, Department of Radiology.

imposed. In the *lateral* position, the radial head is partially superimposed on the coronoid process, facing anteriorly. In the *medial oblique* position, there is even greater superimposition. The *lateral oblique* projection completely separates the proximal radius and ulna, projecting the radial head, neck, and tuberosity free of superimposition with the proximal ulna. (*Ballinger & Frank, vol 1, p 105*)

75. **(B)** The tangential projection projects the sesamoid bones separate from adjacent structures. The patient is best examined in the prone position, as this places the parts of interest closest to the IR. The affected foot is dorsiflexed so as to place its plantar surface 15° to 20° with the vertical. The CR is directed perpendicular to the posterior surface of the foot (near the metatarsophalangeal joints). The dorsoplantar and oblique positions of the foot will demonstrate the sesamoid bones superimposed on adjacent bony structures. (*Bontrager, p 217*)

76. **(D)** The tangential axial projections of the patella are also often referred to as "*sunrise*" or "*skyline*" views. The supine flexion 45° (Merchant) position requires a special apparatus, and the patellae can be examined bilaterally.

This position also requires patient comfort without muscle tension—muscle tension can cause a subluxed patella to be pulled into the intercondyler sulcus, giving the appearance of a normal patella. The two prone positions differ according to the degree of flexion employed. The 90° flexion (Settegast) position must not be employed with suspected patellar fracture. (*Bontrager, pp 240, 241*)

77. **(C)** For the PA projection of the skull, the OML is adjusted perpendicular to the IR, and the MSP must be perpendicular to the IR. The central ray is directed so as to exit the nasion. In this position, the petrous pyramids should completely *fill* the orbits. When caudal angulation is used with this position, the petrous pyramids are projected in the *lower portion*, or out of, the orbits. If cephalad angulation is employed with this position, the petrous pyramids are projected up toward the occipital region (as in the nuchofrontal projection). (*Ballinger & Frank, vol 2, p 242*)

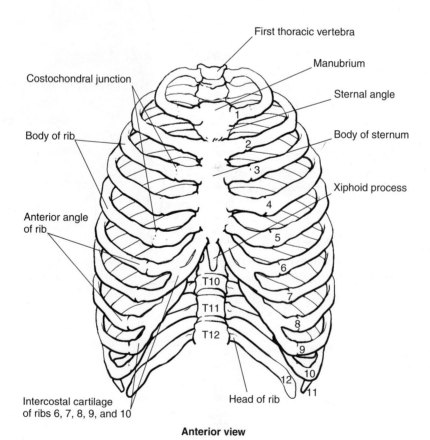

Anterior view

Figure 2–47. Reproduced with permission from Saia DA. *Radiography: Program Review and Examination Preparation*, 2nd ed. Stamford, CT: Appleton & Lange, 1999.

78. (C) The bony thorax consists of *12 pairs of ribs* and the structures to which they are attached anteriorly and posteriorly: the *sternum* and the *thoracic vertebrae* (Fig. 2–47). These structures form a bony cage that surrounds and protects the vital organs within (the heart, lungs, and great vessels). The scapulae, together with the clavicles, form the shoulder (pectoral) girdle of the upper extremity. *(Bontrager, p 336)*

79. (D) Venous blood is returned to the right atrium via the superior (from the upper body) and inferior (from the lower body) vena cava (Fig. 2–48). *During atrial systole, blood passes through the tricuspid valve into the right ventricle.* During ventricular systole, the pulmonary artery (the only artery to carry deoxygenated blood) carries blood to the lungs for oxygenation. Blood is returned via the pulmonary veins (the only veins to carry oxygenated blood) to the left atrium. *During atrial systole,* *blood passes through the mitral (bicuspid) valve into the left ventricle.* During ventricular systole, oxygenated blood is pumped through the aortic semilunar valve into the aorta. *(Tortora & Derrickson, p 718)*

80. (D) A PA projection of the chest is pictured. Adequate *inspiration* is demonstrated by visualization of 10 posterior ribs above the diaphragm. The shoulders are rolled forward, removing the scapulae from the lung fields. *Rotation* of the chest is demonstrated by unequal distance between the sternum and medial extremities of the clavicles. *Pulmonary apices* and *costophrenic angles* are demonstrated adequately. An *air-filled* trachea is seen in the lower cervical and upper thoracic region as a midline area of increased density. Adequate *long scale contrast* has been achieved, as indicated by visualization of pulmonary vascular markings. *(Bontrager, p 75)*

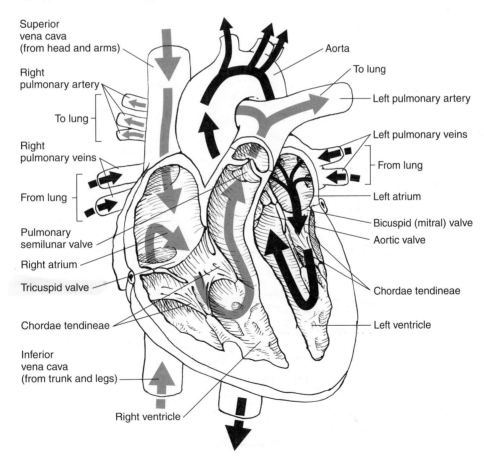

Figure 2–48. Reproduced with permission from Saia DA. *Radiography: Program Review and Examination Preparation*, 2nd ed. Stamford, CT: Appleton & Lange, 1999.

81. (A) A PA projection of the chest is pictured. Adequate *inspiration* is demonstrated by visualization of 10 posterior ribs above the diaphragm. *Rotation* of the chest is demonstrated by asymmetric sternoclavicular joints. The apices and costophrenic angles should be included on every chest radiograph. The letter *A* indicates a left posterior rib, *B* represents a left anterior rib, and *C* represents the right costophrenic angle. *(Ballinger & Frank, vol 1, pp 525–526)*

82. (C) The axial trauma lateral (Coyle) is described. If routine elbow projections in extension are not possible because of limited part movement, this position can be used to demonstrate the coronoid process and/or radial head. With the elbow flexed *90°* and the CR directed to the elbow joint at an angle of *45°* medially (ie, toward the shoulder), the joint space between the *radial head* and capitulum should be revealed. With the elbow flexed *80°* and the CR directed to the elbow joint at an angle of 45° laterally (ie, from the shoulder toward the elbow), the elongated *coronoid process* will be visualized. *(Bontrager, p 160)*

83. (B) The carpal scaphoid is a curved, boat-shaped, bone, and is therefore superimposed on itself ("self-superimposition") in a routine PA projection. Since the scaphoid is the most frequently fractured carpal, special projections have been developed to help overcome self-superimposition. Stecher (in 1937) recommended elevating the hand and wrist 20° and using a perpendicular CR directed to the scaphoid. Effective variations of this position include employing ulnar deviation and angling the CR 20° *proximally* (toward the elbow). The 20° tube angulation would be used in place of the elevated hand/wrist. *(Bontrager, pp 147–149)*

84. (C) The thoracic *apophyseal joints* are 70° to the midsagittal plane and are demonstrated in a steep (70°) oblique position. The thoracic *intervertebral foramina*, formed by the vertebral notches of the pedicles, are 90° to the MSP. They are therefore well demonstrated in the lateral position. The *intervertebral foramina* of the thoracic and lumbar vertebrae are also demon-

strated in the lateral position. *(Ballinger & Frank, vol 1, p 361)*

85. (A) The dome of the acetabulum lies midway between the ASIS and the symphysis pubis. On an adult of average size, a line perpendicular to this point will parallel the plane of the femoral neck. In an AP projection of the hip, the central ray should be directed to a point approximately 2 inches down that perpendicular line, so as to enter the distal portion of the femoral head. *(Ballinger & Frank, vol 1, pp 274, 286)*

86–87. (86, B; 87, B) Figure 2–12 illustrates an anatomic lateral view of the paranasal sinuses. Number 1 points to the *frontal* sinuses and number 2 to the *ethmoidal* sinuses; both can be visualized using the PA axial projection (Caldwell method). Number 3 is the *sphenoidal* sinuses, which are well demonstrated in the SMV projection. Number 4 is the *maxillary* sinuses, which are best demonstrated using the parietoacanthial projection (Waters' method). The lateral projection demonstrates the four pairs of paranasal sinuses superimposed on each other. *(Bontrager, pp 416–418)*

88. (C) With inspiration, the diaphragm moves inferiorly and depresses the abdominal viscera. The ribs and sternum are elevated. As the ribs are elevated, their angle is decreased. Radiographic density can vary considerably in appearance depending on the phase of respiration during which the exposure is made. *(Bontrager, p 74)*

89. (C) The illustrated radiograph is that of a *medial oblique foot*. With the foot rotated medially, so that the plantar surface forms a *30°* oblique with the image receptor, the *sinus tarsi*, the *tuberosity* of the fifth metatarsal, and several articulations should be demonstrated: the *articulations* between the talus and the navicular, between the calcaneus and the cuboid, between the cuboid and the bases of the fourth and fifth metarsals, and between the cuboid and the lateral (third) cuneiform. *(Ballinger & Frank, vol 1, pp 244–245)*

90. (B) Figure 2–14 shows a PA projection of the mandible. The head is positioned PA with the

OML perpendicular to the IR. The mandibular body is well demonstrated in this position. With the patient in the PA position, the rami can be better demonstrated with 20° to 25° cephalad angulation. A caudal angle could be employed if the skull was positioned in the AP position. *(Ballinger & Frank, vol 2, p 382)*

91. **(C)** When the elbow is placed in acute flexion with the posterior aspect of the humerus adjacent to the image receptor and a perpendicular CR is used, the olecranon process of the ulna is seen in profile. The coronoid process is best visualized in the medial oblique position. The coracoid and glenoid are associated with the scapula. *(Ballinger & Frank, vol 1, p 138)*

92. **(B)** Chest positioning must be correct and accurate; thoracic structures are easily distorted. To avoid *superimposition on the upper medial apices*, the patients chin should be sufficiently elevated. Movement of the diaphragm to its lowest position is a function of the erect position and of making the exposure after the second inspiration. The MSP is perpendicular to the IR in the PA projection and parallel to the IR in the lateral projection. The position of the chin has little to do with the MSP. *(Bontrager, p 75)*

93. **(A)** Long bones are composed of a shaft, or diaphysis, and two extremities. The *diaphysis* is referred to as the *primary ossification center*. In the growing bone, the cartilaginous *epiphyseal plate* (located at the extremities of long bones) is gradually replaced by bone. For this reason, the epiphyses are referred to as the secondary ossification centers. The ossified growth area of long bones is the *metaphysis*. *Apophysis* refers to vertebral joints formed by articulation of superjacent articular facets. *(Bontrager, p 9)*

94. **(B)** To reduce anxiety prior to the examination, the radiographer should give the patient a full explanation of the enema procedure. This explanation should include keeping the anal sphincter tightly contracted, relaxing the abdominal muscles, and deep breathing. The barium suspension should be either just below body temperature (at 85° to 90°F) to prevent injury and bowel irritation *or* cold (at 41°F) to pro-

duce less colonic irritation and to stimulate contraction of the anal sphincter. *(Bontrager, p 497)*

95. **(A)** The 45° oblique position of the lumbar spine is generally performed for demonstration of the apophyseal joints. In a correctly positioned oblique lumbar spine, "scotty dog" images are demonstrated. The scotty's ear corresponds to the superior articular process, his nose to the transverse process, his eye to the pedicle, his neck to the pars interarticularis, his body to the lamina, and his front foot to the inferior articular process (Fig. 2–49). *(Saia, p 131)*

96. **(C)** The illustration shows the patient positioned on his left side, with the cassette behind his back. This is a *left lateral decubitus* position. The x-ray beam is directed horizontally in decubitus positions to demonstrate air–fluid levels. Air or fluid levels will be clearly delineated only if the central ray is directed parallel to them. If the patient were lying on the right side, it would be a *right lateral decubitus* position. If the patient were lying on his or her back with a horizontal x-ray beam, it would be a *dorsal decubitus* position. Lying prone with a horizontal x-ray beam is termed a *ventral decubitus* position. *(Bontager, p 20)*

97. **(A)** The medial oblique projection requires that the leg be rotated medially until the plantar surface of the foot forms a 30° angle with the cassette. This position demonstrates the navicular with minimal bony superimposition. The lateral oblique projection of the foot superimposes much of the navicular on the cuboid. The navicular is also superimposed on the

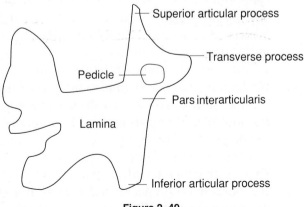

Figure 2–49.

cuboid in the lateral projections. *(Ballinger & Frank, p 245)*

98. **(D)** The common carotid arteries function to supply oxygenated blood to the head and neck. Major branches of the common carotid arteries (internal carotids) function to supply the anterior brain, while the posterior brain is supplied by the vertebral arteries (branches of the subclavian). The carotid arteries bifurcate into internal and external carotid arteries at the level of C4. The foramen magnum and pharynx are superior to the level of bifurcation, and the larynx is inferior to the level of bifurcation. *(Ballinger & Frank, vol 2, p 15)*

99. **(D)** With the patient in the erect position, barium moves inferiorly and air rises to provide double-contrast visualization of the hepatic and splenic flexures. The LAO and RPO positions are used to demonstrate especially the hepatic flexure; the splenic flexure generally appears self-superimposed in this position. A left lateral decubitus position will demonstrate a double-contrast visualization of right-sided bowel structures—that is, the right side of the ascending colon, the right side of the sigmoid and rectum, and so on. The lateral position offers a singularly valuable view of the rectum. *(Ballinger & Frank, vol 2, p 146)*

100–101. **(100, A; 101, C)** Figure 2–16 illustrates the *biliary system.* Bile leaves the liver through the right and left *hepatic ducts* (number 5), which join to form the *common hepatic duct* (number 6). Bile enters the gallbladder through the *cystic duct* (number 7). The *neck* of the gallbladder is indicated by the number 4, its *body* by the number 3, and its *fundus* by the number 2. The gallbladder stores and concentrates bile, and when it contracts, bile flows out through the cystic duct and down the *common bile duct* (number 8). The common bile duct and *pancreatic duct* (number 9) unite to form the short *hepatopancreatic ampulla* (of Vater), which empties into the *duodenum* (number 1). *(Tortora & Derrickson, p 917)*

102. **(B)** The fingers must be supported parallel to the IR (eg, on a "finger sponge") in order that the joint spaces parallel the x-ray beam. When

the fingers are flexed or resting on the cassette, the relationship between the joint spaces and the IR changes, and the joints appear "closed." *(Ballinger & Frank, vol 1, pp 76–77)*

103. **(C)** Hysterosalpingography involves the introduction of a radiopaque contrast medium through a uterine cannula into the uterus and uterine (Fallopian) tubes. This examination is often performed to document patency of the uterine tubes in cases of infertility. A retrograde pyelogram requires cystoscopy and involves introduction of contrast through the vesicoureteral orifices and into the renal collecting system. A voiding cystourethrogram also requires cystoscopy and involves filling the bladder with contrast and documenting the voiding mechanism. A myelogram is performed to investigate the spinal canal. *(Ballinger & Frank, vol 2, p 199)*

104. **(C)** Perhaps the most important prerequisite to a successful BE examination is a thoroughly clean large bowel. Any retained fecal material can simulate pathology. A single-contrast examination demonstrates the anatomy and contour of the large bowel, as well as anything that may project out from the bowel wall (eg, diverticula). In a double-contrast examination, the bowel wall is coated with barium and then the lumen filled with air. This enables visualization of any intraluminal lesions such as polyps and tumor masses. *(Bontrager, p 493)*

105. **(D)** To better visualize the joint space in the lateral projection of the knee, 20° to 30° flexion is recommended. The femoral condyles are superimposed so as to demonstrate the patellofemoral joint and the articulation between the femur and the tibia. The correct degree of forward or backward body rotation is responsible for visualization of the patellofemoral joint. Cephalad tube angulation of 5° to 7° is responsible for demonstrating the articulation between the femur and the tibia (by removing the magnified medial femoral condyle from superimposition on the joint space). *(Ballinger & Frank, p 293)*

106. **(A)** When the shoulders are relaxed, the clavicles are usually carried below the pulmonary

apices. To examine the portions of the lungs lying behind the clavicles, the central ray is directed cephalad 15° to 20° to project the clavicles above the apices when the patient is examined in the AP position. *(Ballinger & Frank, vol 1, p 472)*

107. **(C)** The inferosuperior axial (nontrauma, Lawrence method) projection of the shoulder demonstrates the glenohumeral joint and adjacent structures. The patient is supine with arm abducted 90°, and in *external rotation*. The (horizontal) CR is directed medially 25° to 30° through the axilla. The *coracoid process and lesser tubercle* are seen in profile. *(Bontrager, p 179)*

108. **(D)** Double-contrast studies of the stomach or large intestine involve coating the organ with a thin layer of barium sulfate, then introducing air. This permits seeing through the organ to structures behind it and, most especially, allows visualization of the *mucosal lining* of the organ. A barium-filled stomach or large bowel demonstrates the position, size, and shape of the organ and any lesion that projects *out* from its walls, such as diverticula. Polypoid lesions, which project *inward* from the wall of an organ, may go unnoticed unless a double-contrast examination is performed. *(Ballinger & Frank, vol 2, p 104)*

109. **(A)** Sternoclavicular joints should be performed PA whenever possible to keep the object-to-image receptor distance (OID) to a minimum. The *oblique* position (about 15°) opens the joint *closest* to the image receptor. The erect position may be used, but is not required. Weight-bearing images are not recommended for sternoclavicular joints as they often are for acromioclavicular joints. *(Ballinger & Frank, vol 1, p 485)*

110. **(A)** An *RPO* position is illustrated. The oblique IVU projections should be approximately *30°*; this position significantly changes the position of the kidneys. When the abdomen is obliqued, the kidney of the *"down"* side is *perpendicular* to the IR; the kidney of the *"up"* side is *parallel* to the IR. *(Ballinger & Frank, vol 2, p 218)*

111. **(D)** Operative cholangiography plays a vital role in biliary tract surgery. The contrast medium is injected, and imaging occurs *following* a cholecystectomy. This procedure is used to investigate the patency of the bile ducts, the function of the hepatopancreatic sphincter (of Oddi), and previously undetected biliary tract calculi. *(Ballinger & Frank, vol 2, p 76)*

112. **(C)** The PA axial projection (Camp–Coventry method) of the *intercondyloid fossa ("tunnel view")* is pictured. The knee is flexed about 40°, and the central ray is directed caudally 40° and perpendicular to the tibia (Fig. 2–50). The patella and patellofemoral articulation are demonstrated in the axial/tangential view of the patella. *(Saia, pp 112–113)*

113. **(C)** The parietoacanthial projection (Waters' method) demonstrates a distorted view of the frontal and ethmoidal sinuses. The *maxillary sinuses* (number 4) are well demonstrated, projected free of the petrous pyramids. This is also the best single position for the demonstration of *facial bones*. The *mandibular angle* is illustrated by the number 1, the *zygomatic arch* by 2, and the *coronoid process* by 3. *(Bontrager, p 430)*

114. **(C)** *Diarthrotic*, or synovial, joints, such as the knee and the TMJ, are freely movable. Most diarthrotic joints are associated with a joint capsule containing synovial fluid. Diarthrotic joints are the most numerous in the body and

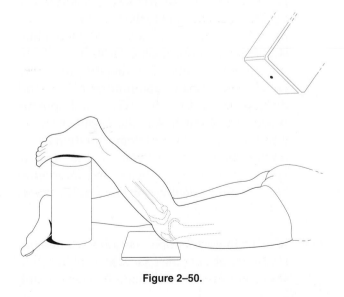

Figure 2–50.

are subdivided according to *type* of movement. *Amphiarthrotic* joints are partially movable joints whose articular surfaces are connected by cartilage, such as intervertebral joints. *Synarthrotic* joints, such as the cranial sutures, are immovable. *(Bontrager, pp 10–13)*

115. **(B)** Oral administration of barium sulfate is used to demonstrate the upper digestive tract: the esophagus; the fundus, body, and pylorus of the stomach; and the small bowel, consisting of duodenum, jejunum, and *ileum*. Consistent care must be taken to read and record patient information accurately and correctly. The large bowel is usually demonstrated via rectal administration of barium. *(Bontrager, pp 442–443)*

116. **(B)** Figure 2–20 shows an AP projection of the shoulder. A plane passing through the epicondyles is parallel to the IR (and perpendicular to the CR). To project the coracoid process with less self-superimposition, the CR must be angled cephalad between 15° and 45°. The amount of cephalad angulation depends on the degree of thoracic kyphosis; the greater the drgree of kyphosis, the greater the degree of cephalad angulation required. A 30° angle is used for the average patient. *(Ballinger & Frank, vol 1, p 220)*

117–118. **(117, D; 118, A)** Four positions for the lumbar spine are illustrated. Number 1 is an *RPO*, and number 2 an *LAO*. The *posterior oblique* positions (LPO and RPO) demonstrate the *apophyseal joints closer* to the IR, while the *anterior oblique* positions (LAO and RAO) demonstrate the apophyseal joints *further* from the IR (Fig. 2–51). Number 3 is the *AP* projection, which demonstrates the lumbar bodies and disk spaces and the transverse and spinous processes. Number 4 is the *lateral* position, which provides the best demonstration of the lumbar bodies, intervertebral disk spaces, spinous processes, pedicles, and intervertebral foramina. *(Bontrager & Frank, vol 1, pp 431, 434–435)*

119. **(C)** The thoracic apophyseal joints are demonstrated by placing the patient in an oblique position with the coronal plane 70° to the IR (MSP

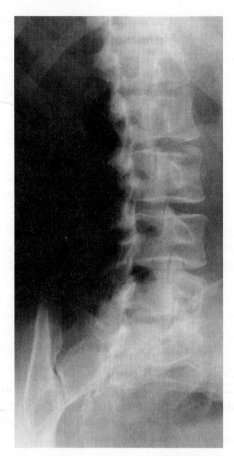

Figure 2–51. Courtesy of Stamford Hospital, Department of Radiology.

20° to the IR). This may be accomplished by first placing the patient lateral, then obliquing the patient 20° "off lateral." The apophyseal joints closest to the IR are demonstrated in the PA oblique, and those remote from the IR in the AP oblique. Comparable detail is obtained using either method, because the OID is about the same. *(Ballinger & Frank, vol 1, p 327)*

120. **(D)** The *scapular Y* projection is an oblique projection of the shoulder and is used to demonstrate anterior or posterior shoulder dislocation. The *inferosuperior axial* projection may be used to evaluate the glenohumeral joint when the patient is able to abduct the arm. The *transthoracic lateral* projection is used to evaluate the glenohumeral joint and upper humerus when the patient is unable to abduct the arm. *(Ballinger & Frank, vol 1, p 142)*

121. **(A)** During lower-limb venography, tourniquets are applied above the knee and ankle to

suppress filling of the more superficial veins and coerce filling of the deep veins. The anterior tibial vein may be blocked when tourniquets are used. The patient is positioned so that the table is tilted with the head up to slow the transit time of the contrast medium, in order that images may be obtained of the entire lower-limb and pelvic area. *(Ballinger & Frank, vol 2, p 542)*

122. **(A)** Breast tissue is most dense, glandular, and radiographically homogeneous in appearance in the postpubertal adolescent. Following pregnancy and lactation, changes occur within the breast that reduce the glandular tissue and replace it with fatty tissue (a process called fatty infiltration). Menopause causes further atrophy of glandular tissue. *(Ballinger & Frank, vol 2, pp 429–431)*

123. **(C)** Accurate *positioning skills* include a knowledge of *anatomy* (the position of the structure with respect to the image receptor) and *geometric principles* (how the x-ray tube angle will project or distort the anatomic structure). *Shape distortion* is related to the *alignment* of the x-ray tube, the object being examined, and the image receptor. When all three are parallel to one another, shape distortion is minimal. If one or more are out of alignment, shape distortion occurs. The two types of shape distortion are *foreshortening* and *elongation*. *Foreshortening* occurs as a result of the anatomic structure within the body being at an angle with the image receptor. For example, in the supine position, the kidneys are not parallel to the image receptor: Their lower pole is anterior to their upper pole. Another example is the curved carpal scaphoid: Its full length will not be appreciated in the PA projection, as because of its curve, it will be self-superimposed and foreshortened. *Elongation* occurs as a result of x-ray tube angulation. Elongation is often used intentionally to see structures better. The axial projection of the sigmoid colon during BE "opens" the S-shaped sigmoid to allow visualization of its entire length. The AP axial skull (Townes/Grashey) projects the facial bones inferiorly to better see the occipital bone. *The greater the tube angulation, the greater the elongation (distortion) produced.* *(Shephard, pp 228–232)*

124. **(D)** IVU images should indicate the amount of *time* elapsed postinjection. Tomographic images should indicate the *fulcrum level*. Abdominal survey images should be marked according to *body position* (such as erect or decubitus). *(Bontrager, p 31)*

125. **(D)** To demonstrate the radius and ulna free of superimposition, the forearm must be radiographed in the AP position, with the hand supinated. Pronation of the hand causes overlapping of the proximal radius and ulna. Two views, at right angles to each other, are generally required for each examination. Therefore, AP and lateral is the usual routine for an examination of the forearm. *(Ballinger & Frank, vol 1, p 98)*

126. **(A)** The four types of body habitus describe differences in visceral shape, position, tone, and motility. One body type is *hypersthenic*, characterized by the very large individual with short, wide heart and lungs; high transverse stomach and gallbladder; and peripheral colon. The *sthenic individual* is the average, athletic, most predominant type. The *hyposthenic* patient is somewhat thinner and a little more frail, with organs positioned somewhat lower. The *asthenic* type is smaller in the extreme, with a long thorax; a very long, almost pelvic stomach; and a low medial gallbladder. The colon is medial and redundant. Hypersthenic patients usually demonstrate the greatest motility. *(Saia, p 73)*

127. **(A)** An *avulsion* fracture is a small bony fragment pulled from a bony process as a result of a forceful pull of the attached ligament or tendon. A *comminuted* fracture is one in which the bone is broken or splintered into pieces. A *torus* fracture is a greenstick fracture with one cortex buckled and the other intact. A *compound* fracture is an open fracture in which the fractured ends have perforated the skin. *(Saia, pp 119–120)*

128. **(D)** The term *proximal* refers to structures closer to the point of attachment. For example, the elbow is described as being *proximal* to the wrist; that is, the elbow is closer to the point of attachment (the shoulder) than the

wrist is. Referring to the question, then, the interphalangeal joints (both proximal and distal) and the metacarpals are both *distal* to the carpal bones. The radial styloid process is *proximal* to the carpals. *(Bontrager, p 23)*

129. **(B)** The scapular Y projection requires that the coronal plane be about 60° to the IR, thus resulting in an *oblique* projection of the shoulder. The vertebral and axillary borders of the scapula are superimposed on the humeral shaft, and the resulting relationship between the glenoid fossa and humeral head will demonstrate anterior or posterior dislocation. Lateral or medial dislocation is evaluated on the AP projection. *(Ballinger & Frank, vol 1, p 179)*

130. **(C)** When the arm is placed in the *AP* position, the epicondyles are parallel to the plane of the cassette and the shoulder is placed in *external rotation.* In this position, an AP projection of the humerus, elbow, and forearm can be obtained; it places the greater tubercle of the humerus in profile. For the *lateral* projection of the humerus, the arm is *internally* rotated, elbow somewhat flexed, with the back of the hand against the thigh and the epicondyles superimposed and perpendicular to the IR. The lateral projections of the humerus, elbow, and forearm all require that the epicondyles be perpendicular to the plane of the cassette. *(Ballinger & Frank, pp 161, 164)*

131. **(A)** The fifth metacarpal is located on the *medial* aspect of the hand. Remember to always view a part in its *anatomic position*. With the arm in the anatomic position, the fifth metacarpal and the ulna lie medially. *(Bontrager, p 23)*

132. **(B)** With the patient in the PA position, the *rami* are well visualized with a perpendicular ray or with 20° to 25° cephalad angulation. A portion of the mandibular body is demonstrated in this position, but most of it is superimposed over the cervical spine. *(Ballinger & Frank, vol 2, p 382)*

133. **(B)** The kidneys lie obliquely in the posterior portion of the trunk, with their superior portion angled posteriorly and their *inferior portion and ureters angled anteriorly.* Therefore, to facilitate filling of the most anteriorly placed structures, the patient is examined in the prone position. Opacified urine then flows to the most dependent part of the kidney and ureter: *the ureteropelvic region, inferior calyces, and ureters. (Saia, p 191)*

134. **(B)** The *median sagittal,* or *midsagittal,* plane passes vertically through the midline of the body, dividing it into left and right halves. Any plane parallel to the MSP is termed a *sagittal* plane. The *midcoronal* plane is perpendicular to the MSP and divides the body into anterior and posterior halves. A *transverse* plane passes through the body at right angles to a sagittal plane. These planes, especially the MSP, are very important reference points in radiographic positioning (Fig. 2–52). *(Saia, p 75)*

135. **(A)** In the AP projection of the shoulder, there is superimposition of the humeral head and glenoid fossa. With the patient obliqued 45° toward the affected side, the glenohumeral joint is open, and the glenoid fossa is seen in profile. The patient's arm is abducted somewhat and placed in internal rotation. *(Ballinger & Frank, vol 1, pp 182–183)*

136. **(B)** The radiograph illustrated shows the odontoid process superimposed on the base of the skull. The maxillary teeth can be seen significantly superior to the base of the skull. A diagnostic image of C1–2 depends on adjusting the flexion of the neck *so that the maxillary occlusal plane and the base of the skull are superimposed* (see the dotted lines in Fig. 2–53). Accurate adjustment of these structures will usually allow good visualization of the odontoid process and the atlantoaxial articulation. Too much flexion superimposes the teeth on the odontoid process; too much extension superimposes the base of the skull on the odontoid process. *(Ballinger & Frank, vol 1, pp 388–389)*

137. **(C)** Myelography is used to demonstrate encroachment on and compression of the spinal cord as a result of disk herniation, tumor growth, or posttraumatic swelling of the cord. This is accomplished by placing positive or

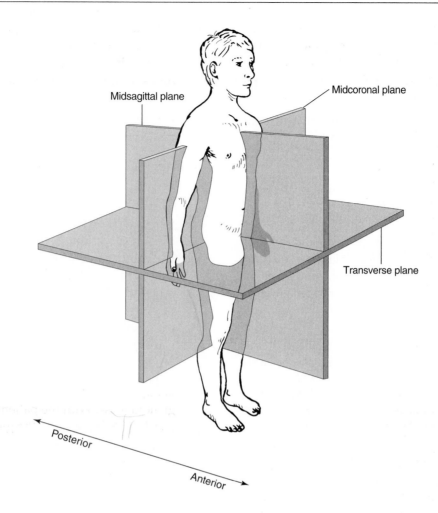

Figure 2–52. Reproduced with permission from Saia DA. *Radiography: Program Review and Examination Preparation,* 2nd ed. Stamford, CT: Appleton & Lange, 1999.

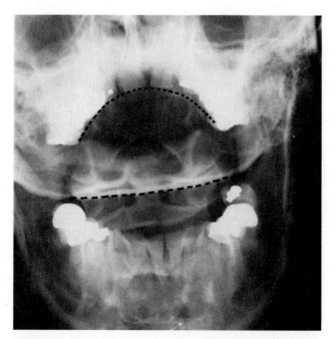

Figure 2–53. Courtesy of Stamford Hospital, Department of Radiology.

negative contrast medium into the subarachnoid space. Myelography will demonstrate posterior protrusion of herniated intervertebral disks or spinal cord tumors. Anterior protrusion of a herniated intervertebral disk does not impinge on the spinal cord and is not demonstrated in myelography. Internal disk lesions can be demonstrated only by injecting contrast medium into the individual disks *(diskography). (Saia, p 198)*

138. **(C)** In the PA position, portions of the barium-filled hypersthenic stomach superimpose upon themselves. Thus, patients with a hypersthenic body habitus usually present a high transverse stomach, with poorly defined curvatures. If the PA stomach is projected with a *35° to 45° cephalad* central ray, the stomach "opens up." That is, the curvatures, the

antral portion, and the duodenal bulb all appear as a sthenic habitus stomach would appear. A 35° to 40° *RAO* position is used to demonstrate many of these structures in the average, or sthenic, body habitus. A *lateral* position is used to demonstrate the anterior and posterior gastric surfaces and retrogastric space. *(Bontrager, pp 450–451)*

139. **(C)** In the dorsoplantar projection of the foot, the central ray may be directed perpendicularly or angled 10° posteriorly. Angulation serves to "open" the tarsometatarsal joints that are not well visualized on the dorsoplantar projection with perpendicular ray. Inversion and eversion of the foot do not affect the tarsometatarsal joints. *(Ballinger & Frank, vol 1, p 242)*

140. **(B)** The central cavity of a long bone is the medullary canal. It contains *yellow* bone marrow, the most abundant type of marrow in the body. *Red* marrow is found within the cancellous tissue forming the extremities of long bones. *(Saia, pp 87, 89)*

141. **(A)** The routine AP projection of the lumbar spine demonstrates the intervertebral disk spaces between the first four lumbar vertebrae. The space between L5 and S1, however, is angled with respect to the other disk spaces. Therefore, the central ray must be directed 30° to 35° cephalad to parallel the disk space, and thus project it open onto the IR. *(Ballinger & Frank, vol 1, p 440)*

142. **(B)** The most prominent part of the greater trochanter is at the same level as the pubic symphysis—both are valuable positioning landmarks. The ASIS is in the same transverse plane as S2. The ASIS and the pubic symphysis are the bony landmarks used to locate the hip joint, which is located midway between the two points. *(Saia, p 77)*

143. **(C)** Patients are instructed to remove all jewelry, hair clips, metal prostheses, coins, and credit cards, before entering the room for an MRI scan. MRI does not use radiation to produce images, but instead uses a very strong magnetic field. All patients must be screened

prior to entering the magnetic field to be sure that they do not have any metal on or within them. Proper screening includes questioning the patient about any eye injury involving metal, cardiac pacemakers, aneurysm clips, insulin pumps, heart valves, shrapnel, or any metal in the body. This is extremely important, and if there is any doubt, the patient should be rescheduled for a time after it has been determined that it is safe for him or her to enter the room. Patients who have done metalwork or welding are frequently sent to diagnostic radiology for screening images of the orbits to ensure that there are no metal fragments near the optic nerve. Any external metallic objects, such as bobby pins, hair clips, or coins in the pocket, must be removed, or they will be pulled by the magnet and can cause harm to the patient. Credit cards and any other plastic cards with a magnetic strip will be wiped clean if they come in contact with the magnetic field. *(Torres et al, pp 362–363)*

144. **(D)** These are all terms used to describe particular body movements. *Eversion* refers to movement of the foot caused by turning the ankle outward. *Inversion* is foot motion caused by turning the ankle inward. *Abduction* is movement of a part away from the midline. *Adduction* is movement of a part toward the midline. *(Bontrager, p 26)*

145. **(B)** The radiograph shown in Figure 2–23 is a *PA recumbent* projection. If the patient was AP, barium would be located in the fundus of the stomach because the fundus is more posterior, and barium would flow down to fill the posterior structure. If the patient was in the *Trendelenburg* position, barium flow to the fundus would be even more facilitated. If the patient was *erect*, air–fluid levels would be clearly defined. Additionally, the barium-filled stomach tends to spread more horizontally in the PA position (as is seen in the radiograph). *(Ballinger & Frank, vol 2, p 102)*

146. **(D)** The *lordotic* curves are *secondary* curves; that is, they develop sometime after birth. The cervical and lumbar vertebrae form lordotic curves. The *thoracic* and *sacral* vertebrae exhibit

the *primary kyphotic* curves, those that are present at birth. *(Saia, p 123)*

147. (B) In the lateral position of the skull, the *midsagittal plane* must be parallel to the IR and the interpupillary line vertical. Flexion of the head is adjusted until the *IOML* is parallel to the IR. The central ray should enter about *2 inches superior* to the EAM. *(Ballinger & Frank, vol 2, p 307)*

148. (B) The *first metacarpal*, on the lateral side of the hand, articulates with the most lateral carpal of the distal carpal row, the greater multangular/*trapezium*. This articulation forms a rather unique and very versatile *saddle joint*, named for the shape of its articulating surfaces. *(Saia, pp 87–88)*

149. (A) The position of the gallbladder varies with the body habitus of the patient. *Hypersthenic* patients are more likely to have their gallbladder located *high and lateral*. The *asthenic* patient's gallbladder is most likely to occupy a *low and medial* position, occasionally superimposed on the vertebrae or iliac fossa. The *LAO* position is most often used to move the gallbladder away from the spine. The erect position would make the gallbladder move even more inferior and medial. *(Ballinger & Frank, vol 2, p 62)*

150. (A) The abdomen is divided into nine regions. The upper lateral regions are the left and right hypochondriac, with the epigastric separating them. The middle lateral regions are the left and right lumbar, with the umbilical region between them. The lower lateral regions are the left and right iliac, with the hypogastric region between them. The *ileocecal valve*, cecum, and appendix (if present) are located in the lower right abdomen—therefore, the *right iliac region. (Saia, p 77)*

151. (B) Evaluation of the acromioclavicular joints requires *bilateral* AP or PA *erect* projections *with and without the use of weights*. Weights are used to emphasize the minute changes within a joint caused by *separation or dislocation*. Weights should be anchored from the patient's wrists rather than held in the patient's

hands, as this encourages tightening of the shoulder muscles and obliteration of any small separation. *(Ballinger & Frank, vol 1, p 200)*

152. (B) Air or fluid levels will be clearly demonstrated only if the central ray is directed *parallel* to them. Therefore, to demonstrate air or fluid levels, the erect or decubitus position should be used. Small amounts of *fluid* are best demonstrated in the lateral decubitus position, affected side *down*. Small amounts of *air* are best demonstrated in the lateral decubitus position, affected side *up*. Dorsal and ventral decubitus positions made with a horizontal x-ray beam can also be used to demonstrate air or fluid levels. *(Ballinger & Frank, vol 3, pp 248–249)*

153. (B) The ankle mortise, or ankle joint, is formed by the articulation of the tibia, fibula, and talus (Fig. 2–54). Two articulations form

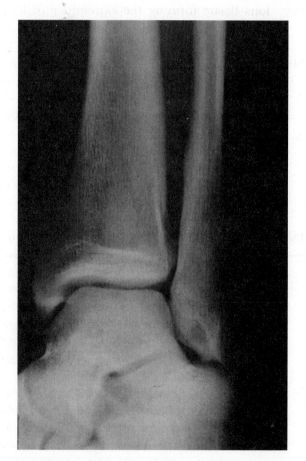

Figure 2–54. Courtesy of Stamford Hospital, Department of Radiology.

the ankle mortise, the talotibial and talofibular. The calcaneus is not associated with the formation of the ankle mortise. *(Ballinger & Frank, vol 1, p 228)*

154. **(D)** The *SMV* projection is made with the patient's head resting on the vertex and the central ray directed perpendicular to the IOML. This position may be used as part of a sinus survey to demonstrate the sphenoidal sinuses or as a view of the cranial base for the basal foramina (especially the foramina ovale and spinosum). It also demonstrates the bony part of the auditory (eustachian) tubes. *AP or PA axial* projections are frequently used to demonstrate the occipital region or evaluate the sellar region. A *lateral* projection is usually part of a routine skull evaluation. The *parietoacanthial* projection is the single best position to demonstrate facial bones. *(Ballinger & Frank, vol 1, p 277)*

155. **(A)** The radiograph in Figure 2–24 illustrates a *lateral* projection of the *scapula*. The axillary and vertebral borders are superimposed. The *acromion* and *coracoid* process are visualized; the coracoid process is partially superimposed on the axillary portion of the third rib. A *scapular Y* projection is often performed to demonstrate shoulder dislocation, but the affected arm is left to rest at the patient's side; the arm in the illustrated radiograph is abducted somewhat to better view the body of the scapula. *(Ballinger & Frank, vol 1, p 166)*

156. **(B)** The femur is the longest and strongest bone in the body. The femoral shaft is bowed slightly anteriorly and presents a long, narrow ridge posteriorly, called the *linea aspera*. The proximal femur consists of a head that is received by the pelvic *acetabulum*. The femoral neck, which joins the head and shaft, normally angles upward about 120° and forward (in anteversion) about 15°. The *greater* and *lesser trochanters* are large processes on the posterior proximal femur. The *intertrochanteric crest* runs obliquely between the trochanters; the *intertrochanteric line* parallels the intertrochanteric crest on the *anterior* femoral surface. The *intercondyloid fossa*, a deep notch, found on the distal posterior femur between the large femoral

condyles, and the *popliteal surface* is a smooth surface just superior to the intercondyloid fossa. The *intertubercular groove* is found on the proximal humerus between the humeral tubercles. *(Ballinger & Frank, vol 1, p 234)*

157. **(C)** An *intrathecal* injection is one made within the meninges. A myelogram requires an intrathecal injection to introduce contrast medium into the subarachnoid space. An IVU requires an IV injection; a retrograde pyelogram requires that contrast be introduced into the ureters by way of cystoscopy. An arthrogram requires that contrast medium be introduced into a joint space. *(Saia, p 199)*

158. **(A)** The typical vertebra is divided into two portions, the *body* (anteriorly) and the *vertebral arch* (posteriorly). The vertebral arch supports seven processes: two transverse, one spinous (number 3), two superior articular processes (number 4), and two inferior articular processes (number 2). The superior articular processes and the superjacent inferior articular processes join to form apophyseal joints. Pedicles (number 5) project posteriorly from the vertebral body (number 6). Their upper and lower surfaces form vertebral notches. Superjacent vertebral notches form intervertebral foramina. The *lamina* is represented by number 1. The transverse and spinous processes serve as attachments for muscles, or articulation for ribs in the thoracic region. The superior and inferior surfaces of the vertebral body are covered with articular cartilage, and between the vertebral bodies lie the intervertebral disks. *(Ballinger & Frank, vol 1, p 402)*

159. **(A)** In the PA projection of the chest, there should be no rotation, as evidenced by *symmetrical* sternoclavicular joints. The shoulders are rolled forward to remove the scapulae from the lung fields. Inspiration should be adequate to demonstrate 10 *posterior* ribs above the diaphragm (the anterior ribs angle downward; the tenth anterior rib is the last attached to the sternum and is very unlikely to be imaged on inspiration). The sternum should be seen lateral without rotation in the *lateral* position of the chest. *(Ballinger & Frank, vol 1, pp 404, 455)*

160. (C) The coronoid process is located on the proximal anterior ulna. The *medial oblique* projection of the elbow demonstrates the coronoid process in profile, as well as the ulnar olecranon process within the humeral olecranon fossa. The *lateral oblique* elbow projects the proximal radius and ulna free of superimposition. The coracoid *process* is located on the scapula. *(Ballinger & Frank, vol 1, p 134)*

161. (C) In the lateral projection of the ankle, the tibia and fibula are superimposed and the foot is somewhat dorsiflexed to better demonstrate the talotibial joint. The talofibular joint is not visualized because of superimposition with other bony structures. It may be well visualized in the medial oblique projection of the ankle. *(Ballinger & Frank, vol 1, p 230)*

162. (B) A double-contrast examination of the large bowel is performed to see through the bowel to its posterior wall and to visualize any intraluminal lesions or masses. Oblique projections are used to "open up" the flexures: the RAO for the hepatic flexure and the LAO for the splenic flexure. To view the redundant S-shaped sigmoid in the AP position, the central ray is directed 30° to 40° cephalad. The central ray is reversed when the patient is PA; that is, the central ray is 30° to 40° caudal with the patient PA. *(Ballinger & Frank, vol 2, pp 134, 139)*

163. (C) Radiographic examinations of the large bowel generally include the AP or PA axial position to "open" the S-shaped sigmoid colon, the lateral position especially for the rectum, and the LAO and RAO (or LPO and RPO) to "open" the colic flexures. The left and right decubitus positions are usually employed only in double-contrast barium enemas to better demonstrate double contrast of the medial and lateral walls of the ascending and descending colon. *(Ballinger & Frank, vol 2, pp 132, 137)*

164. (A) Because sinus examinations are performed to evaluate the presence or absence of fluid, they must be performed in the *erect position with a horizontal x-ray beam*. The PA axial (Caldwell) projection demonstrates the frontal and ethmoidal sinus groups, and the parietoacanthial projection (Waters' method) shows the maxillary sinuses. The lateral position demonstrates all the sinus groups, and the SMV is frequently used to demonstrate the sphenoidal sinuses. *(Ballinger & Frank, vol 2, p 361)*

165. (B) Statement 1 describes the PA axial (Camp-Coventry) projection, and statement 2 describes the AP axial (Beclere) projection, for demonstration of the intercondyloid fossa. The positions are actually the reverse of each other. Statement 3 describes the method of obtaining a PA projection of the patella. *(Ballinger & Frank, vol 1, pp 302–305)*

166. (A) The visualization of the scapular spine indicates that this is a view of the *posterior* aspect of the scapula. The scapula's *anterior*, or *costal*, surface is that which is adjacent to the ribs. The scapula has no sternal articulation. *(Tortora & Derrickson, p 234)*

167–168. (167, A; 168, D) Figure 2–27 depicts a posterior view of the right scapula and its articulation with the humerus (number 4). The scapula presents two borders: the lateral or axillary border (number 7) and the medial or vertebral border (number 9). It also presents three angles: the inferior angle (number 8), the superior angle (number 12), and the lateral angle (number 6). The processes of the scapula are the coracoid (number 2), the acromion (number 3), and the scapular spine (number 13). The scapula has a (supra) scapular notch (number 1), a supraspinatus fossa (number 11), and an infraspinatus fossa (number 10). *(Tortora & Derrickson, p 234)*

169. (C) After forceful eversion or inversion injuries of the ankle, *AP stress studies* are valuable to confirm the presence of a ligament tear. Keeping the ankle in an AP position, the physician guides the ankle into inversion and eversion maneuvers. Characteristic changes in the relationship of the talus, tibia, and fibula will indicate ligament injury. Inversion stress demonstrates the lateral ligament, while eversion stress demonstrates the medial ligament. A fractured ankle would not be manipulated in this manner. *(Ballinger & Frank, vol 1, p 233)*

170. **(D)** A PA axial projection of the skull with a 15° caudad angle will show the petrous pyramids in the lower third of the orbits. If *no* angulation is used, the petrous pyramids will fill the orbits. Either PA projection should demonstrate symmetrical petrous pyramids and an equal distance from the lateral border of the skull to the lateral border of the orbit on both sides. This determines that there is no rotation of the skull. *(Ballinger & Frank, vol 2, p 244)*

171. **(B)** For the lateral projection of the knee, the patient is turned onto the affected side. This places the lateral femoral condyle *closest* to the IR and the medial femoral condyle *remote* from the IR. Consequently, there is significant magnification of the medial femoral condyle and, unless the central ray is angled slightly cephalad, subsequent obliteration of the joint space. *(Ballinger & Frank, vol 1, p 293)*

172. **(D)** Surface landmarks, prominences, and depressions are very useful to the radiographer in locating anatomic structures that are not visible externally. The *costal margin* is at about the same level as L3. The *umbilicus* is at approximately the same level as the L3–4 interspace. The *xiphoid tip* is at about the same level as T10. The *fourth lumbar vertebra* is at approximately the same level as the iliac crest. *(Saia, p 77)*

173. **(C)** The stomach and spleen are both normally located in the LUQ. The cecum is the most distal end of the large bowel and is normally located in the RLQ. *(Ballinger & Frank, vol 1, p 39)*

174. **(B)** The cervical intervertebral foramina lie 45° to the midsagittal plane and 15° to 20° to a transverse plane. When the *posterior oblique* position (LPO or RPO) is used, the cervical intervertebral foramina demonstrated are those *further* from the IR. There is therefore some magnification of the foramina. In the anterior oblique position (LAO or RAO), the foramina disclosed are those *closer* to the IR. *(Ballinger & Frank, vol 1, p 341)*

175. **(C)** The parietoacanthial (Waters' method) projection demonstrates the *maxillary* sinuses. The PA axial with a caudal central ray (Caldwell) demonstrates the *frontal and ethmoidal* sinus groups. The lateral projection, with the central ray entering 1 inch posterior to the outer canthus, demonstrates *all* the paranasal sinuses. X-ray examinations of the sinuses should always be performed *erect*, to demonstrate leveling of any fluid present. *(Bontrager, p 428)*

176. **(C)** A lateral projection of the scapula superimposes its medial and lateral borders (vertebral and axillary, respectively). The coracoid and acromion processes should be readily identified separately (not superimposed) in the lateral projection. The erect position is probably the most comfortable position for a patient with scapula pain. *(Ballinger & Frank, vol 1, p 205)*

177. **(C)** The pictured radiograph is an *RAO* position of the sternum. The sternum is projected to the *left* side of the thorax, over the heart and other mediastinal structures, in the RAO position, thus promoting more uniform density. Although the upper limits of the sternum are well demonstrated in the figure, not all of the xiphoid process is seen, because the central ray was directed somewhat too superiorly. The central ray should be directed midway between the jugular (manubrial) notch and the xiphoid process. *(Ballinger & Frank, vol 1, pp 274–277)*

178. **(C)** In the lateral projection of the knee, the joint space is obscured by the magnified medial femoral condyle unless the central ray is angled 5° to 7° cephalad. The degree of flexion of the knee is important when evaluating the knee for possible transverse patellar fracture. In such a case, the knee should not be flexed more than 10°. The knee should normally be flexed 20° to 30° in the lateral position. *(Ballinger & Frank, vol 1, p 293)*

179. **(B)** The AP projection of the cervical spine demonstrates the bodies and intervertebral spaces of the last five vertebrae (C3–7). The cervical apophyseal joints are 90° to the midsagittal plane and are therefore demonstrated in the lateral projection. *(Ballinger & Frank, vol 1, pp 394–395)*

180. **(C)** Long bones are composed of a shaft, or diaphysis, and two extremities, or epiphyses. In the growing bone, the cartilaginous *epiphyseal plate* is gradually replaced by bone. The ossified growth area of long bones is the *metaphysis. Apophysis* refers to vertebral joints formed by articulation of superjacent articular facets. *(Saia, p 87)*

181. **(D)** The PA axial (Caldwell) projection of the paranasal sinuses is used to demonstrate the frontal and ethmoidal sinuses. The central ray is angled caudally 15° to the OML. This projects the petrous pyramids into the lower one third of the orbits, thus permitting optimal visualization of the frontal and ethmoidal sinuses. *(Ballinger & Frank, vol 1, pp 366–367)*

182. **(D)** The respiratory passageways include the nose, pharynx, larynx (upper respiratory structures), trachea, bronchi, and lungs (lower structures). If obstruction of the breathing passageways occurs in the upper respiratory tract, above the larynx (ie, in the nose or pharynx), *tracheotomy* may be performed to order to restore breathing. *Intubation* can be made into the lower structures, larynx and trachea, moving aside any soft obstruction and restoring the breathing passageway. *(Tortora & Derrickson, p 856)*

183. **(D)** To clearly demonstrate the atlas and axis without superimposition of the teeth or the base of the skull, a line between the maxillary occlusal plane (edge of upper teeth) and mastoid tip must be vertical. If the head is flexed too much, the teeth will be superimposed. If the head is extended too much, the cranial base will be superimposed on the area of interest. A line between the mentum and the mastoid tip is used to demonstrate the odontoid process only through the foramen magnum (Fuchs method). *(Ballinger & Frank, vol 1, p 292)*

184. **(A)** Air or fluid levels will be clearly delineated only if the central ray is directed parallel to them. Therefore, the erect or decubitus position should be used. Small amounts of *fluid* within the peritoneal cavity are best demonstrated in the lateral decubitus position, *affected side down*. Small amounts of *air* within

the peritoneal cavity are best demonstrated in the lateral decubitus position, *affected side up.* *(Ballinger & Frank, vol 2, pp 40–41)*

185. **(A)** Lateral projections of the barium-filled stomach (Fig. 2–55) may be performed recumbent or upright for the demonstration of the retrogastric space. With the patient in the (usually right) lateral position, the central ray is directed to a point midway between the midcoronal line and the anterior surface of the abdomen, at the level of L1. When the patient is in the LPO or RAO position, the central ray should be directed midway between the vertebral column and lateral border of the abdomen. For the PA projection, the central ray is directed perpendicular to the IR at the level of L2. *(Ballinger & Frank, vol 2, pp 114–115)*

186. **(A)** The oblique projection of the hand should demonstrate minimal overlap of the third, fourth, and fifth metacarpals. Excessive overlap of these metacarpals is caused by obliquing the hand *more than 45°*. The use of a 45° foam wedge ensures that the fingers will be extended and parallel to the IR, thus permitting visualization of the interphalangeal joints and avoiding foreshortening of the phalanges. Clenching of the fist and ulnar flexion are

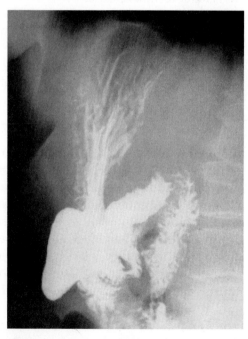

Figure 2–55. Courtesy of Stamford Hospital, Department of Radiology.

maneuvers used to better demonstrate the carpal scaphoid. *(Ballinger & Frank, vol 1, p 107)*

187. **(D)** Patients who are able to cooperate are usually able to control *voluntary* motion. However, certain body functions and responses create *involuntary* motion that is not controllable by the patient. Severe pain, muscle spasm, and chills all cause involuntary movements. Peristaltic activity of the intestinal tract and motion caused by contraction of the heart muscle are other sources of involuntary motion. *(Ballinger & Frank, vol 1, p 12)*

188. **(C)** In the tangential ("sunrise") projection of the patella, the central ray is directed parallel to the longitudinal plane of the patella, thereby demonstrating a vertical fracture and providing the best view of the patellofemoral articulation. The AP knee could demonstrate a vertical fracture through the superimposed femur, but it does not demonstrate the patellofemoral articulation. The "tunnel" view of the knee is used to demonstrate the intercondyloid fossa. *(Ballinger & Frank, vol 1, pp 314–315)*

189–190. **(189, A; 190, B)** The radiograph shown is a lateral projection of the cervical spine taken in flexion. *Flexion and extension* views are useful in certain cervical injuries, such as *whiplash,* to indicate the degree of anterior and posterior motion. The structure labeled 1 is an *apophyseal joint;* because apophyseal joints are positioned 90° to the MSP, they are well visualized in the lateral projection. The structure labeled 2 is a *vertebral body. (Ballinger & Frank, vol 1, pp 398, 399)*

191. **(C)** The erect position in IV urography may be part of the departmental routine, but more often than not it is requested as a supplemental view to rule out nephroptosis. With the patient erect, the kidneys normally change position, dropping no more than 2 inches. More marked dropping of the kidney is termed *nephroptosis,* a condition that is actually due to loss of the surrounding perinephric fat. *(Ballinger & Frank, vol 2, p 170)*

192. **(C)** Scoliosis is a lateral curvature of the spine and is typically noted in early adolescence.

These young patients usually return for follow-up studies, and it is imperative to limit their radiation dose as much as possible. Examining the patient in the PA position is frequently advisable, because the gonadal dose is significantly reduced and there is usually no appreciable loss of detail. Thyroid and breast shields are also a valuable protection, especially for the patient who requires follow-up examinations. Bending images would not be performed on a patient with suspected subluxation or spondylolisthesis, as further serious injury could result. *(Ballinger & Frank, vol 1, p 396)*

193. **(C)** The AP projection demonstrates superimposition of the distal fibula on the talus; the joint space is not well seen. The 15° to 20° medical oblique position shows the entire mortise joint; the talofibular joint is well visualized, as well as the talotibial joint. There is considerable superimposition of the talus and fibula in the lateral and lateral oblique projections. *(Ballinger & Frank, vol 1, p 280)*

194. **(A)** The erect position is most often employed to demonstrate air–fluid levels in the chest or abdomen or both. However, patients having traumatic injuries must frequently be examined in the recumbent position. The recumbent position will not demonstrate air–fluid levels unless it is a decubitus position. If free air is being questioned, we will look for that quantity of air on the "up" side because air rises. However, because liver tissue is so homogeneous, a small amount of air will be more easily perceived superimposed on it, rather than on left-sided structures. Thus, an AP projection obtained in the left lateral decubitus position will best demonstrate small amount of free air because that air will be superimposed on the liver. *(Ballinger & Frank, vol 2, p 20)*

195. **(A)** Blood is oxygenated in the lungs and carried to the left atrium by the four pulmonary veins. From the left atrium, blood flows through the bicuspid (mitral) valve into the left ventricle. Blood leaving the left ventricle is bright red, oxygenated blood that travels through the systemic circulation, delivering oxygenated blood via arteries and returning deoxygenated blood to the lungs via veins. From the left ventricle, blood first goes through the largest arteries, then goes to progressively smaller arteries (arterioles), to the capillaries, to the smallest veins (venules), and on to progressively larger veins. *(Tortora & Derrickson, p 737)*

196. **(C)** On the *AP projection* of the elbow, the radial head and ulna are normally somewhat superimposed. The *lateral oblique* demonstrates the radial head free of ulnar superimposition. The *lateral projection* demonstrates the olecranon process in profile. The *medial oblique* demonstrates considerable overlap of the proximal radius and ulna, but should clearly demonstrate the coronoid process free of superimposition and the olecranon process within the olecranon fossa. *(Saia, p 96)*

197. **(D)** Acromioclavicular joints are usually examined when separation or dislocation is suspected. They must be examined in the erect position, because in the recumbent position, a separation appears to reduce itself. Both AC joints are examined simultaneously for comparison, because separations may be minimal. *(Ballinger & Frank, vol 1, p 152)*

198. **(C)** Myelography is the radiologic examination of the structures within the spinal canal. Opaque contrast medium is usually used. Following injection, the contrast medium is distributed to the vertebral region of interest by *gravity;* the *table* is angled Trendelenburg for visualization of the cervical region and in Fowler's position for visualization of the thoracic and lumbar regions. Although the table is Trendelenburg, care must be taken that the patient's neck be kept in acute *extension* to compress the cisterna magna and keep contrast medium from traveling into the ventricles of the brain. *(Saia, pp 197–198)*

199. **(C)** There are many terms (with which the radiographer must be familiar) that are used to describe radiographic positioning techniques. *Cephalad* refers to that which is toward the head, and *caudad* to that which is toward the feet. Structures close to the source or begin-

ning are said to be *proximal,* while those lying close to the midline are said to be *medial.* *(Bontrager, p 23)*

200. **(C)** The parietoacanthial projection (Waters' position) provides an oblique frontal projection of the facial bones. The maxilla (and antra), zygomatic arches, and orbits are well demonstrated. The patient is positioned PA with the head resting on the extended chin so that the OML forms a 37° angle with the IR. The position may be reversed if the patient is AP and the central ray is directed 30° cephalad to the IOML. This position is not preferred, however, because the facial bones are significantly magnified as a result of increased object–IR distance. *(Saia, p 146)*

201. **(B)** Inhalation of a foreign substance such as water or food particles into the airway and/or bronchial tree is called *aspiration. Asphyxia* is caused by deprivation of oxygen as a result of interference with ventilation, from trauma, electric shock, etc. *Atelectasis* is incomplete expansion of a lung or portion of a lung. *Asystole* is cardiac standstill—failure of heart muscle to contract and pump blood to vital organs. *(Tortora & Derrickson, p 889)*

202. **(B)** ERCP may be performed to investigate abnormalities of the biliary system or pancreas. The patient's throat is treated with a local anesthetic in preparation for the passage of the endoscope. The hepatopancreatic ampulla (of Vater) is located, and a cannula is passed through it so that contrast medium may be introduced into the common bile duct. Spot images of the common bile duct and pancreatic duct are frequently taken in the oblique position. Direct injection of barium mixture into the duodenum occurs during an enteroclysis procedure of the small bowel. *(Ballinger & Frank, vol 2, p 80)*

203. **(C)** A Colles' fracture is usually caused by a fall onto an outstretched (extended) hand, to "brake" a fall. The wrist then suffers an impacted transverse fracture of the *distal* inch of the *radius,* with an accompanying chip fracture of the *ulnar* styloid process. Because of the hand position at the time of the fall, the fracture is usually *displaced backward* approximately 30°. (*Bontrager, pp 130, 598*)

204. **(C)** *Full* or *forced expiration* is used to elevate the diaphragm and demonstrate the ribs *below* the diaphragm to best advantage (with exposure adjustment). *Deep inspiration* is used to depress the diaphragm and demonstrate as many ribs *above the diaphragm* as possible. Shallow breathing is occasionally used to visualize the ribs above the diaphragm, while obliterating pulmonary vascular markings. (*Ballinger & Frank, vol 1, p 472*)

205. **(A)** The architectural features of the female pelvis are designed to accommodate childbearing. The female pelvis as a whole is broader and more shallow than its male counterpart, having a wider and more circular pelvic outlet. The ischial tuberosities and acetabula are further apart. The sacrum is wider and extends more sharply posteriorly. The pubic arch of the man is significantly narrower than that of the woman. (*Saia, pp 106–108*)

206. **(B)** Radiologic interventional procedures function to *treat* pathologic conditions, as well as provide diagnostic information. PTA uses an inflatable balloon catheter, under fluoroscopic guidance, to increase the diameter of a plaque-stenosed vessel. A *stent* is a cage-like metal device that can be placed in the vessel to provide support to the vessel wall. A *peripherally insulated central catheter* (PICC line) is also placed under fluoroscopic control. It is simply a venous access catheter that can be left in place for several months. It provides convenient venous access for patients requiring frequent blood tests, chemotherapy, or large amounts of antibiotics. (*Bontrager, pp 692–693*)

207. **(C)** All traumatic injuries require the radiographer to be particularly alert and observant. Patient status must be continually observed and monitored. The radiographer must speak calmly to the patient, *explaining the procedure* even if the patient appears unconscious or unresponsive. In the case of an injured limb, *both joints must be supported* if any movement is required. *Both joints must also be included* when examining long bones. The injured limb need

not be placed in exact AP and lateral positions, but any two views of the part *at right angles to each* other must be obtained. (*Ballinger & Frank, vol 2, p 27*)

208. **(C)** The *ileocecal valve* is located at the terminal ileum, where it meets the first portion of the large bowel, the cecum. Most small-bowel examinations are performed following oral administration of barium sulfate suspension. The first small-bowel radiograph is taken 15 minutes after the first swallow of barium, with subsequent radiographs made every 15 to 30 minutes, depending on how quickly the barium is moving through the small bowel. Each image is shown to the radiologist, and a decision is made regarding the time of the next image. When the barium reaches the terminal ileum, fluoroscopy may be performed and compression spot images taken of the *ileocecal valve*. (*Ballinger & Frank, vol 2, p 116*)

209. **(C)** As the heart contracts and relaxes while functioning to pump blood from the heart, those arteries that are large and those that are in closest proximity to the heart will feel the effect of the heart's forceful contractions in their walls. The arterial walls pulsate in unison with the heart's contractions. This movement may be detected with the fingers in various parts of the body and is referred to as the *pulse*. (*Saia, p 199*)

210. **(C)** Placing the patient in a 20° to 30° AP Trendelenburg position during an upper GI examination helps demonstrate the presence of a *hiatal hernia*. A 10° to 15° Trendelenburg position with the patient rotated slightly to the right will also help demonstrate regurgitation and hiatal hernia. Filling of the *duodenal bulb* and demonstration of the *duodenal loop* are best seen in the RAO position. *Congenital hypertrophic pyloric stenosis* is caused by excessive thickening of the pyloric sphincter. It is noted in infancy and characterized by projectile vomiting. The pyloric valve will let very little pass through, and as a result the stomach becomes enlarged (hypertrophied). (*Ballinger & Frank, vol 2, p 99*)

211. **(D)** The AP projection will give a general survey and show medial/lateral and inferior/

superior joint relationaships. The scapular Y position (LAO or RAO) is employed to demonstrate anterior (subcoracoid) or posterior (subacromial) humeral dislocation. The humerus is normally superimposed on the scapula in this position; any deviation from this may indicate dislocation. Rotational views must be avoided in cases of suspected fracture. The AP and scapular Y combination is the closest to two views at right angles to each other. *(Ballinger & Frank, vol 1, pp 164, 180)*

212. **(C)** In the *AP* projection, the proximal fibula is at least partially superimposed on the lateral tibial condyle. *Medial rotation* of 45° will "open" the proximal tibiofibular articulation. *Lateral rotation* will obscure the articulation even more. *(Ballinger & Frank, vol 1, p 297)*

213. **(D)** The acetabulum is the bony socket that receives the head of the femur to form the hip joint. The *upper two fifths* of the acetabulum is formed by the ilium, the *lower anterior one fifth* is formed by the pubis, and the *lower posterior two-fifths* is formed by the ischium. Thus, the acetabulum is formed by all three of the bones that form the pelvis: the ilium, the ischium, and the pubis. *(Ballinger & Frank, vol 1, pp 325–326)*

214. **(B)** Retrograde urography requires ureteral catheterization so that a contrast medium can be introduced directly into the pelvicalyceal system. This procedure provides excellent opacification and structural information but does not demonstrate the function of these structures. IV studies such as the IVU demonstrate function. Cystourethrography is an examination of the bladder and urethra, frequently performed during voiding. Nephrotomography is performed after IV administration of a contrast agent; it may be used to evaluate small intrarenal lesions and renal hypertension. *(Ballinger & Frank, vol 2, p 179)*

215. **(A)** The AP projection of the sacrum requires a 15° cephalad angle centered at a point *midway between* the pubic symphysis and the ASIS. The AP projection of the coccyx requires the central ray to be directed 10° caudally and centered 2 inches superior to the pubic symphysis. *(Saia, p 132)*

216. **(C)** Arthritic changes in the knee result in changes in the joint bony relationships. These bony relationships are best evaluated in the AP position. *Narrowing of the joint spaces* is readily detected more on AP *weight-bearing* projections than on recumbent projections. *(Ballinger & Frank, vol 1, p 294)*

217. **(C)** The articular facets (apophyseal joints) of the L5–S1 articulation form a 30° angle with the MSP; they are therefore well demonstrated in a 30° oblique position. The 45° oblique demonstrates the apophyseal joints of L1 through L4. *(Ballinger & Frank, vol 1, p 372)*

218. **(D)** When the shoulder is placed in *internal rotation*, a greater portion of the glenoid fossa is superimposed by the humeral head and the *lesser tubercle* is visualized, as in image B. The *external rotation* position (image A) removes the humeral head from a large portion of the glenoid fossa and better demonstrates the *greater tubercle. (Saia, p 96)*

219. **(C)** The decubitus position is used to describe the patient who is recumbent (prone, supine, or lateral) with the central ray directed horizontally. When the patient is recumbent with the head lower than the feet, he or she is said to be in the Trendelenburg position. In the Fowler's position, the patient's head is positioned higher than the feet. The Sims' position is the (LAO) position assumed for enema tip insertion. *(Bontrager, p 20)*

220. **(C)** Ureteral reflux is best demonstrated during voiding. It can occur even when the bladder is only partially filled with a contrast medium. The *vesicourethral* orifice, as well as other sphincter muscles, relaxes during urination; however, the *vesicoureteral* orifices may also relax and cause reflux. *(Ballinger & Frank, vol 2, p 182)*

221. **(D)** The patient is supine with the leg *abducted* (drawn away from the midline) approximately 40°. This 40° abduction from the vertical places the long axis of the femoral neck parallel to the IR. *Adduction* is drawing the extremity closer to the midline of the body. *(Ballinger & Frank, vol 1, p 338)*

222. **(B)** Typically, traumatic injury to the hip requires a cross-table (axiolateral) lateral projection, as well as an AP projection of the entire pelvis. Both of these are performed using minimal manipulation of the affected extremity, reducing the possibility of further injury. A physician should perform any required manipulation of the traumatized hip. *(Ballinger & Frank, vol 1, pp 287, 290)*

223. **(A)** The hypersthenic body type is large and heavy. The thoracic cavity is short, the lungs are short with broad bases, and the heart is usually in an almost transverse position. The diaphragm is high; the stomach and gallbladder are high and transverse. The large bowel is positioned high and peripheral (and often requires that 14 × 17 cassettes be placed crosswise for imaging a BE). *(Ballinger & Frank, vol 1, p 41)*

224. **(D)** Prior to the start of an IVU, the patient should be instructed to empty the bladder. This is advised to avoid dilution of the contrast agent. Diluted contrast within the bladder will not affect the diagnosis of *renal* abnormalities, but it may obscure bladder abnormalities. The patient's allergy history should be reviewed to avoid the possibility of a severe reaction to the contrast agent. The patient's creatinine level and blood urea nitrogen (BUN) should be checked; significant elevation of these blood chemistry levels often suggests renal dysfunction. The normal BUN level is 8 to 25 mg/100 mL; normal creatinine range is 0.6 to 1.5 mg/100 mL. *(Ballinger & Frank, vol 2, p 168)*

225. **(D)** Although routine elbow projections may be essentially negative, conditions may exist (such as an elevated fat pad) that seem to indicate the presence of a small fracture of the radial head. To demonstrate the entire circumference of the radial head, four exposures are made with the elbow flexed 90° and with the humeral epicondyles superimposed and perpendicular to the cassette: one with the hand supinated as much as possible, one with the hand lateral, one with the hand pronated, and one with the hand in internal rotation, thumb down. Each maneuver changes the position of the radial head, and a different surface is pre-

sented for inspection. *(Ballinger & Frank, vol 1, pp 102–103)*

226. **(B)** The pictured radiograph was made in the right lateral decubitus position. It is part of a series of radiographs made during an air-contrast (double-contrast) BE examination. A double-contrast examination of the large bowel is performed to see *through* the bowel to its posterior wall and to visualize any *intraluminal* (eg, polypoid) *lesions* or *masses*. Various body positions are used to redistribute the barium and air. To demonstrate the medial and lateral walls of the bowel, decubitus positions are performed. The radiograph presents a right lateral decubitus position, because the *barium has gravitated* to the right side (the side of the hepatic flexure). The *air rises* and delineates the medial side of the ascending colon and the lateral side of the descending colon. The posterior wall of the rectum could be visualized using the ventral decubitus position and a horizontal beam lateral of the rectum. *(Ballinger & Frank, vol 2, pp 149–151)*

227. **(D)** Generally, contrast medium is injected into the subarachnoid space between the third and fourth lumbar vertebrae (Fig. 2–56). Because the spinal cord ends at the level of the first or second lumbar vertebra, this is considered to be a relatively safe injection site. The cisterna magna can be used, but the risk of contrast entering the ventricles and causing side effects increases. Diskography requires injection of contrast medium into the individual intervertebral disks. *(Saia, pp 197–198)*

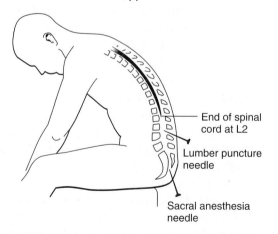

Figure 2–56. Reproduced with permission from deGroot, Correlative Neuroanatomy, 21st ed. Norwalk, CT: Appleton & Lange, 1991.

228. **(C)** *Hydronephrosis* is a collection of urine in the renal pelvis due to obstructed outflow, as from a stricture or obstruction. If the obstruction occurs at the level of the bladder or along the course of the ureter, it will be accompanied by the condition of hydroureter above the level of obstruction. These conditions may be demonstrated during IV urography. The term *pyelonephrosis* refers to some condition of the renal pelvis. *Nephroptosis* refers to drooping or downward displacement of the kidneys. This may be demonstrated using the erect position during IV urography. *Cystourethritis* is inflammation of the bladder and urethra. *(Taber's, p 1022)*

229. **(D)** Spinal column studies are often required for evaluation of adolescent scoliosis, thus presenting a twofold problem: radiation exposure to youthful gonadal and breast tissues, and significantly differing tissue densities/thicknesses. The use of a high-speed film–screen combination helps reduce the exposure required for the examination. Exposure dose concerns can also be resolved with the use of a compensating filter (for uniform density) that incorporates lead shielding for the breasts and gonads (Fig. 2–57). *(Ballinger & Frank, vol 1, pp 456–457)*

230. **(B)** *Diarthrodial* joints are freely movable joints that distinctively contain a joint capsule. Contrast is injected into this joint capsule to demonstrate the menisci, articular cartilage, bursae, and ligaments of the joint under investigation. *Synarthrodial* joints are immovable joints, composed of either cartilage or fibrous connective tissue. *Amphiarthrodial* joints allow only slight movement. *(Ballinger & Frank, vol 1, p 65)*

231. **(B)** The laryngeal prominence, or "Adam's Apple," is formed by the *thyroid cartilage*—the principal cartilage of the larynx. The thyroid *gland*, one of the endocrine glands, is lateral and inferior to the thyroid cartilage. The *vocal cords* are within the laryngeal cavity. Portions of the *pharynx* serve are passage for both air and food. *(Ballinger & Frank, vol 2, p 52)*

232. **(B)** To demonstrate the ankle joint space to best advantage, the plantar surface of the foot

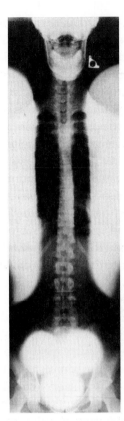

Figure 2–57. Courtesy of Nuclear Associates.

should be vertical in the AP projection of the ankle. Note that the fibula is the more distal of the two long bones of the lower leg, and forms the lateral malleolus. The calcaneus is not well visualized in this projection because of superimposition with other tarsals. *(Ballinger & Frank, vol 1, p 275)*

233. **(D)** Soft tissue neck studies can be performed for a number of reasons including to determine presence of foreign body or to evaluate the swallowing mechanism following a stroke event. Phonation of various vowel sounds, with or contrast media opacification, can help demonstrate the vocal cords. Performance of the Valsalva maneuver fills the larynx and trachea with air, which is then well demonstrated on soft tissue study. Pharyngeal structures are demonstrated during swallowing motion. *(Ballinger and Frank, vol 2, p 67)*

234. **(A)** The PA projection can be easily modified by redirecting the central ray to demonstrate a variety of structures. The central ray can be directed (1) 25° to 30° caudad for the rotundum foramina, (2) 20° to 25° caudad for the superior orbital fissures, or (3) 20° to 25° cephalad for the inferior orbital fissures. *(Ballinger & Frank, vol 2, p 242)*

235. **(C)** Deoxygenated (venous) blood from the *upper* body (head, neck, thorax, and upper extremities) empties into the *superior vena cava.* Deoxygenated (venous) blood from the *lower* body (abdomen, pelvis, and lower extremities) empties into the *inferior vena cava.* The superior and inferior venae cavae empty into the right atrium. The coronary sinus, which returns venous blood from the heart, also empties into the right atrium. Deoxygenated blood passes from the right atrium through the tricuspid valve into the right ventricle. From the right ventricle, blood is pumped (during ventricular systole) through the pulmonary semilunar valve into the pulmonary artery—the only artery that carries deoxygenated blood. From the pulmonary artery, blood travels to the lungs, picks up oxygen, and is carried by the four pulmonary veins (the only veins carrying oxygenated blood) to the left atrium. The oxygenated blood passes through the mitral (or bicuspid) valve during atrial systole and into the left ventricle. During ventricular systole, oxygenated blood from the left ventricle passes through the aortic semilunar valve into the aorta, and into the systemic circulation. *(Tortotra & Derrickson, p 758)*

236. **(B)** Whenever a part is being radiographed for demonstration of air–fluid levels, the central ray *must* be directed parallel to the floor. In this example, the patient was unable to tolerate the 90° tilt of the x-ray table. If the radiographer were to compensate for this by directing the central ray perpendicular to the IR (angling 20° caudad), it is very possible that any air–fluid level would be blurred and indistinct, and would go unrecognized. Remember that air or fluid always levels out parallel to the floor. Thus, if the air–fluid level needs to be demonstrated, the *central ray must also be parallel to the floor. (Ballinger & Frank, vol 2, p 376)*

237. **(D)** Standard radiographic protocols may be reduced to include two views, at right angles to each other, in emergency and trauma radiography. Department policy and procedure manuals include protocols for radiographic examinations. In the best interest of the patient, and to enable the radiologist to make an accurate diagnosis, standard radiographic protocols should be followed. If the radiographer must deviate from the protocol or believes that additional projections might be helpful, then this should be discussed with the radiologist. Emergency and trauma radiography is occasionally an exception to this rule. If the emergency department physician's request varies from the department protocol, the radiographer must respect this. A note should be added to the request so that the radiologist is informed of the reason for a change in protocol. For example, a patient who has been involved in a motor vehicle accident may need many radiographic studies, but the emergency department physician may order an AP chest and an AP and cross-table lateral C-spine only. Standard protocol may include a lateral chest and a cone-down view of the atlas and axis as well as cervical oblique views. The emergency department physician has made a decision the basis on of experience and expertise that overrules standard protocols. At a later time, when the patient has been stabilized, the patient may be sent back to radiology for additional views. *(Dowd & Wilson, vol 2, pp 1056–1057)*

238. **(C)** Blood pressure in the pulmonary circulation is relatively low, and therefore pulmonary vessels can easily become blocked by blood clots, air bubbles, or fatty masses, resulting in a *pulmonary embolism.* If the blockage stays in place, it results in an extra strain on the right ventricle, which is now unable to pump blood. This occurrence can result in congestive heart failure. *Pneumothorax* is air in the pleural cavity. *Atelectasis* is a collapsed lung or part of a lung. *Hypoxia* is a condition of low tissue oxygen. *(Tortora & Derrickson, p 685)*

239. **(B)** About 30 minutes after the ingestion of fatty foods, cholecystokinin is released from the duodenal mucosa and absorbed into the bloodstream. As a result, the gallbladder is

stimulated to contract, releasing bile into the intestine. *(Ballinger & Frank, vol 2, p 64)*

240. **(C)** In the direct PA projection of the wrist, the carpal pisiform is superimposed on the carpal triquetrum. The AP oblique projection (medial surface adjacent to the IR) separates the pisiform and triquetrum and projects the pisiform as a separate structure. The pisiform is the smallest and most palpable carpal. *(Ballinger & Frank, vol I, p 127)*

241. **(D)** The four body types (from largest to smallest) are hypersthenic, sthenic, hyposthenic, and asthenic. The abdominal viscera of the asthenic person are generally located quite low, vertical, and toward the midline. The opposite is true of the hypersthenic individual: Organs are located high, transverse, and lateral. *(Saia, p 76)*

242. **(C)** A zonogram is a thick tomographic section, or "cut"; it appears more similar to conventional radiography. A thick tomographic slice is produced by using a short exposure amplitude (arc), resulting in limited blurring of the radiographic image. Pluridirectional tomography produces maximal blurring of the radiographic image and generally uses a long exposure amplitude, resulting in a thin tomographic section or "cut." *(Ballinger & Frank, vol 3, pp 46–47)*

243. **(D)** A trimalleolar fracture involves three separate fractures. The lateral malleolus is fractured in the "typical" fashion, but the medial malleolus is fractured on both its medial and posterior aspects. The trimalleolar fracture is frequently associated with subluxation of the articular surfaces. *(Laudicina, p 184)*

244. **(C)** The *skeleton's* design functions to *protect* vital internal organs such as the heart and lungs. Bone stores important *minerals* (eg, calcium, phosphorus) and releases them into the blood as needed. Yellow bone marrow is composed mainly of fat cells and stores triglycerides for use as an energy reserve. The endocrine system is associated with hormone production; the integumentary system includes the skin that is important in protection and excretion; the muscular system is responsible for movement and heat production. *(Tortora & Derrickson, p 172)*

245. **(C)** Major branches of the common carotid arteries (internal carotids) function to supply the anterior brain, while the posterior brain is supplied by the vertebral arteries (branches of the subclavian). The brachiocephalic (innominate) artery is unpaired and is one of the three branches of the aortic arch, from which the right common carotid artery is derived. The left common carotid artery comes directly off the aortic arch. *(Tortora & Derrickson, pp 760, 764)*

246. **(A)** The base of the first metatarsal articulates with the first (medial) cuneiform. The base of the second metatarsal articulates with the second (intermediate) cuneiform; the third base of the metatarsal articulates with the third (lateral) cuneiform. The bases of the fourth and fifth metatarsals articulate with the cuboid. The navicular articulates with the first and second cuneiforms anteriorly and the talus posteriorly. *(Bontrager, p 198)*

247. **(B)** *Intussusception* is the telescoping of one part of the intestinal tract into another. It is a major cause of bowel obstruction in children, usually in the region of the ileocecal valve, and is much less common in the adult. Radiographically, intussusception appears as the classic "coil spring," with barium trapped between folds of the telescoped bowel. The diagnostic BE procedure can occasionally reduce the intussusception, although care must be taken to avoid perforation of the bowel. *Appendicitis* occurs when an obstructed appendix becomes inflamed. Distention of the appendix occurs and, if the appendix is left untended, gangrene and perforation can result. *Regional enteritis* (Crohn's disease) is a chronic granulomatous inflammatory disorder that can affect any part of the GI tract but generally involves the area of the terminal ileum. Ulceration and formation of fistulous tracts often occur. *Ulcerative colitis* occurs most often in the young adult; its etiology is unknown, although psychogenic or autoimmune factors seem to be involved. *(Bontrager, p 107)*

248. **(C)** An oblique projection of the lumbar spine is illustrated. This is a 45° LPO position demonstrating the apophyseal joints closest to the IR. The apophyseal joints are formed by the articulation of the inferior articular facets of one vertebra with the superior articular facets of the vertebra below. Note the "scotty dog" images that appear in the oblique lumbar spine. Intervertebral foramina are best visualized in the lateral lumbar position. (*Bontrager, p 320*)

249. **(A)** The chest should be examined in the upright position whenever possible to demonstrate any air–fluid levels. For the *lateral* projection, the patient elevates the arms and flexes and grasps the elbows. The midsagittal and midcoronal planes must remain vertical to avoid distortion of the heart. In the *PA* projection, the shoulders should be relaxed and depressed to move the clavicles below the lung apices, and the shoulders should be rolled forward to move the scapulae out of the lung fields. (*Ballinger & Frank, vol 1, pp 528–529*)

250. **(B)** A cross-sectional image of the abdomen is pictured in Figure 2–34. The large structure on the right, labeled 1, is the liver. The gallbladder is seen as a somewhat darker density on the medial border of the liver. The left kidney is labeled 4; the right kidney is clearly seen on the other side. The vertebra is labeled number 5, and the psoas muscles are seen just posterior to the vertebra. Just anterior to the body of the vertebra is the circular aorta, labeled 3 (some calcification can be seen as brighter densities). The somewhat flattened inferior vena cava (number 2) is seen to the left of, and slightly anterior to, the aorta. (*Bontrager, p 100*)

251. **(A)** The knee (tibiofemoral joint) is the largest joint of the body, formed by the articulation of the femur and tibia. However, it actually consists of three articulations: the patellofemoral joint, the lateral tibiofemoral joint (lateral femoral condyle with tibial plateau), and the medial tibiofemoral joint (medial femoral condyle with tibial plateau). Although the knee is classified as a synovial (diarthrotic) hinge-type joint, the patellofemoral joint is actually a gliding joint, and the medial and

lateral tibiofemoral joints are hinge-type. (*Ballinger & Frank, vol 1, p 226*)

252. **(A)** Femoral necks are nonpalpable bony landmarks. The ASIS, pubic symphysis, and greater trochanter are palpable bony landmarks used in radiography of the pelvis and for localization of the femoral necks. (*Ballinger & Frank, vol 1, p 274*)

253. **(C)** The full length of the nasal septum is best demonstrated in the parietoacanthial (Waters' method) projection. This is also the single best view for facial bones. The PA axial (Caldwell method) projection superimposes the petrous structures over the nasal septum, while the lateral projection superimposes and obscures good visualization of the septum. The AP axial projection is used to demonstrate the occipital bone. (*Ballinger & Frank, vol 2, pp 316–317*)

254. **(A)** The knee joint is formed by the femur, tibia, and patella. The most superior aspect of the tibia is the *tibial plateau*—formed by the *tibial condyles just distal* to it. The proximal tibia also presents the *tibial tuberosity* on its anterior surface, just distal to the condyles. *Proximal* to the tibial plateau, and articulating with it, are the *femoral condyles*. The term *proximal* refers to a part located closer to the point of attachment; the term *distal* refers to a part located farther away from the point of attachment. (*Bontrager, pp 202–203*)

255. **(D)** A successful oral cholecystogram depends on the ability of the liver to remove contrast from the portal bloodstream and to excrete it with bile. A healthy gallbladder should concentrate and store bile as well as contrast medium. With a functioning gallbladder and liver, an opacified gallbladder should result. The pancreas plays an integral part in the digestive process, but it is not in the biliary system. (*Ballinger & Frank, vol 2, p 58*)

256. **(C)** In the *AP* projection of the elbow, the radial head and ulna are normally somewhat superimposed. The *lateral oblique* demonstrates the radial head free of superimposition with the ulna. The *lateral* projection demonstrates the olecranon process in profile. The *medial oblique* position demonstrates considerable overlap of the proximal ulna, but should clearly demonstrate the coronoid process free of superimposition and the olecranon process within the olecranon fossa. *(Saia, p 98)*

257. **(C)** The *posterior oblique* positions of the cervical spine (LPO and RPO) require that the central ray be directed 15° to C4. The posterior obliques demonstrate the intervertebral foramina *farther* away from the IR. The *anterior* oblique positions require a 15° caudal angulation and demonstrate the intervertebral foramina *closest* to the IR. *(Ballinger & Frank, vol 1, pp 402–403)*

258. **(C)** The degree of anterior and posterior motion is occasionally diminished with a "whiplash"-type injury. Anterior (forward, flexion) and posterior (backward, extension) motion is evaluated in the lateral position, with the patient assuming the best possible flexion and extension. Left- and right-bending images of the thoracic and lumbar vertebrae are frequently obtained when evaluating scoliosis. *(Saia, p 126)*

259. **(A)** When one cheekbone is depressed, a tangential projection is required to "open up" the zygomatic arch and draw it away from the overlying cranial bones. This is accomplished by placing the patient in the *SMV* position, rotating the head 15° toward the affected side, and centering to the zygomatic arch. A 30 rotation places the mandibular shadow over the zygomatic arch. *(Ballinger & Frank, vol 2, pp 328–329)*

260. **(B)** In the prone oblique positions (RAO and LAO), the flexure disclosed is the one closer to the IR. Therefore, the LAO position will "open up" the splenic flexure, and the RAO will demonstrate the hepatic flexure. The AP oblique positions (RPO and LPO) demonstrate the side farther from the IR. *(Bontrager, p 510)*

261. **(C)** The SMV (Schüller method) projection of the skull requires that the patient's neck be extended, placing the vertex adjacent to the IR holder/upright Bucky, so that the *IOML* is parallel with the IR. This projection is useful for demonstrating the ethmoidal and sphenoidal sinuses, pars petrosae, mandible, and foramina ovale and spinosum. In the illustration, line 1 represents the *glabellomeatal* line (GML), line 2 is the *orbitomeatal* line (OML), line 3 is the *infraorbitomeatal* line (IOML), and line 4 is the *acanthomeatal* line (AML). Accurate positioning of the skull requires the use of several baselines. The *OML* and the *IOML* are usually separated by 7°. The orbitomeatal line and the glabellomeatal line are usually separated by 8° (therefore, there is 15° between the GML and the IOML). It is useful to remember these differences, because central ray angulation must be adjusted when using a baseline other than the one recommended for a particular position. For example, if it is recommended that the central ray be angled *30° to the OML*, then the central ray would be angled *37° to the IOML*. *(Bontrager, p 407)*

262. **(C)** The lateral projection of the skull requires that the patient be in the prone oblique position with the MSP parallel to the IR and the interpupillary line perpendicular to the IR. The *IOML* (line 3) must be parallel to the long axis of the IR. The supraorbital margins, anterior clinoid processes, and posterior clinoid processes should be superimposed. *(Saia, p 144)*

263. **(A)** Radiographic measurement of long bone length can be required on adults or children having extremity length (especially leg) discrepancies. This can be most easily performed with the use of the metallic *Bell–Thompson scale* secured to the x-ray tabletop adjacent to the limb being examined (or between both limbs for simultaneous bilateral examination. A 14 × 17 cassette is in the Bucky tray and 3 well-collimated exposures are made: at the hip joint, the knee joint, and the ankle joint. A *cannula* is a tube placed in a cavity to introduce or withdraw material. A *speculum* is an instrument for examining canals or hollow organs, for example, a vaginal speculum used in hysterosalpingograms. *(Bontrager, p 743)*

264. **(C)** The forward slipping of one vertebra on the one below it is called *spondylolisthesis*. *Spondylolysis* is the breakdown of the pars interarticularis; it may be unilateral or bilateral

and results in forward slipping of the involved vertebra—the condition of spondylolisthesis. Inflammation of one or more vertebrae is called *spondylitis. Spondylosis* refers to degenerative changes occurring in the vertebra. *(Ballinger & Frank, vol 1, p 321)*

265. **(C)** The patient is placed in a true lateral position, and the central ray is directed perpendicular to a point 3/4 in distal to the nasion. An 8 × 10 cassette divided in half may be used for this procedure. *(Ballinger & Frank, vol 2, p 315)*

266. **(B)** A *frontal* projection (AP or PA) demonstrates the medial and lateral relationship of structures. A *lateral* projection demonstrates the anterior and posterior relationship of structures. Two views, at right angles to each other, are generally taken of most structures. *(Saia, pp 80, 82)*

267. **(A)** The posterior oblique positions (LPO and RPO) of the lumbar vertebrae demonstrate the apophyseal joints closer to the IR. The left apophyseal joints are demonstrated in the *LPO* position, while the right apophyseal joints are demonstrated in the *RPO* position. The *lateral* position is useful to demonstrate the intervertebral disk spaces, intervertebral foramina, and spinous processes. *(Saia, p 131)*

268. **(B)** Blowout fractures of the orbital floor are well demonstrated by using Waters' method [parietoacanthial (PA) projection] and by using tomographic studies. A PA with the OML perpendicular and the central ray angled 30° caudad will demonstrate the orbital floor in profile. Sweet's localization method shows the exact placement of foreign bodies within the eye. *(Ballinger & Frank, vol 2, p 270)*

269. **(D)** The phase of respiration is exceedingly important in thoracic radiography, as lung expansion and the position of the diaphragm strongly influence the appearance of the finished radiograph. Inspiration and expiration radiographs of the chest are taken to demonstrate air in the pleural cavity (*pneumothorax*), to demonstrate *atelectasis* (partial or complete collapse of one or more pulmonary lobes) or the degree of *diaphragm excursion*, or to detect

the presence of a *foreign body.* The expiration image will require a somewhat greater exposure (6 to 8 kV more) to compensate for the diminished quantity of air in the lungs. *(Ballinger & Frank, vol 1, p 444)*

270. **(B)** Shoulder arthrograms (Fig. 2–58) are used to evaluate rotator cuff tear, glenoid labrum (a ring of fibrocartilaginous tissue around the glenoid fossa), and frozen shoulder. Acromioclavicular joint separation is demonstrated on erect AP images with and without the use of weights. Routine radiographs demonstrate arthritis, and the addition of a transthoracic humerus or scapular Y would demonstrate dislocation. *(Ballinger & Frank, vol 1, p 496)*

271. **(C)** In the parieto-orbital projection, the patient is PA with the acanthomeatal line perpendicular to the IR. The head rests on the zygoma, nose, and chin, and the MSP should form a 53° angle with the IR (37° with the central ray). Radiographically, the optic canal should appear in the *lower outer quadrant* of the orbit. Incorrect rotation of the MSP results in lateral displacement, and incorrect positioning of the baseline results in longitudinal displacement. *(Ballinger & Frank, vol 2, pp 290–291)*

272. **(B)** Changes in hormone levels affect changes in the glandular tissue of the breast. These

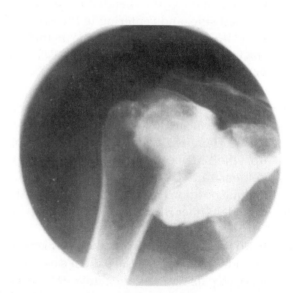

Figure 2–58. Courtesy of Stamford Hospital, Department of Radiology.

breast tissue changes are seen during breast development, during pregnancy and lactation, and during menopause. Women at higher risk of developing breast cancer include those having experienced early menses (before age 12 years), late menopause (after age 52 years), and nulliparity (no full- or late-term pregnancies). Risks other than hormonal include family and personal history and age. The greatest single risk factor for breast cancer is gender—being female. Although occurrence of breast cancer in men is not unknown, it is fairly rare. *(Peart, p. 1)*

273. **(C)** There are several surface landmarks and localization points that can help the radiographer in positioning various body structures. The *jugular notch*, located at the superior aspect of the manubrium, is approximately opposite the T2–3 interspace. The *sternal angle* is located opposite the T4–5 interspace. The *xiphoid* (or ensiform) *process* is located opposite T10. *(Saia, p 77)*

274. **(D)** With the patient in the AP position, the scapula and upper thorax are normally superimposed. With the arm abducted, the elbow flexed, and the hand supinated, much of the scapula is drawn away from the ribs. The patient should not be rotated toward the affected side, as this causes superimposition of ribs on the scapula. The exposure is made during quiet breathing to obliterate pulmonary vascular markings. *(Ballinger & Frank, vol 1, pp 202–203)*

275. **(D)** The typical vertebra has two parts, the body and the vertebral arch. The body is the dense, anterior bony mass. Posteriorly attached is the vertebral arch, a ringlike structure. The vertebral arch is formed by two pedicles (short, thick processes projecting posteriorly from the body) and two laminae (broad, flat processes projecting posteriorly and medially from the pedicles). *(Saia, p 123)*

276. **(D)** The mediastinum is the space between the lungs that contains the heart, great vessels, trachea, esophagus, and thymus gland. It is bounded anteriorly by the sternum and posteriorly by the vertebral column and extends from the upper thorax to the diaphragm. *(Ballinger & Frank, vol 1, p 511)*

277. **(D)** This is a modification of the parietoacanthial projection (Waters' method) in which the patient is requested to open the mouth, and then the skull is positioned so that the OML forms a 37° angle with the IR. The central ray is directed through the sphenoidal sinuses and exits the open mouth. The routine parietoacanthial projection (with mouth closed) is used to demonstrate the maxillary sinuses projected above the petrous pyramids. The frontal and ethmoidal sinuses are best visualized in the PA axial position (modified Caldwell method). *(Saia, p 150)*

278. **(C)** The ribs below the diaphragm are best demonstrated with the diaphragm elevated. This is accomplished by placing the patient in a recumbent position and by taking the exposure at the end of exhalation. Conversely, the ribs above the diaphragm are best demonstrated with the diaphragm depressed. Placing the patient in the erect position and taking the exposure at the end of deep inspiration accomplishes this. *(Ballinger & Frank, vol 1, p 428)*

279. **(D)** The *exact axial* projection is performed by placing the patient in a lordotic position, leaning against the vertical grid device. This places the clavicle at right angles, or nearly so, to the plane of the IR. The central ray is directed to enter the inferior border of the clavicle, at right angles to its coronal plane. Other *axial* projections may include a prone position with a 25° to 30° caudal angle. However, none of these produce an exact axial projection of the clavicle. *(Ballinger & Frank, vol 1, p 159)*

280. **(B)** An axial *dorsoplantar* projection of the calcaneus is described; the central ray enters the dorsal surface of the foot and exits the plantar surface. The *plantodorsal* projection is done *supine* and requires cephalad angulation. The central ray enters the plantar surface and exits the dorsal surface. *(Ballinger & Frank, vol 1, p 263)*

281. **(D)** During GI radiography, the position of the stomach may vary depending on the respiratory phase, the body habitus, and the patient position. *Inspiration* causes the lungs to fill with air and the diaphragm to descend,

thereby pushing the abdominal contents downward. On *expiration*, the diaphragm will rise, allowing the abdominal organs to ascend. Body *habitus* is an important factor in determining the size and shape of the stomach. An asthenic patient may have a long, J-shaped stomach, while the stomach of a hypersthenic patient may be transverse. The body habitus is an important consideration in determining the positioning and placement of the cassette. The patient *position* can also alter the position of the stomach. If a patient turns from the RAO position into the AP position, the stomach will move into a more horizontal position. Although the cardiac sphincter and the pyloric sphincter are relatively fixed, the fundus is quite mobile and will vary in position. *(Dowd & Wilson, vol 2, p 778)*

282. **(A)** With a patient in the PA position and the OML perpendicular to the table, a 15° to 20° caudal angulation would place the petrous ridges in the lower third of the orbit. To achieve the same result in a baby or a small child, it is necessary for the radiographer to decrease the angulation or modify the angulation to 10° to 15° caudal. The reason for this can be understood by examining the baselines for skull positioning. In the adult skull, the OML and IOML are about 7° apart. In a baby or small child, the difference is larger, about 15° apart. Remember that in adults, the head makes up about one seventh the length of the body. In children, the head is about one fourth the length of the body. These differences must be considered in radiographic examination of the skull for babies. *(Ballinger & Frank, vol 3, p 26)*

283. **(B)** The patient position for operative cholangiography is 15° to 20° RPO. Remember that the gallbladder lies in the right upper quadrant. Because the radiographs are obtained while the patient has an indwelling T-tube, they must be obtained with the patient in the supine rather than the prone position. A slight oblique (15° to 20°) will allow visualization of the biliary tract free of superimposition from the vertebrae. The LPO would place the biliary vessels over the spine. A 45° oblique is too steep for visualization of the gallbladder and biliary tree. *(Ballinger & Frank, vol 2, p 76)*

284. **(D)** The brain is generally described as having three divisions. The *forebrain* is composed of the cerebrum, the thalamus, and the hypothalamus. The *midbrain* is a short, constricted portion connecting the forebrain to the hindbrain, containing the corpora quadrigemina and Aqueduct of Sylvius. The *hindbrain* is composed of the pons, medulla oblongata, and cerebellum. *The brain stem is defined as the midbrain, pons, and medulla oblongata. (Bontrager, p 706)*

285. **(A)** Knee arthrography may be performed to demonstrate torn meniscus (cartilage), Baker's cyst, loose bodies, and ligament damage. A torn rotator cuff would be demonstrated on a shoulder, not a knee arthrogram. *(Bontrager, p 726)*

286. **(A)** The tangential axial projections of the patella are also often referred to as *"sunrise"* or *"skyline"* views. The supine flexion 45° (Merchant) position requires a *special apparatus*, and the patellae can be examined bilaterally. This position also requires patient comfort *without muscle tension*—muscle tension can cause a subluxed patella to be pulled into the intercondyler sulcus, giving the appearance of a normal patella. The two prone positions differ according to the degree of flexion employed. The 90° flexion (Settegast) position must not be employed with suspected patellar fracture. *(Bontrager, pp 240, 241)*

287. **(B)** When the foot is positioned for a lateral projection, the plantar surface should be perpendicular to the IR, so as to superimpose the metatarsals. This may be accomplished with the patient lying on either the affected or the unaffected side (usually the affected), that is, mediolateral or lateromedial. The talofibular articulation is best demonstrated in the medial oblique projection of the ankle. *(Ballinger & Frank, vol 1, p 251)*

288. **(D)** Hysterosalpingography may be performed for demonstration of uterine tubal patency, mass lesions in the uterine cavity, and uterine position. Although hysterosalpingography is often performed to check tubal patency, the uterine anatomy, position, and morphology are also exhibited. In addition, polyps, fibroids,

or space-occupying lesions within the uterus are well demonstrated. *(Ballinger & Frank, vol 2, pp 218–219)*

289. **(D)** A fluoroscopic unit with spot device and tilt table should be used for endoscopic retrograde pancreatography. The Trendelenburg position is sometimes necessary to fill the interhepatic ducts, and a semierect position may be necessary to fill the lower end of the common bile duct. Also necessary are a fiberoptic endoscope for locating the hepatopancreatic ampulla and polyethylene catheters for the introduction of contrast media. *(Ballinger & Frank, vol 2, p 80)*

290. **(D)** Radiography of pediatric patients with a myelomeningocele defect should be performed in the prone position, rather than the routine supine position. The supine position would put unnecessary pressure on the protrusion of the meninges and spinal cord. All of the other statements in the question are true. The anatomic dimensions of children are different from those of adults, and this must be kept in mind when performing pediatric radiography. The liver occupies a larger area of the abdominal cavity in a child than in an adult. This causes the kidneys to be in a lower position. Generally, the kidneys will be midway between the diaphragm and the symphysis pubis. Chest radiography for the pediatric patient varies depending on the age of the child. Neonates are routinely radiographed in the supine position. Although infants may also be examined in the supine position, it is preferable to examine them by placing the infant securely in a support device to obtain a good PA erect radiograph. Exceptions to this rule are made if the infant is in respiratory distress. To avoid aggravating the respiratory distress, an erect AP radiograph is usually obtained. *(Dowd & Wilson, vol 2, pp 1004–1005, 1013)*

291. **(D)** Operative cholangiography may be performed to visualize biliary stones or a neoplasm, determine the function of the hepatopancreatic ampulla, and examine the patency of the biliary tract. Any strictures or obstructions may be localized when contrast medium is introduced into the catheter and

images are obtained. It is important that no air bubbles are introduced into the biliary tract because they can imitate radiolucent stones. The radiographer can coordinate the time of exposure with the anesthesiologist to obtain the radiographs during suspended respiration. *(Ballinger & Frank, vol 2, pp 76–77)*

292. **(A)** The axial trauma lateral (Coyle) is described. If routine elbow projections in extension are not possible because of limited part movement, this position can be used to demonstrate the coronoid process and/or radial head. With the elbow flexed 90° and the CR directed to the elbow joint at an angle of 45° medially (ie, toward the shoulder), the joint space between the *radial head* and capitulum should be revealed. With the elbow flexed *80°* and the CR directed to the elbow joint at an angle of 45° laterally (ie, from the shoulder toward the elbow), the elongated *coronoid process* will be visualized. *(Bontrager, p 160)*

293. **(C)** The foot is composed of the 7 tarsal bones, 5 metatarsals, and 14 phalanges. The metatarsals and phalanges are miniature long bones; each has a shaft, base (proximal), and head (distal). The bases of the first to third metatarsals articulate with the three cuneiforms. The bases of the fourth and fifth metatarsals articulate with the cuboid. The heads of the metatarsals articulate with the bases of the first row of phalanges. *(Bontrager, p 196)*

294. **(C)** Arthrography requires the use of local, rather than general, anesthesia. Sterile technique should be employed to avoid introducing infection into the joint. Other possible complications of arthrography include pain, trauma to nearby structures, and capsular rupture. It is recommended that contrast agents with meglumine salts, rather than sodium salts, be used, as they have been found to be less painful when introduced into joint spaces. Fluoroscopy is used for proper placement of the needle and to obtain images immediately after the introduction of contrast medium. *(Ballinger & Frank, vol 1, pp 560–561)*

295. **(C)** The contrast media of choice for use in myelography are nonionic water-soluble. For years, Pantopaque, a non–water-soluble (ethyl ester) contrast agent, was used for radiographic demonstration of the spinal canal. Because it was nonsoluble, it had to be removed after the procedure. Metrizamide was the first nonionic contrast agent introduced for use in myelography, but it has been replaced with iohexol and iopamidol, which are cheaper and safer and do not dissipate as quickly. Ionic contrast media are not used for intrathecal injections because they are too toxic, and gas or air does not provide adequate demonstration. *(Bontrager, p 135)*

296. **(B)** The cephalic, basilic, and subclavian veins should be demonstrated on an upper-limb venogram. Venography of the upper limb is usually performed to rule out venous obstruction or thrombosis. The injection site is usually in the hand or wrist, and images should be obtained up to the area of the superior vena cava. *(Ballinger & Frank, vol 2, p 540)*

297. **(C)** Neither an antishock garment nor a pneumatic splint should be removed by the radiographer prior to performing radiographic examination. A *ring* may certainly be removed whenever possible before performing a hand radiograph. An *antishock* garment is used when a patient has suffered a traumatic incident and is suffering from internal bleeding; it functions to slow the rate of bleeding. An *air cast* may be used to temporarily support a fractured limb until surgery and/or a more permanent cast is in place. Both antishock garments and air splints are *radiolucent;* most rings are radiopaque. *(Adler & Carlton, pp 165–166)*

298. **(A)** The sacroiliac joints angle posteriorly and medially 25° to the MSP. Therefore, to demonstrate the sacroiliac joints with the patient in the *AP* position, the *affected* side must be elevated 25°. This places the joint space perpendicular to the IR and parallel to the central ray. Therefore, the *RPO* position will demonstrate the *left sacroiliac joint*, and the *LPO* position will demonstrate the *right sacroiliac joint*. When the examination is performed with the patient *PA*, the *unaffected* side will be elevated 25°. *(Ballinger & Frank, vol 1, pp 442–443)*

299. **(C)** When imaging a patient with a possible traumatic spine injury, it is appropriate to either maneuver the x-ray tube head or, if the patient must be moved, to use the log-rolling method. This cannot be done by one person; the radiographer must summon assistance. If the patient is on a backboard and in a neck collar, as most patients with suspected spine injury are, it is never appropriate to ask the patient to turn, scoot, or slide over. The only movement that should be permitted is movement of the entire spine, body, and head together, as in log rolling. Any twisting could cause severe and permanent damage to the spinal cord, resulting in paralysis or even death. *(Torres et al, pp 77–79)*

300. **(B)** The type of fracture in which the splintered ends of bone are forced through the skin is a *compound* fracture. In a *closed* fracture, no bone protrudes through the skin. *Compression* fractures are seen in stressed areas, such as the vertebrae. A *depressed* fracture would not protrude, but rather would be pushed in. *(Bontrager, p 596)*

Subspecialty List

168. Extremity imaging
169. Extremity imaging
170. Cranium imaging
171. Extremity imaging
172. General procedural considerations
173. Abdomen and GI studies
174. Spine and pelvis imaging
175. Cranium imaging
176. Extremity imaging
177. Thorax imaging
178. Extremity imaging
179. Spine and pelvis imaging
180. Extremity imaging
181. Cranium imaging
182. Thorax imaging
183. Spine and pelvis imaging
184. Abdomen and GI studies
185. Abdomen and GI studies
186. Extremity imaging
187. General procedural considerations
188. Extremity imaging
189. Extremity imaging
190. Spine and pelvis imaging
191. Urologic studies
192. Spine and pelvis imaging
193. Extremity imaging
194. Abdomen and GI studies
195. Other procedures
196. Extremity imaging
197. Extremity imaging
198. Other procedures
199. General procedural considerations
200. Cranium imaging
201. Thorax imaging
202. Abdomen and GI studies
203. Extremity imaging
204. Thorax imaging
205. Spine and pelvis imaging
206. Other procedures
207. Extremity imaging
208. Abdomen and GI studies
209. Other procedures
210. Abdomen and GI studies
211. Extremity imaging
212. Extremity imaging
213. Spine and pelvis imaging
214. Urologic studies
215. Spine and pelvis imaging
216. Extremity imaging
217. Spine and pelvis imaging
218. Extremity imaging
219. General procedural considerations
220. Urological studies
221. Spine and pelvis imaging
222. Extremity imaging
223. General procedural considerations
224. Urologic studies
225. Extremity imaging
226. Abdomen and GI studies
227. Other procedures
228. Urological studies
229. Spine and pelvis imaging
230. Other procedures
231. Thorax imaging
232. Extremity imaging
233. Thorax imaging
234. Cranium imaging
235. Thorax imaging
236. Abdomen and GI studies
237. General procedural considerations
238. Cardiovascular/neurologic/miscellaneous imaging
239. Abdomen and GI studies
240. Extremity imaging
241. Abdomen and GI studies
242. Urological studies
243. Extremity imaging
244. Extremity imaging
245. Other procedures
246. Extremity imaging
247. Abdomen and GI studies
248. Spine and pelvis imaging
249. Thorax imaging
250. Other procedures
251. Extremity imaging
252. Spine and pelvis imaging
253. Cranium imaging
254. Extremity imaging
255. Abdomen and GI studies
256. Extremity imaging
257. Spine and pelvis imaging
258. Spine and pelvis imaging
259. Cranium imaging
260. Abdomen and GI studies
261. Cranium imaging
262. Cranium imaging
263. Extremity imaging
264. Spine and pelvis imaging
265. Cranium imaging
266. Extremity imaging
267. Spine and pelvis imaging
268. Head and neck imaging

269. Thorax imaging
270. Extremity imaging
271. Cranium imaging
272. Other procedures
273. Extremity imaging
274. Extremity imaging
275. Spine and pelvis imaging
276. Thorax imaging
277. Cranium imaging
278. Thorax imaging
279. Extremity imaging
280. Extremity imaging
281. Abdomen and GI studies
282. Cranium imaging
283. Abdomen and GI studies
284. Cranium imaging
285. Extremity imaging
286. Extremity imaging
287. Extremity imaging
288. Other procedures
289. Abdomen and GI studies
290. Other procedures
291. Abdomen and GI studies
292. Extremity imaging
293. Extremity imaging
294. Other procedures
295. Other procedures
296. Other procedures
297. General procedural considerations
298. Spine and pelvis imaging
299. Spine and pelvis imaging
300. Extremity imaging

Radiation Protection
Questions

1. Late effects of radiation, whose incidence is dose related and for which there is no threshold dose, are referred to as

   (A) nonstochastic.
   (B) stochastic.
   (C) chromosomal aberration.
   (D) hematologic depression.

2. Acording to the NCRP, the annual occupational dose equivalent limit to the lens of the eye is

   A. 1 mSv.
   B. 50 mSv.
   C. 150 mSv.
   D. 500 mSv.

3. How is the intensity of an x-ray photon affected after each time it scatters?

   (A) Its intensity increases 4 times.
   (B) Its intensity increases 1000 times.
   (C) Its intensity decreases 4 times.
   (D) Its intensity decreases 1000 times.

4. If the exposure rate to an individual standing 2.0 m from a source of radiation is 15 R/min, what will be the dose received after 2 minutes at a distance of 5 m from the source?

   (A) 1.2 R
   (B) 2.4 R
   (C) 4.8 R
   (D) 9.6 R

5. All of the following statements regarding mobile radiographic equipment are true, *except*

   (A) the exposure cord must permit the operator to stand at least 4 feet from the patient, x-ray tube, and useful beam.
   (B) exposure switches must be the "dead man" type.
   (C) a lead apron should be carried with the unit and worn by the radiographer during exposure.
   (D) the radiographer must alert individuals in the area before making the exposure.

6. Late or long-term effects of radiation exposure are generally represented by which of the following dose–response curves?

   (A) Linear threshold
   (B) Linear nonthreshold
   (C) Nonlinear threshold
   (D) Nonlinear nonthreshold

7. If the exposure rate to a body standing 5 feet from a radiation source is 10 mR/min, what will be the dose to that body at a distance of 8 feet from the source?

(A) 25.6 mR/min
(B) 16 mR/min
(C) 6.25 mR/min
(D) 3.9 mR/min

8. The use of which of the following intensifying screen phosphor materials can help in reducing patient dose?

1. Calcium tungstate
2. Gadolinium
3. Lanthanum

(A) 1 only
(B) 1 and 2 only
(C) 2 and 3 only
(D) 1, 2, and 3

9. What is the approximate entrance skin exposure (ESE) for the average AP supine lumbar spine radiograph?

A. 350 rad
B. 350 mrad
C. 35 rad
D. 35 mrad

10. The use of which of the following devices helps reduce patient dose?

1. Grid
2. Collimator
3. Gonad shield

(A) 1 only
(B) 1 and 2 only
(C) 2 and 3 only
(D) 1, 2, and 3

11. How will x-ray photon intensity be affected if the SID is doubled?

(A) Its intensity increases two times.
(B) Its intensity increases four times.
(C) Its intensity decreases two times.
(D) Its intensity decreases four times.

12. What is the established fetal dose limit guideline for pregnant radiographers during the entire gestation period?

(A) 100 mrem
(B) 250 mrem
(C) 500 mrem
(D) 1000 mrem

13. Some patients, such as infants and children, are unable to maintain the necessary radiographic position without assistance. If mechanical restraining devices cannot be used, which of the following should be requested or permitted to hold this patient?

(A) Transporter
(B) Patient's father
(C) Patient's mother
(D) Student radiographer

14. Sources of natural background radiation contributing to whole-body radiation dose include

1. terrestrial radionuclides.
2. internal radionuclides.
3. nuclear medicine.

(A) 1 only
(B) 1 and 2 only
(C) 2 and 3 only
(D) 1, 2, and 3

15. Irradiation of water molecules within the body, and their resulting breakdown, is termed

(A) epilation.
(B) radiolysis.
(C) proliferation.
(D) repopulation.

16. Which of the following is (are) important for patient protection during fluoroscopic procedures?

    1. Intermittent fluoroscopy
    2. Fluoroscopic field size
    3. Focus-to-table distance

    (A) 1 and 2 only
    (B) 1 and 3 only
    (C) 2 and 3 only
    (D) 1, 2, and 3

17. What is used to account for the differences in ionizing characteristics of various radiations, when determining their effect on biologic material?

    1. Radiation weighting factors (W_r)
    2. Tissue weighting factors (W_t)
    3. Absorbed dose

    (A) 1 only
    (B) 1 and 2 only
    (C) 2 and 3 only
    (D) 1, 2, and 3

18. The x-ray interaction with matter that is responsible for the majority of scattered radiation reaching the IR is

    (A) the photoelectric effect.
    (B) Compton scatter.
    (C) classical scatter.
    (D) Thompson scatter.

19. If a patient received 2000 mrad during a 10-minute fluoroscopic examination, what was the dose rate?

    (A) 0.2 rad/min
    (B) 2.0 rad/min
    (C) 5 rad/min
    (D) 200 rad/min

20. With mA increased to maintain output intensity, how is the ESE affected as the SSD is increased?

    (A) The ESE increases.
    (B) The ESE decreases.
    (C) The ESE remains unchanged.
    (D) ESE is unrelated to SSD.

21. Sources of natural background radiation exposure include

    1. the food we eat.
    2. air travel.
    3. medical and dental x-rays.

    (A) 1 only
    (B) 1 and 2 only
    (C) 2 and 3 only
    (D) 1, 2, and 3

22. Each time an x-ray beam scatters, its intensity at 1 m from the scattering object is what fraction of its original intensity?

    (A) 1/10
    (B) 1/100
    (C) 1/500
    (D) 1/1000

23. According to the NCRP, the annual occupational whole-body dose equivalent limit is

    A. 1 mSv.
    B. 50 mSv.
    C. 150 mSv.
    D. 500 mSv.

24. A thermoluminescent dosimetry system would use which of the following crystals?

    (A) Silver bromide
    (B) Sodium sulfite
    (C) Lithium fluoride
    (D) Aluminum oxide

25. Sources of secondary radiation include

    1. background radiation.
    2. leakage radiation.
    3. scattered radiation.

    (A) 1 only
    (B) 1 and 2 only
    (C) 2 and 3 only
    (D) 1, 2, and 3

26. All of the following affect patient dose *except*

    (A) inherent filtration.
    (B) added filtration.
    (C) source-image distance.
    (D) focal spot size.

27. The photoelectric effect is an interaction between an x-ray photon and

    (A) an inner-shell electron.
    (B) an outer-shell electron.
    (C) a nucleus.
    (D) another photon.

28. Which of the following radiation exposure responses exhibit a nonlinear threshold dose–response relationship?

    1. Skin erythema
    2. Hematologic depression
    3. Lethality

    (A) 1 only
    (B) 1 and 2 only
    (C) 2 and 3 only
    (D) 1, 2, and 3

29. In radiation protection, the product of absorbed dose and the correct modifying factor (rad × QF) is used to determine

    (A) roentgen (C/kg).
    (B) rem (Sv).
    (C) rad (Gy).
    (D) radiation quality.

30. Which of the following are recommended for the pregnant radiographer?

    1. Continue monthly dosimeter readings.
    2. Wear a second dosimeter under the lead apron.
    3. Wear two dosimeters and switch their position periodically.

    (A) 1 only
    (B) 1 and 2 only
    (C) 1 and 3 only
    (D) 2 and 3 only

31. The annual dose limit for medical imaging personnel includes radiation from

    1. medical x-rays.
    2. occupational exposure.
    3. background radiation.

    (A) 1 only
    (B) 2 only
    (C) 2 and 3 only
    (D) 1, 2, and 3

32. What is likely to occur if 25 rad is accidentally delivered to a recently fertilized ovum?

    (A) Skeletal anomalies
    (B) CNS anomalies
    (C) Spontaneous abortion
    (D) Childhood malignancy

33. The symbols $^{130}_{56}Ba$ and $^{138}_{56}Ba$ are examples of which of the following?

    (A) Isotopes
    (B) Isobars
    (C) Isotones
    (D) Isomers

34. Medical and dental radiation accounts for what percentage of the general public's exposure to man-made radiation?

    (A) 10%
    (B) 50%
    (C) 75%
    (D) 90%

35. Which of the following is (are) possible long-term somatic effects of radiation exposure?

1. Nausea and vomiting
2. Carcinogenesis
3. Leukemia

(A) 1 only
(B) 1 and 2 only
(C) 2 and 3 only
(D) 1, 2, and 3

36. How does filtration affect the primary beam?

(A) It increases the average energy of the primary beam.
(B) It decreases the average energy of the primary beam.
(C) It makes the primary beam more penetrating.
(D) It increases the intensity of the primary beam.

37. The skin response to radiation exposure, which appears as reddening of the irradiated skin area, is known as

(A) dry desquamation.
(B) moist desquamation.
(C) erythema.
(D) epilation.

38. An optically stimulated luminescence dosimeter contains which of the following detectors?

(A) Gadolinium
(B) Aluminum oxide
(C) Lithium fluoride
(D) Photographic film

39. Immature cells are referred to as

1. undifferentiated cells.
2. stem cells.
3. genetic cells.

(A) 1 only
(B) 1 and 2 only
(C) 1 and 3 only
(D) 1, 2, and 3

40. The unit of measurement used to express occupational exposure is the

(A) roentgen (C/kg).
(B) rad (Gy).
(C) rem (Sv).
(D) relative biologic effectiveness (RBE).

41. What is the approximate ESE for the average AP cervical spine radiograph?

A. 40 rad
B. 40 mrad
C. 80 rad
D. 80 mrad

42. To be in compliance with radiation safety standards, the fluoroscopy exposure switch must

(A) sound during fluoro-on time.
(B) be on a 6-foot-long cord.
(C) terminate fluoro after 5 minutes.
(D) be the dead-man type.

43. Primary radiation barriers must be *at least* how high?

(A) 5 feet
(B) 6 feet
(C) 7 feet
(D) 8 feet

44. The annual dose limit for occupationally exposed individuals is valid for

(A) alpha, beta, and x-radiations.
(B) x- and gamma radiations only.
(C) beta, x-, and gamma radiations.
(D) all ionizing radiations.

45. The interaction between x-ray photons and matter pictured in Figure 3–1 is associated with

1. high-energy x-ray photons.
2. ionization.
3. characteristic radiation.

(A) 1 only
(B) 1 and 2 only
(C) 1 and 3 only
(D) 2 and 3 only

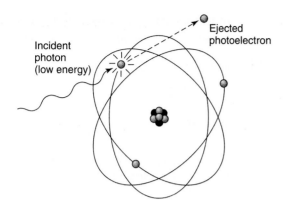

Incident photon (low energy)

Ejected photoelectron

Figure 3–1.

46. Which acute radiation syndrome requires the largest exposure before any effects become apparent?

(A) hematopoietic
(B) gastrointestinal
(C) CNS
(D) skeletal

47. Types of gonadal shielding include which of the following?

1. Flat contact
2. Shaped contact (contour)
3. Shadow

(A) 1 only
(B) 1 and 2 only
(C) 2 and 3 only
(D) 1, 2, and 3

48. The unit of absorbed dose is the

(A) roentgen (C/kg).
(B) rad (Gy).
(C) rem (Sv).
(D) RBE.

49. The law of Bergonié and Tribondeau states that cells are more radiosensitive if they are

1. highly mitotic.
2. undifferentiated.
3. mature cells.

(A) 1 only
(B) 1 and 2 only
(C) 2 and 3 only
(D) 1, 2, and 3

50. For exposure to 1 rad of each of the following ionizing radiations, which would result in the greatest dose to the individual?

(A) External source of 1-MeV x-rays
(B) External source of diagnostic x-rays
(C) Internal source of alpha particles
(D) External source of beta particles

51. The skin response to radiation exposure that appears as hair loss is known as

(A) dry desquamation.
(B) moist desquamation.
(C) erythema.
(D) epilation.

52. Biologic material is *most* sensitive to irradiation under which of the following conditions?

(A) Anoxic
(B) Hypoxic
(C) Oxygenated
(D) Deoxygenated

53. The reduction in the intensity of an x-ray beam as it passes through material is termed

(A) absorption.
(B) scattering.
(C) attenuation.
(D) divergence.

54. Which type of dose–response relationship expresses radiation-induced leukemia?

(A) Nonlinear, nonthreshold
(B) Nonlinear, threshold
(C) Linear, nonthreshold
(D) Linear, threshold

55. A dose of 25 rad to the fetus during the fourth or fifth week of pregnancy is more likely to cause which of the following:

(A) Spontaneous abortion
(B) skeletal anomalies
(C) neurologic anomalies
(D) organogenesis

56. What unit of measurement expresses the amount of energy deposited in tissue?

   (A) Roentgen (C/kg)
   (B) Rad (Gy)
   (C) Rem (Sv)
   (D) RBE

57. The largest dose to the male gonads is most likely to result from which of the following exposures?

   (A) Lateral thoracic spine
   (B) Oblique lumbar spine
   (C) Cross-table lateral hip
   (D) AP axial skull

58. Which of the following is likely to improve image quality *and* decrease patient dose?

   1. Beam restriction
   2. Low kV and high mAs factors
   3. Grids

   (A) 1 only
   (B) 1 and 3 only
   (C) 2 and 3 only
   (D) 1, 2, and 3

59. The largest amount of diagnostic x-ray absorption will occur in which of the following tissues?

   (A) Lung
   (B) Adipose
   (C) Muscle
   (D) Bone

60. According to National Council on Radiation Protection and Measurements (NCRP) regulations, leakage radiation from the x-ray tube must not exceed

   (A) 10 mR/h.
   (B) 100 mR/h.
   (C) 10 mR/min.
   (D) 100 mR/min.

61. Which of the following *most* effectively minimizes radiation exposure to the patient?

   (A) Small focal spot
   (B) Low-ratio grids
   (C) Long source-image distance
   (D) High-speed intensifying screens

62. Isotopes are atoms that have the same

   (A) mass number but a different atomic number.
   (B) atomic number but a different mass number.
   (C) atomic number but a different neutron number.
   (D) atomic number and mass number.

63. The effects of radiation on biologic material are dependent on several factors. If a quantity of radiation is delivered to a body over a long period of time, the effect

   (A) will be greater than if it were delivered all at one time.
   (B) will be less than if it were delivered all at one time.
   (C) has no relation to how it is delivered in time.
   (D) is solely dependent on the radiation quality.

64. Which of the following accounts for the x-ray beam's heterogeneity?
   1. Incident electrons interacting with several layers of tungsten target atoms
   2. Energy differences among incident electrons
   3. Electrons moving to fill different shell vacancies

   (A) 1 only
   (B) 1 and 2 only
   (C) 1 and 3 only
   (D) 1, 2, and 3

65. In the production of Bremsstrahlung radiation, the incident electron

   (A) ejects an inner-shell tungsten electron.
   (B) ejects an outer-shell tungsten electron.
   (C) is deflected, with resulting energy loss.
   (D) is deflected, with resulting energy increase.

66. Diagnostic x-radiation may be correctly described as

   (A) low energy, low LET.
   (B) low energy, high LET.
   (C) high energy, low LET.
   (D) high energy, high LET.

67. Secondary radiation barriers usually require the following thickness of shielding:

   (A) 1/4-inch lead
   (B) 1/8-inch lead
   (C) 1/16-inch lead
   (D) 1/32-inch lead

68. Which of the following illustrates the inverse square law?

   1. Distance is a most effective protection from radiation.
   2. Distance is a rather ineffective protection from radiation.
   3. As distance from the radiation source decreases, radiation decreases.

   (A) 1 only
   (B) 1 and 2 only
   (C) 1 and 3 only
   (D) 2 and 3 only

69. The *rad* may be described as

   (A) disintegrations per second.
   (B) ions produced in air.
   (C) energy deposited in an absorber.
   (D) biologic effects.

70. According to the NCRP, the annual occupational whole-body dose equivalent limit for students under age 18 is

   A. 1 mSv
   B. 50 mSv
   C. 150 mSv
   D. 500 mSv

71. Which of the following is a measurement of dose to biologic tissue?

   (A) Roentgen (C/kg)
   (B) Rad (Gy)
   (C) Rem (Sv)
   (D) RBE

72. Which of the dose–response curve(s) seen in Figure 3–2 illustrate(s) a threshold response to radiation exposure?

   1. Dose–response curve *A*
   2. Dose–response curve *B*
   3. Dose–response curve *C*

   (A) 1 only
   (B) 1 and 2 only
   (C) 2 and 3 only
   (D) 1, 2, and 3

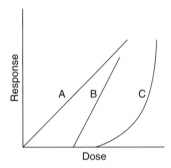

Figure 3–2.

73. What is the intensity of scattered radiation perpendicular to and 1 m from the patient, compared to the useful beam at the patient's surface?

   (A) 0.01%
   (B) 0.1%
   (C) 1.0%
   (D) 10.0%

74. Which of the following formulae is a representation of the inverse square law of radiation and may be used to determine x-ray intensity at different distances?

    (A) $\dfrac{I_1}{I_2} = \dfrac{D_2^2}{D_1^2}$

    (B) $\dfrac{I_1}{I_2} = \dfrac{D_1^2}{D_2^2}$

    (C) $\dfrac{kVp_1}{kVp_2} = \dfrac{D_2^2}{D_1^2}$

    (D) $\dfrac{kVp_1}{kVp_2} = \dfrac{D_1^2}{D_2^2}$

75. The biologic effect on an individual is dependent on which of the following?

    1. Type of tissue interaction(s)
    2. Amount of interactions
    3. Biologic differences

    (A) 1 and 2 only
    (B) 1 and 3 only
    (C) 2 and 3 only
    (D) 1, 2, and 3

76. Aluminum filtration has its greatest effect on

    (A) long wavelength radiation.
    (B) short wavelength radiation.
    (C) low mA factors.
    (D) high mA factors.

77. The amount of time that x-rays are being produced and directed toward a particular wall is referred to as the

    (A) workload.
    (B) use factor.
    (C) occupancy factor.
    (D) controlling factor.

78. The operation of personnel radiation monitoring devices depends on which of the following?

    1. Ionization
    2. Luminescence
    3. Thermoluminescence

    (A) 1 only
    (B) 1 and 2 only
    (C) 2 and 3 only
    (D) 1, 2, and 3

79. Which of the following result(s) from restriction of the x-ray beam?

    1. Less scattered radiation production
    2. Less patient hazard
    3. Less radiographic contrast

    (A) 1 only
    (B) 1 and 2 only
    (C) 2 and 3 only
    (D) 1, 2, and 3

80. Patient dose increases as fluoroscopic

    (A) FOV increases.
    (B) FOV decreases.
    (C) FSS increases.
    (D) FSS decreases.

81. Early symptoms of acute radiation syndrome include

    1. leukopenia.
    2. nausea and vomiting.
    3. Cataracts.

    (A) 1 and 2 only
    (B) 2 only
    (C) 1 and 3 only
    (D) 2 and 3 only

82. Referring to the nomogram in Figure 3–3, what is the approximate patient ESE from an AP projection of the abdomen made at 105 cm using 70 kVp, 300 mA, 0.2-second, and 2.5 mm Al total filtration?

    (A) 5 mR
    (B) 166 mR
    (C) 245 mR
    (D) 288 mR

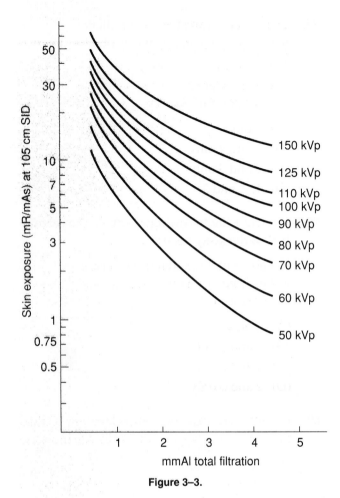

Figure 3–3.

85. Which of the following contributes *most* to occupational exposure?

   (A) The photoelectric effect
   (B) Compton scatter
   (C) Classical scatter
   (D) Thompson scatter

86. Which type of personnel radiation monitor can provide an immediate reading?

   (A) TLD
   (B) OSL
   (C) film badge
   (D) ionization chamber

87. Which of the following is (are) features of fluoroscopic equipment that are designed especially to eliminate unnecessary radiation to patient and personnel?

   1. Protective curtain
   2. Filtration
   3. Collimation

   (A) 1 only
   (B) 1 and 2 only
   (C) 1 and 3 only
   (D) 1, 2, and 3

83. What is the term used to describe x-ray photon interaction with matter and the transference of part of the photon's energy to matter?

   (A) Absorption
   (B) Scattering
   (C) Attenuation
   (D) Divergence

84. If 600 rad or more is received as a whole-body dose in a short period of time, certain symptoms will occur; these are referred to as

   (A) short-term effects.
   (B) long-term effects.
   (C) lethal dose.
   (D) acute radiation syndrome.

88. The *most* efficient type of male gonadal shielding for use during fluoroscopy is

   (A) flat contact.
   (B) shaped contact (contour).
   (C) shadow.
   (D) cylindrical.

89. Which of the following statements is/are true with respect to radiation safety in fluoroscopy?

   1. Tabletop radiation intensity must not exceed 2.1 R/min/mA.
   2. Tabletop radiation intensity must not exceed 10 R/min.
   3. In high-level fluoroscopy, tabletop intensity up to 20 R/min is permitted.

   (A) 1 only
   (B) 1 and 2 only
   (C) 2 and 3 only
   (D) 1, 2, and 3

90. What is the annual dose-equivalent limit for the skin and hands of an occupationally exposed individual?

(A) 5 rem
(B) 25 rem
(C) 50 rem
(D) 100 rem

91. If an individual receives an exposure of 150 mR/hr at a distance of 2 feet from a radiation source, what will be their dose after 30 minutes at a distance of 5 feet from the source?

(A) 60 mR
(B) 30 mR
(C) 24 mR
(D) 12 mR

92. Factors that determine the amount of scattered radiation produced include

1. radiation quality.
2. field size.
3. pathology.

(A) 1 only
(B) 1 and 2 only
(C) 2 and 3 only
(D) 1, 2, and 3

93. The focal spot-to-table distance, in mobile fluoroscopy, must be

(A) a minimum of 15 inches.
(B) a maximum of 15 inches.
(C) a minimum of 12 inches.
(D) a maximum of 12 inches.

94. The automatic exposure device that is located immediately under the x-ray table is the

(A) ionization chamber.
(B) scintillation camera.
(C) photomultiplier.
(D) photocathode.

95. LET is best defined as

1. a method of expressing radiation quality.
2. a measure of the rate at which radiation energy is transferred to soft tissue.
3. absorption of polyenergetic radiation.

(A) 1 only
(B) 1 and 2 only
(C) 1 and 3 only
(D) 1, 2, and 3

96. It is necessary to question a female patient of childbearing age regarding the

1. date of her last menstrual period.
2. possibility of her being pregnant.
3. number of children she presently has.

(A) 1 only
(B) 1 and 2 only
(C) 1 and 3 only
(D) 2 and 3 only

97. In 1906, Bergonié and Tribondeau established their law, which states that cells are more radiosensitive if they

1. are young.
2. are stem cells.
3. have a low proliferation rate.

(A) 1 only
(B) 1 and 2 only
(C) 2 and 3 only
(D) 1, 2, and 3

98. What is the effect on RBE as LET increases?

(A) As LET increases, RBE increases.
(B) As LET increases, RBE decreases.
(C) As LET increases, RBE stabilizes.
(D) LET has no effect on RBE.

99. Which of the following would *most* likely result in the greatest skin dose?

(A) Short SID
(B) High kVp
(C) Increased filtration
(D) Increased mA

100. The NCRP recommends an annual effective occupational dose equivalent limit of

(A) 2.5 rem (25 mSv).
(B) 5 rem (50 mSv).
(C) 10 rem (100 mSv).
(D) 20 rem (200 mSv).

101. Which of the following ionizing radiations is described as having an RBE of 1.0?

A. 10 MeV protons
B. 5 MeV alpha particles
C. Diagnostic x-rays
D. Fast neutrons

102. If an individual receives 50 mR while standing 4 feet from a source of radiation for 2 minutes, which of the options listed below will *most* effectively reduce his or her radiation exposure to that source of radiation?

(A) Standing 3 feet from the source for 2 minutes
(B) Standing 8 feet from the source for 2 minutes
(C) Standing 5 feet from the source for 1 minutes
(D) Standing 6 feet from the source for 2 minutes

103. Which of the following tissues or organs is the *most* radiosensitive?

(A) Rectum
(B) Esophagus
(C) Small bowel
(D) Central nervous system (CNS)

104. How do fractionation and protraction affect radiation dose-effects?

1. They reduce the effect of radiation exposure.
2. They permit cellular repair.
3. They allow tissue recovery.

A. 1 only
B. 1 and 2 only
C. 2 and 3 only
D. 1, 2, and 3

105. The photoelectric effect is the interaction between x-ray photons and matter that is largely responsible for patient dose. The photoelectric effect is likely to occur under which of the following conditions?

1. With absorbers of high atomic number
2. With low-energy incident photons
3. With the use of positive contrast media

(A) 1 and 2 only
(B) 1 and 3 only
(C) 2 and 3 only
(D) 1, 2, and 3

106. Filters used in radiographic x-ray tubes are generally composed of

(A) aluminum.
(B) copper.
(C) tin.
(D) lead.

107. The use of all of the following will function to reduce patient dose *except*

(A) collimation.
(B) high-kVp, low-mAs factors.
(C) a grid.
(D) fast intensifying screens.

108. Which of the following factors will affect both the quality and the quantity of the primary beam?

1. HVL
2. kV
3. mA

(A) 1 only
(B) 1 and 2 only
(C) 1 and 3 only
(D) 1, 2, and 3

109. An increase in total filtration of the x-ray beam will increase

A. patient skin dose.
B. beam HVL.
C. image contrast.
D. mR output.

110. Which of the following is considered the unit of exposure in air?

    (A) Roentgen (C/kg)
    (B) Rad (Gy)
    (C) Rem (Sv)
    (D) RBE

111. Which of the following are considered especially radiosensitive tissues?

    1. Blood-forming organs
    2. Reproductive organs
    3. Lymphocytes

    (A) 1 only
    (B) 1 and 2 only
    (C) 2 and 3 only
    (D) 1, 2, and 3

112. How many HVLs are required to reduce the intensity of a beam of monoenergetic photons to less than 10% of its original value?

    (A) 2
    (B) 3
    (C) 4
    (D) 5

113. Which of the following has (have) an effect on the amount and type of radiation-induced tissue damage?

    1. Quality of radiation
    2. Type of tissue being irradiated
    3. Fractionation

    (A) 1 only
    (B) 1 and 2 only
    (C) 1 and 3 only
    (D) 1, 2, and 3

114. Radiation dose to personnel is reduced by which of the following exposure control cord guidelines?

    1. Exposure cords on fixed equipment must be very short.
    2. Exposure cords on mobile equipment should be fairly long.
    3. Exposure cords on fixed and mobile equipment should be of the coiled expandable type.

    (A) 1 only
    (B) 1 and 2 only
    (C) 2 and 3 only
    (D) 1, 2, and 3

115. Lead aprons are worn during fluoroscopy to protect the radiographer from exposure to radiation from

    (A) the photoelectric effect.
    (B) Compton scatter.
    (C) classical scatter.
    (D) pair production.

116. Which of the following body parts is (are) included in whole-body dose?

    1. Gonads
    2. Blood-forming organs
    3. Extremities

    (A) 1 only
    (B) 1 and 2 only
    (C) 1 and 3 only
    (D) 1, 2, and 3

117. Which unit of exposure is described as 100 ergs of energy per gram of irradiated absorber?

    A. roentgen
    B. rad
    C. rem
    D. curie

118. Which of the following personnel monitoring devices used in diagnostic radiography is considered to be the *most* sensitive and accurate?

    (A) TLD
    (B) Film badge
    (C) OSL
    (D) Pocket dosimeter

119. Irradiation of macromolecules in vitro can result in

    1. main chain scission.
    2. cross-linking.
    3. point lesions.

    (A) 1 only
    (B) 1 and 2 only
    (C) 2 and 3 only
    (D) 1, 2, and 3

120. What quantity of radiation exposure to the reproductive organs is required to cause temporary infertility?

    A. 100 rad
    B. 200 rad
    C. 300 rad
    D. 400 rad

121. How much protection is provided from a 75-kVp x-ray beam when using a 0.50-mm lead equivalent apron?

    (A) 51%
    (B) 66%
    (C) 88%
    (D) 99%

122. The correct way(s) to check for cracks in lead aprons (are)

    1. to fluoroscope them once a year.
    2. to radiograph them at low kilovoltage twice a year.
    3. by visual inspection.

    (A) 1 only
    (B) 1 and 2 only
    (C) 2 and 3 only
    (D) 1, 2, and 3

123. Radiation safety requirements for fluoroscopic equipment include the following:

    1. SSD at least 38 cm on stationary (fixed) equipment.
    2. SSD at least 30 cm on mobile equipment.
    3. high level/boost mode must have continuous audible signal.

    A. 1 only
    B. 1 and 2 only
    C. 2 and 3 only
    D. 1, 2, and 3

124. Which of the following is (are) associated with Compton scattering?

    1. High-energy incident photons
    2. Outer-shell electrons
    3. Characteristic radiation

    (A) 1 only
    (B) 1 and 2 only
    (C) 2 and 3 only
    (D) 1, 2, and 3

125. Which of the following cells are the *most* radiosensitive?

    (A) Myelocytes
    (B) Erythroblasts
    (C) Megakaryocytes
    (D) Myocytes

126. Which of the following statements regarding the pregnant radiographer is/are true?

    1. She should declare her pregnancy to her supervisor.
    2. She should be assigned a second personnel monitor.
    3. Her radiation history should be reviewed.

    A. 1 only
    B. 1 and 2 only
    C. 2 and 3 only
    D. 1, 2, and 3

127. What is (are) the major effect(s) of deoxyribonucleic acid (DNA) irradiation?

1. Malignant disease
2. Chromosome aberration
3. Cell death

(A) 1 only
(B) 1 and 2 only
(C) 2 and 3 only
(D) 1, 2, and 3

128. Which of the following statements regarding the human gonadal cells is (are) true?

1. The female oogonia reproduce only during fetal life.
2. The male spermatogonia reproduce continuously.
3. Both male and female stem cells reproduce only during fetal life.

(A) 1 only
(B) 2 only
(C) 1 and 2 only
(D) 3 only

129. Which of the following statements is (are) true with respect to the dose–response curve shown in Figure 3–4?

1. The quantity of radiation is directly related to the dose received.
2. No threshold is required for effects to occur.
3. A minimum amount of radiation is required for manifestation of effects.

(A) 1 only
(B) 1 and 2 only
(C) 1 and 3 only
(D) 2 and 3 only

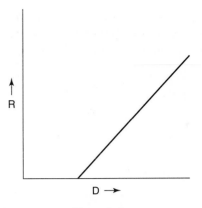

Figure 3–4.

130. Reducing the number of repeat images is an important way to decrease patient exposure and can be accomplished by

1. good patient communication.
2. accurate positioning skills.
3. using AEC.

A. 1 only
B. 1 and 2 only
C. 2 and 3 only
D. 1, 2, and 3

131. In the production of characteristic radiation at the tungsten target, the incident electron

(A) ejects an inner-shell tungsten electron.
(B) ejects an outer-shell tungsten electron.
(C) is deflected, with resulting energy loss.
(D) is deflected, with resulting energy increase.

132. Which of the following defines the gonadal dose that, if received by every member of the population, would be expected to produce the same total genetic effect on that population as the actual doses received by each of the individuals?

(A) Genetically significant dose
(B) Somatically significant dose
(C) Maximum permissible dose
(D) Lethal dose

133. The likelihood of adverse radiation effects to any radiographer whose dose is kept below the recommended guideline is

    (A) very probable.
    (B) possible.
    (C) very remote.
    (D) zero.

134. The term *effective dose* refers to

    (A) whole-body dose.
    (B) localized organ dose.
    (C) genetic effects.
    (D) somatic and genetic effects.

135. Which of the following is (are) composed of nondividing, differentiated cells?

    1. Neurons and neuroglia
    2. Epithelial tissue
    3. Lymphocytes

    (A) 1 only
    (B) 1 and 2 only
    (C) 1 and 3 only
    (D) 1, 2, and 3

136. The operation of personal radiation monitoring can be based on stimulated luminescence. Which of the following personal radiation monitors function(s) in that manner?

    1. OSL
    2. TLD
    3. Pocket dosimeter

    (A) 1 only
    (B) 1 and 2 only
    (C) 1 and 3 only
    (D) 1, 2, and 3

137. The exposure rate to a body 4 feet from a source of radiation is 16 R/hr. What distance from the source would be necessary to decrease the exposure to 6 R/hr?

    (A) 5 feet
    (B) 7 feet
    (C) 10 feet
    (D) 14 feet

138. Biologic material irradiated under hypoxic conditions is

    (A) more sensitive than when irradiated under oxygenated conditions.
    (B) less sensitive than when irradiated under anoxic conditions.
    (C) less sensitive than when irradiated under oxygenated conditions.
    (D) unaffected by the presence or absence of oxygen.

139. From which of the following primary beam sizes, all other factors remaining constant, will the greatest radiation exposure result?

    A. 8×10
    B. 10×12
    C. 11×14
    D. 14×17

140. What is the single most important scattering object in both radiography and fluoroscopy?

    (A) The x-ray table
    (B) The x-ray tube
    (C) The patient
    (D) The IR

141. All of the following statements regarding TLDs are true *except*

    (A) TLDs are reusable.
    (B) TLDs store energy.
    (C) The TLD's response is proportional to the quantity of radiation received.
    (D) Following x-ray exposure, TLDs are exposed to light and emit a quantity of heat in response.

142. A student radiographer who is under 18 years of age must not receive an annual occupational dose greater than

    (A) 0.1 rem (1 mSv).
    (B) 0.5 rem (5 mSv).
    (C) 5 rem (50 mSv).
    (D) 10 rem (100 mSv).

143. What is the approximate ESE for the average upright PA chest radiograph, using 115 kVp and a grid?

    A. 20 rad
    B. 20 mrad
    C. 200 rad
    D. 200 mrad

144. Classify the following tissues in order of *increasing* radiosensitivity.

    1. Liver cells
    2. Intestinal crypt cells
    3. Muscle cells

    (A) 1, 3, 2
    (B) 2, 3, 1
    (C) 2, 1, 3
    (D) 3, 1, 2

145. Types of secondary radiation barriers include

    1. the control booth.
    2. lead aprons.
    3. the x-ray tube housing.

    (A) 2 only
    (B) 1 and 2 only
    (C) 2 and 3 only
    (D) 1, 2, and 3

146. Any wall that the useful x-ray beam can be directed toward is called a

    (A) secondary barrier.
    (B) primary barrier.
    (C) leakage barrier.
    (D) scattered barrier.

147. A test radiograph like the one pictured in Figure 3–5 would be made by the radiation safety officer (RSO) or equipment service person and is used to evaluate

    (A) focal spot size.
    (B) linearity.
    (C) collimator alignment.
    (D) spatial resolution.

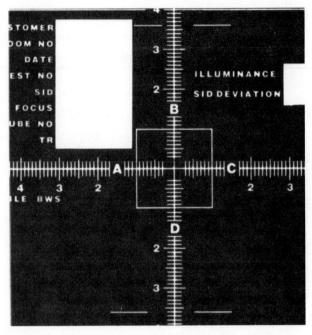

Figure 3–5. Courtesy of Stamford Hospital, Department of Radiology

148. Which of the following can be an effective means of reducing radiation exposure?

    1. Barriers
    2. Distance
    3. Time

    (A) 1 only
    (B) 2 only
    (C) 1 and 2 only
    (D) 1, 2, and 3

149. The effects of radiation to biologic material are dependent on several factors. If a large quantity of radiation is delivered to a body over a short period of time, the effect

    (A) will be greater than if it were delivered in increments.
    (B) will be less than if it were delivered in increments.
    (C) has no relation to how it is delivered in time.
    (D) is solely dependent on the radiation quality.

150. *Somatic effects* of radiation refer to effects that are manifested

   (A) in the descendants of the exposed individual.

   (B) during the life of the exposed individual.

   (C) in the exposed individual and his or her descendants.

   (D) in the reproductive cells of the exposed individual.

151. What minimum total amount of filtration (inherent plus added) is required in x-ray equipment operated above 70 kVp?

   (A) 2.5 mm Al equivalent

   (B) 3.5 mm Al equivalent

   (C) 2.5 mm Cu equivalent

   (D) 3.5 mm Cu equivalent

152. The dose of radiation that will cause a noticeable skin reaction is referred to as the

   (A) linear energy transfer (LET).

   (B) source-to-skin distance (SSD).

   (C) skin erythema dose (SED).

   (D) source-image distance (SID).

153. Which of the following radiation-induced conditions is most likely to have the *longest* latent period?

   (A) Leukemia

   (B) Temporary infertility

   (C) Erythema

   (D) Acute radiation lethality

154. The recommendation of "elective booking" states that elective abdominal radiographic examinations on women of reproductive age should be limited to the

   (A) 10 days following the menses.

   (B) 10 days following the onset of menses.

   (C) 10 days before the onset of menses.

   (D) last 10 days of the menstrual cycle.

155. A *controlled area* is defined as one

   1. that is occupied by people trained in radiation safety.
   2. that is occupied by people who wear radiation monitors.
   3. whose occupancy factor is 1.

   (A) 1 and 2 only

   (B) 2 only

   (C) 1 and 3 only

   (D) 1, 2, and 3

156. Which of the following terms refers to the period between conception and birth?

   (A) Gestation

   (B) Congenital

   (C) Neonatal

   (D) In vitro

157. Which of the following are features of fluoroscopic equipment that are designed especially to eliminate unnecessary radiation exposure to the patient and/or personnel?

   1. Bucky slot cover
   2. Exposure switch/foot pedal
   3. Cumulative exposure timer

   (A) 1 only

   (B) 1 and 2 only

   (C) 2 and 3 only

   (D) 1, 2, and 3

158. How does the use of rare earth intensifying screens contribute to lowering the patient dose?

   1. It permits the use of lower mAs.
   2. It permits the use of lower kVp.
   3. It eliminates the need for patient shielding.

   (A) 1 only

   (B) 1 and 2 only

   (C) 1 and 3 only

   (D) 2 and 3 only

159. In which type of monitoring device do photons release electrons by their interaction with air?

    (A) Film badge
    (B) Thermoluminescent dosimeter (TLD)
    (C) Pocket dosimeter
    (D) Optically stimulated luminescence (OSL) dosimeter

160. The advantages of beam restriction include the following:

    1. less scattered radiation is produced.
    2. Less biologic material is irradiated.
    3. less total filtration will be necessary.

    (A) 1 only
    (B) 1 and 2 only
    (C) 2 and 3 only
    (D) 1, 2, and 3

161. The person responsible for ascertaining that all radiation guidelines are adhered to and that personnel understand and employ radiation safety measures is the

    (A) radiology department manager.
    (B) radiation safety officer.
    (C) chief radiologist.
    (D) chief technologist.

162. The dose–response curve that appears to be valid for genetic and some somatic effects is the

    1. linear.
    2. nonlinear.
    3. nonthreshold.

    (A) 1 only
    (B) 1 and 3 only
    (C) 2 and 3 only
    (D) 1, 2, and 3

163. Which of the following contributes *most* to patient dose?

    (A) The photoelectric effect
    (B) Compton scatter
    (C) Classical scatter
    (D) Thompson scatter

164. Protective devices such as lead aprons function to protect the user from

    1. scattered radiation.
    2. the primary beam.
    3. remnant radiation.

    (A) 1 only
    (B) 1 and 2 only
    (C) 1 and 3 only
    (D) 1, 2, and 3

165. The primary function of filtration is to reduce

    (A) patient skin dose.
    (B) operator dose.
    (C) image noise.
    (D) scattered radiation.

166. Which of the following factors can affect the amount or the nature of radiation damage to biologic tissue?

    1. Radiation quality
    2. Absorbed dose
    3. Size of irradiated area

    (A) 1 only
    (B) 2 only
    (C) 1 and 2 only
    (D) 1, 2, and 3

167. Methods of reducing radiation exposure to patients and/or personnel include

    1. beam restriction.
    2. shielding.
    3. high-kV, low-mAs factors.

    (A) 1 only
    (B) 1 and 2 only
    (C) 2 and 3 only
    (D) 1, 2, and 3

168. Which of the following tissues is (are) considered to be particularly radiosensitive?

    1. intestinal mucous membrane
    2. epidermis of extremities
    3. optic nerves

    (A) 1 only
    (B) 1 and 2 only
    (C) 2 and 3 only
    (D) 1, 2, and 3

169. Which of the following groups of exposure factors will deliver the *least* amount of exposure to the patient?

    (A) 400 mA, 0.25 second, 100 kVp
    (B) 600 mA, 0.33 second, 90 kVp
    (C) 800 mA, 0.5 second, 80 kVp
    (D) 800 mA, 1.0 second, 70 kVp

170. Stochastic effects of radiation are those that

    1. have a threshold.
    2. may be described as "all-or-nothing" effects.
    3. are late effects.

    (A) 1 only
    (B) 1 and 2 only
    (C) 2 and 3 only
    (D) 1, 2, and 3

171. To within what percentage of the SID must the collimator light and actual irradiated area be accurate?

    (A) 2%
    (B) 5%
    (C) 10%
    (D) 15%

172. Under what circumstances might a radiographer be required to wear two dosimeters?

    1. During pregnancy
    2. While performing vascular procedures
    3. While performing mobile radiography

    (A) 1 and 2 only
    (B) 2 only
    (C) 2 and 3 only
    (D) 1, 2, and 3

173. Which of the following radiation situations is potentially the *most* harmful?

    (A) A large dose to a specific area all at once
    (B) A small dose to the whole body over a period of time
    (C) A large dose to the whole body all at one time
    (D) A small dose to a specific area over a period of time

174. Which of the following personnel radiation monitors will provide an immediate reading?

    (A) TLD
    (B) Film badge
    (C) Lithium fluoride chips
    (D) Pocket dosimeter

175. The tabletop exposure rate during fluoroscopy shall *not* exceed

    (A) 5 mR/min.
    (B) 10 R/min.
    (C) 10 mR/hr.
    (D) 5 R/hr.

176. Patient exposure can be minimized by using which of the following?

    1. Accurate positioning
    2. High-kV, low-mAs factors
    3. Rare earth screens

    (A) 1 only
    (B) 1 and 2 only
    (C) 1 and 3 only
    (D) 1, 2, and 3

177. If the exposure rate at 3 feet from the fluoroscopic table is 40 mR/hr, what will be the exposure rate for 30 minutes at a distance of 5 feet from the table?

    (A) 7 mR
    (B) 12 mR
    (C) 14 mR
    (D) 24 mR

178. Which of the following are radiation protection measures that are appropriate for mobile radiography?

1. The radiographer must be at least 6 feet from the patient and the x-ray tube during the exposure.
2. The radiographer must announce in a loud voice that an exposure is about to be made and wait for personnel, visitors, and patients to temporarily leave the area.
3. The radiographer must try to use the shortest practical SID.

(A) 1 and 2 only
(B) 1 and 3 only
(C) 2 and 3 only
(D) 1, 2, and 3

179. Radiation that passes through the tube housing in directions other than that of the useful beam is termed

(A) scattered radiation.
(B) secondary radiation.
(C) leakage radiation.
(D) remnant radiation.

180. The presence of ionizing radiation may be detected in which of the following ways?

1. Ionizing effect on air
2. Photographic effect on film emulsion
3. Fluorescent effect on certain crystals

(A) 1 only
(B) 1 and 2 only
(C) 1 and 3 only
(D) 1, 2, and 3

181. Which of the following refers to a regular program of evaluation that ensures the proper functioning of x-ray equipment, thereby protecting both radiation workers and patients?

(A) Sensitometry
(B) Densitometry
(C) Quality assurance
(D) Modulation transfer function

182. What should be the radiographer's main objective regarding personal radiation safety?

(A) Not to exceed his or her dose limit
(B) To keep personal exposure as far below the dose limit as possible
(C) To avoid whole-body exposure
(D) To wear protective apparel when "holding" patients for exposures

183. Radiographers use monitoring devices to record their monthly exposure to radiation. The types of devices suited for this purpose include the

1. pocket dosimeter.
2. TLD.
3. OSL dosimeter.

(A) 1 only
(B) 1 and 2 only
(C) 2 and 3 only
(D) 1, 2, and 3

184. Guidelines for the use of protective shielding state that gonadal shielding should be used

1. if the patient has reasonable reproductive potential.
2. when the gonads are within 5 cm of the collimated field.
3. when tight collimation is not possible.

(A) 1 only
(B) 1 and 2 only
(C) 1 and 3 only
(D) 2 and 3 only

185. Which of the following types of radiation is (are) considered electromagnetic?

1. X-ray
2. Gamma
3. Beta

(A) 1 only
(B) 1 and 2 only
(C) 2 and 3 only
(D) 1, 2, and 3

186. Somatic effects resulting from radiation exposure can

1. have possible consequences on the exposed individual.
2. have possible consequences on future generations.
3. cause temporary infertility.

A. 1 only
B. 1 and 3 only
C. 2 and 3 only
D. 1, 2, and 3

187. Radiation output from a diagnostic x-ray tube is measured in which of the following units of measurement

A. rad
B. rem
C. roentgen
D. becqueral

188. The purpose of filters in a film badge is

(A) to eliminate harmful rays.
(B) to measure radiation quality.
(C) to prevent exposure by alpha particles.
(D) as a support for the film contained within.

189. What safeguards are taken to prevent inadvertent irradiation in early pregnancy?

1. Patient postings
2. Patient questionnaire
3. Elective booking

(A) 1 and 2 only
(B) 1 and 3 only
(C) 2 and 3 only
(D) 1, 2, and 3

190. The interaction between x-ray photons and tissue that is responsible for radiographic contrast but that also contributes significantly to patient dose is

(A) the photoelectric effect.
(B) Compton scatter.
(C) coherent scatter.
(D) pair production.

191. Which of the following is (are) acceptable way(s) to monitor the radiation exposure of those who are occupationally employed?

1. TLD
2. OSL
3. Quarterly blood cell count

(A) 1 only
(B) 1 and 2 only
(C) 1 and 3 only
(D) 1, 2, and 3

192. A fluoroscopic examination requires 3 minutes of exposure on time. If the exposure rate for the examination is 250 mR/hr, what is the approximate radiation exposure for the radiologic staff present in the fluoroscopy room during the examination?

(A) 83.3 R
(B) 83.3 mR
(C) 12.5 R
(D) 12.5 mR

193. According to the NCRP, the total gestational dose equivalent limit for the pregnant radiographer is

A. 1 mSv
B. 5 mSv
C. 15 mSv
D. 50 mSv

194. Which of the following interactions between x-ray photons and matter involves a high-energy photon and the ejection of an outer shell electron?

(A) Photoelectric effect
(B) Coherent scatter
(C) Compton scatter
(D) Pair production

195. Occupational radiation monitoring is required when it is likely that an individual will receive more than what fraction of the annual dose limit?

(A) 1/2
(B) 1/4
(C) 1/10
(D) 1/40

196. When an image intensifier's magnification mode is used,

1. output screen gain is increased.
2. resolution increases.
3. patient dose increases.

(A) 1 only
(B) 1 and 2 only
(C) 2 and 3 only
(D) 1, 2, and 3

197. Which of the following terms is correctly used to describe x-ray beam quality?

(A) mA
(B) HVL
(C) Intensity
(D) Dose rate

198. Which of the following has/have been identified as sources of radon exposure?

1. indoors, in houses
2. smoking cigarettes
3. radiology departments

(A) 1 only
(B) 1 and 2 only
(C) 2 and 3 only
(D) 1, 2, and 3

199. What is the relationship between LET and RBE?

A. As LET increases, RBE increases
B. As LET increases, RBE decreases
C. As LET decreases, RBE increases
D. There is no direct relationship between LET and RBE.

200. An increase of 1.0 mm added aluminum filtration of the x-ray beam would have the following effect:

1. Increase average energy of the beam
2. Increase patient skin dose
3. Increase mR output

(A) 1 only
(B) 1 and 2 only
(C) 2 and 3 only
(D) 1, 2, and 3

Answers and Explanations

1. **(B)** *Late or long-term effects* of radiation can occur in tissues that have survived a previous irradiation months or years earlier. These late effects, such as carcinogenesis and genetic effects, are "all-or-nothing" effects—either the organism develops cancer or it does not. Most late effects *do not have a threshold dose;* that is, any dose, however small, can induce an effect. Increasing that dose will increase the *likelihood* of the occurrence, but will not affect its severity; these effects are termed *stochastic. Nonstochastic effects* are those that will not occur below a particular threshold dose and that increase in severity as the dose increases. *Early* effects of radiation exposure are in response to relatively high radiation doses. These should never occur in diagnostic radiology; they occur only in response to doses much greater than those used in diagnostic radiology. One of the effects that may be noted in such a circumstance is the hematologic effect—reduced numbers of white blood cells, red blood cells, and platelets in the circulating blood. Immediate local tissue effects can include effects on the gonads (temporary infertility) and on the skin (epilation, erythema). Acute radiation lethality, or radiation death, occurs after an acute exposure and results in death in weeks or days. (*Ballinger & Frank, vol 1, p 41*)

2. **(C)** According to the NCRP, the annual occupational *whole-body* dose equivalent limit is 50 mSv (5 rem or 5000 mrem). The annual occupational whole-body dose equivalent limit for *students* under the age of 18 years is 1 mSv (100 mrem or 0.1 rem). The annual occupational dose equivalent limit for the *lens of the eye*, a particularly radiosensitive organ, is 150 mSv (15 mrem or 0.015 rem). The annual occupational dose equivalent limit for the *skin and extremities* is 500 mSv (50 mrem or 0.05 rem). The total gestational dose equivalent limit for embryo/fetus of a pregnant radiographer is 5 mSv (500 mrem or 0.5 rem). (*Ballinger & Frank, vol 1, p 46*)

3. **(D)** One of the radiation protection guidelines for the occupationally exposed is that the x-ray beam must scatter twice before reaching the operator. *Each time the x-ray beam scatters, its intensity at 1 m from the scattering object is approximately 0.1% of the intensity of the primary beam*, that is, *one thousandth* of its original intensity. That is why, in terms of radiation protection, the patient is considered the most important source of scatter. Of course, the operator should be behind a shielded booth while making the exposure, but multiple scatterings further reduce danger of exposure from scatter radiation. Other scattering objects include the x-ray table, the Bucky-slot cover, and the control booth wall. (*Dowd & Tilson, p 199*)

4. **(C)** The relationship between x-ray intensity and distance from the source is expressed in

the inverse square law of radiation. The formula is

$$\frac{I_1}{I_2} = \frac{D_2^2}{D_1^2}$$

Substituting known values:

$$\frac{15}{x} = \frac{25}{4}$$
$$25\,x = 60$$
$$x = 2.4 \text{ R/minute at 2 m} = 4.8 \text{ R after}$$
$$\text{2 minutes}$$

Distance has a profound effect on dose received and therefore is one of the cardinal rules of radiation protection. As distance from the source increases, dose received decreases. (*Bushong, pp 68–70*)

5. **(A)** NCRP Report No. 102 states that the exposure switch on mobile radiographic units shall be so arranged that the operator can stand at least 2 m (*6 feet*) from the patient, the x-ray tube, and the useful beam. An appropriately long exposure cord accomplishes this requirement. The fluoroscopic and/or radiographic exposure switch or switches must be of the *"dead man"* type, that is, the exposure will terminate, should the switch be released. A lead apron should be carried with every mobile x-ray unit for the operator to wear during the exposure. Lastly, the radiographer must be certain to alert individuals in the area, enabling unnecessary occupants to move away, before making the exposure. (*NCRP Report No. 102, p 25*)

6. **(B)** Late or long-term effects of radiation can occur in tissues that have survived a previous irradiation months or years earlier. These late effects, such as carcinogenesis and genetic effects, are "all-or-nothing" effects—either the organism develops cancer or it does not. Most late effects *do not have a threshold dose;* that is, *any* dose, however small, theoretically can induce an effect. Increasing that dose will increase the likelihood of the occurrence, but will not affect its severity; these effects are termed *stochastic. Nonstochastic effects* are those that will not occur below a particular threshold

dose and that increase in severity as the dose increases. (*Bushong, p 4*)

7. **(D)** The relationship between x-ray intensity and distance from the source is expressed in the inverse square law of radiation. The formula is

$$\frac{I_1}{I_2} = \frac{D_2^2}{D_1^2}$$

Substituting known values,

$$\frac{10 \text{ mR/min}}{x \text{ mR/min}} = \frac{64}{25}$$
$$64\,x = 250$$
$$x = 3.9 \text{ mR/min at 8 feet from}$$
$$\text{the source}$$

Note the inverse relationship between distance and dose. *As distance from the source of radiation increases, dose rate significantly decreases.* (*Bushong, pp 68–70*)

8. **(C)** The use of "fast" intensifying screen phosphors enables the radiographer to decrease the required mAs. Since mAs is x-ray *quantity*, the lower the mAs the lower the patient dose. Gadolinium, lanthanum, and yttrium are *rare earth phosphors;* they are much faster than calcium tungstate. The use of rare earth phosphors enables the radiographer to use a significantly lower mAs, thereby decreasing patient exposure. (*Bushong p 228*)

9. **(B)** Patients will occasionally question the radiographer regarding the amount of radiation they are receiving during their examination. Most of these patients are merely curious because they have heard a recent news report about x-rays, or have perhaps studied about x-rays in school recently. It is a good idea for radiographers to have some knowledge of average exposure doses for patients who desire this information. The curious patient can also be referred to the medical physicist for more detailed information. The average AP supine lumbar spine radiograph delivers an ESE of about 350 mrad (0.35 rad). The average AP supine abdomen delivers about 300 mrad; the

average AP cervical spine is about 80 mrad. (*Dowd & Tilson, p 247*)

10. **(C)** Collimators or other kinds of *beam restrictors* limit the amount of tissue being irradiated and, therefore, can significantly reduce patient dose. The use of *gonadal shielding* protects the reproductive organs from unnecessary radiation exposure and should be employed whenever possible. *Grids* function to absorb scattered radiation before it reaches the image to cause fog. Grids improve our radiographic image considerably, but their use requires a significant *increase in mAs*—ie, patient dose. (*Ballinger & Frank, vol 1, p 50*)

11. **(D)** Source-to-image-receptor distance (SID) has a significant impact on x-ray beam *intensity* (other terms we could use are *exposure rate* and *dose*). *As the distance between the x-ray tube and image receptor increases, exposure rate/intensity/dose (and therefore radiographic density) decreases according to the inverse square law.*

     According to the inverse square law, the exposure rate is *inversely* proportional to the *square* of the distance; that is, if the SID is doubled, the resulting beam intensity will be one fourth the original intensity; if the SID is cut in half, the resulting beam intensity will be four times the original intensity. (*Dowd & Tilson, p 199*)

12. **(C)** The pregnant radiographer poses a special radiation protection consideration, for the safety of the unborn individual must be considered. It must be remembered that the developing fetus is particularly sensitive to radiation exposure. Therefore, established guidelines state that the occupational radiation exposure to the fetus must not exceed 0.5 rem (500 mrem or 5 mSv) during the entire gestation period. (*Bushong, p 557*)

13. **(B)** If mechanical restraint is impossible, a friend or relative accompanying the patient should be requested to hold the patient. If a parent is to perform this task, it is preferable to elect the father so as to avoid the possibility of subjecting a newly fertilized ovum to even scattered radiation. If a friend or relative is not available, a nurse or transporter may be asked

for help. Protective apparel, such as lead apron and gloves, must be provided to the person(s) holding the patient. *Radiology personnel must never assist in holding patients, and the individual assisting must never be in the path of the primary beam.* (*Thompson et al, p 484*)

14. **(B)** The entire population of the world is exposed to varying amounts of background (environmental) radiation. Sources of background radiation are either *natural* or *man-made*. Exposure to *natural* background radiation is a result of cosmic radiation from space, naturally radioactive elements *within the earth's crust (terrestrial)* and *our own bodies (internal radionuclides)*. Naturally, the closer we are to the *cosmic radiations* from space, the greater our personal exposure will be; living at higher elevations and air travel expose us to greater amounts of radiation. Living or working in a building made of materials derived from the ground exposes us to some background radiation from the naturally radioactive elements found in the earth's crust. The food we eat, the water we drink, and the air we breathe, all contribute to the quantity of radiation we ingest and inhale. Man-made radiation, however, is the type of background radiation over which we have some control. Medical and dental x-rays, and nuclear medicine, contribute to our exposure to *man-made* background radiation. (*Selman, p 501*)

15. **(B)** *Radiolysis* has to do with the irradiation of water molecules and the formation of free radicals. Free radicals contain enough energy to damage other molecules some distance away. They can migrate to and damage a DNA molecule (indirect hit theory). (*Bushong, pp 506, 507*)

16. **(D)** The fluoroscopist should release his or her foot from the exposure pedal at frequent intervals, thus reducing total patient exposure, as the image will fade from the screen only slowly. Field size plays an important role in controlling patient dose in fluoroscopy (as in radiography). Focus-to-table distance is extremely important in controlling patient exposure; the law states that this distance must be a minimum of 12 inches (preferably 15 inches) to decrease patient dose. (*Bushong, p 569*)

17. **(A)** The *Tissue Weighting Factor* (W_t) represents the relative tissue radiosensitivity of irradiated material (eg, muscle vs intestinal epithelium vs bone, etc). The *Radiation Weighting Factor* (W_r) is a number assigned to different types of ionizing radiations in order to better determine their effect on tissue (eg, x-ray vs alpha particles). The W_r of different ionizing radiations is dependent on the LET of that particular radiation. The following formula is used to determine *Effective Dose (E):*

Effective Dose (E) = Radiation Weighting Factor (W_r) × Tissue Weighting Factor (W_t) × Absorbed Dose

(Bushong, p 556)

18. **(B)** In the *photoelectric effect*, a relatively low-energy photon uses all its energy to eject an inner-shell electron, leaving a vacancy. An electron from the shell above drops down to fill the vacancy, and in doing so gives up a characteristic ray. This type of interaction is most harmful to the patient, as all the photon energy is transferred to tissue. In *Compton scatter*, a high-energy incident photon ejects an outer-shell electron. In doing so, the incident photon is deflected with reduced energy, but it *usually retains most of its energy and exits the body as an energetic scattered ray.* This scattered ray will either contribute to image fog or pose a radiation hazard to personnel, depending on its direction of exit. In *classical scatter*, a low-energy photon interacts with an atom but causes no ionization; the incident photon disappears into the atom, and is then immediately released as a photon of identical energy but changed direction. *Thompson scatter* is another name for classical scatter. *(Bushong, pp 176–178)*

19. **(A)** Two thousand mrad is equal to 2 rad. If 2 rad was delivered in 10 minutes, then the dose rate must be 0.2 rad/min:

$$\frac{2 \text{ rad}}{10 \text{ min}} = \frac{x \text{ rad}}{1 \text{ min}}$$
$$10x = 2$$
$$x = 0.2 \text{ rad/min}$$

(Selman, p 117)

20. **(A)** Although increasing the SSD would decrease ESE, the resulting image would be adversely affected because of decreased density. So if *mA is increased to maintain output intensity* (and resulting radiographic density), *patient dose (ESE) will be also increased. (Bushong, p 569)*

21. **(B)** The entire population of the world is exposed to varying amounts of background (environmental) radiation. Sources of background radiation are either natural or man-made. Exposure to *natural* background radiation is a result of cosmic radiation from space, naturally radioactive elements within the earth's crust, and our own bodies. Naturally, the closer we are to the cosmic radiations from space, the greater our personal exposure will be; living at higher elevations and air travel expose us to greater amounts of radiation. Living or working in a building made of materials derived from the ground exposes us to some background radiation from the naturally radioactive elements found in the earth's crust. The food we eat, the water we drink, and the air we breathe, all contribute to the quantity of radiation we ingest and inhale. Man-made radiation, however, is the type of background radiation over which we have some control. Medical and dental x-rays contribute to our exposure to *man-made* background radiation. *(Selman, p 501)*

22. **(D)** One of the radiation protection guidelines for the occupationally exposed is that the x-ray beam should scatter twice before reaching the operator. Each time the x-ray beam scatters, its intensity at 1 m from the scattering object is *one one thousandth* of its original intensity. Of course, the operator should be behind a shielded booth while making the exposure, but multiple scatterings further reduce the danger of exposure from scattered radiation. *(Bushong, p 572)*

23. **(B)** According to the NCRP, the annual occupational *whole-body* dose equivalent limit is 50 mSv (5 rem or 5000 mrem). The annual occupational whole-body dose equivalent limit for *students* under the age of 18 years is 1 mSv (100 mrem or 0.1 rem). The annual occupational dose equivalent limit for the *lens of the eye*, a particularly radiosensitive organ, is 150 mSv

(15 mrem or 0.015 rem). The annual occupational dose equivalent limit for the *skin and extremities* is 500 mSv (50 mrem or 0.05 rem). The total gestational dose equivalent limit for embryo/fetus of a pregnant radiographer is 5 mSv (500 mrem or 0.5 rem). (*Ballinger & Frank, vol 1, p 46*)

24. **(C)** TLDs are personnel radiation monitors that use *lithium fluoride* crystals. Once exposed to ionizing radiation and then heated, these crystals give off light proportional to the amount of radiation received. TLDs are very accurate personal monitors. Even more accurate are optically stimulated luminescence dosimeters (OSLs). OSLs use *aluminum oxide* as their sensitive crystal. (*Bushong, p 593*)

25. **(C)** *Secondary* radiation consists of *leakage and scattered* radiation. Leakage radiation can be emitted when a defect exists in the tube housing. A significant quantity of scattered radiation is generated within, and emitted from, the patient. *Background* radiation is naturally occurring radiation that is emitted from the earth and that also exists within our bodies. (*Sherer et al, p 190*)

26. **(D)** Inherent filtration is provided by materials that are a permanent part of the tube housing, that is, the glass envelope of the x-ray tube and the oil coolant. Added filtration, usually thin sheets of aluminum, is present to make a total of 2.5 mm Al equivalent for equipment operated above 70 kVp. Filtration is used to decrease patient dose by removing the weak x-rays that have no value but contribute to the skin dose. According to the inverse square law of radiation, exposure dose increases as distance from the source decreases, and vice versa. The effect of focal spot size is principally on radiographic sharpness; it has no effect on patient dose. (*Bushong, pp 137, 138*)

27. **(A)** In the *photoelectric effect,* a relatively low-energy incident photon uses all of its energy to eject an inner-shell electron, leaving a vacancy. An electron from the next shell will drop to fill the vacancy, and *a characteristic ray is given up* in the transition. This type of interaction is more

harmful to the patient, as all the photon energy is transferred to tissue. (*Bushong, pp 176–178*)

28. **(D)** The genetic effects of radiation and some somatic effects, like leukemia, are plotted on a *linear* dose–response curve. The linear dose–response curve has *no threshold;* that is, *there is no dose below which radiation is absolutely safe.* The *nonlinear/sigmoidal* dose–response curve has a *threshold* and is thought to be generally correct for most *somatic* effects—such as *skin erythema, hematologic depression,* and *radiation lethality* (death). (*Ballinger & Frank, vol 1, p 45*)

29. **(B)** *Rem (dose-equivalent) is the only unit of measurement that expresses the dose–effect relationship.* The product of rad (absorbed dose) and the quality factor appropriate for the radiation type is expressed as rem or DE (dose equivalent), and may be used to predict the type and extent of response to radiation. (*Sherer et al, p 43*)

30. **(B)** Special arrangements are required for occupational monitoring of the pregnant radiographer. The pregnant radiographer will wear two dosimeters: one in its usual place at the collar, and the other, a "baby/fetal dosimeter," worn over the abdomen and *under* the lead apron during fluoroscopy. The baby/fetal dosimeter must be identified as such and must always be worn in the same place. Care must be taken not to mix the position of the two dosimeters. The dosimeters are read monthly, as usual. (*Bushong, p 560*)

31. **(B)** Occupationally exposed individuals are required to use devices that will record and provide documentation of the radiation they receive over a given period of time, traditionally 1 month. The most commonly used personal dosimeters are the film badge, the TLD, and the OSL. These devices must be worn *only* for documentation of occupational exposure. They must not be worn for any medical or dental x-rays one receives as a patient, and they are not used to measure naturally occurring background radiation. (*Thompson et al, p 459*)

32. **(C)** Irradiation during *pregnancy,* especially in early pregnancy, is avoided because the fetus

is particularly radiosensitive during the first trimester. Especially high-risk examinations include pelvis, hip, femur, lumbar spine, cystograms and urograms, upper gastrointestinal (GI) series, and barium enema examinations. During the 2nd to 10th week of pregnancy (ie, during major organogenesis), fetal anomalies can be produced. *Skeletal and/or organ anomalies* can appear if irradiation occurs early on, and *neurologic anomalies* can be formed in the latter part; *mental retardation* childhood *malignant diseases* can also result from irradiation during the first trimester. Fetal irradiation during the second and third trimester, with sufficient dose, can cause some type of childhood malignant disease. Fetal irradiation during the first 2 weeks of gestation will most likely result in *embryonic resorption or spontaneous abortion.*

It must be emphasized that the likelihood of producing fetal anomalies at doses below 20 rad is exceedingly small and that most general diagnostic examinations are likely to deliver fetal doses of less than 1 to 2 rad. *(Bushong, p 561)*

33. **(A)** $^{130}_{56}$Ba and $^{138}_{56}$Ba are isotopes of the same element, barium (Ba), because they have the *same atomic number* but different mass numbers (numbers of neutrons). *Isobars* are atoms with the same mass number but different atomic numbers. *Isotones* have the *same number of neutrons* but different atomic numbers. *Isomers* have the *same atomic number and mass number;* they are identical atoms existing at different energy states. *(Bushong, p 49)*

34. **(D)** Artificial/man-made sources of radiation include radioactive fallout, industrial radiation, and medical and dental x-rays. About 90% of the general public's exposure to artificial radiation is from medical and dental x-rays. It is our professional obligation, therefore, to keep our patient's radiation dose to a minimum. *(Bushong, p 6)*

35. **(C)** *Somatic effects* are those induced in the irradiated body. *Genetic effects* of ionizing radiation are those that may not appear for many years (generations) following exposure. Formation of cataracts or cancer (such as leukemia) and embryologic damage are all possible *long-term*

somatic effects of radiation exposure. A fourth is life-span shortening. Nausea and vomiting are early effects of exposure to large quantities of ionizing radiation. *(Bushong, pp 533–534)*

36. **(A)** X-rays produced at the tungsten target make up a heterogeneous primary beam. Filtration serves to eliminate the softer, less penetrating photons, leaving an x-ray beam of higher average energy. Filtration is important in patient protection because unfiltered, low-energy photons that are not energetic enough to reach the IR stay in the body and contribute to total patient dose. *(Bushong, p 157)*

37. **(C)** The first noticeable skin response to excessive irradiation would be *erythema,* a reddening of the skin very much like sunburn. *Dry desquamation,* a dry peeling of the skin, may follow. *Moist desquamation* is peeling with associated puslike fluid. *Epilation,* or hair loss, may be temporary or permanent depending on sensitivity and dose. *(Bushong, p 521)*

38. **(B)** There are different types of monitoring devices available for the occupationally exposed. The film badge has *photographic film;* the pocket dosimeter contains an ionization chamber; TLDs use *lithium fluoride crystals.* *OSL dosimeetters* are personnel radiation monitors that use *aluminum oxide* crystals. These crystals, once exposed to ionizing radiation and then subjected to a laser, give off luminescence proportional to the amount of radiation received. *(Bushong, p 594)*

39. **(B)** Cells are frequently identified by their stage of development. *Immature* cells may be referred to as *undifferentiated* or *stem* cells. Immature cells are much more radiosensitive than mature cells. *(Bushong, pp 591, 592)*

40. **(C)** *Roentgen* is the unit of exposure; it measures the quantity of ionizations in air. *Rad* is an acronym for radiation *a*bsorbed *d*ose; it measures the energy deposited in any material. *Rem* is an acronym for radiation equivalent man; it includes the RBE specific to the tissue irradiated, and therefore is a valid unit of measurement for the *dose to biologic material.* *(Bushong, pp 24–25)*

41. **(D)** Patients will occasionally question the radiographer regarding the amount of radiation they are receiving during their examination. Most of these patients are merely curious because they have heard a recent news report about x-rays, or have perhaps studied about x-rays in school recently. It is a good idea for radiographers to have some knowledge of average exposure doses for patients who desire this information. The curious patient can also be referred to the medical physicist for more detailed information. The average AP cervical spine is about 80 mrad (0.080 rad). The average AP supine lumbar spine radiograph delivers an ESE of about 350 mrad (0.35 rad). The average AP supine abdomen delivers about 300 mrad. *(Dowd & Tilson, p 247)*

42. **(D)** For radiation safety, the fluoroscopy exposure switch must be of the *dead-man type.* When the foot is removed from the fluoro pedal, the dead-man switch will terminate the exposure immediately. There must also be a fluoroscopy timer that will either sound or interrupt exposure after 5 minutes of fluoroscopy. *(Bushong, p 570)*

43. **(C)** Radiation protection guidelines have established that primary radiation barriers must be 7 feet high. Primary radiation barriers are walls that the primary beam might be directed toward. They usually contain 1.5mm lead (1/16 inch), but this may vary depending on use factor, etc. *(Bushong, pp 571–572)*

44. **(C)** The occupational dose limit is valid for beta, x-, and gamma radiations. Because alpha radiation is so rapidly ionizing, traditional personnel monitors will not record alpha radiation. However, because alpha particles are capable of penetrating only a few centimeters of air, they are practically harmless as an external source. *(Bushong, p 596)*

45. **(D)** Diagnostic x-ray photons interact with tissue in a number of ways, but most frequently they are involved in the *photoelectric effect* or in the production of *Compton scatter.* The photoelectric effect is pictured in Figure 3–6; it occurs when a relatively *low-energy* x-ray photon *uses all its energy* to eject an *inner-shell elec-*

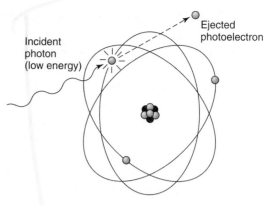

Figure 3–6.

tron. That electron is ejected (photoelectron), leaving a "hole" in the K shell and producing a positive ion. An L-shell electron then drops down to fill the K vacancy, and in doing so emits a *characteristic ray* whose energy is equal to the difference between the binding energies of the K and L shells. The photoelectric effect occurs with high-atomic-number absorbers such as bone and positive contrast media, and is responsible for the production of contrast. Therefore, its occurrence is helpful for the production of the radiographic image, but it contributes significantly to the dose received by the patient (because it involves complete absorption of the incident photon). Scattered radiation, which produces a radiation hazard to the radiographer (as in fluoroscopy), is a product of the Compton scatter interaction occurring with higher-energy x-ray photons. *(Selman, pp 125–126)*

46. **(C)** Radiation effects that appear days or weeks following exposure (early effects) are in response to high radiation doses; this is called acute radiation syndrome. These effects should never occur in diagnostic radiology; they occur only in response to much greater doses. Sufficient exposure of the *hematologic* system to ionizing radiation can result in nausea, vomiting, diarrhea, decreased blood cells count, and infection. Very large exposure of the *GI system* (1000–5000 rad) causes severe damage to the (stem) cells lining the GI tract. This can result in nausea, vomiting, diarrhea, blood changes, and hemorrhage. Exposure greater than 5000 rad are required to affect the normally resilient CNS. *(Bushong, pp 517–518)*

47. **(D)** Gonadal shielding should be used whenever appropriate and possible during radiographic and fluoroscopic examinations. *Flat contact* shields are useful for simple recumbent (AP, PA) studies, but when the examination necessitates obtaining oblique, lateral, or erect projections, they become less efficient. *Shaped contact (contour)* shields are best because they enclose the male reproductive organs and remain in position in oblique, lateral, and erect positions. *Shadow* shields that attach to the tube head are particularly useful for surgical sterile fields. *(Sherer et al, pp 156–160)*

48. **(B)** *Rad* is an acronym for *radiation absorbed dose*; it measures the energy deposited in any material. *Roentgen* is the unit of exposure; it measures the quantity of ionizations in air. *Rem* is an acronym for *radiation equivalent man*; it includes the RBE specific to the tissue irradiated and therefore is a valid unit of measurement for the *dose to biologic tissue*. *(Bushong, p 23)*

49. (B) Bergonié and Tribondeau were French scientists who, in 1906, theorized what has now become verified law. Cells are more radiosensitive if they are *immature* (undifferentiated or stem) cells, if they are *highly mitotic* (having a high rate of proliferation), and if the irradiated tissue is young. Cells and tissues that are still undergoing development are more radiosensitive than fully developed tissues. *(Bushong, p 495)*

50. **(C)** Electromagnetic radiations such as x-rays and gamma rays are considered low LET-radiations because they produce fewer ionizations than the highly ionizing particulate radiations such as alpha particles. *Alpha particles* are large and heavy (two protons and two neutrons), and although they possess a great deal of kinetic energy (approximately 5 MeV), their energy is rapidly lost through multiple ionizations (approximately 40,000 atoms/cm of air). As an *external* source, alpha particles are almost harmless, because they ionize the air very quickly and never reach the individual. As *internal sources*, however, they ionize tissues and are potentially the most harmful. It may be stated that the alpha particle has one

of the highest LETs of all ionizing radiations. *(Bushong, p 496)*

51. **(D)** The various skin responses to irradiation include all four choices. The first noticeable response would be *erythema*, a reddening of the skin very much like sunburn. *Dry desquamation* may follow; it is a dry peeling of the skin. *Moist desquamation* is peeling with associated puslike fluid. *Epilation* is hair loss; it may be temporary or permanent, depending on sensitivity and dose. *(Bushong, p 522)*

52. **(C)** Tissue is most sensitive to radiation when it is *oxygenated*. *Anoxic* refers to tissue without oxygen; *hypoxic* refers to tissue with little oxygen. Anoxic and hypoxic tumors are typically avascular (with little or no blood supply) and therefore more radioresistant. *(Bushong, pp 496–497)*

53. **(C)** The reduction in the intensity (quantity) of an x-ray beam, as it passes through matter as a result of absorption and scatter, is called *attenuation*. *Absorption* occurs when an x-ray photon interacts with matter and disappears, as in the *photoelectric effect*. *Scattering* occurs when there is partial transfer of energy to matter, as in the *Compton effect*. *(Bushong, pp 185–186)*

54. **(C)** Radiation-induced malignancy, leukemia, and genetic effects are late effects (or stochastic effects) of radiation exposure. These can occur years after survival of an acute radiation dose, or after exposure to low levels of radiation over a long period of time. Radiation workers need to be especially aware of the late effects of radiation because their exposure to radiation is usually low-level over a long period of time. Occupational radiation protection guidelines are therefore based on late effects of radiation according to a linear, nonthreshold dose–response curve. *(Bushong, p 499)*

55. **(B)** During the first trimester, specifically the 2 to 8 week of pregnancy (during major organogenesis), if the radiation dose is at least 20 rad, fetal anomalies can be produced. *Skeletal anomalies* usually appear if irradiation occurs in the early part of this time period, and *neurologic anomalies* are formed in the latter

part; mental retardation and childhood malignant diseases, such as cancers or leukemia, can also result from irradiation during the first trimester. Fetal irradiation during the second and third trimester is not likely to produce anomalies, but rather, with sufficient dose, some type of childhood malignant disease. Fetal irradiation during the first 2 weeks of gestation can result in *spontaneous abortion*.

It must be emphasized that the likelihood of producing fetal anomalies at doses below 20 rad is exceedingly small and that most general diagnostic examinations are likely to deliver fetal doses of less than 1 to 2 rad. *(Bushong, p 546)*

56. **(B)** The *rad* is the unit of absorbed dose. It is equal to *100 ergs of energy per gram of any absorber*. The roentgen measures quantity of ionization in air. The rem and RBE express radiation dose to biologic material. *(Bushong, p 23)*

57. **(C)** The *cross-table lateral hip* will bring the primary beam in closest proximity to the male reproductive organs. A grid is required, and gonadal shielding is most likely not possible. Close, accurate collimation is recommended to keep exposure to a minimum, but the cross-table lateral hip will deliver the greatest dose to the male reproductive organs. *(Bontrager, p 267)*

58. **(A)** The use of beam restrictors limits the amount of tissue being irradiated, thus decreasing patient dose *and* decreasing the production of scattered radiation. High mAs factors increase patient dose. Patient dose is reduced by using high-kVp and *low*-mAs combinations. Although the use of a grid improves image quality by decreasing the amount of scattered radiation reaching the IR, it always requires an increase in exposure factor (usually mAs) and therefore results in increased patient dose. *(Bushong, p 236, 238)*

59. **(D)** Our bodies contain a variety of tissues, having a variety of *tissue densities*. These tissues densities afford differing degrees of resistance to the passage of x-ray photons. Tissues having *greater density absorb more* of the x-ray beam (recall photoelectric effect). Soft tissues are fairly easity penetrated to varying degrees; that is, lung and adipose are easier to penetrate than muscle. *Bone* has much higher tissue mass density and therefore absorbs more of the x-ray beam. *(Bushong p 183)*

60. **(B)** X-ray photons produced in the x-ray tube can radiate in directions other than the one desired. The *tube housing* is therefore constructed so that very little of this leakage radiation is permitted to escape. The regulation states that leakage radiation must not exceed 100 mR/hour at 1 m while the tube is operated at maximum potential. *(Bushong, p 130)*

61. **(D)** Focal spot size affects recorded detail and x-ray tube heat limits—it has no effect on patient dose. Low-ratio grids, although they require less mAs than high-ratio grids, are not a means of patient protection. Long source-image distances usually require the use of higher mAs and so would not be an effective means of patient protection. The use of high-speed intensifying screens enables the use of lower mAs values and is therefore an important consideration in limiting patient dose. Limiting the irradiated field size, through collimation or other beam restriction, is perhaps the most effective way of controlling patient exposure dose. *(Bushong, p 12)*

62. **(B)** *Isotopes* are atoms of the same element (the same atomic number or number of protons) but a different mass number. They differ, therefore, in the number of neutrons. Atoms with the same mass number but different atomic number are *isobars*. Atoms with the same atomic number but different neutron number are *isotones*. Atoms with the same atomic number and mass number are *isomers*. *(Bushong, p 47)*

63. **(B)** The effects of a quantity of radiation delivered to a body are dependent on the amount of radiation received, the size of the irradiated area, and how the radiation is delivered in time. If the radiation is delivered in portions over a period of time, it is said to be fractionated and has a less harmful effect than if it were delivered all at once, as cells have an opportunity to repair and some recovery occurs between doses. *(Bushong, p 496)*

64. **(D)** The x-ray photons produced at the tungsten target make up a heterogeneous beam, a spectrum of photon energies. This is accounted for by the fact that the incident electrons have differing energies. Also, the incident electrons travel through several layers of tungsten target material, lose energy with each interaction, and therefore produce increasingly weaker photons. During characteristic x-ray production, vacancies may be filled in the *K, L,* or *M* shells, which differ from each other in binding energies, and therefore photons with varying amounts of energy are emitted. (*Bushong, pp 144–146*)

65. **(C)** Bremsstrahlung (or Brems) radiation is one of the two kinds of x-rays produced at the tungsten target of the x-ray tube. The incident high-speed electron, passing through a tungsten atom, is attracted by the positively charged nucleus and therefore is *deflected from its course, with a resulting loss of energy.* This energy loss is given up in the form of an x-ray photon. (*Bushong, p 151–152*)

66. **(A)** X-radiation used for diagnostic purposes is of relatively *low energy.* Kilovoltages of up to 150 are used, as compared with radiations having energies of up to several million volts. LET (linear energy transfer) refers to the rate at which energy is transferred from ionizing radiation to soft tissue. Particulate radiations, such as alpha particles, have mass and charge, and therefore lose energy rapidly as they penetrate only a few centimeters of air. X- and gamma radiations, having no mass or charge, are *low-LET* radiations. (*Bushong, p 495*)

67. **(D)** Examples of *primary* barriers are the lead walls and doors of a radiographic room, that is, any surface that could be struck by the useful beam. Primary protective barriers of typical installations generally consist of walls with *1/16 inch* (1.5 mm) lead thickness and 7 feet high.

Secondary radiation is defined as leakage and/or scattered radiation. The x-ray tube housing protects from leakage radiation as stated previously. The patient is the source of most scattered radiation. *Secondary radiation barriers* include that portion of the walls *above*

7 feet in height; this area requires only *1/32-inch lead.* The control booth is also a secondary barrier, toward which the primary beam must never be directed. (*Bushong, p 572*)

68. **(A)** The inverse square law of radiation states that the intensity or exposure rate of radiation at a given distance from a point source is inversely proportional to the square of the distance. This means that if the distance from a radiation source is doubled, the dose received will be one fourth the original intensity (quantity). Distance, therefore, can be a very effective means of protection from radiation exposure. (*Bushong, pp 56–66*)

69. **(C)** The *curie* is the unit of radioactivity, describing *disintegrations per second.* The *roentgen* is the unit of exposure; it measures the quantity of *ionization in air. Rad* is an acronym for radiation absorbed dose; it measures the *energy deposited in any material. Rem* is an acronym for radiation equivalent man; it includes the relative biologic effectiveness *(RBE)* specific to the tissue irradiated, and therefore is a valid unit of measure for the *dose to biologic material.* (*Bushong, p 24*)

70. **(A)** According to the NCRP, the annual occupational *whole-body* dose equivalent limit is 50 mSv (5 rem or 5000 mrem). The annual occupational whole-body dose equivalent limit for *students* under the age of 18 years is 1 mSv (100 mrem or 0.1 rem). The annual occupational dose equivalent limit for the *lens of the eye,* a particularly radiosensitive organ, is 150 mSv (15 mrem or 0.015 rem). The annual occupational dose equivalent limit for the *skin and extremities* is 500 mSv (50 mrem or 0.05 rem). The total gestational dose equivalent limit for embryo/fetus of a pregnant radiographer is 5 mSv (500 mrem or 0.5 rem). (*Ballinger & Frank, vol 1, p 46*)

71. **(C)** *Roentgen* is the unit of exposure; it measures the quantity of ionization in air. *Rad* is an acronym for radiation absorbed dose; it measures the energy deposited in any material. *Rem* is an acronym for radiation equivalent man; it includes the *RBE* specific to the tissue irradiated, and therefore is a valid unit of

measurement for the dose to biologic material. *(Bushong, p 24)*

72. **(C)** Figure 3–2 illustrates three dose–response curves. *Curve A* begins at zero, indicating that there is no safe dose, that is, *no threshold.* Even one x-ray photon can, theoretically, cause a response. It is a straight *(linear)* line, indicating that *response is proportional to dose.* That is, as dose increases, response increases. *Curve B* is another linear curve, but this one illustrates a situation in which a particular dose of radiation must be received before the response will occur. That is, there is a *threshold dose,* and this is a linear threshold curve. *Curve C* is another threshold curve, but this curve is nonlinear. It illustrates that once the minimum dose is received, a response initially occurs slowly, then increases sharply as exposure increases. *(Bushong, p 499)*

73. **(B)** The patient is the most important radiation scatterer during both radiography and fluoroscopy. In general, at 1 m from the patient, *the intensity is reduced by a factor of 1000,* to about 0.1% of the original intensity. Successive scatterings can render the intensity to unimportant levels. *(Bushong, p 572)*

74. **(A)** As an x-ray source moves away from a detector, the x-ray intensity (quantity) decreases. Conversely, as the source of x-rays moves closer to the detector, the intensity increases. This is a predictable relationship that may be calculated using the inverse square law, which states that the intensity (exposure rate) of radiation at a given distance from a point source is inversely proportional to the square of the distance. For example, if the distance from an x-ray source were doubled, the intensity of x-rays at the detector would be one fourth of its original value. This relationship is represented by the formula:

$$\frac{I_1}{I_2} = \frac{D_2^2}{D_1^2}$$

(Bushong, pp 68–70)

75. **(D)** Photoelectric interaction in tissue involves complete absorption of the incident photon,

whereas Compton interactions involve only partial transfer of energy. The larger the quantity of radiation and the greater the number of photoelectric interactions, the greater the patient dose. Radiation to more radiosensitive tissues such as gonadal tissue or blood-forming organs is more harmful than the same dose to muscle tissue. *(Selman, pp 513–514)*

76. **(A)** X-ray photons emerging from the focal spot comprise a *heterogeneous* primary beam. There are many low energy x-rays that, if not removed, would contribute significantly to patient *skin dose.* These low-energy photons are too weak to penetrate the patient and expose the image receptor; they simply penetrate a small thickness of tissue before being absorbed. Filters, usually made of aluminum, are used in radiography to reduce patient dose by removing this low energy radiation (ie, *decreased* beam *intensity*), and resulting in an x-ray beam of *higher average energy. Total filtration* is composed of *inherent filtration* plus *added filtration.* *(Bushong, p 165)*

77. **(B)** *Use factor* describes the percentage of time that the primary beam is directed toward a particular wall. The use factor is one of the factors considered in determining protective barrier thickness. Another is *workload,* which is determined by the number of x-ray exposures made per week. *Occupancy factor* is a reflection of who occupies particular areas (radiation workers or nonradiation workers) and is another factor used in determining radiation barrier thickness. *(Bushong, p 573)*

78. **(D)** *Ionization* is the fundamental principle of operation of both the film badge and the pocket dosimeter. In the film badge, the film's silver halide emulsion is ionized by x-ray photons. The pocket dosimeter contains an ionization chamber, and the number of ionizations taking place may be equated to the exposure dose. TLDs contain lithium fluoride crystals that undergo characteristic changes upon irradiation. When the crystals are subsequently *heated,* they emit a quantity of visible *(thermo)luminescence/light* in proportion to the amount of radiation absorbed. OSLs contain aluminum oxide crystals that also undergo

characteristic changes upon irradiation. When the Al_2O_3 crystals are *stimulated by a laser,* they emit *(optically stimulated) luminescence/light* in proportion to the amount of radiation absorbed. *(Bushong, p 593)*

79. **(B)** As the size of the irradiated field decreases, scattered radiation production and patient hazard decrease. If the amount of scattered radiation decreases, then radiographic contrast is higher (shorter scale). *(Selman, p 247)*

80. **(B)** During fluoroscopic procedures, as FOV (field of view) decreases, magnification of the output screen image increases and contrast and resolution improve. The focal point on an image intensifier's 6-inch field/mode is further away from the output phosphor than the focal point on the normal mode; therefore, the output image is magnified. Because less minification takes place, the *image is not as bright. Exposure factors are automatically increased to compensate for the loss in brightness with smaller FOVs.* FSS (focal spot size) is unrelated to patient dose. *(Fosbinder, p 285)*

81. **(A)** Occupationally exposed individuals generally receive small amount of low-energy radiation over a long period of time. These individuals are therefore concerned with the potential *long-term* effects of radiation, such as *carcinogenesis* (including *leukemia*) and *cataractogenesis.* However, if a large amount of radiation is delivered to the whole body at one time, the short-term early somatic effects must be considered. If the whole body receives 600 rad at one time, *acute radiation syndrome* is likely to occur. Early signs of acute radiation syndrome include *nausea, vomiting, diarrhea, fatigue,* and *leukopenia* (decreased white blood cells count); these occur in the first *(prodromal)* stage of acute radiation syndrome. *(Bushong, p 524)*

82. **(D)** An approximate ESE can be determined using the illustrated nomogram. First, mark 2.5 mm Al on the *x*/horizontal axis. Next, mark where a line drawn up from that point intersects the 70-kVp line. Draw a line straight across to the *y*/vertical axis; this should approximately reach the 4.8 mR/mAs point.

Because 60 mAs was used for the exposure, the approximate entrance skin dose is 288 mR (60 × 4.8). *(Bushong, p 587)*

83. **(B)** *Scattering* occurs when there is partial transfer of the proton's energy to matter, as in the Compton effect. *Absorption* occurs when an x-ray photon interacts with matter and disappears, as in the photoelectric effect. The reduction in the intensity (quantity) of an x-ray beam, as it passes through matter, is termed *attenuation. Divergence* refers to a directional characteristic of the x-ray beam, as it is emitted from the focal spot. *(Bushong, p 241)*

84. **(D)** Radiation is most hazardous when it is received in a large dose, all at one time, to the whole body. When 600 rad or more is received as a whole-body dose in a short time, biologic effects will appear within minutes to weeks (depending on the dose received). These immediate effects are known as *acute radiation syndrome. (Bushong, p 524)*

85. **(B)** In the *photoelectric effect,* a relatively low-energy photon uses all its energy to eject an inner-shell electron, leaving a vacancy. An electron from the shell above drops down to fill the vacancy, and in doing so gives up a characteristic ray. This type of interaction is most harmful to the patient, as all the photon energy is transferred to tissue. In *Compton scatter,* a high-energy incident photon uses some of its energy to eject an outer-shell electron. In doing so, the incident photon is deflected with reduced energy, but it usually retains most of its energy and exits the body as an energetic scattered ray. *This scattered ray will either contribute to image fog or pose a radiation hazard to personnel,* depending on its direction of exit; thus, Compton scatter contributes the most to occupational exposure. In *classical scatter,* a low-energy photon interacts with an atom but causes no ionization; the incident photon disappears into the atom, and then is immediately released as a photon of identical energy but with changed direction. *Thompson scatter* is another name for classical scatter. *(Selman, p 128)*

86. **(D)** The pocket dosimeter, or *pocket ionization chamber,* resembles a penlight. Within the

dosimeter is a thimble ionization chamber. In the presence of ionizing radiation, a particular quantity of air will be ionized and cause the fiber indicator to register radiation quantity in milliroentgen (mR). The self-reading type may be "read" by holding the dosimeter up to the light and, looking through the eyepiece, observing the fiber indicator, which indicates a quantity of 0 to 200 mR. Although it provides an immediate reading, while the other personnel monitors require "processing," the disadvantage of the pocket dosimeter is that it does not provide a permanent legal record of exposure. (*Ballinger & Frank, vol 1, p 54*)

87. **(D)** The *protective curtain*, which is usually made of leaded vinyl with at least 0.25 mm Pb equivalent, must be positioned between the patient and the fluoroscopist to greatly reduce the exposure of the fluoroscopist to energetic scatter from the patient. As with overhead equipment, fluoroscopic total *filtration* must be at least 2.5 mm Al equivalent to reduce excessive exposure to soft radiation. *Collimator/beam alignment* must be accurate to within 2%. (*Bushong, p 570*)

88. **(B)** Gonadal shielding should be used whenever appropriate and possible during radiographic and fluoroscopic examinations. *Flat contact* shields are useful for simple recumbent studies, but when the examination necessitates obtaining that oblique, lateral, or erect projections, they are easily displaced and become less efficient. *Shaped contact* (contour) shields are best because they enclose the male reproductive organs and remain in position for oblique, lateral, and erect projections. *Shadow* shields that attach to the tube head are particularly useful for surgical sterile fields. (*Bushong, pp 598–599*)

89. **(D)** In fluoroscopy, the source of x-rays is 12–15 inches below the x-ray tabletop. Since the SOD is so short, patient skin dose can be quite high. Consequently, the x-ray intensity at the tabletop is limited to keep patient dose (ESE) within safe limits. The radiation protection guidelines state that x-ray intensity at tabletop must not exceed *2.1 R/min/mA at 80 kVp*. In equipment without *high-level fluo-*

roscopy capability, the guideline can be expressed as *10 R/min* tabletop limit. In equipment with high-level fluoroscopy capability, the tabletop limit is *20 R/min. (Bushong, p 570)*

90. **(C)** The dose-equivalent limit for the hands and skin of an occupationally exposed individual is 50 rem. The dose-equivalent limit for the lens of the eye is 5 rem. An occupationally exposed individual may receive up to 3 rem in a given calendar quarter, or 13-week period. However, that individual may not exceed 5 rem in that particular year. If, for example, one received 3 rem during the first 3 months of a year, that individual must not receive more than 2 rem in the remaining 9 months. (*Bushong, p 557*)

91. **(D)** The relationship between x-ray intensity and distance from the source is expressed in the *inverse square law of radiation*. The formula is

$$\frac{I_1}{I_2} = \frac{D_2^2}{D_1^2}$$

Substituting known values:

$$\frac{150}{x} = \frac{25}{4}$$
$$25x = 600$$
$$x = 24 \text{ mR in 60 minutes, therefore}$$
$$12 \text{ mR in 30 minutes}$$

Distance has a profound effect on dose received and therefore is one of the cardinal rules of radiation protection. *As distance from the source increases, dose received decreases.* (*Bushong, pp 68–70*)

92. **(D)** The amount of scattered radiation produced is dependent first on the kilovoltage (beam quality) selected; *the higher the kVp*, the more the scattered radiation produced. The size of the irradiated field has a great deal to do with the amount of scattered radiation produced; *the larger the field size*, the greater the amount of scattered radiation. Thickness and condition of tissue are important considerations; *the thicker and/or more dense the tissue*, the more scatter produced. If the condition of the tissue is such that *pathology* makes it more

difficult to penetrate, more scattered radiation will be produced. *(Thompson et al, pp 280, 282)*

93. **(C)** Lead and distance are the two most important ways to protect from radiation exposure. Fluoroscopy can be particularly hazardous because the *SID* is so much shorter than in overhead radiography. Therefore, it has been established that *fixed* (stationary) *and mobile* fluoroscopic equipment must provide at least 12 inches (30 cm) source-to-tabletop/skin distance for the protection of the patient. *(Bushong, p 569)*

94. **(A)** Automatic exposure control (AEC) devices are used in today's equipment and serve to produce consistent and comparable radiographic results. In one type of AEC, there is an *ionization chamber* just beneath the tabletop above the cassette. The part to be examined is centered on it (the sensor) and radiographed. When a predetermined quantity of ionization has occurred (equal to the correct density), the exposure terminates automatically. In the other type of AEC, the *phototimer/photomultiplier,* a small fluorescent screen is positioned beneath the cassette. When remnant radiation emerging from the patient exposes the IR and exits the cassette, the fluorescent screen emits light. Once a predeter-mined amount of fluorescent light is "seen" by the photocell sensor, the exposure is terminated. A *scintillation camera* is used in nuclear medicine. A *photocathode* is an integral part of the image intensification system. *(Bushong, p 116)*

95. **(B)** When biologic material is irradiated, there are a number of modifying factors that determine what kind and how much response will occur in the material. One of these factors is *LET,* which expresses *the rate at which particulate or photon energy is transferred to the absorber.* Because different kinds of radiation have different degrees of penetration in different materials, it is also a useful way of expressing the quality of the radiation. *(Thompson et al, p 419)*

96. **(B)** It is our ethical responsibility to minimize radiation exposure to ourselves and our patients, particularly during early pregnancy. One way to do this is to inquire about the pos-

sibility of our female patients being pregnant, or for the date of their last menstrual period (to determine the possibility of irradiating a newly fertilized ovum). The safest time for a woman of childbearing age to have elective radiographic examinations is during the first 10 days following the onset of menstruation. *(Thompson et al, p 487)*

97. (B) The Law of Bergonié and Tribondeau states that stem cells (which give rise to a specific type of cell, as in hematopoiesis) are particularly radiosensitive, as are *young cells* and tissues. It also states that *cells with a high rate of proliferation* (mitosis) are more sensitive to radiation. This law is historically important in that it was the first to recognize that some tissues have greater radiosensitivity than others (such as the fetus). *(Bushong, p 495)*

98. **(A)** LET expresses the rate at which photon or particulate energy is transferred to (absorbed by) biologic material (through ionization processes); it is dependent on the type of radiation and the characteristics of the absorber. RBE describes the degree of response or amount of biologic change one can expect of the irradiated material. *As the amount of transferred energy (LET) increases* (from interactions occurring between radiation and biologic material), *the amount of biologic effect/damage will also increase. (Thompson et al, pp 419–420)*

99. **(A)** *The shorter the SID, the greater the skin dose.* That is why there are specific source-to-skin distance restrictions in fluoroscopy. High kVp produces more penetrating photons, thereby decreasing skin dose. Filtration is used to remove the low-energy photons from the primary beam, which contribute to skin dose. *(Thompson et al, pp 293–294)*

100. **(B)** In the past few decades, ICRP and NCRP studies have indicated that radiation-induced cancer risks are greater than radiation-induced genetic risks—contrary to previous thought. Their philosophy then grew to be concerned with the probability of radiation-induced cancer mortality in the occupational radiation industry in comparison with annual accidental mortality in "safe" (radiation free) industries.

The NCRP reexamined its 1987 recommendations, and in NCRP report 116 reiterates its *annual effective occupational dose limit as 50 mSv (5 rem)*. *(NCRP Report 116, pp 1, 4, 12)*

101. **(C)** LET increases with the *ionizing* potential of the radiation, for example, alpha particles are more ionizing than x-radiation, therefore they have a higher LET. As ionizations and LET increase, there is greater possibility of an effect on living tissue; therefore, the RBE increases. The *RBE* (sometimes called QF—Quality Factor) *of diagnostic x-rays is 1*; the RBE of fast neutrons is 10; the RBE of 5 MeV alpha particles is 20, and the RBE of 10 MeV protons is 5.0. *(Bushong, p 496)*

102. **(B)** A quick survey of the distractors reveals that option A will increase exposure dose and thus is eliminated as a possible correct answer. Options B, C, and D will serve to reduce radiation exposure, as in each case either time is decreased or distance is increased. It remains to be seen, then, which is the more effective. Using the inverse square law of radiation, at a distance of 8 feet, the individual will receive *12.5 mR in 2 minutes* (double distance from source = one fourth of the original intensity).

At 5 feet, the individual will receive 16 mR in 1 minutes:

$$\frac{50\ (I_1)}{x\ (I_2)} = \frac{25\ D_2^2}{16\ (D_1^2)}$$
$$25\ x = 800$$
$$x = 32 \text{ mR in 2 minutes; therefore,}$$
$$\qquad 16 \text{ mR in 1 minutes at 5 feet.}$$

At 6 feet, the individual will receive 22.2 mR in 2 minutes:

$$\frac{50\ (I_1)}{x\ (I_2)} = \frac{36\ (D_2^2)}{16\ (D_1^2)}$$
$$36\ x = 800$$
$$x = 22.22 \text{ mR in 2 minutes at 6 feet}$$

Therefore, the most effective option is B, *12.5 mR in 2 minutes at 8 feet. (Bushong, p 66)*

103. **(C)** The most radiosensitive portion of the GI tract is the small bowel. Projecting from the lining of the small bowel are villi, from the crypts of Lieberkühn, which are responsible for the absorption of nutrients into the bloodstream. Because the cells of the villi are continually being cast off, new cells must continually arise from the crypts of Lieberkühn. Being highly mitotic, undifferentiated stem cells, they are very radiosensitive. Thus, the small bowel is the most radiosensitive portion of the GI tract. In the adult, the CNS is the most radioresistant system. *(Dowd & Tilson, p 155)*

104. **(D)** Fractionation and protraction influence the effect of radiation on tissue. Larger quantities, of course, increase tissue effect. The energy (quality, penetration) of the radiation determines whether the effects will be superficial (erythema) or deep (organ dose). Certain tissues (such as blood-forming organs, the lens, and the gonads) are more radiosensitive than others (such as muscle and nerve). If the dose is delivered in *portions (fractionation)*, and/or delivered over a *length of time (protraction)*, the *less the tissue effects. (Bushong, p 496)*

105. **(D)** The photoelectric effect occurs when a relatively low-energy photon uses all its energy to eject an inner-shell electron. That electron flies off into space, leaving a hole in, for example, the K shell. An L-shell electron then drops down to fill the K vacancy, and in doing so emits a characteristic ray whose energy equals the difference in binding energies for the K and L shells. The photoelectric effect occurs with high-atomic-number absorbers such as bone and with positive contrast media. *(Bushong, p 176)*

106. **(A)** Filters are used in radiography to remove soft (low-energy) radiation that contributes only to patient dose. The filters are usually made of aluminum. Equipment operating above 70 kVp must have *total filtration* of 2.5 mm aluminum equivalent (inherent + added). *(Bushong, p 11)*

107. **(C)** The use of a *grid* requires an increase in mAs and, therefore, patient dose; the higher the grid ratio, the greater the increase in mAs required. *Collimation* restricts the amount of tissue being irradiated and therefore reduces patient dose. *High kVp* reduces the amount of radiation absorbed by the patient's tissues

(recall the photoelectric effect), and low mAs reduces the quantity of radiation delivered to the patient. The higher the speed (fast) of the *intensifying screens*, the less the required mAs. (*Bushong, pp 11, 248*)

108. **(B)** Kilovoltage (kV) and the HVL (half-value layer) effect a change in both the quantity and the quality of the primary beam. *The principal qualitative factor of the primary beam is kV*, but an increase in kV will also increase the *number* of photons produced at the target. HVL, defined as *the amount of material necessary to decrease the intensity of the beam to one half*, therefore changes both beam quality and beam quantity. Milliamperage is directly proportional to x-ray intensity (quantity) but is unrelated to the quality of the beam. (*Thompson et al, p 405*)

109. **(B)** Aluminum filters are used to decrease patient skin dose by absorbing the low energy photons (therefore *decreased* mR output) that *do not contribute to the image* but *do contribute to patient skin dose*. HVL is defined as that thickness of any absorber that will decrease the intensity of a particular beam to one half of its original value. As filtration of an x-ray beam is increased, the overall *average energy of the resulting beam is greater* (because the low energy photons have been removed)—and therefore the HVL thickness required would be greater. (*Bushong, p 165*)

110. **(A)** The *roentgen measures ionization in air and is referred to as the unit of exposure*. Rad is an acronym for radiation absorbed dose, and rem is an acronym for radiation equivalent man. RBE is used to determine biologic damage in living tissue. (*Thompson et al, p 456*)

111. **(D)** All of the tissues listed are considered especially radiosensitive tissues. Excessive radiation to the *reproductive organs* can cause genetic mutations or sterility. Excessive radiation to the *blood-forming organs* can cause leukemia or life span shortening. *Lymphocyte* cells are the most radiosensitive cells in the body. (*Bushong, p 492*)

112. **(C)** An *HVL* may be defined as the amount and thickness of absorber necessary to reduce the radiation intensity to half its original value. Thus, the first HVL would reduce the intensity to 50% of its original value, the second to 25%, the third to 12.5%, and the fourth to 6.25% of its original value. (*Bushong, p 54*)

113. **(D)** All the factors listed influence the effect of radiation on tissue. Larger *quantities*, of course, increase tissue effect. The *energy* (quality, penetration) of the radiation determines whether the effects will be superficial (erythema) or deep (organ dose). *Certain tissues* (such as blood-forming organs, the lens, and the gonads) are more radiosensitive than others (such as muscle and nerve). The *length of time* over which the exposure is spread *(fractionation)* is important; the longer the period of time, the less the tissue effects. (*Bushong, pp 496–497*)

114. **(B)** Radiographic and fluoroscopic equipment is designed to help decrease the exposure dose to patient and operator. One of the design features is the exposure cord. Exposure cords on *fixed* equipment must be short enough to prevent the exposure from being made outside the control booth. Exposure cords on *mobile* equipment must be long enough to permit the operator to stand at least 6 feet from the x-ray tube. (*Bushong, p 569*)

115. **(B)** In the *photoelectric effect*, a relatively low-energy photon uses all its energy to eject an inner-shell electron, leaving a vacancy. An electron from the shell above drops down to fill the vacancy and in doing so gives up a characteristic ray. This type of interaction is most harmful to the patient, as all the photon energy is transferred to tissue. In *Compton scatter*, a high-energy incident photon ejects an outer-shell electron. The incident photon is deflected with reduced energy, but it usually retains most of its energy and exits the body as an energetic scattered ray. This scattered ray will either contribute to image fog or *pose a radiation hazard to personnel*, depending on its direction of exit. In *classical* scatter, a low-energy photon interacts with an atom but causes no ionization; the incident photon disappears into the atom, and is then immediately released as a photon of identical energy but changed direction. *Pair production* is an interaction that

occurs only at energies of 1.02 MeV, and therefore it does not occur in diagnostic radiography. *(Bushong, pp 174–175)*

116. **(B)** Whole-body dose is calculated to include all the especially radiosensitive organs. The gonads, the lens of the eye, and the blood-forming organs are particularly radiosensitive. Some body parts, such as the skin and extremities, have a higher annual dose limit. *(Bushong, p 555)*

117. **(B)** *Rad* is an acronym for *radiation absorbed dose*; it measures the energy deposited in any material; that is, It is equal to *100 ergs of energy per gram of any absorber. Roentgen* is the unit of exposure; it measures the quantity of ionizations in air. *Rem* is an acronym for *radiation equivalent man*; it includes the RBE specific to the tissue irradiated and therefore is a valid unit of measurement for the *dose* to biologic tissue. *(Bushong, p 24)*

118. **(C)** Ionization is the fundamental principle of operation of both the film badge and pocket dosimeter. In the film badge, the film's silver halide emulsion is ionized by x-ray photons. The pocket dosimeter contains an ionization chamber, and the number of ionizations taking place may be equated to exposure dose; it is accurate, but it is used only to detect larger amounts of radiation exposure. The *TLD* can measure exposures as low as 5 mrem, whereas *film badges* will measure a minimum exposure only as low as 10 mrem. TLDs contain lithium fluoride crystals that undergo characteristic changes upon irradiation. When the crystals are subsequently *heated*, they emit a quantity of visible *(thermo)luminescence/light* in proportion to the amount of radiation absorbed. The relatively new *OSLs* contain aluminum oxide crystals that also undergo characteristic changes upon irradiation. When the Al_2O_3 crystals are *stimulated by a laser*, they emit *(optically stimulated) luminescence/light* in proportion to the amount of radiation absorbed. *OSLs can measure exposures as low as 1 mrem. (Thompson et al, p 461)*

119. **(D)** Irradiation damage is a result of either the effects of irradiation on water (radiolysis) or its effects on macromolecules. Effects on macromolecules include main chain scission, cross-linking, and point lesions. Main chain scission breaks the DNA molecule into two or more pieces. Cross-linking is incorrect joining of broken DNA fragments. A point lesion is the disruption of a single chemical bond as a result of irradiation. Because 80% of the body is made up of water, radiolysis of water is the predominant radiation interaction in the body. *(Bushong, p 503)*

120. **(B)** The reproductive cells are considered among the most radiosensitive cells in the body. The immature female sex cells are the oogonia; they mature to ova. The immature male sex cells are the spermatogonia; they mature to sperm. Different amounts of ionizing radiation to these cells can cause differing levels/degrees of response. Doses as low as 10 rad can cause menstrual changes in the woman and decrease the number of sperm in the man. At 200 rad temporary infertility is likely, and at 500 rad sterility will result. *(Bushong, p 523)*

121. **(C)** Lead aprons are worn by occupationally exposed individuals during fluoroscopic procedures. Lead aprons are available with various lead equivalents; 0.25, 0.5, and 1.0 mm are the most common. The *1.0-mm* lead equivalent apron will provide close to 100% protection at most kVp levels, but it is rarely used because it weighs anywhere from 12 to 24 lb. *A 0.25-mm* lead equivalent apron will attenuate about 97% of a 50-kVp x-ray beam, 66% of a 75-kVp beam, and 51% of a 100-kVp beam. *A 0.5-mm* apron will attenuate about 99% of a 50-kVp beam, 88% of a 75-kVp beam, and 75% of a 100-kVp beam. *(Thompson et al, p 457)*

122. **(A)** Lead aprons require certain maintenance and care if they are to continue to provide protection from ionizing radiation. They can be kept clean with a damp cloth. It is very important that they be hung when not in use, rather than being folded or left in a heap between examinations. A folded or crumpled position encourages the formation of cracks in the leaded vinyl. Lead aprons should be *fluoroscoped* (at about 120 kVp) at least *once a year* to check for development of any cracks. *(Bushong, p 464)*

123. **(D)** Fluoroscopy is potentially a high patient dose procedure. The principal reason is that the source of x-ray photons is much closer to the patient than in overhead radiography. There are recommendations that provide guidelines for minimum SSD, maximum tube output, collimation, timer, exposure switch specifications, and others. *SSD must be at least 38 cm (15 inches)* in *stationary* (fixed) fluoroscopic equipment, and *at least 30 cm (12 inches)* for *mobile* fluoroscopic equipment. The tabletop intensity of the fluoroscopic beam must be less than 10 R/min. A cumulative timing device must be available to signal the fluoroscopist (audibly, visibly, or both) when a maximum of 5 minutes of fluoroscopy time has elapsed. High level mode requires continuous manual activation and audible signal. (*Dowd and Tilson, p 175*)

124. **(B)** Compton scattering occurs when a relatively high-energy incident photon uses *part* of its energy to eject an outer-shell electron, and in doing so changes its direction (is scattered). The energy retained by the scattered photon depends on the angle formed by the ejected electron and the scattered photon: The greater the angle of deflection, the less the retained energy. Compton scatter is very energetic scatter. It emerges from the patient and is responsible for scattered radiation reaching the image in the form of fog. Characteristic radiation is associated with the photoelectric effect. (*Bushong, pp 174–176*)

125. **(B)** Bergonié and Tribondeau theorized in 1906 that all precursor cells are particularly radiosensitive (eg, stem cells found in bone marrow). There are several types of stem cells in bone marrow, and the different types differ in degree of radiosensitivity. Of these, red blood cell precursors, or erythroblasts, are the most radiosensitive. White blood cell precursors, or myelocytes, follow. Platelet precursor cells, or megakaryocytes, are the least radiosensitive. Myocytes are mature muscle cells and are fairly radioresistant. (*Bushong, p 495*)

126. **(D)** The pregnant radiographer *should declare her pregnancy* to her supervisor; at that time her radiation exposure history can be reviewed and appropriate assignments made. Special arrangements are required for occupational monitoring of the pregnant radiographer. The pregnant radiographer will wear two dosimeters: one in its usual place at the collar, and the other, a "baby/fetal dosimeter," worn over the abdomen and *under* the lead apron during fluoroscopy. The baby/fetal dosimeter must be identified as such and must always be worn in the same place. Care must be taken not to mix the position of the two dosimeters. The dosimeters are read monthly, as usual. (*Bushong, p 560*)

127. **(D)** *Chromosome aberration, cell death, and malignant disease* are major effects of DNA irradiation, often as a result of abnormal metabolic activity. If the damage happens to the DNA of a germ cell, the radiation response may not occur until one or more generations later. (*Bushong, pp 404–405*)

128. **(C)** The development of male and female reproductive stem cells has important radiation protection implications. Male stem cells reproduce continuously. However, the female stem cells develop only during fetal life; females are born with all the reproductive cells they will ever have. It is exceedingly important to shield children whenever possible, as they have their reproductive futures ahead of them. (*Bushong, p 522*)

129. **(C)** Figure 3–4 illustrates a linear threshold dose–response curve. Its linear aspect indicates that the response/effect is directly related to the dose received, that is, as the dose increases, the response increases. The fact that this is a threshold curve indicates that a particular dose is required before any response/effect will occur. (*Bushong, p 498*)

130. **(D)** The best way to ensure patient cooperation is through effective *communication*. A patient who understands what the examination entails, who knows what to expect, and what will be expected of him or her is better able to cooperate with the radiographer. This patient is more likely to be able to maintain the required position and suspend their respiration when required—thereby avoiding a repeated image. Radiographers who use their knowledge along with patience and critical thinking

skills are more apt to obtain good images the *first* time around, thus avoiding repeat examinations. The use of *AEC* also helps avoid repeat radiographs; AEC will adjust the exposure—compensating for position, habitus, or pathology, and reducing the likelihood of repeat radiographs. (*Dowd & Tilson, p 243*)

131. **(A)** Characteristic radiation is one of two kinds of x-rays produced at the tungsten target of the x-ray tube. The incident, or incoming, high-speed electron ejects a K-shell tungsten electron. This leaves a hole in the K shell, and an L-shell electron drops down to fill the K vacancy. Because L electrons are at a higher energy level than K-shell electrons, the L-shell electron gives up the difference in binding energy in the form of a photon, a "characteristic x-ray" (characteristic of the K shell). (*Selman, p 115*)

132. **(A)** The genetically significant dose (GSD) illustrates that large exposures to a few people are cause for little concern when diluted by the total population. On the other hand, we all share the burden of that radiation received by the total population, especially as the use of medical radiation increases, and so each individual's share of the total exposure increases. (*Selman, pp 386–387*)

133. **(C)** The likelihood of radiation effects to occupationally exposed individuals whose dose is kept below the recommended limits is very remote. Exposure to ionizing radiation always carries some risk, but studies have indicated that the risk is a very small one if established guidelines are followed. Potential hazards must be understood and proper precautions taken. (*Bushong, p 555*)

134. **(A)** Every radiographic examination involves an *ESE*, which can be determined fairly easily. It also involves a gonadal dose and marrow dose, which if needed, can be calculated by the radiation physicist. If the ESE of a particular examination was calculated to determine the *equivalent whole-body dose*, this is termed the *effective dose*. For example, the ESE of a PA chest is approximately 70 mrem, while the effective dose is 10 mrem. The effective (whole-

body) dose is much less because much of the body is not included in the primary beam. (*Fosbinder & Kelsey, p 390*)

135. **(A)** Nondividing, differentiated cells are specialized, mature cells that *do not undergo mitosis*. Having these qualities, they are rendered radioresistant, according to the theory proposed by Bergonié and Tribondeau. The adult nervous system is composed of nondividing, differentiated cells, and thus is the most radioresistant system in the adult. Epithelial tissue and lymphocytes contain many precursor stem cells, and hence are among the most radiosensitive cells in the body. (*Bushong, p 492*)

136. **(B)** Occupationally exposed individuals are required to use devices to record and document the radiation they receive over a given period of time, traditionally 1 month. The most commonly used personal dosimeters are the OSL, the TLD, and the film badge. These devices are worn *only* for documentation of occupational exposure, not for any medical or dental x-rays received as a patient. *TLDs* are personnel radiation monitors that use lithium fluoride crystals. Once exposed to ionizing radiation and then heated, these crystals *give off light* proportional to the amount of radiation received. *OSL dosimeters* are personnel radiation monitors that use aluminum oxide crystals. These crystals, once exposed to ionizing radiation and then subjected to a laser, and *give off luminescence* proportional to the amount of radiation received. The *pocket dosimeter* contains an ionization chamber (containing *air*), and the number of ions formed (of either sign) is equated to exposure dose. (*Bushong, p 594*)

137. **(B)** The relationship between x-ray intensity and distance from the source is expressed in the inverse square law of radiation. The formula is

$$\frac{I_1}{I_2} = \frac{D_2^2}{D_1^2}$$

Substituting known values,

$$\frac{16 \text{ R/hr}}{6 \text{ R/hr}} = \frac{x^2}{16}$$
$$6\,x^2 = 256$$

$$x^2 = 42.66$$
$$x = 6.5 \text{ feet (necessary to decrease}$$
$$\text{the exposure to 6 R/hr)}$$

Note that in order for the exposure rate to decrease, the distance from the source of radiation must increase. (*Bushong, pp 68*)

138. **(C)** Biologic tissue is more sensitive to radiation when it is in an oxygenated state. A characteristic of many avascular (and therefore hypoxic) tumors is their resistance to treatment with radiation. Hyperbaric (high-pressure oxygen) therapy is used in some therapy centers in an effort to increase the sensitivity of the tissues being treated. (*Bushong, pp 496–497*)

139. **(D)** Limiting the irradiated field size, through collimation or other beam restriction, is perhaps the most effective way of controlling patient exposure dose. The smaller the irradiated area, the smaller the patient dose; the larger the irradiated area, the larger the patient dose. Therefore, the 14 × 17 primary beam size will result in the greatest patient exposure dose.

With greater beam restriction, less biologic material is irradiated, thereby reducing the possibility of harmful effects. Additionally, if less tissue is irradiated, less scattered radiation is produced, resulting in improved contrast and image quality. (*Dowd & Tilson, p 231*)

140. **(C)** The patient, as the first scatterer, is the most important scatterer. At 1 m from the patient, the intensity of the scattered beam is 0.1% of the intensity of the primary beam. Compton scatter emerging from the patient is almost as energetic as the primary beam entering the patient. (*Selman, p 535*)

141. **(D)** A TLD is a sensitive and accurate device used in radiation dosimetry. It may be used as a personal dosimeter or to measure patient dose during radiographic examinations and therapeutic procedures. The TLD utilizes a thermoluminescent phosphor, usually lithium fluoride. When used as a personal monitor, the TLD is worn for 1 month. During this time, it stores information regarding the radiation to which it has been exposed. It is then returned to the commercial supplier. In the laboratory, the phosphors are heated. They respond by emitting a particular quantity of light (not heat) that is in proportion to the quantity of radiation delivered to it. After they are cleared of stored information, they are returned for reuse. (*Bushong, p 580*)

142. **(A)** Because the established dose-limit formula guideline is used for occupationally exposed persons 18 years of age and older, guidelines had to be established to cover the event that a student entered the clinical component of a radiography educational program prior to age 18. The guideline states that the occupational dose limit for students *under age 18* is *0.1 rem* (100 mrem or 1 mSv) in any given year. It is important to note that this 0.1 rem *is included* in the 0.5-rem dose limit allowed for the student as a member of the general public. (*Bushong, p 557*)

143. **(B)** Patients will occasionally question the radiographer regarding the amount of radiation they are receiving during their examination. Most of these patients are merely curious because they have heard a recent news report about x-rays, or have perhaps studied about x-rays in school recently. It is a good idea for radiographers to have some knowledge of average exposure doses for patients who desire this information. The curious patient can also be referred to the medical physicist for more detailed information. The average high kVp chest with grid delivers an ESE of about 20 mrad (0.020 rad). The same chest done without grid at 80 kVp would deliver an ESE of about 12 mrad (0.012 rad). The average AP supine lumbar spine radiograph delivers an ESE of about 350 mrad (0.35 rad). The average AP supine abdomen delivers about 300 mrad; the average AP cervical spine is about 80 mrad. (*Dowd & Tilson, p 247*)

144. **(D)** According to Bergonié and Tribondeau, the most radiosensitive cells are undifferentiated, rapidly dividing cells, such as lymphocytes, intestinal crypt (of Lieberkühn) cells, and spermatogonia. Liver cells are among the types of cells that are somewhat differentiated and capable of mitosis. These characteristics

render them somewhat radiosensitive. Muscle cells, as well as nerve cells and red blood cells, are highly differentiated and do not divide. Therefore, in order of *increasing* sensitivity (from least to greatest sensitivity), the cells are muscle, liver, and then intestinal crypt cells. *(Selman, pp 374–375)*

145. **(D)** *Secondary* radiation includes *leakage and scattered* radiation. The control booth wall is a secondary barrier; therefore, the primary beam must never be directed toward it. The x-ray tube housing must reduce leakage radiation to less than 100 mR/hour at a distance of 1 m from the housing. Lead aprons, lead gloves, portable x-ray barriers, and so on are also designed to protect the user from exposure to *scattered* radiation and will not protect her or him from the primary beam. *(Selman, p 403)*

146. **(B)** Protective barriers are classified as either primary or secondary. Primary barriers protect from the useful, or primary, x-ray beam and consist of a certain thickness of lead. They are located anywhere that the primary beam can possibly be directed, for example, the walls of the x-ray room. The walls of the x-ray room usually require a 1/16-inch (1.5-mm) thickness of lead and should be 7 feet high. Secondary barriers protect from secondary (scattered and leakage) radiation. Secondary barriers are control booths, lead aprons, and gloves, and the wall of the x-ray room *above 7 feet*. Secondary barriers require much less lead than primary barriers. *(Bushong, p 571)*

147. **(C)** The radiograph illustrates testing done to evaluate the x-ray beam and light beam alignment. Light-localized collimators must be tested periodically and must be accurate to within 2% of the SID. Linearity means that a given mA, using different mA stations with appropriate exposure time adjustments, will provide consistent intensity. A star pattern would be used to evaluate focal spot resolution, and a parallel line-type resolution pattern could also be used to evaluate spatial resolution. *(Bushong, p 568)*

148. **(D)** As the amount of time one spends in a controlled area decreases, radiation exposure

should decrease. Radiation exposure is affected considerably by one's proximity to the radiation source, as defined by the inverse square law. Barriers (shielding) are an effective means of reducing radiation exposure; primary barriers, such as walls, protect one from the primary beam, and secondary barriers, such as lead aprons, are used to protect one from secondary radiation. *(Bushong, p 557)*

149. **(A)** The effects of a quantity of radiation delivered to a body is dependent on a few factors, including the amount of radiation received, the size of the irradiated area, and how the radiation is delivered in time. If the radiation is delivered in portions over a period of time, it is said to be fractionated and has a less harmful effect than if the radiation was delivered all at once. Cells have an opportunity to repair and some recovery occurs between doses. *(Bushong, p 496)*

150. **(B)** *Somatic effects* of radiation refer to those effects experienced directly by the exposed individual, such as erythema, epilation, and cataracts. *Genetic effects* of radiation exposure are caused by irradiation of the reproductive cells of the exposed individual and are transmitted from one generation to the next. *(Selman, p 382)*

151. **(A)** The x-ray tube's glass envelope and oil coolant are considered inherent ("built-in") filtration. Thin sheets of aluminum are added to make *a total of at least 2.5 mm Al equivalent filtration in equipment operated above 70 kVp.* This is done to remove the low-energy photons that serve only to contribute to patient skin dose. *(Bushong, p 168)*

152. **(C)** *Erythema* is the reddening of skin as a result of exposure to large quantities of ionizing radiation. It was one of the first somatic responses to irradiation demonstrated to the early radiology pioneers. The effects of radiation exposure to the skin follow a *nonlinear, threshold dose–response relationship.* An individual's response to skin irradiation depends on the dose received, the period of time over which it was received, the size of the area irradiated, and the individual's sensitivity. The dose that it takes to bring about a noticeable erythema is referred to as the *SED*. *(Bushong, p 521)*

153. **(A)** Radiation effects that appear days or weeks following exposure (early effects) are in response to relatively high radiation doses. These should never occur in diagnostic radiology today; they occur only in response to doses much greater than those used in diagnostic radiology. One of the effects that may be noted in such a circumstance is the hematologic effect—reduced numbers of white blood cells, red blood cells, and platelets in the circulating blood. Immediate local tissue effects can include effects on the gonads (temporary infertility) and on the skin (epilation, erythema). Acute radiation lethality, or radiation death, occurs after an acute exposure and results in death in weeks or days. Radiation-induced malignancy, leukemia, and genetic effects are late effects (or stochastic effects) of radiation exposure. These can occur years after survival of an acute radiation dose, or after exposure to low levels of radiation over a long period of time. Radiation workers need to be especially aware of the late effects of radiation because their exposure to radiation is usually low-level over a long period of time. Occupational radiation protection guidelines are therefore based on late effects of radiation according to a linear, nonthreshold dose–response curve. *(Bushong, p 537)*

154. **(B)** We must be particularly careful to avoid radiating a newly fertilized ovum. This is precisely the time when a pregnancy may be unsuspected and fetal irradiation could be most damaging. The ICRP used to recommend use of the "10-day rule." Current protocol now recommends its use along with elective booking, patient questionnaires, and patient postings. Elective booking recommends that discretionary abdominal radiography on women of childbearing age should be limited to the first 10 days following the onset of menses, a time when pregnancy is most improbable. *(Selman, p 389)*

155. **(D)** A controlled area is one that is occupied by radiation workers who are trained in radiation safety and who wear radiation monitors.

The exposure rate in a *controlled area* must not exceed 100 mR per week; its occupancy factor is considered to be 1, indicating that the area may always be occupied, and therefore requires maximum shielding. An *uncontrolled area* is one occupied by the general population; the exposure rate there must not exceed 10 mR per week. Shielding requirements vary according to several factors, one being *occupancy factor. (Bushong, p 573)*

156. **(A)** The length of time from conception to birth, that is, pregnancy, is referred to as *gestation.* The term *congenital* refers to a condition existing at birth. Neonatal relates to the time immediately after birth and the first month of life. *In vitro* refers to something living outside a living body (as in a test tube), as opposed to *in vivo* (within a living system). *(Bushong, p 544)*

157. **(D)** The *bucky slot cover* shields the opening at the side of the table, as the bucky tray is parked at the end of the table for the fluoroscopy procedure; this is important because the opening created would otherwise allow scattered radiation to emerge at approximately the level of the operator's gonads. The *exposure switch* (usually a foot pedal) must be of the dead-man type; that is, when the foot is released from the switch, there is immediate termination of exposure. The *cumulative exposure timer* sounds or interrupts the exposure after 5 minutes of fluoro time, thus making the fluoroscopist aware of accumulated fluoro time. In addition, *source-to-tabletop distance* is restricted to at least 15 inches for stationary equipment and at least 12 inches for mobile equipment. Increased source-to-tabletop distance increases source-to-patient distance, thereby decreasing patient dose. *(Bushong, p 570)*

158. **(A)** The faster the intensifying screens used, the less the required mAs. Decreasing the intensity (mAs, quantity) of photons significantly contributes to reducing total patient dose. Decreasing the kilovoltage would increase patient dose because the primary beam would be made up of less penetrating photons, and so the mAs would have to be increased. The importance of patient shielding is never diminished. *(Bushong, p 222)*

159. **(C)** There are different types of monitoring devices available for the occupationally exposed. Ionization is the fundamental principle of operation of both the film badge and the pocket dosimeter. In the *film badge*, the film's silver halide emulsion is ionized by x-ray photons. The *pocket dosimeter* contains an ionization chamber (containing *air*), and the number of ions formed (of either sign) is equated to exposure dose. *TLDs* are personnel radiation monitors that use lithium fluoride crystals. Once exposed to ionizing radiation and then heated, these crystals give off light proportional to the amount of radiation received. *OSL dosimeters* are personnel radiation monitors that use aluminum oxide crystals. These crystals, once exposed to ionizing radiation and then subjected to a laser, give off luminescence proportional to the amount of radiation received. *(Selman, p 400)*

160. **(B)** With greater beam restriction, less biologic material is irradiated, thereby reducing the possibility of harmful effects. If less tissue is irradiated, less scattered radiation is produced, resulting in improved IR contrast. The total filtration is not a function of beam restriction, but rather is a radiation protection guideline aimed at reducing patient skin dose. *(Selman, p 247)*

161. **(B)** Radiation safety guidelines are valuable only if they are followed by radiation personnel. The RSO is responsible for being certain that established guidelines are enforced and that personnel understand and employ radiation safety measures to protect themselves and their patients. The RSO is also responsible for performing routine equipment checks to ensure that all equipment meets radiation safety standards. *(NCRP Report No. 405, p 34)*

162. **(B)** The genetic effects of radiation and some somatic effects, like leukemia, are plotted on a linear dose–response curve. The linear dose–response curve has *no threshold*; that is, *there is no dose below which radiation is absolutely safe.* The nonlinear/sigmoidal dose–response curve has a threshold and is thought to be generally correct for most somatic effects. *(Bushong, p 498)*

163. **(A)** In the *photoelectric effect*, a relatively low-energy photon uses all its energy to eject an inner-shell electron, leaving a vacancy. An electron from the shell above drops down to fill the vacancy, and in doing so emits a characteristic ray. This type of interaction is most harmful to the patient, as *all the photon energy is transferred to tissue.* In *Compton scatter*, a high-energy incident photon uses some of its energy to eject an outer-shell electron. In doing so, the incident photon is deflected with reduced energy, but usually retains most of its energy and exits the body as an energetic scattered ray. The scattered radiation will either contribute to image fog or pose a radiation hazard to personnel, depending on its direction of exit. In *classical scatter*, a low-energy photon interacts with an atom but causes no ionization; the incident photon disappears in the atom, then immediately reappears and is released as a photon of identical energy but changed direction. *Thompson scatter* is another name for classical scatter. *(Bushong, p 176)*

164. **(A)** Protective apparel functions to protect the occupationally exposed person *from scattered radiation only.* Lead aprons and lead gloves do not protect from the primary beam. No one in the radiographic room except the patient must ever be exposed to the primary beam. The occupationally exposed and those (family and friends) who might assist a patient during an examination must wear protective apparel and keep out of the way of the primary beam. *(Bushong, p 596)*

165. **(A)** It is our ethical responsibility to minimize the radiation dose to our patients. X-rays produced at the tungsten target make up a heterogeneous primary beam. There are many "soft" (low-energy) photons that, if not removed by filters, would only contribute to greater patient skin dose. They are too weak to penetrate the patient and contribute to the image-forming radiation; they penetrate a small thickness of tissue and are absorbed. *(Bushong, p 11)*

166. **(D)** *Radiation quality* determines degree of penetration and the amount of energy transferred to the irradiated tissue (LET). Certainly, the larger the absorbed radiation dose, the greater the effect. Biologic effect is increased as the size of the irradiated area is increased. The nature of the effect is influenced by the location of irradiated tissue (bone marrow vs gonads and so on). *(Bushong, pp 520–521)*

167. **(D)** *Beam restriction* is probably the single best method of protecting your patient from excessive radiation. It is also an important factor in obtaining high-quality radiographs because there will be less fog from scattered radiation. *Shielding* areas not included in the radiograph, especially particularly radiosensitive areas, is another effective means of reducing patient dose. If the patient is subjected to less radiation exposure, then so is the operator. *Shielding, distance,* and *time* are the three cardinal rules of radiation protection. *High-kV, low-mAs* exposure factors employ the use of fewer and more penetrating x-rays. *(Bontrager, p 58)*

168. **(A)** The most radiosensitive portion of the GI tract is the small bowel. Projecting from the lining of the small bowel are villi, from the crypts of Lieberkühn, which are responsible for the absorption of nutrients into the bloodstream. Because the cells of the villi are continually being cast off, new cells must continually arise from the crypts of Lieberkühn. Being highly mitotic, undifferentiated stem cells, they are very radiosensitive. Thus, the small bowel is the most radiosensitive portion of the GI tract. In the adult, the CNS is the most radioresistant system and the epidermis is composed of mature, postmitotic cells—making them both radioresistant. *(Dowd & Tilson, p 155)*

169. **(A)** mAs regulates the quantity of radiation delivered to the patient, and kVp regulates the quality (penetration) of the radiation delivered to the patient. Therefore, higher energy (more penetrating) radiation (which is more likely to exit the patient), accompanied by lower mAs, is the safest combination for the patient. *(Thompson et al, p 275)*

170. **(C)** Late effects of radiation can occur in cells that have survived a previous irradiation months or years earlier. These late effects, such as carcinogenesis and genetic effects, are "all-or-nothing" effects—either the organism develops cancer or it does not. Most late effects do not have a threshold dose; that is, *any* dose, however small, theoretically can induce an effect. Increasing that dose *will* increase the *likelihood* of the occurrence, but *will not* affect its *severity*; these effects are termed *stochastic*. *Nonstochastic effects* are those that will not occur below a particular threshold dose and that increase in severity as the dose increases. *(Bushong, p 532)*

171. **(A)** Restriction of field size is one important method of patient protection. However, the accuracy of the light field must be evaluated periodically as part of a QA program. Guidelines for patient protection state that the collimator light and actual irradiated area must be accurate to within 2% of the source-image distance. *(Thompson et al, p 403)*

172. **(A)** Radiographers are usually required to wear one dosimeter, positioned at their collar and worn *outside* a lead apron. Special circumstances, however, warrant the use of a second monitor. During pregnancy, a second "baby monitor" is worn at the abdomen, *under* any lead apron. During special vascular procedures, the dose to the radiographer can increase significantly. This is because the leaded protective curtain is often absent from the fluoro tower and because of the extensive use of cineradiography. As a result, the radiographer's upper extremities can receive a greater exposure (eg, when assisting during catheter introduction), and a *ring or bracelet badge* is often recommended. A second dosimeter is not required when performing mobile radiography. *(Bushong, p 525)*

173. **(C)** The greatest effect–response from irradiation is brought about by a *large dose of radiation to the whole body delivered all at one time*. Whole-body radiation can depress many body functions. With a fractionated dose, the effects would be less severe because the body would have an opportunity to repair between doses. *(Bushong, p 464)*

174. **(D)** A *TLD* is used to measure monthly exposure to radiation, as is the *film badge*. *Lithium fluoride chips* are the thermoluminescent material

used in TLDs. A *pocket dosimeter* (a small personal ionization chamber) measures the quantity of ionizations occurring during the period worn and reads out in mrem; it is used primarily when working with large quantities of radiation. *(Selman, p 400)*

175. **(B)** It is important to limit tabletop exposure during fluoroscopy, because the SSD is so much less than in overhead radiography, so that a much higher skin dose is delivered to the patient. For this reason, the tabletop exposure rate during fluoroscopy shall not exceed 10 R/min. *(Selman, p 415)*

176. **(D)** *Accurate positioning* helps decrease the number of retakes. The use of *high-kV* and *low-mAs* exposure factors limits the quantity of radiation delivered to the patient. Use of *rare earth screens* can enable the technologist to reduce mAs by as much as four to eight times. *Patient shielding* should be used whenever appropriate and possible. *(Selman, p 413)*

177. **(A)** The intensity/exposure rate of radiation at a given distance from a point source is inversely proportional to the square of the distance. This is the inverse square law of radiation, and it is expressed in the following equation:

$$\frac{I_1}{I_2} = \frac{D_2^2}{D_1^2}$$

Substituting known values,

$$\frac{40\text{ mR/hr}}{x\text{ mR/hr}} = \frac{25}{9}$$
$$25\,x = 360$$
$$x = 14.4\text{ mR/hr, } \textit{therefore, 7.2 mR}$$
$$\textit{in 30 minutes}$$

(Bushong, pp 68–70)

178. **(A)** Mobile radiography (along with fluoroscopy and special procedures) is an area of *higher occupational exposure*. With no lead barrier to retreat behind, distance becomes the best source of protection. The exposure switch of mobile equipment must be manufactured to allow the technologist to stand *at least 6 feet* away from the patient and the x-ray tube. Hospital personnel, visitors, and patients must also be protected from unnecessary radiation exposure. Therefore, the radiographer must request that these people leave the immediate area until after the exposure is made, and *announce* in a loud voice when the exposure is about to be made, allowing time for individuals to leave the area. The use of a short SID increases patient exposure and produces poor recorded detail. *(Carlton & Adler, p 523)*

179. **(C)** *Scattered and secondary radiations* are those that have deviated in direction while passing through a part. *Leakage radiation* is radiation that emerges from the leaded tube housing in directions other than that of the useful beam. Tube head construction must keep leakage radiation to less than 0.1 R/hr at 1 m from the tube. *Remnant radiation* is the radiation that emerges from the patient to form the radiographic image. *(Bushong, p 130)*

180. **(D)** The presence of ionizing radiation may be detected in several ways. It has an *ionizing* effect on air, which is the basic principle of the roentgen as unit of measurement. X-rays have a *photographic* effect on film emulsion, which is readily observable on radiographic images. The *fluorescent* effect on certain crystals, such as calcium tungstate and lanthanum, accounts for our use of these phosphors in intensifying screens. Radiation's *physiologic* effects have been demonstrated to be genetic damage, erythema, and cataractogenesis; many of these were noted by the early radiology pioneers. *(Selman, pp 115, 116)*

181. **(C)** *Sensitometry* and *densitometry* are used in evaluation of the film processor; they are just one portion of a complete *quality assurance* (QA) program. *Modulation transfer function* (MTF) is used to express spatial resolution—another component of the QA program. A complete QA program includes testing of all components of the imaging system: processors, focal spot, x-ray timers, filters, intensifying screens, beam alignment, and so on. *(Thompson et al, pp 399–400)*

182. **(B)** Even the smallest exposure to radiation can be harmful. It must, therefore, be every radiographer's objective to keep his or her

occupational exposure as far below the dose limit as possible. Radiology personnel should never hold patients during an x-ray examination. *(Bushong, pp 9–10)*

183. **(C)** The OSL is rapidly becoming the most commonly used personnel monitor today. Film badges and TLDs have been used successfully for years. A pocket dosimeter is used primarily when working with large amounts of radiation and when a daily reading is desired. *(Bushong, p 594)*

184. **(B)** It is our professional responsibility to minimize exposure dose to both patients and ourselves, and one of the most important ways is with a closely collimated radiation field. Gonadal shielding should be used when the patient is of reproductive age or younger, when the gonads are in or near the collimated field, and when the clinical objectives will not be compromised. *(Ballinger & Frank, vol 1, p 45)*

185. **(B)** *Alpha and beta radiation are particulate radiations;* alpha is composed of two protons and two neutrons, and beta is identical to an electron. *Gamma and x-radiation are electromagnetic,* having wavelike fluctuations like other radiations of the electromagnetic spectrum (visible light, radio waves, etc). *(Bushong, p 60)*

186. **(B)** It is well established that sufficient quantities of ionizing radiation can cause a number of serious *somatic* and/or *genetic* effects. *Somatic effects* of radiation are those that affect the *irradiated body itself.* Somatic effects are described as being *early* or *late,* depending on the length of time between irradiation and manifestation of effects. The human reproductive organs are particularly radiosensitive. *Fertility* and *heredity* are greatly affected by the *germ cells* produced within the testes (*spermatogonia*) and ovaries (*oogonia*). Excessive radiation exposure to the gonads can cause *temporary or permanent infertility,* and/or *genetic mutations.* Infertility is somatic because it affects the exposed individual; genetic mutations affect future generations. *(Dowd & Tilson, p 117)*

187. **(C)** As x-ray photons emerge from the x-ray tube, they immediately encounter air—before being intercepted by any material. The *Roentgen* is the unit of exposure; it measures the quantity of ionizations in air. The Roentgen is, therefore, the unit of choice for measuring x-ray tube output—and an ion chamber dosimeter instrument is used for that purpose. *Rad* is an acronym for *radiation absorbed dose;* it measures the energy deposited in any material. *Rem* is an acronym for *radiation equivalent man;* it includes the relative biologic effectiveness Becqueral is the SI unit of measurement for radioactivity. *(Bushong, p 588)*

188. **(B)** The filters (usually aluminum and copper) serve to help measure radiation quality (energy). Only the most energetic radiation will penetrate the copper; radiation of lower levels of energy will penetrate the aluminum, and the lowest energy radiation will pass readily through the unfiltered area. Thus, radiation of different energy levels can be recorded, measured, and reported. *(Bushong, p 593)*

189. **(D)** Elective booking of a radiologic examination after inquiring about the patient's previous menstrual cycle is the most effective means of preventing accidental exposure of a recently fertilized ovum. Patient questionnaires obtain that information from the patient and are often also used in an informed consent form. Patient postings in waiting and changing areas alert patients to advise the radiographer if there is any chance of pregnancy. These three safeguards replace the earlier "10-day rule," which is now obsolete. *(Bushong, p 559)*

190. **(A)** In the photoelectric effect, the incident (low-energy) photon is completely absorbed, and thus is responsible for producing contrast and contributing to patient dose. The photoelectric effect is the interaction between x-ray and tissue that predominates in the diagnostic range. In Compton scatter, only partial absorption occurs, and most energy emerges as scattered photons. In coherent scatter, no energy is absorbed by the part; it all emerges as scattered photons. Pair production occurs only at very high energy levels, at least 1.02 MeV. *(Bushong, p 176)*

191. **(B)** The OSL and TLD are frequently used to measure the radiation exposure of radiographers. The pocket dosimeter may be employed by those radiation workers who are exposed to higher doses of radiation and need a daily reading. A blood test is an unacceptable method of monitoring radiation dose effects, as a very large dose would have to be received before blood changes would occur. *(Sherer et al, p 594)*

192. **(D)** If the exposure rate for the examination is 250 mR/hour (60 minutes), then a 3-minute examination would be proportionally less—as the equation below illustrates:

$$\frac{250 \ (\text{mR})}{60 \ (\text{min})} = \frac{x \ (\text{mR})}{3 \ (\text{min})}$$

$$60 \ x = 750$$

$$x = 12.5 \ \text{mR, dose in 3 minutes}$$

(Bushong, p 570)

193. **(B)** According to the NCRP, the annual occupational *whole-body* dose equivalent limit is 50 mSv (5 rem or 5000 mrem). The *total gestational dose equivalent* limit for embryo/fetus of a *pregnant radiographer* is 5 mSv (500 mrem or 0.5 rem); the *monthly* dose equivalent limit is 0.5 mSv (50 mrem or 0.05rem). The annual occupational whole-body dose equivalent limit for *students* under the age of 18 years is 1 mSv (100 mrem or 0.1 rem). The annual occupational dose equivalent limit for the *lens of the eye*, a particularly radiosensitive organ, is 150 mSv (15 mrem or 0.015 rem). The annual occupational dose equivalent limit for the *skin and extremities* is 500 mSv (50 mrem or 0.05 rem). *(Ballinger & Frank, vol 1, p 46)*

194. **(C)** *Compton* scattering occurs when a relatively *high-energy* incident photon uses *part* of its energy to eject an *outer* shell electron, and in doing so changes its direction (is scattered). The energy retained by the scattered photon depends on the angle formed by the ejected electron and the scattered photon: The greater the angle of deflection, the less the retained energy. Compton scatter is very energetic scatter. It emerges from the patient and is responsible for scatter radiation reaching the image in the form of fog. In the *photoelectric effect*, a relatively *low energy* photon uses *all* its energy to eject an *inner* shell electron, leaving a vacancy. An electron from the shell above drops down to fill the vacancy, and in doing so gives up a characteristic ray. This type of interaction contributes most to patient dose, as all the photon energy is transferred to tissue. In *coherent* scatter, no energy is absorbed by the part; it all emerges as scattered photons. *Pair production* occurs only at very high energy levels, at least 1.02 MeV. *(Bushong, p 174)*

195. **(C)** There are different types of monitoring devices available for the occupationally exposed and anyone who might receive more than *1/10 the annual dose limit* must be monitored. Ionization is the fundamental principle of operation of both the film badge and the pocket dosimeter. In the *film badge,* the film's silver halide emulsion is ionized by x-ray photons. The *pocket dosimeter* contains an ionization chamber (containing *air*), and the number of ions formed (of either sign) is equated to exposure dose. *TLDs* are personnel radiation monitors that use lithium fluoride crystals. Once exposed to ionizing radiation and then heated, these crystals give off light proportional to the amount of radiation received. *OSL dosimeters* are personnel radiation monitors that use aluminum oxide crystals. These crystals, once exposed to ionizing radiation and then subjected to a laser, give off luminescence proportional to the amount of radiation received. *(Bushong, p 593)*

196. **(C)** During fluoroscopic procedures, as FOV decreases, magnification of the output screen image increases and *contrast and resolution improve*. The focal point on an image intensifier's 6-inch field/mode, is further away from the output phosphor than the focal point on the normal mode; therefore, the output image is magnified. Because less minification takes place, the *image is not as bright. Exposure factors are automatically increased* to compensate for the loss in brightness that occurs with smaller FOVs used in magnification mode. *(Fosbinder, p 285)*

197. **(B)** Kilovoltage (kV) and the HVL effect a change in both the quantity and the quality of the primary beam. *The principal qualitative factor of the primary beam is kV,* but an increase in kV will also increase the *number* of photons produced at the target. HVL, defined as *the amount of material necessary to decrease the intensity of the beam to one half,* therefore changes both beam quality and beam quantity. Milliamperage is directly proportional to x-ray intensity (quantity/dose rate) but is unrelated to the quality of the beam. *(Bushong, p 165)*

198. **(B)** Because minerals in rocks and the earth can emanate radioactivity, high levels of radon gas inside homes have been of recent concern. Another source of radon gas is from burning cigarettes, whether as a smoker or as passive exposure. Uranium miners have been identified with a much higher incidence of lung cancer; many of these individuals were also smokers. Radiology departments are not known as a source of radon gas exposure. *(Dowd & tilson, p 147)*

199. **(A)** LET increases with the *ionizing* potential of the radiation, for example, alpha particles are more ionizing than x-radiation; therefore, they have a higher LET. As ionizations and LET increase, there is greater possibility of an effect on living tissue; therefore, the RBE increases. The *RBE* (sometimes called QF—Quality Factor) *of diagnostic x-rays is 1*; the RBE of fast neutrons is 10; the RBE of 5 MeV alpha particles is 20. *(Bushong, p 496)*

200. **(A)** Aluminum filters are used to *decrease* patient skin dose by absorbing the low-energy photons (therefore *decreased* mR output) that *do not contribute to the image* but *do contribute to patient skin dose.* HVL is defined as that thickness of any absorber that will decrease the intensity of a particular beam to one half of its original value. As filtration of an x-ray beam is increased, the overall *average energy of the resulting beam is greater* (because the low-energy photons have been removed)—and therefore the HVL thickness required would be greater. *(Bushong, p 165)*

Subspecialty List

67. Personnel protection
68. Personnel protection
69. Radiation exposure and monitoring
70. Radiation exposure and monitoring
71. Radiation exposure and monitoring
72. Biological aspects of radiation
73. Personnel protection
74. Personnel protection
75. Biological aspects of radiation
76. Minimizing patient exposure
77. Personnel protection
78. Radiation exposure and monitoring
79. Minimizing patient exposure
80. Minimizing patient exposure
81. Biological aspects of radiation
82. Minimizing patient exposure
83. Biological aspects of radiation
84. Biological aspects of radiation
85. Personnel protection
86. Radiation exposure and monitoring
87. Minimizing patient exposure
88. Minimizing patient exposure
89. Minimizing patient exposure
90. Radiation exposure and monitoring
91. Personnel protection
92. Personnel protection
93. Minimizing patient exposure
94. Minimizing patient exposure
95. Biological aspects of radiation
96. Minimizing patient exposure
97. Biological aspects of radiation
98. Biological aspects of radiation
99. Minimizing patient exposure
100. Radiation exposure and monitoring
101. Biological aspects of radiation
102. Personnel protection
103. Biological aspects of radiation
104. Biological aspects of radiation
105. Biological aspects of radiation
106. Minimizing patient exposure
107. Minimizing patient exposure
108. Minimizing patient exposure
109. Minimizing patient exposure
110. Radiation exposure and monitoring
111. Biological aspects of radiation
112. Minimizing patient exposure
113. Minimizing patient exposure
114. Personnel protection
115. Personnel protection
116. Personnel protection
117. Radiation exposure and monitoring
118. Radiation exposure and monitoring
119. Biological aspects of radiation
120. Minimizing patient exposure
121. Personnel protection
122. Personnel protection
123. Minimizing patient exposure
124. Minimizing patient exposure
125. Biological aspects of radiation
126. Personnel protection
127. Biological aspects of radiation
128. Biological aspects of radiation
129. Biological aspects of radiation
130. Minimizing patient exposure
131. Personnel protection
132. Biological aspects of radiation
133. Personnel protection
134. Radiation exposure and monitoring
135. Biological aspects of radiation
136. Radiation exposure and monitoring
137. Personnel protection
138. Biological aspects of radiation
139. Minimizing patient exposure
140. Personnel protection
141. Radiation exposure and monitoring
142. Personnel protection
143. Minimizing patient exposure
144. Minimizing patient exposure
145. Radiation exposure and monitoring
146. Radiation exposure and monitoring
147. Minimizing patient exposure
148. Personnel protection
149. Biological aspects of radiation
150. Biological aspects of radiation
151. Minimizing patient exposure
152. Biological aspects of radiation
153. Biological aspects of radiation
154. Minimizing patient exposure
155. Personnel protection
156. Biological aspects of radiation
157. Personnel protection
158. Minimizing patient exposure
159. Radiation exposure and monitoring
160. Minimizing patient exposure
161. Radiation exposure and monitoring
162. Biological aspects of radiation
163. Minimizing patient exposure
164. Personnel Protection
165. Minimizing patient exposure
166. Biological aspects of radiation
167. Minimizing patient exposure
168. Minimizing patient exposure

169. Minimizing patient exposure
170. Biological aspects of radiation
171. Radiation exposure and monitoring
172. Personnel protection
173. Minimizing patient exposure
174. Radiation exposure and monitoring
175. Radiation exposure and monitoring
176. Minimizing patient exposure
177. Personnel protection
178. Personnel protection
179. Personnel protection
180. Radiation exposure and monitoring
181. Radiation exposure and monitoring
182. Personnel protection
183. Radiation exposure and monitoring
184. Minimizing patient exposure

185. Biological aspects of radiation
186. Biological aspects of radiation
187. Radiation exposure and monitoring
188. Radiation exposure and monitoring
189. Minimizing patient exposure
190. Minimizing patient exposure
191. Radiation exposure and monitoring
192. Minimizing patient exposure
193. Radiation exposure and monitoring
194. Minimizing patient exposure
195. Personnel protection
196. Minimizing patient exposure
197. Minimizing patient exposure
198. Biological aspects of radiation
199. Biological aspects of radiation
200. Minimizing patient exposure

CHAPTER 4

Image Production and Evaluation
Questions

DIRECTIONS (Questions 1 through 250): Each of the numbered items or incomplete statements in this section is followed by answers or by completions of the statement. Select the *one* lettered answer or completion that is *best* in each case.

1. When a slow screen–film system is used with a fast screen–film automatic exposure control system, the resulting images

   (A) are too light.
   (B) are too dark.
   (C) have improved detail.
   (D) have poor detail.

2. What pixel size has a 2048 × 2048 matrix with a 80-cm FOV?

   A. 0.04 mm
   B. 0.08 mm
   C. 0.2 mm
   D. 0.4 mm

3. With all other factors constant, as digital image matrix size increases,

   1. pixel size decreases.
   2. resolution increases.
   3. pixel size increases.

   (A) 1 only
   (B) 2 only
   (C) 1 and 2 only
   (D) 2 and 3 only

4. The conversion of the invisible latent image into a visible manifest image takes place in the

   (A) developer.
   (B) stop bath.
   (C) first half of the fixer process.
   (D) second half of the fixer process.

5. The chest radiograph shown in Figure 4–1 demonstrates

   (A) motion.
   (B) focal spot blur.
   (C) double exposure.
   (D) poor screen–film contact.

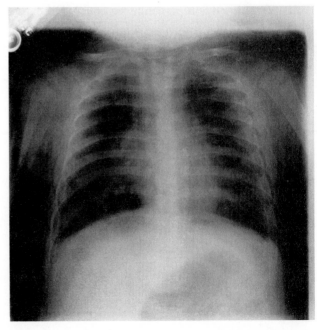

Figure 4–1. Courtesy of Stamford Hospital, Department of Radiology.

6. The absorption of useful radiation by a grid is called

   (A) grid selectivity.
   (B) contrast improvement factor.
   (C) grid cutoff.
   (D) latitude.

7. Most laser film must be handled

   (A) under a Wratten 6B safelight.
   (B) in total darkness.
   (C) under a GBX safelight.
   (D) with high-temperature processors.

8. The exposure factors used for a particular nongrid radiograph were 400 mA, 0.02 second, and 90 kVp. Another radiograph using an 8:1 grid is requested. Which of the following groups of factors is *most* appropriate?

   (A) 400 mA, 0.02 second, 110 kVp
   (B) 200 mA, 0.08 second, 90 kVp
   (C) 300 mA, 0.05 second, 100 kVp
   (D) 400 mA, 0.08 second, 90 kVp

9. Which of the lines indicated in Figure 4–2 represents the dynamic range offered by CR/DR?

   (A) Line A is representative of CR/DR.
   (B) Line B is representative of CR/DR.
   (C) Neither line is representative of CR/DR.
   (D) Both lines are representative of CR/DR.

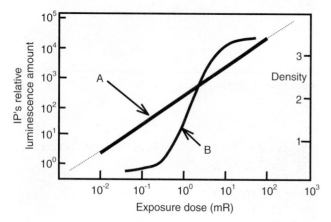

Figure 4–2. Courtesy FUJIFILM Medical Systems USA, Inc.

10. Which of the following are methods of limiting the production of scattered radiation?

    1. Using moderate ratio grids
    2. Using the prone position for abdominal examinations
    3. Restricting the field size to the smallest practical size

    (A) 1 and 2 only
    (B) 1 and 3 only
    (C) 2 and 3 only
    (D) 1, 2, and 3

11. Screen–film imaging is one example of a (n)

    (A) analog system.
    (B) digital system.
    (C) electromagnetic system.
    (D) direct-action radiation system.

12. The three radiographs illustrated in Figure 4–3 were made with identical exposures, but one was developed at 90°F, one at the usual 95°F, and one at 100°F. Which is the radiograph made at 100°F?

    (A) Film A
    (B) Film B
    (C) Film C

13. Decreasing field size from 14 × 17 into 8 × 10 inches will

    (A) decrease radiographic density and decrease the amount of scattered radiation generated within the part.
    (B) decrease radiographic density and increase the amount of scattered radiation generated within the part.
    (C) increase radiographic density and increase the amount of scattered radiation generated within the part.
    (D) increase radiographic density and decrease the amount of scattered radiation generated within the part.

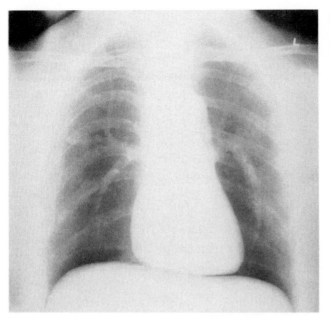

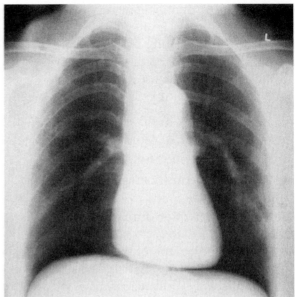

A

B

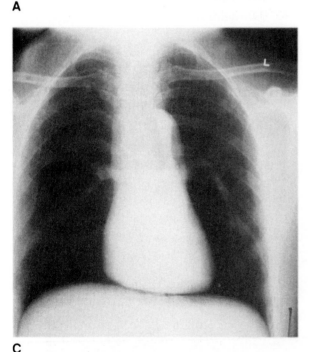

C

Figure 4–3. From the American College of Radiology Learning File. Courtesy of the ACR.

14. Which of the following groups of exposure factors will produce the greatest radiographic density?

(A) 100 mA, 0.30 second

(B) 200 mA, 0.10 second

(C) 400 mA, 0.03 second

(D) 600 mA, 0.03 second

15. That portion of a CR cassette that records the radiologic image is the

(A) emulsion.

(B) helium–neon laser.

(C) photostimulable phosphor.

(D) scanner–reader.

16. The left and right oblique cervical spine radiographs seen in Figure 4–4**A** and **B** were performed using automatic exposure control (AEC) during a particular examination. Which of the following most likely accounts for the difference in radiographic density between the images?

    (A) Focused grid placed upside down
    (B) Incorrect photocell selected
    (C) Incorrect positioning of the part being imaged
    (D) Patient motion during exposure

17. A lateral radiograph of the cervical spine was made at 40 inches using 100 mA and 0.1-second exposure. If it is desired to increase the distance to 72 inches, what should be the new mA, all other factors remaining the same?

    (A) 100
    (B) 200
    (C) 300
    (D) 400

18. All of the following statements regarding dual x-ray absorptiometry are true, *except*

    1. two x-ray photon energies are used.
    2. radiation dose is considerable.
    3. photon attenuation by bone is calculated.

    (A) 1 only
    (B) 1 and 2 only
    (C) 1 and 3 only
    (D) 1, 2, and 3

19. The violet light emited by the photostimulable phosphor (PSP) is transformed into the image seen on the CRT by the

    (A) PSP.
    (B) scanner–reader.
    (C) ADC.
    (D) helium-neon laser.

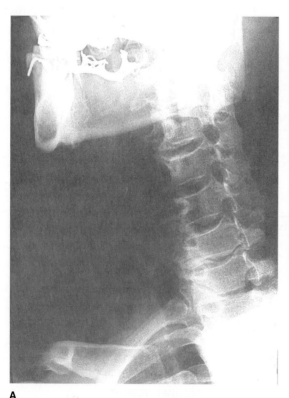

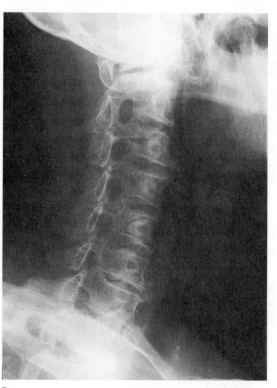

A   B

Figure 4–4. Courtesy of Stamford Hospital, Department of Radiology.

20. A grid is usually employed in which of the following circumstances?

   1. When radiographing a large or dense body part
   2. When using high kilovoltage
   3. When a lower patient dose is required

(A) 1 only
(B) 3 only
(C) 1 and 2 only
(D) 1, 2, and 3

21. If the quantity of black metallic silver on a particular radiograph is such that it allows 1% of the illuminator light to pass through the film, that film has a density of

(A) 0.01.
(B) 0.1.
(C) 1.0.
(D) 2.0.

22. The process of "leveling and windowing" of digital images determines the image

(A) spatial resolution.
(B) contrast.
(C) pixel size.
(D) matrix size.

23. Exposure factors of 90 kVp and 4 mAs are used for a particular nongrid exposure. What should be the new mAs if an 8:1 grid is added?

(A) 8
(B) 12
(C) 16
(D) 20

24. What pixel size has a 1024 × 1024 matrix with a 35-cm FOV?

A. 30 mm
B. 0.35 mm
C. 0.15 mm
D. 0.03 mm

25. In a PA projection of the chest being used for cardiac evaluation, the heart measures 15.2 cm between its widest points. If the magnification factor is known to be 1.3, what is the actual diameter of the heart?

(A) 9.7 cm
(B) 11.7 cm
(C) 19.7 cm
(D) 20.3 cm

26. Unopened boxes of radiographic film should be stored away from radiation and

(A) in the horizontal position.
(B) in the vertical position.
(C) stacked with the oldest on top.
(D) stacked with the newest on top.

27. Which of the following pathologic conditions would require a decrease in exposure factors?

(A) Congestive heart failure
(B) Pneumonia
(C) Emphysema
(D) Pleural effusion

28. Factors that contribute to film fog include

   1. the age of the film.
   2. excessive exposure to safelight.
   3. processor chemistry.

(A) 1 only
(B) 1 and 2 only
(C) 1 and 3 only
(D) 1, 2, and 3

29. X-ray photon energy is inversely related to

   1. photon wavelength.
   2. applied mA.
   3. applied kVp.

(A) 1 only
(B) 1 and 2 only
(C) 1 and 3 only
(D) 1, 2, and 3

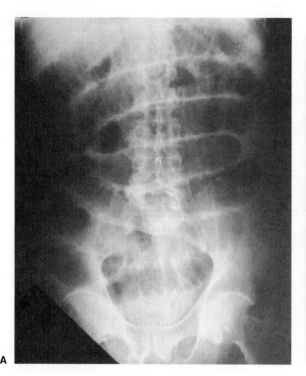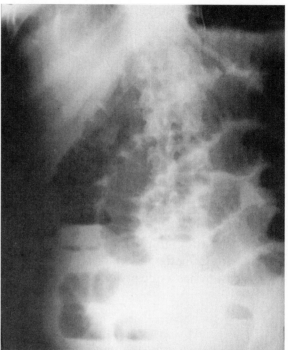

A

B

Figure 4–5. From the American College of Radiology Learning File. Courtesy of the ACR.

30. Which of the radiographs in Figure 4–5 most likely required a greater exposure?

   (A) Image A
   (B) Image B
   (C) No difference in exposure was required

31. Characteristics of digital radiographic imaging include

   1. solid state detector receptor plates.
   2. direct-capture imaging system.
   3. immediate image display.

   (A) 1 only
   (B) 1 and 3 only
   (C) 2 and 3 only
   (D) 1, 2, and 3

32. Compared to a low ratio grid, a high ratio grid will

   1. absorb more primary radiation.
   2. absorb more scattered radiation.
   3. allow more centering latitude.

   (A) 1 only
   (B) 1 and 2 only
   (C) 2 and 3 only
   (D) 1, 2, and 3

33. How is the mAs adjusted in an AEC system as the film–screen speed combination is decreased?

   (A) The mAs increases as film–screen speed decreases.
   (B) Both the mAs and the kVp increase as film–screen speed decreases.
   (C) The mAs decreases as film–screen speed decreases.
   (D) The mAs remains unchanged as film–screen speed decreases.

34. Using a short (25–30 inches) SID with a large size (14 × 17 inches) image receptor is likely to

    (A) increase the scale of contrast.
    (B) increase the anode heel effect.
    (C) cause malfunction of the AEC.
    (D) cause premature termination of the exposure.

35. To be suitable for use in intensifying screens, a phosphor should have which of the following characteristics?

    1. High conversion efficiency
    2. High x-ray absorption
    3. High atomic number

    (A) 1 only
    (B) 3 only
    (C) 1 and 2 only
    (D) 1, 2, and 3

36. Resolution in computed radiography increases as

    1. laser beam size decreases
    2. monitor matrix size decreases
    3. PSP crystal size decreases

    (A) 1 only
    (B) 1 and 2 only
    (C) 1 and 3 only
    (D) 1, 2, and 3

37. The purpose of the automatic processor's circulation system is to

    (A) monitor and adjust temperature.
    (B) agitate, mix, and filter solutions.
    (C) move the film and change its direction.
    (D) monitor the solution and replace it as necessary.

38. In radiography of a large abdomen, which of the following is (are) effective way (s) to minimize the amount of scattered radiation reaching the IR?

    1. Use of close collimation
    2. Use of compression devices
    3. Use of a low-ratio grid

    (A) 1 only
    (B) 1 and 2 only
    (C) 1 and 3 only
    (D) 1, 2, and 3

39. The reduction in x-ray photon intensity as the photon passes through material is termed

    (A) absorption.
    (B) scattering.
    (C) attenuation.
    (D) divergence.

40. The changes between the images observed in Figure 4–6 A, B, and C represent changes made to

    (A) pixel size.
    (B) matrix size..
    (C) window width.
    (D) window level.

41. A radiograph made using 300 mA, 0.1 second, and 75 kVp exhibits motion unsharpness, but otherwise satisfactory technical quality. The radiograph will be repeated using a shorter exposure time. Using 86 kV and 500 mA, what should be the new exposure time?

    (A) 0.12 second
    (B) 0.06 second
    (C) 0.03 second
    (D) 0.01 second

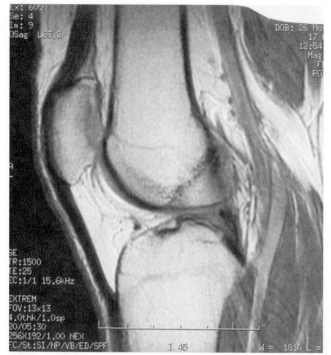

A

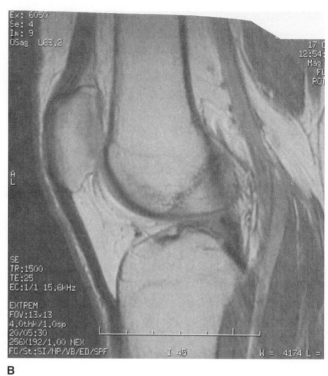

B

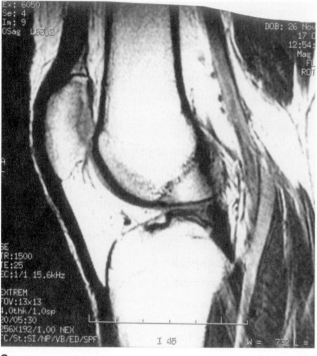

C

Figure 4–6.

42. In general, as the intensification factor increases,

    1. radiographic density increases.
    2. screen resolution increases.
    3. recorded detail increases.

    (A) 1 only
    (B) 1 and 2 only
    (C) 2 and 3 only
    (D) 1, 2, and 3

43. When green-sensitive rare earth screens are properly matched with the correct film, what type of safelight should be used in the darkroom?

    (A) Wratten 6B
    (B) GBX
    (C) Amber
    (D) None

44. What grid ratio is represented in Figure 4–7?

    (A) 3:1
    (B) 5:1
    (C) 10:1
    (D) 16:1

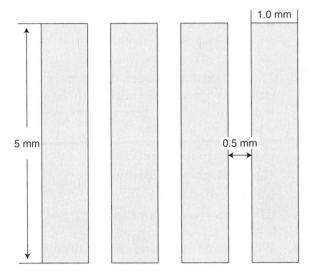

1.0 mm

5 mm   0.5 mm

Figure 4–7.

45. A 3-inch object to be radiographed at a 36-inch SID lies 4 inches from the image recorder. What will be the image width?

    (A) 2.6 inches
    (B) 3.3 inches
    (C) 26 inches
    (D) 33 inches

46. In comparison to 60 kVp, 80 kVp will

    1. permit greater exposure latitude.
    2. produce longer scale contrast.
    3. produce more scattered radiation.

    (A) 1 only
    (B) 2 only
    (C) 1 and 2 only
    (D) 1, 2, and 3

47. If the developer temperature in the automatic processor is higher than normal, what will be the effect on the finished radiograph?

    1. Loss of contrast
    2. Increased density
    3. Wet, tacky films

    (A) 1 only
    (B) 1 and 2 only
    (C) 2 and 3 only
    (D) 1, 2, and 3

48. Misalignment of the tube–part–IR relationship results in

    (A) shape distortion.
    (B) size distortion.
    (C) magnification.
    (D) blur.

49. Which of the following have an effect on recorded detail?

    1. Focal spot size
    2. Type of rectification
    3. SID

    (A) 1 and 2 only
    (B) 1 and 3 only
    (C) 2 and 3 only
    (D) 1, 2, and 3

50. Which of the following statements are true with respect to the radiograph shown in Figure 4–8?

1. The radiograph exhibits long-scale contrast.
2. The radiograph exhibits a clothing artifact.
3. The radiograph demonstrates motion blur.

(A) 1 and 2 only
(B) 1 and 3 only
(C) 2 and 3 only
(D) 1, 2, and 3

51. Which of the following can impact the visibility of the anode heel effect?

1. SID
2. Image recorder size
3. Screen speed

(A) 1 only
(B) 1 and 2 only
(C) 2 and 3 only
(D) 1, 2, and 3

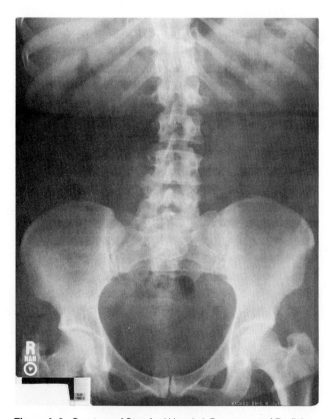

Figure 4–8. Courtesy of Stamford Hospital, Department of Radiology.

52. Which of the following groups of technical factors will produce the greatest radiographic density?

(A) 400 mA, 0.010 second, 94 kVp, 100-speed screens
(B) 500 mA, 0.008 second, 94 kVp, 200-speed screens
(C) 200 mA, 0.040 second, 94 kVp, 50-speed screens
(D) 100 mA, 0.020 second, 80 kVp, 200-speed screens

53. The line focus principle expresses the relationship between

(A) the actual and the effective focal spot.
(B) exposure given the IR and resultant density.
(C) SID used and resultant density.
(D) grid ratio and lines per inch.

54. Greater latitude is available to the radiographer in which of the following circumstances?

1. Using high-kVp technical factors
2. Using a slow film–screen combination
3. Using a low-ratio grid

(A) 1 only
(B) 1 and 2 only
(C) 2 and 3 only
(D) 1, 2, and 3

55. The relationship between the intensity of light striking a film and the intensity of light transmitted through the film is an expression of which of the following?

(A) Radiographic contrast
(B) Radiographic density
(C) Recorded detail
(D) Radiographic filtration

56. With a given exposure, as intensifying screen speed decreases, how is radiographic density affected?

(A) Decreases
(B) Increases
(C) Remains unchanged
(D) Is variable

57. Using a 48-inch SID, how much object-image distance (OID) must be introduced to magnify an object two times?

   (A) 8-inch OID
   (B) 12-inch OID
   (C) 16-inch OID
   (D) 24-inch OID

58. How is SID related to exposure rate and radiographic density?

   (A) As SID increases, exposure rate increases and radiographic density increases.
   (B) As SID increases, exposure rate increases and radiographic density decreases.
   (C) As SID increases, exposure rate decreases and radiographic density increases.
   (D) As SID increases, exposure rate decreases and radiographic density decreases.

59. What determines the quantity of fluorescent light emitted from a fluorescent screen?

   1. Thickness of the phosphor layer
   2. Type of phosphor used
   3. kV range used for exposure

   (A) 1 only
   (B) 1 and 2 only
   (C) 2 and 3 only
   (D) 1, 2, and 3

60. Which of the following is *most* likely to produce a radiograph with a long scale of contrast?

   (A) Increased photon energy
   (B) Increased screen speed
   (C) Increased mAs
   (D) Increased SID

61. Which of the following technical changes would *best* serve to remedy the effect of widely different tissue densities?

   (A) Use of high-speed screens
   (B) Use of a high-ratio grid
   (C) High kVp exposure factors
   (D) High mAs exposure factors

62. When an automatic processor is started up at the beginning of the day, or restarted after an extended standby period, the technologist should process an

   (A) unexposed, undeveloped 14 × 17 inches film.
   (B) exposed and developed 14 × 17 inches film.
   (C) unexposed and developed 14 × 17 inches film.
   (D) unexposed or unexposed and developed 14 × 17 inches film.

63. An increase in kVp will have which of the following effects?

   1. More scattered radiation will be produced.
   2. The exposure rate will increase.
   3. Radiographic contrast will increase.

   (A) 1 only
   (B) 1 and 2 only
   (C) 2 and 3 only
   (D) 1, 2, and 3

64. The radiograph shown in Figure 4–9 is an example of

   (A) linear tomography.
   (B) computed tomography (CT).
   (C) grid cutoff.
   (D) poor screen–film contact.

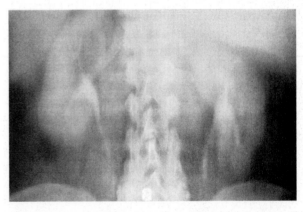

Figure 4–9. From the American College of Radiology Learning File. Courtesy of the ACR.

65. SID affects recorded detail in which of the following ways?

(A) Recorded detail is directly related to SID.
(B) Recorded detail is inversely related to SID.
(C) As SID increases, recorded detail decreases.
(D) SID is not a detail factor.

66. Which of the two film emulsions illustrated in Figure 4–10 requires less exposure to produce a density of 2.0?

(A) Number 1 requires less exposure to produce a density of 2.0.
(B) Number 2 requires less exposure to produce a density of 2.0.
(C) Emulsions 1 and 2 are of identical speed.
(D) Speed cannot be predicted from the illustration.

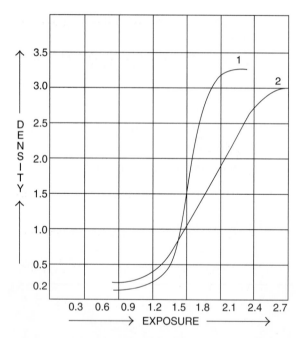

Figure 4–10.

67. The function(s) of the fixer in film processing is (are) to

1. remove the unexposed silver bromide crystals.
2. change the unexposed silver bromide crystals to black metallic silver.
3. harden the emulsion.

(A) 1 only
(B) 1 and 3 only
(C) 2 and 3 only
(D) 1, 2, and 3

68. A film emerging from the automatic processor exhibits excessive density. This may be attributable to which of the following?

1. Developer temperature too high
2. Chemical fog
3. Underreplenishment

(A) 1 only
(B) 1 and 2 only
(C) 2 and 3 only
(D) 1, 2, and 3

69. Types of moving grid mechanisms include

1. oscillating.
2. reciprocating.
3. synchronous.

(A) 1 only
(B) 1 and 2 only
(C) 1 and 3 only
(D) 2 and 3 only

70. All of the following are related to recorded detail *except*

(A) mA.
(B) focal spot size.
(C) screen speed.
(D) OID.

71. An exposure was made of a part using 300 mA and 0.06 second and using a 100-speed film–screen combination. An additional radiograph is requested using a 400-speed system to reduce motion unsharpness. Using 200 mA, all other factors remaining constant, what should be the new exposure time?

    (A) 0.02 second
    (B) 0.04 second
    (C) 0.45 second
    (D) 0.80 second

72. Of the following groups of exposure factors, which will produce the greatest radiographic density?

    (A) 200 mA, 0.03 second, 72-inch source-image distance (SID)
    (B) 100 mA, 0.03 second, 36-inch SID
    (C) 100 mA, 0.06 second, 36-inch SID
    (D) 200 mA, 0.06 second, 72-inch SID

73. Which of the following groups of exposure factors will produce the *longest scale of contrast?*

    (A) 200 mA, 0.08 second, 95 kVp, 12:1 grid
    (B) 500 mA, 0.03 second, 81 kVp, 8:1 grid
    (C) 300 mA, 0.05 second, 95 kVp, 8:1 grid
    (D) 600 mA, 1/40 second, 70 kVp, 6:1 grid

74. What will result from using single-emulsion film in an image receptor having a two intensifying screens?

    (A) Double exposure
    (B) Decreased density
    (C) Increased recorded detail
    (D) Greater latitude

75. A particular radiograph was produced using 6 mAs and 110 kVp with an 8:1 ratio grid. The radiograph is to be repeated using a 16:1 ratio grid. What should be the new mAs?

    (A) 3
    (B) 6
    (C) 9
    (D) 12

76. Which of the following factors influence(s) the production of scattered radiation?

    1. Kilovoltage level
    2. Tissue density
    3. Size of field

    (A) 1 only
    (B) 1 and 2 only
    (C) 1 and 3 only
    (D) 1, 2, and 3

77. A 15% increase in kVp accompanied by a 50% decrease in mAs will result in a(n)

    (A) shorter scale of contrast.
    (B) increase in exposure latitude.
    (C) increase in radiographic density.
    (D) decrease in recorded detail.

78. Which of the following is (are) causes of grid cutoff when using reciprocating grids?

    1. Inadequate SID
    2. X-ray tube off-center with the long axis of the lead strips
    3. Angling the beam in the direction of the lead strips

    (A) 1 only
    (B) 1 and 2 only
    (C) 2 and 3 only
    (D) 1, 2, and 3

79. Foreshortening of an anatomic structure means that
    (A) it is projected on the IR smaller than its actual size.
    (B) its image is more lengthened than its actual size.
    (C) it is accompanied by geometric blur.
    (D) it is significantly magnified.

80. Focal spot blur is greatest

    (A) directly along the course of the central ray.
    (B) toward the cathode end of the x-ray beam.
    (C) toward the anode end of the x-ray beam.
    (D) as the SID is increased.

81. A particular mAs, regardless of the combination of mA and time, will reproduce the same radiographic density. This is a statement of the

(A) line focus principle.
(B) inverse square law.
(C) reciprocity law.
(D) law of conservation of energy.

82. Cassette front material can be made of which of the following?

1. Carbon fiber
2. Magnesium
3. Lead

(A) 1 only
(B) 1 and 2 only
(C) 1 and 3 only
(D) 1, 2, and 3

83. Treelike, branching black marks on a radiograph are usually the result of

(A) bending the film acutely.
(B) improper development.
(C) improper film storage.
(D) static electricity.

84. The continued emission of light by a phosphor after the activating source has ceased is termed

(A) fluorescence.
(B) phosphorescence.
(C) image intensification.
(D) quantum mottle.

85. Which of the following is (are) method(s) that would enable the radiographer to reduce the exposure time required for a particular radiograph?

1. Use higher mA.
2. Use higher kVp.
3. Use faster film–screen combination.

(A) 1 only
(B) 1 and 2 only
(C) 2 and 3 only
(D) 1, 2, and 3

86. If 82 kVp, 300 mA, and 0.05 second were used for a particular exposure using 3-phase, 12-pulse equipment, what mAs would be required, using single-phase equipment, to produce a similar radiograph?

(A) 7.5
(B) 20
(C) 30
(D) 50

87. Which of the following materials may be used as grid interspace material?

1. Lead
2. Plastic
3. Aluminum

(A) 1 only
(B) 1 and 2 only
(C) 2 and 3 only
(D) 1, 2, and 3

88. The radiograph in Figure 4–11 demonstrates an example of

(A) tree static.
(B) underexposure.
(C) processing artifact.
(D) exposure artifact.

89. Materials that emit light when stimulated by x-ray photons are called

(A) ions.
(B) electrodes.
(C) phosphors.
(D) crystals.

90. In which of the following examinations should 70 kVp *not* be exceeded?

(A) Upper GI (UGI)
(B) Barium enema (BE)
(C) Intravenous urogram (IVU)
(D) Chest

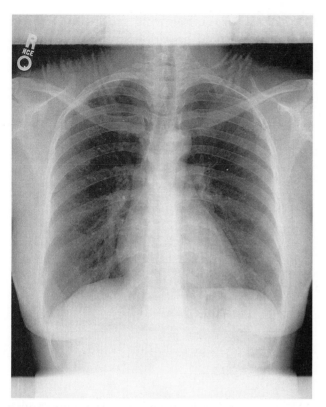

Figure 4–11. Courtesy of Stamford Hospital, Department of Radiology.

91. The term *spectral matching* refers to the fact that film sensitivity must be matched with the

    (A) proper color screen fluorescence.
    (B) correct kVp level.
    (C) correct mA level.
    (D) proper developer concentration.

92. Which of the following is the correct order of radiographic film processing?

    (A) Developer, wash, fixer, dry
    (B) Fixer, wash, developer, dry
    (C) Developer, fixer, wash, dry
    (D) Fixer, developer, wash, dry

93. If the radiographer is unable to achieve a short OID because of the structure of the body part or patient condition, which of the following adjustments can be made to minimize magnification distortion?

    (A) A smaller focal spot size should be used.
    (B) A longer SID should be used.
    (C) Faster intensifying screens should be used.
    (D) A lower-ratio grid should be used.

94. The variation in photon distribution between the anode and cathode ends of the x-ray tube is known as

    (A) the line focus principle.
    (B) the anode heel effect.
    (C) the inverse square law.
    (D) Bohr's theory.

95. A compensating filter is used to

    (A) absorb the harmful photons that contribute only to patient dose.
    (B) even out widely differing tissue densities.
    (C) eliminate much of the scattered radiation.
    (D) improve fluoroscopy.

96. Which of the following contribute to the radiographic contrast present on the finished radiograph?

    1. Atomic number of tissues radiographed
    2. Any pathologic processes
    3. Degree of muscle development

    (A) 1 and 2 only
    (B) 1 and 3 only
    (C) 2 and 3 only
    (D) 1, 2, and 3

97. Which of the following pathologic conditions will probably require a decrease in exposure factors?

    (A) Osteomyelitis
    (B) Osteoporosis
    (C) Osteosclerosis
    (D) Osteochondritis

98. An unexposed and processed film will have a density of about

    (A) zero.
    (B) 0.1.
    (C) 1.0.
    (D) 2.5.

99. Foreshortening can be caused by

    (A) the radiographic object being placed at an angle to the IR.
    (B) excessive distance between the object and the IR.
    (C) insufficient distance between the focus and the IR.
    (D) excessive distance between the focus and the IR.

100. If a lateral projection of the chest is being performed on an asthenic patient and the outer photocells are selected, what is likely to be the outcome?

    (A) Decreased density
    (B) Increased density
    (C) Scattered radiation fog
    (D) Motion blur

101. If 300 mA has been selected for a particular exposure, what exposure time would be required to produce 60 mAs?

    (A) 1/60 second
    (B) 1/30 second
    (C) 1/10 second
    (D) 1/5 second

102. What are the effects of scattered radiation on the radiographic image?

    1. It produces fog.
    2. It increases contrast.
    3. It increases grid cutoff.

    (A) 1 only
    (B) 2 only
    (C) 1 and 2 only
    (D) 1, 2, and 3

103. Which of the following groups of exposure factors would be *most* appropriate to control involuntary motion?

    (A) 400 mA, 0.03 second
    (B) 200 mA, 0.06 second
    (C) 600 mA, 0.02 second
    (D) 100 mA, 0.12 second

104. Which of the following terms refers to light being reflected from one intensifying screen, through the film, to the opposite emulsion and screen?

    (A) Reflectance
    (B) Crossover
    (C) Scatter
    (D) Filtration

105. Types of shape distortion include

    1. magnification.
    2. elongation.
    3. foreshortening.

    (A) 1 only
    (B) 1 and 2 only
    (C) 2 and 3 only
    (D) 1, 2, and 3

106. Although the stated focal spot size is measured directly under the actual focal spot, focal spot size really varies along the length of the x-ray beam. At which portion of the x-ray beam is the effective focal spot the largest?

    (A) At its outer edge
    (B) Along the path of the central ray
    (C) At the cathode end
    (D) At the anode end

107. The radiograph pictured in Figure 4–12 demonstrates

    (A) overdevelopment.
    (B) quantum noise.
    (C) scattered radiation fog.
    (D) grid cutoff.

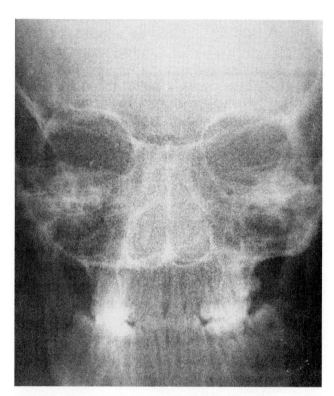

Figure 4–12. From the American College of Radiology Learning File. Courtesy of the ACR.

108. Which of the following can affect the amount of developer replenisher delivered per film in an automatic processor?

(A) Developer temperature
(B) Amount of film exposure
(C) Film size
(D) Processor capacity

109. The squeegee assembly in an automatic processor

1. functions to remove excess solution from films.
2. is located near the crossover rollers.
3. helps establish the film's rate of travel.

(A) 1 only
(B) 2 only
(C) 1 and 2 only
(D) 1, 2, and 3

110. Because of the anode heel effect, the intensity of the x-ray beam is greatest along the

(A) path of the central ray.
(B) anode end of the beam.
(C) cathode end of the beam.
(D) transverse axis of the IR.

111. Underexposure of a radiograph can be caused by all of the following *except* insufficient

(A) mA.
(B) exposure time.
(C) kVp.
(D) SID.

112. Which of the following is performed to check the correctness of the developing parameters?

(A) Densitometry
(B) A thorough cleaning of rollers
(C) A warm-up procedure
(D) Sensitometry

Questions 113 and 114

An AP radiograph of the hip was made using 400 mA, 0.05 second, 76 kVp, 40-inch SID, 1.2-mm focal spot, and a 400 speed film–screen system.

113. Referring to the given information, and with all other factors remaining constant, which of the following exposure times would be required to maintain radiographic density at a 36-inch SID using the 500-mA station, and with an increase to 87 kVp?

(A) 0.04 second
(B) 0.08 second
(C) 0.016 second
(D) 0.032 second

114. Referring to the original factors, and with all other factors remaining constant, which of the following exposure times would be required to maintain radiographic density using 400 mA and a 200 speed film–screen system, and with the addition of an 8:1 grid?

    (A) 0.12 second
    (B) 0.18 second
    (C) 0.4 second
    (D) 0.6 second

115. The sensitometric curve may be used to

    1. identify automatic processing problems.
    2. determine film sensitivity.
    3. illustrate screen speed.

    (A) 1 only
    (B) 1 and 2 only
    (C) 2 and 3 only
    (D) 1, 2, and 3

116. Using fixed-mAs and variable-kVp technical factors, each centimeter increase in patient thickness requires what adjustment in kilovoltage?

    (A) Increase 2 kVp
    (B) Decrease 2 kVp
    (C) Increase 4 kVp
    (D) Decrease 4 kVp

117. Bone densitometry is often performed to

    1. measure degree of bone (de) mineralization.
    2. evaluate results of osteoporosis treatment/therapy.
    3. evaluate condition of soft tissue adjacent to bone.

    (A) 1 only
    (B) 1 and 2 only
    (C) 2 and 3 only
    (D) 1, 2, and 3

118. Factor(s) that can be used to regulate radiographic density is (are)

    1. milliamperage.
    2. exposure time.
    3. kilovoltage.

    (A) 1 only
    (B) 2 only
    (C) 1 and 2 only
    (D) 1, 2, and 3

119. Which of the following errors is illustrated in Figure 4–13?

    (A) Patient not centered to IR
    (B) X-ray tube not centered to grid
    (C) Inaccurate collimation
    (D) Unilateral grid cutoff

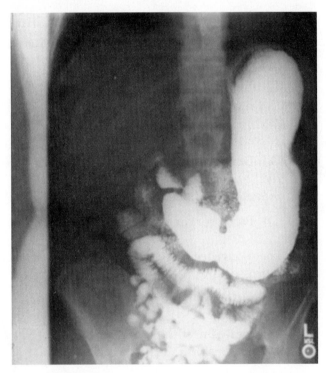

Figure 4–13. Courtesy of Stamford Hospital, Department of Radiology.

120. Which of the following can result from improper film storage or darkroom conditions?

   1. Safelight fog
   2. Background radiation fog
   3. Screen lag

   (A) 1 only
   (B) 1 and 2 only
   (C) 2 and 3 only
   (D) 1, 2, and 3

121. What is the purpose of the thin layer of lead that is often located behind the rear intensifying screen in a image receptor?

   (A) To prevent crossover
   (B) To increase screen speed
   (C) To diffuse light photons
   (D) To prevent scattered radiation fog

122. Which of the following will result if developer replenishment is inadequate?

   (A) Images with excessively high contrast
   (B) Images with excessively low contrast
   (C) Images with excessively high density
   (D) Dry, brittle films

123. What combination of exposure factors and image receptor speed would best function to reduce quantum mottle?

   (A) Decreased mAs, decreased kVp, fast-speed screens
   (B) Increased mAs, decreased kVp, slow-speed screens
   (C) Decreased mAs, increased kVp, fast-speed screens
   (D) Increased mAs, increased kVp, fast-speed screens

124. Acceptable method(s) of minimizing motion unsharpness is (are)

   1. suspended respiration.
   2. short exposure time.
   3. patient instruction.

   (A) 1 only
   (B) 1 and 2 only
   (C) 1 and 3 only
   (D) 1, 2, and 3

125. Which of the following possesses the widest dynamic range?

   A. high-speed screens
   B. slow-speed screens
   C. AEC
   D. CR

126. Which of the following quantities of filtration is most likely to be used in mammography?

   (A) 0.5 mm Mo
   (B) 1.5 mm Al
   (C) 1.5 mm Cu
   (D) 2.0 mm Cu

127. The device shown in Figure 4–14 is used for

   (A) tomographic quality assurance (QA) testing.
   (B) timer and rectifier testing.
   (C) mammography QA testing.
   (D) kV calibration testing.

128. Which of the following can be used to determine the sensitivity of a particular film emulsion?

   (A) Sensitometric curve
   (B) Dose–response curve
   (C) Reciprocity law
   (D) Inverse square law

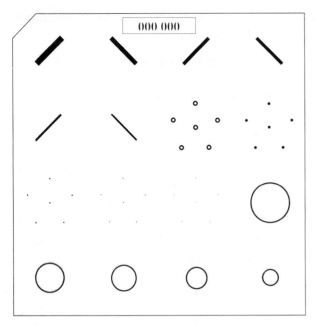

Figure 4–14. Reproduced with permission from, compliments of, Gammex/RMI, 2500 West Beltline Highway, Middletown, WI 53562.

129. A wire mesh test is performed to diagnose screen

(A) lag.
(B) contact.
(C) resolution.
(D) intensification.

130. The exposure factors of 300 mA, 0.017 second, and 72 kVp produce an mAs value of

(A) 5.
(B) 50.
(C) 500.
(D) 5000.

131. All of the following statements regarding CR cassettes are true, *except*

(A) CR cassettes do not contain radiographic film.
(B) CR cassettes use no intensifying screens.
(C) CR cassettes must exclude all white light.
(D) CR cassettes function to protect the IP (image plate).

132. The radiographic accessory used to measure the thickness of body parts in order to determine optimum selection of exposure factors is the:

A. fulcrum
B. caliper
C. densitometer
D. ruler

133. A change from 100 speed screens to 200 speed screens would require what change in mAs?

(A) mAs should be increased by 15%.
(B) mAs should be increased by 30%.
(C) mAs should be doubled.
(D) mAs should be halved.

134. Which of the following is (are) classified as rare earth phosphors?

1. Lanthanum oxybromide
2. Gadolinium oxysulfide
3. Cesium iodide

(A) 1 only
(B) 1 and 2 only
(C) 2 and 3 only
(D) 1, 2, and 3

135. For which of the following examinations can the anode heel effect be an important consideration?

1. Lateral thoracic spine
2. AP femur
3. RAO sternum

(A) 1 only
(B) 1 and 2 only
(C) 1 and 3 only
(D) 1, 2, and 3

136. Which of the following pathologic conditions would require an increase in exposure factors?

(A) Pneumoperitoneum
(B) Obstructed bowel
(C) Renal colic
(D) Ascites

137. A radiograph made with a parallel grid demonstrates decreased density on its lateral edges. This is most likely due to

(A) static electrical discharge.
(B) the grid being off-centered.
(C) improper tube angle.
(D) decreased SID.

138. Which of the two characteristic curves shown in Figure 4–15 will require more exposure to produce a density of 1.5 on the finished radiograph?

(A) Film emulsion 1.
(B) Film emulsion 2.
(C) They require identical exposures.
(D) Insufficient information is provided.

139. How are mAs and radiographic density related in the process of image formation?

(A) mAs and radiographic density are inversely proportional.
(B) mAs and radiographic density are directly proportional.
(C) mAs and radiographic density are related to image unsharpness.
(D) mAs and radiographic density are unrelated.

140. OID is related to recorded detail in which of the following ways?

(A) Radiographic detail is directly related to OID.
(B) Radiographic detail is inversely related to OID.
(C) As OID increases, so does radiographic detail.
(D) OID is unrelated to radiographic detail.

141. Which of the following devices is used to overcome severe variation in patient anatomy or tissue density, providing more uniform radiographic density?

(A) Compensating filter
(B) Grid
(C) Collimator
(D) Intensifying screen

142. The developer temperature in a 90-second automatic processor is usually about

(A) 75° to 80°F.
(B) 80° to 85°F.
(C) 85° to 90°F.
(D) 90° to 95°F.

143. An increase in kilovoltage will serve to

(A) produce a longer scale of contrast.
(B) produce a shorter scale of contrast.
(C) decrease the radiographic density.
(D) decrease the production of scattered radiation.

144. In digital imaging, as the size of the image matrix increases:

1. FOV increases
2. pixel size decreases
3. spatial resolution increases

A. 1 only
B. 1 and 2 only
C. 2 and 3 only
D. 1, 2, and 3

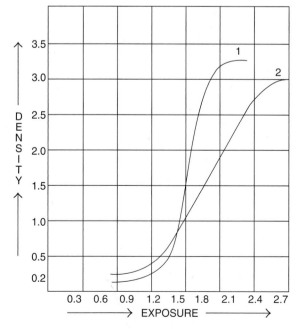

Figure 4–15.

145. Radiographic recorded detail is directly related to

    1. SID.
    2. OID.
    3. imaging-system speed.

    (A) 1 only
    (B) 1 and 2 only
    (C) 2 and 3 only
    (D) 1, 2, and 3

146. Of the following groups of exposure factors, which will produce the shortest scale of radiographic contrast?

    (A) 500 mA, 0.040 second, 70 kVp
    (B) 100 mA, 0.100 second, 80 kVp
    (C) 200 mA, 0.025 second, 92 kVp
    (D) 700 mA, 0.014 second, 80 kVp

147. Which of the following factors contribute(s) to the efficient performance of a grid?

    1. Grid ratio
    2. Number of lead strips per inch
    3. Amount of scatter transmitted through the grid

    (A) 1 only
    (B) 2 only
    (C) 1 and 2 only
    (D) 1, 2, and 3

148. The device used to give a film a predetermined exposure in order to test its response to processing is called the

    (A) sensitometer.
    (B) densitometer.
    (C) step wedge.
    (D) spinning top.

149. The plus-density artifact pictured in Figure 4–16 was probably produced

    1. by careless handling.
    2. after exposure.
    3. before exposure.

    (A) 1 only
    (B) 2 only
    (C) 1 and 2 only
    (D) 1 and 3 only

150. Image receptors/cassettes frequently have a lead foil layer behind the rear screen that functions to

    (A) improve penetration.
    (B) absorb backscatter.
    (C) preserve resolution.
    (D) increase the screen speed.

151. Which of the following conditions would require an increase in exposure factors?

    1. Congestive heart failure
    2. Pleural effusion
    3. Emphysema

    (A) 1 only
    (B) 1 and 2 only
    (C) 1 and 3 only
    (D) 1, 2, and 3

152. Focusing distance is associated with which of the following?

    (A) Computed tomography
    (B) Chest radiography
    (C) Magnification radiography
    (D) Grids

153. The steeper the straight-line portion of a characteristic curve for a particular film, the

    1. slower the film speed.
    2. higher the film contrast.
    3. greater the exposure latitude.

    (A) 1 only
    (B) 2 only
    (C) 2 and 3 only
    (D) 1, 2, and 3

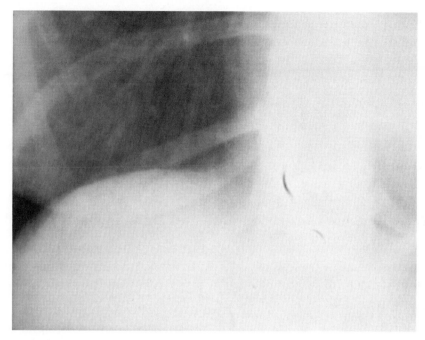

Figure 4–16. From the American College of Radiology Learning File. Courtesy of the ACR.

154. The relationship between the height of a grid's lead strips and the distance between them is referred to as grid

(A) ratio.

(B) radius.

(C) frequency.

(D) focusing distance.

155. Which of the following would be useful for an examination of a patient suffering from Parkinson's disease?

1. High-speed screens
2. Short exposure time
3. Compensating filtration

(A) 1 only

(B) 1 and 2 only

(C) 1 and 3 only

(D) 1, 2, and 3

156. Characteristics of low ratio focused grids include the following:

1. they have a greater focal range
2. they are less efficient in collecting SR
3. they can be used inverted

A. 1 only

B. 1 and 2 only

C. 2 and 3 only

D. 1, 2, and 3

157. A film emulsion having wide latitude is likely to exhibit

(A) high density.

(B) low density.

(C) high contrast.

(D) low contrast.

158. The area of blurriness seen in the upper part of the radiograph shown in Figure 4–17 is *most* likely due to

(A) scattered radiation fog.

(B) patient motion.

(C) poor screen–film contact.

(D) grid cutoff.

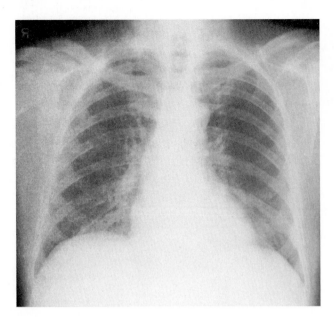

Figure 4–17. From the American College of Radiology Learning File. Courtesy of the ACR.

159. What is the best way to reduce magnification distortion?

(A) Use a small focal spot.
(B) Increase the SID.
(C) Decrease the OID.
(D) Use a slow screen–film combination.

160. Which of the following can cause poor screen–film contact?

1. Damaged image receptor frame
2. Foreign body in image receptor
3. Warped image receptor front

(A) 1 only
(B) 2 only
(C) 1 and 3 only
(D) 1, 2, and 3

161. Which of the following examinations might require the use of 120 kVp?

1. AP abdomen
2. Chest radiograph
3. Barium-filled stomach

(A) 1 only
(B) 2 only
(C) 1 and 2 only
(D) 2 and 3 only

162. Base-plus fog is a result of

1. blue-tinted film base.
2. chemical development.
3. the manufacturing process.

(A) 1 only
(B) 1 and 2 only
(C) 1 and 3 only
(D) 1, 2, and 3

163. A lateral radiograph of the lumbar spine was made using 200 mA, 1-second exposure, and 90 kVp. If the exposure factors were changed to 200 mA, 1/2 second, and 104 kVp, there would be an obvious change in which of the following?

1. Radiographic density
2. Scale of radiographic contrast
3. Distortion

(A) 1 only
(B) 2 only
(C) 2 and 3 only
(D) 1, 2, and 3

164. Which of the following will contribute to the production of longer-scale radiographic contrast?

1. An increase in kV
2. An increase in grid ratio
3. An increase in photon energy

(A) 1 only
(B) 1 and 2 only
(C) 1 and 3 only
(D) 1, 2, and 3

165. The cause of films coming from the automatic processor still damp can be

(A) air velocity too high.
(B) unbalanced processing temperatures.
(C) insufficient hardening action.
(D) underreplenishment.

166. The term *latitude* describes

1. an emulsion's ability to record a range of densities.
2. the degree of error tolerated with given exposure factors.
3. the conversion efficiency of a given intensifying screen.

(A) 1 only
(B) 1 and 2 only
(C) 2 and 3 only
(D) 1, 2, and 3

167. The microswitch for controlling the amount of replenishment used in an automatic processor is located at the

(A) receiving bin.
(B) crossover roller.
(C) entrance roller.
(D) replenishment pump.

168. The radiograph seen in Figure 4–18 illustrates

(A) high contrast.
(B) light fog.
(C) chemical fog.
(D) double exposure.

169. The effect described as differential absorption is

1. responsible for radiographic contrast.
2. a result of attenuating characteristics of tissue.
3. minimized by the use of high kVp.

(A) 1 only
(B) 1 and 2 only
(C) 1 and 3 only
(D) 1, 2, and 3

170. A satisfactory radiograph of the abdomen was made at a 42-inch SID using 300 mA, 0.06-second exposure, and 80 kVp. If the distance is changed to 38 inches, what new exposure time would be required?

(A) 0.02 second
(B) 0.05 second
(C) 0.12 second
(D) 0.15 second

171. Of the following groups of technical factors, which will produce the greatest radiographic density?

(A) 10 mAs, 74 kVp, 44-inch SID
(B) 10 mAs, 74 kVp, 36-inch SID
(C) 5 mAs, 85 kVp, 48-inch SID
(D) 5 mAs, 85 kVp, 40-inch SID

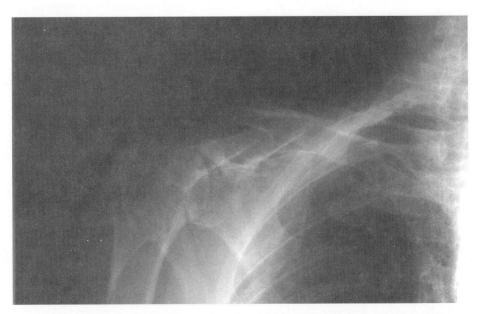

Figure 4–18. From the American College of Radiology Learning File. Courtesy of the ACR.

172. What apparatus is needed for the construction of a sensitometric curve?

1. Penetrometer
2. Densitometer
3. Electrolytic canister

(A) 1 and 2 only
(B) 1 and 3 only
(C) 2 and 3 only
(D) 1, 2, and 3

173. Exposed silver halide crystals are changed to black metallic silver by the

(A) preservative.
(B) reducers.
(C) activators.
(D) hardener.

174. The major function of filtration is to reduce

(A) image noise.
(B) scattered radiation.
(C) operator dose.
(D) patient dose.

175. Why is a very short exposure time essential in chest radiography?

(A) To avoid excessive focal spot blur
(B) To maintain short-scale contrast
(C) To minimize involuntary motion
(D) To minimize patient discomfort

176. The interaction between x-ray photons and matter illustrated in Figure 4–19 is *most* likely to occur

1. in structures having a high atomic number.
2. during radiographic examination of the abdomen.
3. using high kV and low mAs exposure factors.

(A) 1 only
(B) 1 and 2 only
(C) 2 and 3 only
(D) 1, 2, and 3

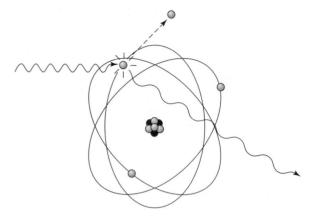

Figure 4–19. Reproduced with permission from Saia DA. *Radiography: Program Review and Examination Preparation*, 2nd ed. Stamford, CT: Appleton & Lange, 1999.

177. Conditions contributing to poor radiographic film archival quality include

1. fixer retention.
2. insufficient developer replenishment.
3. poor storage conditions.

(A) 1 only
(B) 3 only
(C) 2 and 3 only
(D) 1, 2, and 3

178. An exposure was made at a 38-inch SID using 300 mA, a 0.03-second exposure, and 80 kVp with a 400 film–screen combination and an 8:1 grid. It is desired to repeat the radiograph and, in order to improve recorded detail, to use a 42-inch SID and a 200-speed film–screen combination. With all other factors remaining constant, what exposure time will be required to maintain the original radiographic density?

(A) 0.03 second
(B) 0.07 second
(C) 0.14 second
(D) 0.36 second

179. Which of the following is (are) characteristic(s) of a 16:1 grid?

    1. It absorbs a high percentage of scattered radiation.
    2. It has little positioning latitude.
    3. It is used with high-kVp exposures.

    (A) 1 only
    (B) 1 and 3 only
    (C) 2 and 3 only
    (D) 1, 2, and 3

180. Exposure rate increases with an increase in

    1. mA.
    2. kVp.
    3. SID.

    (A) 1 only
    (B) 1 and 2 only
    (C) 2 and 3 only
    (D) 1, 2, and 3

181. If a 4-inch collimated field is changed to a 14-inch collimated field, with no other changes, the radiographic image will possess

    (A) more density.
    (B) less density.
    (C) more detail.
    (D) less detail.

182. Which of the following is an abnormal intensifying screen action?

    (A) Fluorescence
    (B) Luminescence
    (C) Speed
    (D) Lag

183. The advantage(s) of high kilovoltage chest radiography is (are) that

    1. exposure latitude is increased.
    2. it produces long-scale contrast.
    3. it reduces patient dose.

    (A) 1 only
    (B) 1 and 2 only
    (C) 2 and 3 only
    (D) 1, 2, and 3

184. Slow-speed screens are used

    (A) to minimize patient dose.
    (B) to keep exposure time to a minimum.
    (C) to image fine anatomic details.
    (D) in pediatric radiography.

185. Film base is currently made of which of the following materials?

    (A) Cellulose nitrate
    (B) Cellulose acetate
    (C) Polyester
    (D) Glass

186. Which of the following may be used to reduce the effect of scattered radiation on the finished radiograph?

    1. Grids
    2. Collimators
    3. Compression bands

    (A) 1 only
    (B) 1 and 3 only
    (C) 2 and 3 only
    (D) 1, 2, and 3

187. The primary source of scattered radiation is the

    (A) patient.
    (B) tabletop.
    (C) x-ray tube.
    (D) grid.

188. Any images obtained using DXA bone densitometry

    1. are used to evaluate accuracy of the ROI.
    2. are used as evaluation for various bone/joint disorders.
    3. reflect the similar attenuation properties of soft tissue and bone.

    (A) 1 only
    (B) 1 and 2 only
    (C) 1 and 3 only
    (D) 1, 2, and 3

189. Which of the following is (are) tested as part of a QA program?

1. Beam alignment
2. Reproducibility
3. Linearity

(A) 1 only
(B) 1 and 2 only
(C) 1 and 3 only
(D) 1, 2, and 3

190. To produce a just perceptible increase in radiographic density, the radiographer must increase the

(A) mAs by 30%.
(B) mAs by 15 %.
(C) kVp by 15%.
(D) kVp by 30%.

191. All of the following affect the exposure rate of the primary beam *except*

(A) mA.
(B) kVp.
(C) distance.
(D) field size.

192. The radiograph in Figure 4–20 exhibits an artifact caused by

(A) an inverted focused grid.
(B) poor screen–film contact.
(C) a foreign body in the image receptor.
(D) static electricity.

193. The function(s) of automatic beam limitation devices include

1. reducing the production of scattered radiation.
2. increasing the absorption of scattered radiation.
3. changing the quality of the x-ray beam.

(A) 1 only
(B) 2 only
(C) 1 and 2 only
(D) 1, 2, and 3

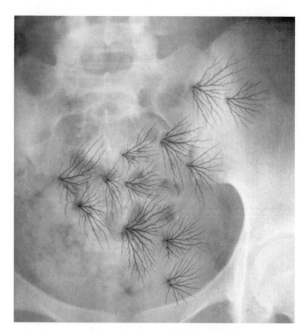

Figure 4–20. From the American College of Radiology Learning File. Courtesy of the ACR.

194. Which of the following statements is true with respect to the diagram in Figure 4–21?

(A) Film emulsion 2 has more sensitivity above the point of intersection.
(B) Film emulsion 1 has more sensitivity below the point of intersection.
(C) Film emulsion 1 has more sensitivity above the point of intersection.
(D) Film emulsion 2 has less sensitivity below the point of intersection.

195. Exposure-type artifacts include

1. motion
2. static electricity marks.
3. pi lines

(A) 1 only
(B) 1 and 2 only
(C) 2 and 3 only
(D) 1, 2, and 3

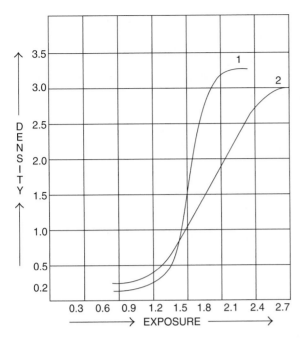

Figure 4–21.

196. When involuntary motion must be considered, the exposure time may be cut in half if the kVp is

(A) doubled.
(B) increased by 15%.
(C) increased by 25%.
(D) increased by 35%.

197. Which of the following groups of exposure factors would be most effective in eliminating prominent pulmonary vascular markings in an RAO position of the sternum?

(A) 500 mA, 1/30 second, 70 kVp
(B) 200 mA, 0.04 second, 80 kVp
(C) 300 mA, 1/10 second, 80 kVp
(D) 25 mA, 7/10 second, 70 kVp

198. A satisfactory radiograph was made using a 40-inch SID, 10 mAs, and a 12:1 grid. If the examination will be repeated at a distance of 48 inches and using an 8:1 grid, what should be the new mAs to maintain the original density?

(A) 5.6
(B) 8.8
(C) 11.5
(D) 14.4

199. The artifacts on the radiograph in Figure 4–22 are called

(A) pi lines.
(B) guide shoe marks.
(C) hesitation marks.
(D) reticulation.

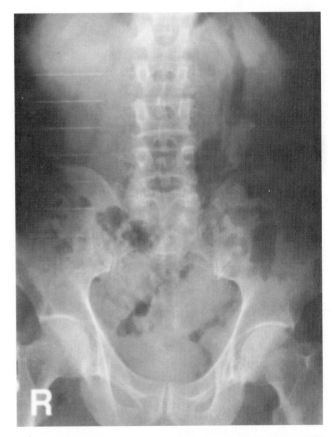

Figure 4–22. Courtesy of Stamford Hospital, Department of Radiology.

200. Radiographic contrast is a result of

  1. differential tissue absorption.
  2. emulsion characteristics.
  3. proper regulation of mAs.

  (A) 1 only
  (B) 1 and 2 only
  (C) 1 and 3 only
  (D) 1, 2, and 3

201. X-ray photon beam attenuation is influenced by

  1. tissue type.
  2. subject thickness.
  3. photon quality.

  (A) 1 only
  (B) 3 only
  (C) 2 and 3 only
  (D) 1, 2, and 3

202. What effect will a stained intensifying screen have on the finished radiograph?

  (A) Blurring
  (B) Magnification
  (C) Decreased density
  (D) Increased density

203. Why are a single intensifying screen and single emulsion film used for select radiographic examinations?

  (A) To decrease patient dose
  (B) To achieve longer-scale contrast
  (C) For better recorded detail
  (D) To decrease fiscal expenses

204. Boxes of film stored in too warm an area may be subject to

  (A) static marks.
  (B) film fog.
  (C) high contrast.
  (D) loss of density.

205. Which of the following will influence recorded detail?

  1. Screen speed
  2. Screen–film contact
  3. Focal spot

  (A) 1 and 2 only
  (B) 1 and 3 only
  (C) 2 and 3 only
  (D) 1, 2, and 3

206. Which of the following chemicals is used in the production of radiographic film emulsion?

  (A) Sodium sulfite
  (B) Potassium bromide
  (C) Silver halide
  (D) Chrome alum

207. Which of the following terms is used to describe unsharp edges of tiny radiographic details?

  (A) Diffusion
  (B) Mottle
  (C) Blur
  (D) Umbra

208. A focal spot size of 0.3 mm or smaller is essential for

  (A) small-bone radiography.
  (B) magnification radiography.
  (C) tomography.
  (D) fluoroscopy.

209. The mottled appearance of the radiograph in Figure 4–23 is most likely representative of

  (A) Paget's disease.
  (B) osteoporosis.
  (C) safelight fog.
  (D) pillow artifacts.

210. As grid ratio is increased,

  (A) the scale of contrast becomes longer.
  (B) the scale of contrast becomes shorter.
  (C) radiographic density increases.
  (D) radiographic distortion decreases.

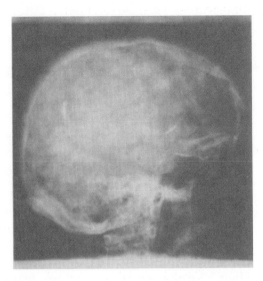

Figure 4–23. Courtesy of Stamford Hospital, Department of Radiology.

211. X-ray film emulsion is most sensitive to safe-light fog

(A) before exposure and development.
(B) after exposure.
(C) during development.
(D) at low humidity.

212. Hardener is added to the developer solution of automatic processors to

1. keep emulsion swelling to a minimum.
2. decrease the possibility of a processor jam-up.
3. remove unexposed silver halide crystals.

(A) 1 only
(B) 1 and 2 only
(C) 2 and 3 only
(D) 1, 2, and 3

213. If a 6-inch OID is introduced during a particular radiographic examination, what change in SID will be necessary to overcome objectionable magnification?

(A) The SID must be increased by 6 inches.
(B) The SID must be increased by 18 inches.
(C) The SID must be decreased by 6 inches.
(D) The SID must be increased by 42 inches.

214. If a particular grid has lead strips 0.40 mm thick, 4.0 mm high, and 0.25 mm apart, what is its grid ratio?

(A) 8:1
(B) 10:1
(C) 12:1
(D) 16:1

215. Chemical fog may be attributed to

1. excessive developer temperature.
2. oxidized developer.
3. excessive replenishment.

(A) 1 only
(B) 1 and 2 only
(C) 2 and 3 only
(D) 1, 2, and 3

216. Which of the following has the greatest effect on radiographic density?

(A) Aluminum filtration
(B) Kilovoltage
(C) SID
(D) Scattered radiation

217. Shape distortion is influenced by the relationship between the

1. x-ray tube and the part to be imaged.
2. part to be imaged and the image recorder.
3. image recorder and the x-ray tube.

(A) 1 only
(B) 1 and 2 only
(C) 1 and 3 only
(D) 1, 2, and 3

218. How can the radiograph in Figure 4–24 be improved?

1. Decrease mAs.
2. Eliminate motion.
3. Lengthen the scale of contrast.

(A) 1 only
(B) 2 only
(C) 1 and 3 only
(D) 1, 2, and 3

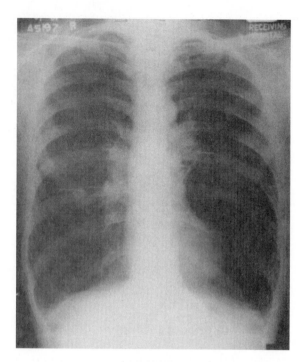

Figure 4–24.

219. Which of the following is (are) associated with subject contrast?

1. Patient thickness
2. Tissue density
3. Kilovoltage

(A) 1 only
(B) 1 and 2 only
(C) 1 and 3 only
(D) 1, 2, and 3

220. If a radiograph exposed using a 12:1 ratio grid exhibits a loss of density at its lateral edges, it is probably because the

(A) SID was too great.
(B) grid failed to move during the exposure.
(C) x-ray tube was angled in the direction of the lead strips.
(D) central ray was off-center.

221. Which combination of exposure factors will most likely contribute to producing the longest-scale contrast?

	mAs	kVp	Film–Screen System	Grid Ratio	Field Size
(A)	10	70	400	5:1	14 × 17 inches
(B)	12	90	200	8:1	14 × 17 inches
(C)	15	90	200	12:1	8 × 10 inches
(D)	20	80	400	10:1	11 × 14 inches

222. High-kilovoltage exposure factors are usually required for radiographic examinations using

1. water-soluble, iodinated media.
2. a negative contrast agent.
3. barium sulfate.

(A) 1 only
(B) 2 only
(C) 3 only
(D) 1 and 3 only

223. Which of the following focal spot sizes should be employed for magnification radiography?

(A) 0.2 mm
(B) 0.6 mm
(C) 1.2 mm
(D) 2.0 mm

224. For which of the following examinations may the use of a grid *not* be necessary in the adult patient?

(A) Hip
(B) Knee
(C) Abdomen
(D) Lumbar spine

225. Grid cutoff due to off - centering would result in

(A) overall loss of density.
(B) both sides of the image being underexposed.
(C) overexposure under the anode end.
(D) underexposure under the anode end.

226. All of the following have an impact on radiographic contrast, *except*

(A) photon energy.

(B) grid ratio.

(C) OID.

(D) focal spot size.

227. The exposure factors of 300 mA, 0.07 second, and 95 kVp were used to produce a particular radiographic density and contrast. A similar radiograph can be produced using 500 mA, 80 kVp, and

(A) 0.01 second.

(B) 0.04 second.

(C) 0.08 second.

(D) 0.16 second.

228. Disadvantage(s) of using low kV technical factors include

1. insufficient penetration.
2. increased patient dose.
3. diminished latitude.

(A) 1 only

(B) 1 and 2 only

(C) 1 and 3 only

(D) 1, 2, and 3

229. Which of the following statements is (are) true regarding Figure 4–25?

1. Image A was made using a higher kVp than image B.
2. Image A was made with a higher ratio grid than image B.
3. Image A demonstrates shorter-scale contrast than image B.

(A) 1 only

(B) 1 and 2 only

(C) 2 and 3 only

(D) 1, 2, and 3

230. Which of the following influences geometric unsharpness?

1. OID
2. Source-object distance
3. SID

(A) 1 only

(B) 1 and 2 only

(C) 1 and 3 only

(D) 1, 2, and 3

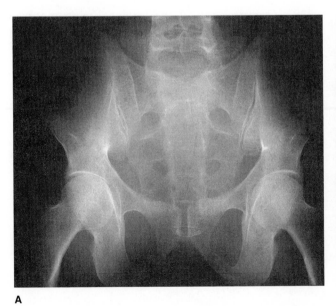
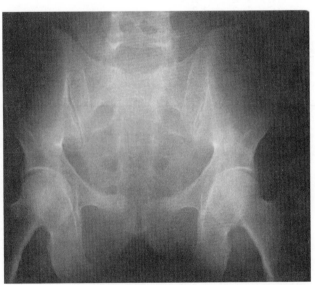

A   B

Figure 4–25. Reproduced with permission from Saia DA. *Radiography: Program Review and Examination Preparation*, 2nd ed. Stamford, CT: Appleton & Lange, 1999.

231. Which of the following affect(s) both the quantity and the quality of the primary beam?

    1. Half-value layer (HVL)
    2. kVp
    3. mA

    (A) 1 only
    (B) 2 only
    (C) 1 and 2 only
    (D) 1, 2, and 3

232. A quality assurance program serves to

    1. keep patient dose to a minimum.
    2. keep radiographic quality consistent.
    3. ensure equipment efficiency.

    (A) 1 only
    (B) 1 and 2 only
    (C) 1 and 3 only
    (D) 1, 2, and 3

233. The darkroom should be constructed and equipped so as to avoid

    1. external light leaks.
    2. film bin light leaks.
    3. safelight fog.

    (A) 1 only
    (B) 2 only
    (C) 1 and 3 only
    (D) 1, 2, and 3

234. What information, located on each box of film, is important to note and has a direct relationship to image quality?

    (A) Number of films in the box
    (B) Manufacturer's name
    (C) Expiration date
    (D) Emulsion lot

235. If 40 mAs and a 50-speed screen–film system were used for a particular exposure, what new mAs value would be required to produce the same density if the screen–film system were changed to 200 speed?

    (A) 10
    (B) 20
    (C) 80
    (D) 160

236. An exposure was made using 12 mAs and 60 kVp. If the kVp was changed to 70 to obtain longer-scale contrast, what should be the new mAs?

    (A) 3
    (B) 6
    (C) 18
    (D) 24

237. Recorded detail can be improved by decreasing

    1. the SID.
    2. the OID.
    3. motion unsharpness.

    (A) 1 only
    (B) 3 only
    (C) 2 and 3 only
    (D) 1, 2, and 3

238. Compression of the breast during mammographic imaging improves the technical quality of the image because

    1. geometric blurring is decreased.
    2. less scattered radiation is produced.
    3. patient motion is reduced.

    (A) 1 only
    (B) 3 only
    (C) 2 and 3 only
    (D) 1, 2, and 3

239. Distortion can be caused by

1. tube angle.
2. the position of the organ or structure within the body.
3. the radiographic positioning of the part.

(A) 1 only
(B) 1 and 2 only
(C) 2 and 3 only
(D) 1, 2, and 3

240. Methods that help reduce the production of scattered radiation include using

1. compression.
2. beam restriction.
3. a grid.

(A) 1 and 2 only
(B) 1 and 3 only
(C) 2 and 3 only
(D) 1, 2, and 3

241. The speed of an intensifying screen is influenced by which of the following factors?

1. Phosphor layer thickness
2. Antihalation backing
3. Phosphor type used

(A) 1 only
(B) 1 and 3 only
(C) 2 and 3 only
(D) 1, 2, and 3

242. If 0.05 second was selected for a particular exposure, what mA would be necessary to produce 30 mAs?

(A) 900
(B) 600
(C) 500
(D) 300

243. The rate of chemical replenishment in automatic processing is based on

(A) solution temperature.
(B) processor speed.
(C) amount of film processed.
(D) solution agitation.

244. If a radiograph exhibits insufficient density, this might be attributed to

1. inadequate kVp.
2. inadequate SID.
3. grid cutoff.

(A) 1 only
(B) 1 and 2 only
(C) 1 and 3 only
(D) 1, 2, and 3

245. An exposure was made using 300 mA, 0.04-second exposure, and 85 kVp. Each of the following changes will decrease the radiographic density by one half *except* a change to

(A) 1/50-second exposure.
(B) 72 kVp.
(C) 10 mAs.
(D) 150 mA.

246. The use of which of the following is (are) essential in magnification radiography?

1. High-ratio grid
2. Fractional focal spot
3. Direct exposure film

(A) 1 only
(B) 2 only
(C) 1 and 3 only
(D) 1, 2, and 3

247. Which of the following are methods used for silver reclamation?

1. Photoelectric method
2. Metallic replacement method
3. Electrolytic method

(A) 1 only
(B) 1 and 2 only
(C) 2 and 3 only
(D) 1, 2, and 3

248. Which of the following groups of technical factors would be most appropriate for the radiographic examination shown in Figure 4–26?

   (A) 400 mA, 1/30 second, 72 kVp

   (B) 300 mA, 1/50 second, 82 kVp

   (C) 300 mA, 1/120 second, 94 kVp

   (D) 50 mA, 1/4 second, 72 kVp

249. An increase in the kilovoltage applied to the x-ray tube increases the

   1. x-ray wavelength.
   2. exposure rate.
   3. patient absorption.

   (A) 1 only

   (B) 2 only

   (C) 2 and 3 only

   (D) 1, 2, and 3

250. Which of the following statements is (are) true regarding the artifact seen in the erect PA projection of the chest shown in Figure 4–27?

   (A) The object is located within the patient.

   (B) The object is located within the cassette.

   (C) The object is located between the patient and the x-ray tube.

   (D) The object is located between the patient and the image receptor.

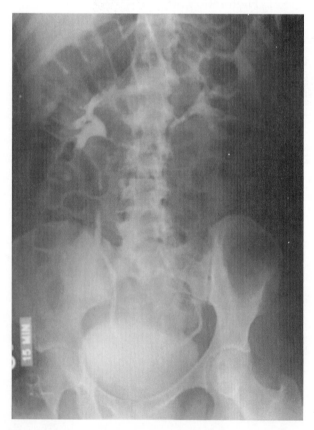

Figure 4–26. Courtesy of Stamford Hospital, Department of Radiology.

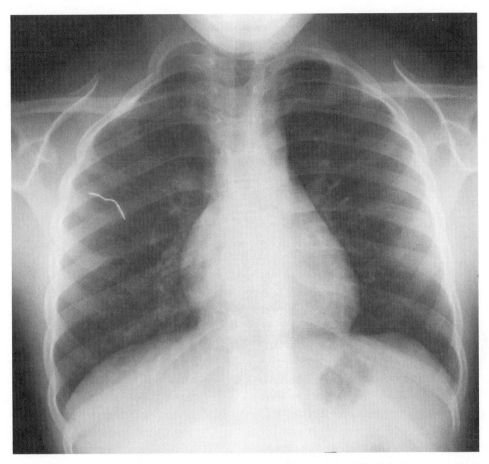

Figure 4–27. Courtesy of Stamford Hospital, Department of Radiology.

Answers and Explanations

1. **(A)** When an AEC (phototimer or ionization chamber) is used, the system is programmed for the use of a particular screen–film speed (eg, 400 speed). If a slower-speed screen image receptor is placed in the bucky tray, the AEC has no way of recognizing it as different, and will time the exposure for the system that it is programmed for. For example, if the AEC is programmed for a 400 screen–film combination, and if a 200-speed screen image receptor is placed in the bucky tray, the resulting radiograph will have half the required radiographic density. (*Shepherd, pp 65–66*)

2. **D.** In digital imaging, pixel size is determined by dividing the field of view (FOV) by the matrix. In this case the FOV is 80 cm; since the answer is expressed in mm, first change 80 cm to 800 mm. Then 800 divided by 2048 equals 0.4 mm.

$$80 \text{ cm} = 800 \text{ mm}$$

$$\frac{800}{2048} = 0.4 \text{ mm}$$

The FOV and matrix size are independent of one another, that is, either can be changed and the other will remain unaffected. However, pixel size is affected by changes in either the FOV or matrix size. For example, if the matrix size is increased, pixel size decreases. If FOV increases, pixel size increases. Pixel size is inversely related to resolution. As pixel size increases, resolution decreases. (*Fosbinder & Kelsey, p 285*)

3. **(C)** A digital image is formed by a *matrix of pixels* (picture elements) in rows and columns. A matrix that has 512 pixels in each row and column is a 512×512 matrix. The term *field of view* is used to describe how much of the patient (eg, 150-mm diameter) is included in the matrix. The matrix and the field of view can be changed independently, without one affecting the other, but changes in either will change pixel size. As in traditional radiography, *spatial resolution* is measured in line pairs per mm (*lp/mm*). As matrix size is increased, there are more and smaller pixels in the matrix, and therefore improved resolution. Fewer and larger pixels result in a poor resolution, "pixelly" image, that is, one in which you can actually see the individual pixel boxes. (*Fosbinder & Kelsey, p 286; Shephard, p 336*)

4. **(A)** The invisible silver halide image is composed of exposed silver grains. These are "reduced" to a visible black metallic silver image in the developer solution. The fixer solution functions to remove *unexposed* silver halide crystals from the film. (*Shephard, pp 97–98*)

5. **(C)** The radiographic image seen in Figure 4–1 demonstrates *double exposure*. Notice the *double image of the ribs, humerus, and clavicle, especially on the left side* of the chest. The anatomic parts and diaphragm are sharply defined, not blurry, as they would be in the case of *motion*. Focal spot *blur* would also cause a slight blur of anatomic details. *Poor screen–film contact* would most likely appear as localized blurriness in

one area; poor contact is unlikely to affect the entire cassette. (*Bushong, p 473*)

6. **(C)** Grids are used in radiography to *absorb scattered radiation* before it reaches the IR, thus improving radiographic contrast. Contrast obtained with a grid compared to contrast without a grid is termed *contrast improvement factor*. The greater the percentage of scattered radiation absorbed compared to absorbed primary radiation, the greater the "selectivity" of the grid. If a grid absorbs an abnormally large amount of useful radiation as a result of improper centering, tube angle, or tube distance, *grid cutoff* occurs. (*Selman, p 370*)

7. **(B)** Most laser film is sensitive to both the Wratten 6B and the GBX (green, blue, x-ray) safelight filters. Laser film will fog if it is handled under these safelight conditions. Most laser film is loaded into a film magazine in total darkness. Processing temperatures for laser film are the same as those for regular x-ray film. (*Shephard, pp 92, 94*)

8. **(D)** The addition of a grid will help clean up the scattered radiation produced by higher kVp, but it requires an *mAs adjustment*. According to the grid conversion factors listed here, the addition of an 8:1 grid requires that the original mAs be multiplied by a factor of 4:

   No grid = 1 × the original mAs
   5:1 grid = 2 × the original mAs
   6:1 grid = 3 × the original mAs
   8:1 grid = 4 × the original mAs
   12:1 (or 10:1) grid = 5 × the original mAs
   16:1 grid = 6 × the original mAs

   The adjustment therefore requires 32 mAs at 90 kVp. (*Saia, p 328*)

9. **(A)** One of the biggest advantages of CR/DR is the *latitude* it offers. The characteristic curve of typical film emulsion has a "range of correct exposure," limited by the toe and shoulder of the curve. In CR/DR, there is a *linear* relationship between the exposure, given the PSP and its resulting luminescence, as it is scanned by the laser, as illustrated in the figure shown. This affords much *greater exposure latitude*; technical inaccuracies can be effectively eliminated.

Overexposure of up to 500% and underexposure of up to 80% are reported as recoverable, thus eliminating most retakes. *This surely affords increased efficiency; however this does not mean that images can be exposed arbitrarily.* The professional radiographer has a responsibility to keep dose reduction to a minimum. The same exposure factors as screen–film systems, or less, are generally recommended for CR/DR. (*Shephard, p 332*)

10. **(C)** If a fairly large patient is turned *prone*, the abdominal measurement will be significantly different from the AP measurement as a result of the effect of *compression*. Thus, the part is essentially "thinner," and less scattered radiation will be produced. If the patient remains supine and a compression band is applied, a similar effect will be produced. *Beam restriction* is probably the single most effective means of reducing the production of scattered radiation. *Grid ratio* affects the *cleanup* of scattered radiation; it has no effect on the *production* of scattered radiation. (*Shephard, p 203*)

11. **(A)** Screen–film imaging consists of an exposure method of converting x-ray energy to light energy, then converting light energy to electrochemical energy in the development process. Processing changes the invisible electrochemical image to a visible/manifest radiographic image. This process ends with *analog* data. *Digital* imaging is an electronic imaging method that allows data capture and manipulation in an electron pattern. The resulting image can be turned into an analog image after going through several energy changes (electron to light to film or TV screen). The *direct action of x-rays* has very little influence on a radiographic image produced with intensifying screens (fluorescent light is responsible for the majority of film exposure). (*Selman, p 310*)

12. **(C)** *Radiograph B* was made of a chest phantom and processed using the recommended 95°F developer temperature. *Radiograph A* was exposed under the same conditions but was processed with a developer temperature of 90°F. The development process slows at the lower temperature, and a much lighter radiograph results. To produce the original density

using a 90°F developer, higher exposure factors would be required. *Radiograph C* was exposed under the same conditions as radiographs A and B but was developed at 100°F; at this temperature, the development process is accelerated and the radiograph is too dark. *(Saia, p 409)*

13. **(A)** Limiting the size of the radiographic field serves to limit the amount of scattered radiation produced within the anatomic part. As the amount of scattered radiation generated within the part decreases, so does the resultant density within the radiographic image. Hence, beam restriction is a very effective means of reducing the quantity of non–information-carrying scattered radiation (fog) produced, resulting in a shorter scale of contrast with fewer radiographic densities. *(Shephard, p 203)*

14. **(A)** The mAs is the exposure factor governing radiographic density. Using the equation milliamperage × time = mAs, determine each mAs: A = 30 mAs; B = 20 mAs; C = 12 mAs; D = 18 mAs. Group A will produce the greatest radiographic density. *(Selman, p 214)*

15. **(C)** Inside the CR cassette is the *photostimulable phosphor (PSP) image plate*, sometimes referred to simply as an *image plate* or *IP*. This PSP or IP with its layer of europium-activated barium fluorohalide serves as the *image receptor* as it is exposed in the traditional manner and receives the latent image. The PSP can *store* the latent image for several hours; after about 8 hours noticable image fading will occur. Once the CR cassette is placed into the CR processor (*scanner* or *reader*), the PSP plate is automatically removed. The latent image on the PSP is changed to a manifest image as it is scanned by a narrow high-intensity *helium-neon laser* to obtain the pixel data. As the plate is scanned in the "reader," it releases a violet light—a process referred to as *photo-* (or light) *stimulated luminescence*. (Carlton & Adler, p 633)

16. **(C)** In the left and right oblique cervical spine radiographs seen in Figure 4–4, radiograph **A** appears lighter than radiograph **B**. The key to their density difference lies in the fact that both were performed *using AEC* during a particular examination. If the focused grid had been placed upside down, only the central portion of the image (along the long axis of the image receptor) would have been imaged. The remainder would demonstrate grid cutoff. Incorrect photocell selection would most likely produce unsatisfactory images in both instances, not just in one of the obliques. The lack of blurriness indicates that this is not a case of patient motion. However, incorrect or different positioning of the part being imaged will cause the AEC photocell (the center cell is selected for the cervical spine) to react differently. When the photocell is "reading" exit radiation emerging from the cervical bodies, one exposure is recorded. When the photocell is "reading" exit radiation emerging from the cervical spinous processes/soft tissue, quite another (much *lower*) exposure is recorded—hence the difference in radiographic density between the two radiographs in this example. This example demonstrates the critical relationship between exact positioning and recorded density when using AEC. *(Carlton & Adler, pp 505–506)*

17. **(C)** When exposure rate decreases (as a result of increased SID), an appropriate increase in mAs is required to maintain the original radiographic density. Unless exposure is increased, the resulting radiograph will be underexposed. The formula used to determine the new mAs *(density maintenance formula)* is

$$\frac{\text{old mAs}}{\text{new mAs}} = \frac{\text{old } D^2}{\text{new } D^2}$$

Substituting known values,

$$\frac{(\text{old mAs}) \ 10}{(\text{new mAs}) \ x} = \frac{(\text{old } D^2) \ 1600}{(\text{new } D^2) \ 5184}$$

$$1600x = 51{,}840$$

$$x = 32.4 = \text{mAs at 72 inches SID}$$

To determine the required mA (mA × s = mAs),

$$0.1x = 32.4$$

$$x = 324 \text{ mA}$$

(Selman, p 214)

18. **(C)** Dual xray absorptiometry (DXA) imaging is used to evaluate bone mineral density (BMD). It is the most widely used method of *bone densitometry*—it is *low dose, precise,* and *uncomplicated* to use/perform. DXA uses *two photon energies*—one for soft tissue and one for bone. Since bone is more dense and attenuates x-ray photons more readily, their *attenuation is calculated* to represent the degree of bone density. Bone densitometry, DXA, can be used to evaluate bone mineral content of the body, or part of it, to diagnosis osteoporosis or to evaluate the effectiveness of treatments for osteoporosis. (*Ballinger & Frank, vol 3, pp 488–489*)

19. **(C)** The exposed CR cassette is placed into the CR scanner reader, where the PSP/imaging plate is automatically removed. The latent image appears as the PSP is scanned by a narrow high-intensity *helium-neon laser* to obtain the pixel data. As the plate is scanned in the CR reader, it releases a violet light—a process referred to as *photo-stimulated luminescence.*

    The luminescent light is converted to electrical energy representing the *analog* image. The electrical energy is sent to an *analog-to-digital converter (ADC)* where it is digitized and becomes the *digital* image that is eventually displayed (after a short delay) on a high-resolution monitor and/or printed out by a laser printer. The digitized images can also be manipulated in postprocessing, electronically transmitted, and stored/archived. (*Carlton & Adler, p 635*)

20. **(C)** Significant scattered radiation is generated within the part when imaging large or dense body parts and when using high kilovoltage. A radiographic grid is made of alternating lead strips and interspace material; it is placed between the patient and the IR to absorb energetic scatter emerging from the patient. Although a grid prevents much of the scattered radiation from reaching the radiograph, its use does necessitate a significant *increase* in patient exposure. (*Saia, p 327*)

21. **(D)** If a film is placed on an illuminator and 100% of the illuminator's light is transmitted through the film, that film must have a density of 0. According to the equation

$$\text{Density} = \log_{10} \frac{\text{incident light intensity}}{\text{transmitted light intensity}}$$

If 10% of the illuminator's light passes through the film, that film has a density of 1. If 1% of the light passes through the film, that film has a density of 2. (*Shephard, p 102*)

22. **(B)** The digital images' *scale of contrast,* or *contrast resolution,* can be changed electronically through leveling and windowing of the image. The *level control* determines the *central or mid density* of the scale of contrast, while the *window control* determines the *total number* of densities/grays (to the right and left of the central/mid density). Matrix and pixel sizes are related to (spatial) resolution of digital images. (*Fosbinder & Kelsey, p 289*)

23. **(C)** To change nongrid to grid exposure or to adjust exposure when changing from one grid ratio to another, it is necessary to recall the factor for each grid ratio:

    No grid = 1 × the original mAs
    5:1 grid = 2 × the original mAs
    6:1 grid = 3 × the original mAs
    8:1 grid = 4 × the original mAs
    12:1 (or 10:1) grid = 5 × the original mAs
    16:1 grid = 6 × the original mAs

    Therefore, to change from nongrid to an 8:1 grid, multiply the original mAs by a factor of 4. A new mAs of 16 is required. (*Saia, p 328*)

24. **B.** In digital imaging, pixel size is determined by dividing the FOV by the matrix. In this case, the FOV is 35 cm; since the answer is expressed in millimeters, first change 35 cm to 350 mm. Then 350 divided by 1024 equals 0.35 mm.

$$35 \text{ cm} = 350 \text{ mm}$$
$$\frac{350}{1024} = 0.35 \text{ mm}$$

The FOV and matrix size are independent of one another, that is, either can be changed and the other will remain unaffected. However, pixel size is affected by changes in either the FOV or matrix size. For example, if the matrix size is increased, pixel size decreases. If FOV increases, pixel size increases. Pixel size is inversely related to resolution. As pixel size increases, resolution decreases. *(Fosbinder & Kelsey, p 285)*

25. **(B)** The formula for *magnification factor* is MF = image size/object size. In the stated problem, the anatomic measurement is 15.2 cm, and the magnification factor is known to be 1.3. Substituting the known factors in the appropriate equation,

$$MF = \frac{\text{image size}}{\text{object size}}$$

$$1.3 = \frac{x}{15.2}$$

$$x = 15.2 \div 1.3$$

$$x = 11.69 \text{ cm (actual anatomic size)}$$

(Fauber, pp 90–92)

26. **(B)** Boxes of x-ray film, especially the larger sizes, should be stored in the vertical (upright) position. If film boxes are stacked upon one another, the sensitive emulsion can be affected by pressure from the boxes above. *Pressure marks* are produced and result in loss of contrast in that area of the radiographic image. When retrieving x-ray film from storage, the oldest should be used first. *(Shephard, p 110)*

27. **(C)** *Emphysema* is abnormal distention of the pulmonary alveoli (or tissue spaces) with air. The presence of abnormal amounts of air makes a decrease from normal exposure factors necessary to avoid excessive density. *Congestive heart failure, pneumonia,* and *pleural effusion,* all involve abnormal amounts of fluid in the chest and would therefore require an *increase* in exposure factors. *(Carlton & Adler, p 258)*

28. **(D)** Film *age* is an important consideration when determining the causes of film fog. Outdated film will exhibit loss of contrast in the form of fog and loss of speed. A *safelight* is "safe" only for practical periods of time required for the necessary handling of film. Films that are left out on the darkroom counter can be fogged by excessive exposure to the safelight. Film emulsion is much more sensitive to safelight fog *after* exposure. The high temperatures required for *automatic processors'* rapid processing are a source of film fog. Daily QA ensures that fog levels do not exceed the upper limit of 0.2 density. *(Shephard, pp 110, 123, 137)*

29. **(A)** As kVp is increased, more high-energy photons are produced and the overall energy of the primary beam is increased. Photon energy is inversely related to wavelength; that is, as photon energy increases, wavelength decrease. An increase in milliamperage serves to increase the number of photons produced at the target, but is unrelated to their energy. *(Selman, p 118)*

30. **(B)** Of the two radiographs illustrated, image A was made recumbent, and image B was made in the erect position; this may be discerned by the presence of clearly defined air–fluid levels in the lower abdomen. Abdominal viscera move to a lower position in the erect position, making the abdomen "thicker" and requiring an increase in exposure (usually the equivalent of about 10 kVp). *(Saia, pp 76, 80, 84)*

31. **(D)** Whereas CR utilizes traditional x-ray devices to enclose and protect the PSP image plate, *digital radiography* requires the use of somewhat different equipment. DR does not use cassettes or a traditional x-ray table; it is a *direct-capture* system of x-ray imaging. DR uses *solid state detector* plates as the x-ray image receptor (instead of a cassette in the Bucky tray) to intercept the collimated x-ray beam and form the latent image. The solid state detector plates are made of barium fluorohalide compounds similar to that used in CR's PSP image plates. DR affords the advantage of *immediate display of the image,*compared to CR's delayed image display. *(Shephard, p 335)*

32. **(B)** *Grid ratio* is defined as the height of the lead strips to the width of the interspace material (Fig. 4–28). The higher the lead strips (or the smaller the distance between the strips),

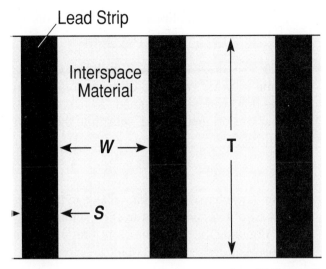

Lead Strip

Interspace Material

W

T

S

Figure 4–28. Reproduced with permission from Wolbarst AB. *Physics of Radiology.* East Norwalk, CT: Appleton & Lange, 1993.

the greater the grid ratio and the greater the percentage of scattered radiation absorbed. However, a grid does absorb some primary radiation as well. The higher the lead strips, the *more* critical the need for accurate centering, as the lead strips will more readily trap photons whose direction do not parallel them. *(Shephard, pp 245, 255)*

33. **(D)** As the speed of the film–screen system decreases, an *increase* in mAs is usually required to maintain radiographic density. *However, when an automatic exposure control (photo-timer or ionization chamber) is used, the system is programmed for the use of a particular film–screen speed.* If a slower-speed screen cassette–image receptor is placed in the bucky tray, the AEC has no way of recognizing it as different and will time the exposure for the system that it is programmed for. For example, if the system is programmed for a 400-speed film–screen combination, and if a 200-speed screen cassette–image receptor was placed in the bucky tray, the resulting radiograph would have half the required radiographic density. *(Saia, p 305)*

34. **(B)** Use of a short SID with a large-size image receptor (and also with anode angles of 10° or less) causes the anode heel effect to be much more apparent. The x-ray beam needs to diverge more to cover a *large-size image re-*

ceptor, and it needs to diverge even more for coverage as the SID decreases. The x-ray beam has no problem diverging toward the cathode end of the beam, but as it tries to diverge toward the anode end of the beam, it is eventually stopped by the anode (x-ray photons are absorbed by the anode). This causes a decrease in beam intensity at the anode end of the beam and is characteristic of the *anode heel effect. (Carlton & Adler, p 120)*

35. **(D)** Intensifying-screen phosphors that have a *high atomic number* are more likely to *absorb* a high percentage of the incident x-ray photons and *convert* x-ray photon energy to fluorescent light energy. How efficiently the phosphors detect and interact with the x-ray photons is termed *quantum detection efficiency.* How effectively the phosphors make this energy conversion is termed *conversion efficiency. (Shephard, p 65)*

36. **(C)** Spatial resolution in *CR* is impacted by the size of the PSP, the size of the scanning laser beam, and monitor matrix size. *High-resolution monitors (2–4 K) are required for high-quality, high-resolution image display. The larger the matrix size, the better the image resolution.* Typical image matrix size (rows and columns) used in chest radiography is 2048 × 2048. As in traditional radiography, *spatial resolution* is measured in line pairs per mm. As matrix size is increased, there are more and smaller pixels in the matrix therefore improved spatial resolution. Other factors contributing to image resolution are the *size of the laser beam* and the *size of the PSP/IP phosphors.* Smaller phosphor size improves resolution in ways similar to that of intensifying screens—anything that causes an increase in light diffusion will result in a decreae in resolution. Smaller phosphors in the PSP plate allow less light diffusion. Additionally, the scanning laser light must be the correct intensity and size. A narrow laser beam is required for optimum resolution. *(Shephard, p 336)*

37. **(B)** The automatic film processor has a number of component systems. The *circulation* system functions to agitate, mix, and filter solutions.

The *transport* system moves film from solution to solution between rollers, changing the direction of the film around critical turns. The *temperature control* system functions to monitor and control solution temperature. The *replenishment* system serves to monitor the solution and replace it as needed. *(Bushong, p 212)*

38. **(B)** One way to minimize scattered radiation reaching the IR is to use optimal kilovoltage; excessive kVp increases the production of scattered radiation. Close *collimation* is also important because the smaller the volume of irradiated material, the less scattered radiation is produced. Using *compression* bands or the prone position in a large abdomen has the effect of making the abdomen "thinner"; it will therefore generate less scattered radiation. *Low*-ratio grids allow a greater percentage of scattered radiation to reach the IR. Use of a *high*-ratio grid will clean up a greater amount of scattered radiation before it reaches the IR. *(Shephard, p 203)*

39. **(C)** *Absorption* occurs when an x-ray photon interacts with matter and disappears, as in the photoelectric effect. *Scattering* occurs when there is partial transfer of energy to matter, as in the Compton effect. The reduction in the intensity of an x-ray beam as it passes through matter is called *attenuation*. *(Bushong, p 185)*

40. **(C)** The radiographer can *manipulate* (change, enhance) digital images displayed on the CRT through *postprocessing*. One way to alter image contrast and/or density is through *windowing*. The term *windowing* refers to some change made to *window width* and/or *window level*. Change in window *width* affects change in the number of gray shades, that is, *image contrast*—as demonstrated in the figures shown (Figure 4–6 A, B, and C). Change in window *level* affects change in the image brightness, that is, *optical density*. Windowing and other postprocessing mechanisms permit the radiographer to affect changes in the image and to produce "special effects" such as edge enhancement, image stitching (useful in

scoliosis examinations), image inversion, rotation, and reversal. *(Shephard, p 346)*

41. **(C)** The mAs formula is milliamperage $\times$ time = mAs. With two of the factors known, the third can be determined. To find the mAs that was originally used, substitute the known values:

$$300 \times 0.1 = 30$$

We have increased the kilovoltage to 86, an increase of 15%, which has an effect similar to that of doubling the mAs. Therefore, only 15 mAs is now required as a result of the kV increase:

$$mA \times s = mAs$$
$$500\,x = 15$$
$$x = 0.03\text{-second exposure}$$

(Selman, p 214)

42. **(A)** Factors that contribute to an increase in the intensification factor generally function to reduce *resolution*. Slow-speed (detail or "extremity") screens resolve more line pairs per millimeter (lp/mm) than much faster screens. The use of fast screens results in some loss of recorded detail. As intensification factor increases, radiographic *density* generally increases. *(Bushong, pp 222–223)*

43. **(B)** The GBX is a red filter that is safe with green-sensitive film emulsion. The amber-colored Wratten 6B filter is safe only for blue-sensitive film. Although using no safelight is possible, it is not a practical way to function. *(Carlton & Adler, p 306)*

44. **(C)** *Grid ratio* is defined as the height of the lead strips compared to (divided by) the width of the interspace material. The width of the lead strips has no bearing on the grid ratio. The height of the lead strips is 5 mm; the width of the interspace material (same as the distance between the lead strips) is 0.5 mm. Therefore, the grid ratio is 5 ÷ 0.5, or a 10:1 grid ratio. *(Bushong, p 250)*

45. **(B)** Magnification is part of every radiographic image. Anatomic parts within the body are at

various distances from the image recorder and therefore have various degrees of magnification. The formula used to determine the amount of image magnification is:

$$\frac{\text{Image Size}}{\text{Object Size}} = \frac{\text{SID}}{\text{SOD}}$$

Substituting known values:

$$\frac{x}{3 \text{ inches}} = \frac{36 \text{ inches SID}}{32 \text{ inches SOD}}$$

$$(\text{SOD} = \text{SID minus OID})$$

$$32x = 108$$

$$x = 3.37 \text{ inches } \textit{image width}$$

(Bushong, p 284)

46. **(D)** The higher the kVp range, the greater the exposure latitude (margin of error in exposure). Higher kVp is more penetrating and produces more grays on the radiograph, lengthening the scale of contrast. As kVp increases, the percentage of scattered radiation also increases. *(Saia, p 360)*

47. **(B)** Higher than normal developing temperatures cause overdevelopment of the less exposed silver halide crystals, producing chemical fog. The resulting radiograph will appear very gray, exhibiting loss of contrast and increased density. Wet, tacky films are usually the result of lower-than-normal dryer temperature or fixer underreplenishment. *(Shephard, p 153)*

48. **(A)** Shape distortion (foreshortening, elongation) is caused by improper alignment of the tube, part, and IR. Size distortion, or magnification, is caused by too great an OID or too short an SID. Focal spot blur is caused by the use of a large focal spot. *(Fauber, p 93)*

49. **(B)** *Focal spot size* affects recorded detail by its effect on focal spot blur: The larger the focal spot size, the greater the blur produced. Recorded detail is significantly affected by distance changes because of their effect on magnification. As *SID* increases, magnification decreases and recorded detail increases.

The method of *rectification* has no effect on recorded detail. Single-phase rectified units produce "pulsed" radiation, whereas three-phase units produce almost constant potential. *(Shephard, p 215)*

50. **(D)** The abdomen radiograph seen in Figure 4–8 demonstrates *motion* blur. This can be seen particularly in the upper abdomen and in the bowel gas patterns. Motion obliterates detail. Patients who are in pain are often unable to cooperate as fully as patients who are not in pain. Careful positioning and patient instruction are often helpful, but it remains useful to employ the shortest exposure time possible. The radiograph also demonstrates good long-scale contrast that enables visualization of many tissue densities. The dark horizontal line across the abdomen is a clothing artifact resulting from a taut elastic underwear waistband. *(Fauber, p 87; Shephard, p 197)*

51. **(B)** Because the focal spot (track) of an x-ray tube is along the anode's beveled edge, photons produced at the target are able to diverge considerably toward the cathode end of the x-ray tube but are absorbed by the heel of the anode at the opposite end of the tube. This results in a greater number of x-ray photons distributed toward the cathode end, which is known as the *anode heel effect*. The effect of this restricting heel is most pronounced when the x-ray photons are required to *diverge* more, as would be the case with *short SID, large-size IRs*, and *steeper (smaller) target angles*. *(Carlton & Adler, p 120; Shephard, p 192)*

52. **(B)** Each mAs is determined (A = 4; B = 4; C = 8; D = 2) and numbered in order of greatest to least density (C = 1; A and B = 2; D = 3). Then the kilovoltages are reviewed and also numbered in order of greatest to least density (A, B, and C = 1; D = 2). Next, screen speeds are numbered from greatest-density-producing to least-density-producing (D and B = 1; A = 2; C = 3). Finally, the numbers assigned to the mAs, kVp, and screen speed are added up for each of the four groups (B = 4; A and C = 5; D = 6); the *lowest* total (B) indicates the group

of factors that will produce the greatest radiographic density. This process is illustrated as follows:

A. 4 mAs (2) + 94 kVp (1) + 100 screens (2) = 5

B. 4 mAs (2) + 94 kVp (1) + 200 screens (1) =4

C. 8 mAs (1) + 94 kVp (1) + 50 screens (3) = 5

D. 2 mAs (3) + 80 kVp (2) + 200 screens (1) = 6

(Shephard, p 179)

53. **(A)** The line focus principle is a geometric principle illustrating that the *actual focal spot is larger than the effective (projected) focal spot*. The actual focal spot (target) is larger, to accommodate heat over a larger area, and is angled so as to *project* a smaller focal spot, thus maintaining recorded detail by reducing blur. The relationship between the exposure given the IR and the resulting density is expressed in the reciprocity law; the relationship between the SID and resulting density is expressed by the inverse square law. Grid ratio and lines per inch are unrelated to the line focus principle. (Selman, p 138; Shephard, pp 218–219).

54. **(D)** In the low kilovoltage ranges, a difference of just a few kVp makes a very noticeable radiographic difference. High-kVp technical factors offer much greater margin for error, as do slow film–screen combinations. Lower-ratio grids offer more tube-centering latitude than high-ratio grids. (Saia, p 360)

55. **(B)** The greater the quantity of black metallic silver deposited on a film, the greater the radiographic density. The greater the degree of radiographic density (degree of blackening), the *less* the quantity of illuminator light transmitted through the film. Therefore, the relationship between the amount of illuminator light striking the film and the amount of light transmitted through the film is an expression of radiographic density. It is expressed by the formula

$$\text{Density} = \log_{10} \frac{\text{incident light intensity}}{\text{transmitted light intensity}}$$

(Bushong, p 279)

56. **(A)** As intensifying-screen speed decreases, less fluorescent light is emitted from the phosphors. If less fluorescent light strikes the film emulsion, a smaller number of silver halide grains are changed to black metallic silver in the developer, and hence there is a decrease in radiographic density. As intensifying-screen speed decreases, so does radiographic density. Intensifying-screen speed and radiographic density are directly related. (Shephard, pp 67–68)

57. **(D)** Magnification radiography may be used to delineate a suspected hairline fracture or to enlarge tiny, contrast-filled blood vessels. It also has application in mammography. To magnify an object to twice its actual size, the part must be placed midway between the focal spot and the IR. (Selman, pp 223–225; Shephard, pp 229–231)

58. **(D)** According to the inverse square law of radiation, the intensity or exposure rate of radiation is inversely proportional to the square of the distance from its source. Thus, as distance from the source of radiation increases, exposure rate decreases. Because exposure rate and radiographic density are directly proportional, if the exposure rate of a beam directed to an IR is decreased, the resultant radiographic density would be decreased proportionally. (Selman, p 117)

59. **(D)** The thicker the *layer* of phosphors, the more fluorescent light is emitted from the screen. Different *types* of phosphors have different *conversion efficiencies*; rare earth phosphors emit more light during a given exposure than do calcium tungstate phosphors. As the *kVp* level is increased, so is the amount of fluoroscopic light emitted by intensifying-screen phosphors. (Selman, pp 181–183)

60. **(A)** An increase in photon energy accompanies an increase in *kilovoltage*. Kilovoltage regulates the penetrability of x-ray photons; it regulates their *wavelength*—the amount of *energy* with which they are associated. The higher the related energy of an x-ray beam, the greater its *penetrability* (kilovoltage and photon energy are directly related; kilovoltage and wavelength

are inversely related). Adjustments in kilovoltage have a big impact on radiographic contrast: As kilovoltage (photon energy) is increased, the number of grays increases, thereby producing a longer scale of contrast. In general, as *screen speed* increases, so does contrast (resulting in a shorter scale of contrast). An increase in *mAs* is frequently accompanied by an appropriate decrease in kilovoltage, which would also shorten the contrast scale. *SID* and radiographic contrast are unrelated. *(Shephard, p 204)*

61. **(C)** When tissue densities within a part vary greatly (eg, chest x-ray), the radiographic result can be unacceptably high contrast. To "even out" these densities and produce a more appropriate scale of grays, exposure factors using high kVp should be employed. Radiographic contrast generally increases with an increase in screen speed. The higher the grid ratio, the higher the contrast. Exposure factors using high mAs generally result in excessive image density, frequently obliterating much of the gray scale. *(Bushong, p 273; Shephard, p 200)*

62. **(A)** After the processor has been turned off overnight, or after it has been on standby for an extended period of time, artifacts can be produced on the first few films processed. "Delay streaks" can be produced and are usually caused by a buildup of oxidized developer on the crossover rack as a result of inadequate ventilation. A "cleanup" film or two should first be processed to rid the rollers of any accumulated foreign particles, such as lint, oxidized developer, and gelatin. It is important that the cleanup film be *unprocessed film* to avoid contamination of the developer with any retained fixer on the film or redepositing of any foreign particles on the rollers. *(Haus & Jaskulski, p 212)*

63. **(B)** An increase in kilovoltage (photon energy) will result in a *greater number* (ie, exposure rate) of scattered photons (Compton interaction). These scattered photons carry no useful information and contribute to radiation *fog*, thus decreasing radiographic contrast. *(Selman, p 117)*

64. **(A)** Body section tomography functions to provide an image of a particular plane (objective plane) of tissues within the body, blurring out everything above and below the plane of interest. The radiograph shown in Figure 4–9 is an example of linear tomography; the x-ray tube moves in one direction, while the x-ray IR moves in the opposite direction. The two pivot at a fixed fulcrum that corresponds to the objective plane and is therefore the level of no motion. A variety of x-ray tube motions (circular, hypocycloidal, etc) is available with more complex tomographic equipment. *(Ballinger & Frank, vol 3, pp 185–188)*

65. **(A)** As the distance from focal spot to IR (SID) increases, so does recorded detail. Because the part is being exposed by more perpendicular (less divergent) rays, less magnification and blur are produced. Although the best recorded detail is obtained using a long SID, the necessary increase in exposure factors and resulting increased patient exposure becomes a problem. An optimal 40-inch SID is used for most radiography, with the major exception being chest examinations. *(Selman, pp 206–207; Shephard, pp 221–222)*

66. **(A)** A characteristic curve is representative of a film emulsion's response to light or x-rays. A slow film emulsion (one with greater latitude and lower contrast) responds more gradually than does a fast film. In general, the more gentle or gradual the slope of a particular film's characteristic curve, the slower the film is, the longer the scale of contrast it will produce, the more latitude it possesses, and the more exposure that is required to produce a particular density. A line is drawn vertically from each curve at a density of 2.0 to where it intersects with the horizontal axis (exposure). Image *1 requires an exposure of about 1.7 to produce a density of 2.0.* Image *2 requires an exposure of about 2.1 to produce a density of 2.0. (Selman, p 221; Shephard, p 105)*

67. **(B)** *Developing* agents change the exposed silver bromide crystals to black metallic silver, thus producing a manifest image. The *fixer* solution removes the unexposed silver bromide crystals from the emulsion and hardens the gelatin emulsion, thus ensuring permanence of the radiograph. *(Fauber, p 167)*

68. **(B)** Excessive radiographic density may be a result of *overdevelopment*. Overdevelopment may be due to *excessive developer temperature*, resulting in *chemical fog*. Excessive density can also be a result of *overreplenishment* as a result of faulty microswitches or of feeding film into the processor "the long way" rather than "the wide way." *(Fauber, p 181; Shephard, pp 151–153)*

69. **(B)** Grids are devices constructed of alternating strips of lead foil and radiolucent interspacing material. They are placed between the patient and the IR, and they function to remove scattered radiation from the remnant beam before it forms the latent image. *Stationary* grids will efficiently remove scattered radiation from the remnant beam; however, their lead strips will be imaged on the radiograph. If the grid is made to *move* (usually in a direction perpendicular to the lead strips) during the exposure, the lead strips will be effectively blurred. The motion of a moving grid, or Potter-Bucky diaphragm, may be *reciprocating* (equal strokes back and forth), *oscillating* (almost circular direction), or *catapult* (rapid forward motion and slow return). *Synchronous* refers to a type of x-ray timer. *(Bushong, p 256)*

70. **(A)** The *focal spot size* selected will determine the amount of focal spot, or geometric, blur produced in the image. Different *screen speeds* will create differing degrees of fluorescent light diffusion, affecting recorded detail. *OID* is responsible for image magnification, and hence recorded detail. The *milliamperage* is unrelated to recorded detail; it affects only the quantity of x-ray photons produced and thus the radiographic density. *(Selman, pp 206–210)*

71. **(A)** High-speed imaging systems are valuable for reducing patient exposure and patient motion. However, some detail will be sacrificed, and quantum mottle can cause further image impairment. In general, *doubling the film–screen speed doubles the radiographic density*, thereby requiring that the mAs be halved to maintain the original radiographic density. Changing from 100 to 400 screens requires halving the mAs value *twice*, to 4.5 mAs. That is, when going from 100- to 200-speed screens, the mAs is changed from 18 to 9; when going from 200- to 400-speed screens, the mAs is changed from 9 to 4.5.

The new exposure time, using 200 mA, is
$200x = 4.5$
$x = 0.225$ second exposure using 200 mA and 400- speed screens.

(Selman, p 181)

72. **(C)** The formula mA $\times$ s = mAs is used to determine each mAs. The greatest radiographic density will be produced by the combination of greatest mAs and shortest SID. The groups in choices B and D should produce *identical radiographic density*, according to the inverse square law, because group D includes twice the distance and four times the mAs of group B. The group A has twice the distance of the group B, but only twice the mAs; therefore, it has *less* density than the groups B and D. The group C has the same distance as the group B and twice the mAs, making group C the group of technical factors that will produce the *greatest radiographic density*. *(Selman, p 214)*

73. **(C)** Of the given factors, kilovoltage and grid ratio will have a significant effect on radiographic contrast. mAs has no effect on contrast. Because a combination of increased kilovoltage and a low-ratio grid would allow the greatest amount of scattered radiation to reach the IR, thereby producing more gray tones, C is the best answer. D also uses a low-ratio grid, but the kilovoltage is too low to produce as many gray tones as C. *(Shephard, pp 305–308)*

74. **(B)** Dual-screen cassettes are made to be used with dual-emulsion film. The fluorescing screens are adjacent to the emulsions. If single-emulsion film is placed in a dual-screen cassette, the emulsion will receive only *one half of the intended exposure*, and the resulting image will exhibit decreased density. *(Carlton & Adler, p 281)*

75. **(C)** To change nongrid exposures to grid exposures, or to adjust exposure when changing

from one grid ratio to another, you must remember the factor for each grid ratio:

No grid = 1 × the original mAs
5:1 grid = 2 × the original mAs
6:1 grid = 3 × the original mAs
8:1 grid = 4 × the original mAs
12:1 grid = 5 × the original mAs
16:1 grid = 6 × the original mAs

To adjust exposure factors, you simply compare the old with the new:

$$\frac{6 \text{ (old mAs)}}{x \text{ (new mAs)}} = \frac{4 \text{ (old grid factor)}}{6 \text{ (new grid factor)}}$$

$$4x = 36$$
$$x = 9 \text{ mAs using 16:1 grid.}$$

(Saia, p 328)

76. **(D)** As *photon energy* (kVp) increases, so does the production of scattered radiation. The greater the *density* of the irradiated tissues, the greater the production of scattered radiation. As the size of the *irradiated field* increases, there is an increase in the volume of tissue irradiated, and the percentage of scatter again increases. Beam restriction is the single most important way to limit the amount of scattered radiation produced. *(Saia, p 322)*

77. **(B)** A 15% increase in kVp with a 50% decrease in mAs serves to produce a radiograph *similar* to the original, but with some obvious differences. The overall blackness *(radiographic density) is cut in half* because of the decrease in mAs. However, the loss of blackness is compensated for by the *addition of grays* (therefore, *longer*-scale contrast) from the increased kVp. The increase in kVp also *increases exposure latitude*; there is a greater margin for error in higher kVp ranges. *Recorded detail* is unaffected by changes in kVp. *(Fauber, pp 59–60)*

78. **(A)** If the SID is above or below the recommended focusing distance, the primary beam will not coincide with the angled lead strips at their lateral edges. Consequently, there will be *absorption of the primary beam*, termed *grid cutoff*. If the central ray is off-center *longitudinally*,

there will be no ill effects. If the central ray is off-center *side-to-side*, the lead strips are no longer parallel with the divergent x-ray beam, and there will be loss of density due to grid cutoff. Central ray angulation *in the direction of* the lead strips is appropriate and will not cause grid cutoff. Central ray angulation *against the direction of* the lead strips will cause grid cutoff. *(Selman, pp 239–242)*

79. **(A)** If a structure of a given length is not positioned parallel to the recording medium (PSP or film), it will be projected smaller than its actual size (foreshortened). An example of this can be a lateral projection of the third digit. If the finger is positioned so as to be parallel to the image receptor, no distortion will occur. If, however, the finger is positioned so that its distal portion rests on the cassette while its proximal portion remains a distance from the IR, foreshortening will occur. *(Shephard, pp 232–233)*

80. **(B)** Focal spot blur, or geometric blur, is caused by photons emerging from a large focal spot. The actual focal spot is always larger than the effective (or projected) focal spot, as illustrated by the line focus principle. In addition, the effective focal spot size varies along the longitudinal tube axis, being greatest in size at the cathode end of the beam and smallest at the anode end of the beam. Because the projected focal spot is greatest at the cathode end of the x-ray tube, geometric blur is also greatest at the corresponding part (cathode end) of the radiograph. *(Bushong, p 287–288)*

81. **(C)** The *reciprocity law* states that a particular mAs, regardless of the mA and exposure time used, will provide identical radiographic density. This holds true with direct exposure techniques, but it does fail somewhat with the use of intensifying screens. However, the fault is so slight as to be unimportant in most radiographic procedures. *(Shephard, p 193)*

82. **(B)** The cassette–image receptor front material must not attenuate the remnant beam, yet must be sturdy enough to withstand daily use. Bakelite was long been used as the material for tabletops and image receptor fronts,

but it has now largely been replaced by *magnesium* and *carbon fiber*. Lead would not be a suitable material, as it would absorb the remnant beam, and no image would be formed. *(Shephard, p 41)*

83. **(D)** X-ray film is sensitive and requires proper handling and storage. Several kinds of artifacts can be produced by careless handling during production of the radiographic image. Treelike, branching black marks on a radiograph are usually due to static electrical discharge. Problems with static electricity are especially prevalent during cold, dry weather and can be produced by simply removing a sweater in the darkroom. *(Selman, p 197)*

84. **(B)** *Fluorescence* occurs when an intensifying screen absorbs x-ray photon energy, emits light, and then *ceases* to emit light as soon as the energizing source ceases. *Phosphorescence* occurs when an intensifying screen absorbs x-ray photon energy, emits light, and *continues* to emit light for a short time after the energizing source ceases. *Quantum mottle* is the freckle-like appearance on some radiographs made using a very fast imaging system. The brightness of a fluoroscopic image is amplified through *image intensification (Bushong, p 221)*

85. **(D)** If it is desired to reduce the exposure time for a particular radiograph, as it might be when radiographing those who are unable to cooperate fully, the *milliamperage* must be *increased* sufficiently to maintain the original mAs, and thus radiographic density. A *higher kilovoltage* could be useful because it would allow further reduction of the mAs (exposure time) according to the 15% rule. Use of a *higher-speed* film–screen combination also helps reduce mAs (exposure time) through more efficient conversion of photon energy to fluorescent light energy. *(Selman, pp 182, 214)*

86. **(C)** With three-phase equipment, the voltage never drops to zero and x-ray intensity is significantly greater. When changing *from single-phase to three-phase, six-pulse equipment, two thirds of the original mAs is required* to produce a radiograph with similar density. When changing *from single-phase to three-phase, 12-pulse*

equipment, only one half of the original mAs is required. In this problem, we are changing from three-phase, 12-pulse to single-phase equipment; therefore, the mAs should be doubled (from 15 to 30 mAs). *(Carlton & Adler, p 98)*

87. **(C)** A grid is composed of alternate strips of lead and interspace material. The lead strips serve to trap scattered radiation before it fogs the IR. The interspace material must be radiolucent; plastic or sturdier aluminum is usually used. Cardboard was formerly used as interspace material, but it had the disadvantage of being affected by humidity (moisture). *(Selman, p 234)*

88. **(D)** The illustrated radiograph is that of an adult PA erect chest. The image is well positioned and exposed, but observe the *braids of hair* that extend past the neck and superimpose on the pulmonary apices. Braided hair should be pinned up or otherwise removed from superimposition on thoracic structures. The braided hair was imaged during the exposure of the PA chest and is therefore referred to as an *exposure artifact*. Examples of *processing* artifacts are guide shoe marks, roller marks, and scratches. *Tree static* appears as black branching lines caused by electrical discharge. It is important to inquire or examine patients for materials that will image radiographically and cast unwanted densities over essential anatomy. *(Bushong, p 474)*

89. **(C)** *Materials that emit light when stimulated by x-ray photons are called phosphors.* Phosphors are used in intensifying screens, where they function to absorb x-ray photon energy and convert it to visible light energy. Typically, for each x-ray photon absorbed, many light photons are emitted; intensifying screens serve to amplify the action of x-rays. *(Carlton & Adler, p 330)*

90. **(C)** The iodine-based contrast material used in intravenous (IV) urography gives optimum opacification at 60 to 70 kVp. Use of higher kVp will negate the effect of the contrast medium; a lower contrast will be produced, and poor visualization of the renal collecting system will result. GI and BE examinations employ high-kVp

exposure factors (about 120 kVp) to penetrate *through* the barium. In chest radiography, high-kVp technical factors are preferred for maximum visualization of pulmonary vascular markings, made visible with long-scale contrast. *(Saia, p 347)*

91. **(A)** Different types of intensifying screens are available for radiographic use, and they can differ greatly. Some intensifying screens emit a blue and others a green fluorescent light. Film emulsions are manufactured to be sensitive to one of these colors. This is termed *spectral matching.* If the film emulsion and intensifying screens are incorrectly matched, speed will be reduced. *(Shephard, pp 65–66)*

92. **(C)** During automatic processing (Fig. 4–29), radiographic film is first immersed in the *developer* solution, which functions to reduce the exposed silver bromide crystals in the film emulsion to black metallic silver (which constitutes the image). Next, the film goes directly into the *fixer,* which functions to remove the *unexposed* silver bromide crystals from the emulsion. The film is then transported to the *wash* tank, where chemicals are removed from the film, and then into the *dryer* section, where it is dried before leaving the processor. *(Fauber, p 162; Shephard, p 134)*

93. **(B)** An *increase in SID* will help decrease the effect of excessive OID. For example, in the lateral projection of the cervical spine, there is normally a significant OID that would result in obvious magnification at a 40-inch SID. This effect is decreased by the use of a 72-inch SID. However, especially with larger body parts, increased SID usually requires a significant increase in exposure factors. Focal spot size, screen speed, and grid ratio are unrelated to magnification. *(Selman, p 224)*

94. **(B)** Because the focal spot (track) of an x-ray tube is along the anode's beveled edge, photons produced at the target are able to diverge toward the cathode end of the tube, but are absorbed by the "heel" of the anode at the opposite anode end of the tube. This results in a greater number of x-ray photons distributed toward the cathode end and is known as the *anode heel effect.* The *line focus principle* is a geometric principle illustrating that the effective focal spot is always smaller than the actual focal spot. The *inverse square law of radiation* deals with the relationship between distance and radiation intensity. *Bohr's theory* refers to an atom's resemblance to the solar system. *(Selman, p 253)*

95. **(B)** A compensating filter is used to make up for widely differing tissue densities. For example,

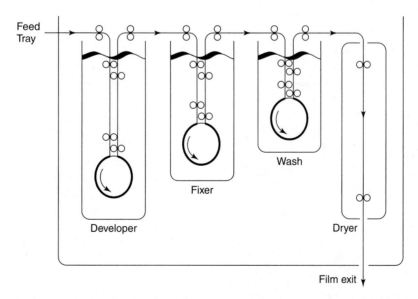

Feed Tray

Developer

Fixer

Wash

Dryer

Film exit

Figure 4–29. Reproduced with permission from Saia DA. *Radiography: Program Review and Examination Preparation,* 2nd ed. Stamford, CT: Appleton & Lange, 1999.

it is difficult to obtain a satisfactory image of the mediastinum and lungs simultaneously without the use of a compensating filter to "even out" the densities. With this device, the chest is radiographed using mediastinal factors, and a trough-shaped filter (thicker laterally) is used to absorb excess photons that would overexpose the lungs. The middle portion of the filter lets the photons pass to the mediastinum almost unimpeded. Filters that absorb the photons contributing to skin dose are inherent and added filters. Compensating filtration is unrelated to elimination of scattered radiation or fluoroscopy. (Selman, p 254)

96. **(D)** The *radiographic subject*, the patient, is composed of many different tissue types that have varying densities, resulting in varying degrees of photon attenuation and absorption. The *atomic number* of the tissues under investigation is directly related to their *attenuation coefficient*. This *differential absorption* contributes to the various shades of gray (scale of radiographic contrast) on the finished radiograph. Normal tissue density may be significantly altered in the presence of *pathologic processes*. For example, destructive bone disease can cause a dramatic decrease in tissue density (and subsequent increase in radiographic density). Abnormal accumulation of fluid (as in ascites) will cause a significant increase in tissue density. *Muscle* atrophy or highly developed muscles will similarly decrease or increase tissue density. (Saia, p 364)

97. (B) *Osteoporosis* is a condition, often seen in the elderly, marked by increased porosity and softening of bone. The bones are much less dense, and thus a decrease in exposure is required. *Osteomyelitis* and *osteochondritis* are inflammatory conditions that usually have no effect on bone density. *Osteosclerosis* is abnormal hardening of the bone, and an increase in exposure factors would be required. (Carlton & Adler, p 258)

98. **(B)** Film that is unexposed and has been processed will not be completely clear. The blue-tinted base contributes a small measure of density. A small but measurable amount of exposure from background radiation can also be present, and processing itself produces a small

amount of density from chemical fog. Together, this is expressed as base-plus fog and should never exceed a density of 0.2. (Fauber, p 198)

99. **(A)** Aligning the x-ray tube, anatomic part, and image recorder so that they are parallel reduces *shape distortion*. Angulation of the long axis of the part with respect to the IR results in *foreshortening* of the object. Tube angulation causes *elongation* of the part. Size distortion (magnification) is inversely proportional to SID and directly proportional to OID. Decreasing the SID and increasing the OID serve to increase size distortion. (Shephard, pp 232–233)

100. **(A)** If a lateral projection of the chest is being performed on an asthenic patient and the outer photocells are incorrectly selected, the outcome is likely to be an underexposed radiograph. The patient is thin, and the lateral cells have no tissue superimposed on them. Therefore, as soon as the lateral photocells detect radiation (which will be immediately), the exposure will be terminated, giving the lateral chest insufficient exposure. (Shephard, pp 280–281)

101. **(D)** The mAs is the exposure factor that regulates radiographic density. The equation used to determine mAs is mA × s = mAs. Substituting the known factors,

$$300x = 60$$
$$x = 0.2 \ (1/5) \ \text{second}$$

(Fauber, p 55)

102. **(A)** Scattered radiation is produced as x-ray photons travel through matter, interact with atoms, and are scattered (change direction). If these scattered rays are energetic enough to exit the body, they will strike the IR from all different angles. They therefore do not carry useful information and merely produce a flat, gray (low-contrast) fog over the image. Grid cutoff *increases* contrast and is caused by an improper relationship between the x-ray tube and the grid, resulting in absorption of some of the useful/primary beam. (Saia, p 322)

103. **(C)** Control of motion, both voluntary and involuntary, is an important part of radiography.

Patients are unable to control certain types of motion, such as heart action, peristalsis, and muscle spasm. In these circumstances, it is essential to use the shortest possible exposure time in order to have a "stop action" effect. *(Carlton & Adler, p 410)*

104. **(B)** If fluorescent light from one intensifying screen passes through the film to the opposite emulsion and intensifying screen, the associated diffusion creates a type of distortion called *crossover*. Intensifying screens do need a degree of *reflectance* to enhance their speed. *Scatter* and *filtration* are unrelated to intensifying screens. *(Selman, p 185)*

105. **(C)** *Size* distortion (magnification) is inversely proportional to SID and directly proportional to OID. Increasing the SID and decreasing the OID decreases size distortion. Aligning the tube, part, and IR so that they are parallel reduces *shape* distortion. There are two types of shape distortion, *elongation* and *foreshortening*. Angulation of the part with relation to the IR results in foreshortening of the object. Tube angulation causes elongation of the object. *(Shephard, pp 228, 231–234)*

106. **(C)** X-ray tube targets are constructed according to the *line focus principle*—the focal spot is angled (usually 12° to 17°) to the vertical (Fig. 4–30). As the actual focal spot is projected downward, it is foreshortened; thus, the effective focal spot is always smaller than the actual focal spot. As it is projected toward the *cathode* end of the x-ray beam, the effective focal spot becomes *larger* and approaches the actual size. As it is projected toward the anode end, it gets smaller because of the anode "heel" effect. *(Selman, p 139)*

107. **(B)** Quantum *noise,* or mottle, is a grainy appearance on a finished radiograph that is seen especially in fast-imaging systems. It is very similar in appearance to a photograph taken with fast film and enlarged; it has a spotted or freckled appearance. Fast film and screens with low mAs and high kVp factors are most likely to be the cause of quantum noise/mottle. *Overdevelopment* makes a radiograph appear very dark, and sometimes gray. *Scattered radiation fog* gives the radiograph a flat, gray appearance. *Grid cutoff* is absorption of the primary beam by the grid and usually results

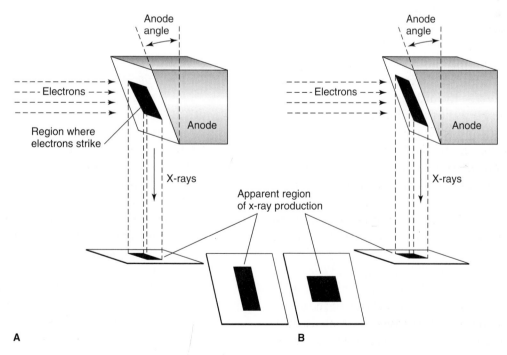

Figure 4–30. Reproduced with permission from Saia DA. *Radiography: Program Review and Examination Preparation,* 2nd ed. Stamford, CT: Appleton & Lange, 1999.

in loss of density and visibility of grid lines. (*Selman, p 211*)

108.   **(C)** The film processor is automated, and replenishment quantities are preset. A microswitch is activated as a film enters the processor at the entrance rollers. Replenisher is added according to the length of the x-ray film—for as long as the detector senses the presence of film. Once the back end of the film passes the entrance roller sensor, replenishment stops. When films are fed into the processor the "long way," too much replenishment occurs, and the image can exhibit excessive density. (*Shephard, p 146*)

109.   **(C)** An exposed radiographic film contains an invisible (latent) image. Only through processing can this image be converted to a permanent, visible (manifest) image. As the film exits the developer section, it passes through the crossover assembly, and before it enters the fixer section, it passes through the squeegee assembly. The squeegee assembly rollers function to remove excess developer solution from the emulsion before the film enters the fixer. This process helps maintain fixer strength/activity. The rate of travel through the processor is determined by the transport mechanism, that is, the speed of the rollers as established at time of manufacture. (*Shephard, p 143*)

110.   **(C)** Because the anode's focal track is beveled (angled, facing the cathode), x-ray photons can freely diverge toward the cathode end of the x-ray tube. However, the "heel" of the focal track prevents x-ray photons from diverging toward the anode end of the tube. This results in varying intensity from anode to cathode, with fewer photons at the anode end and more photons at the cathode end. *The anode heel effect is most noticeable when using large IR sizes, short SIDs, and steep target angles.* (*Saia, p 298*)

111.   **(D)** Insufficient milliamperage and/or exposure time will result in lack of radiographic density. Insufficient kVp will result in underpenetration and excessive contrast. Insufficient SID, however, will result in increased exposure rate and radiographic *overexposure*. (*Selman, pp 214–215*)

112.   **(D)** *Sensitometry* is a method of quality control for daily monitoring of the automatic film processor. A *densitometer* is a device used to read optical density. Crossover rollers should be *cleaned daily* to prevent the buildup of crystallized solution on the rollers. A *warm-up* procedure is performed on an x-ray tube for safe operation after prolonged disuse. (*Selman, pp 292–293*)

113.   **(C)** The original mAs was 20 (400 mA × 0.05 s). Using the *density maintenance formula*, the new mAs must be determined for the distance change from 40 to 36 inches of SID:

$$\frac{\text{(old mAs) } 20}{\text{(new mAs) } x} = \frac{\text{(old } D^2) \, 40^2}{\text{(new } D^2) \, 36^2}$$

$$1600x = 25{,}920$$
$$x = 16.2 \text{ mAs at 36 inches SID}$$

A 15% increase in kilovoltage was made, increasing the kilovoltage to 87. Because the kilovoltage change effectively doubles the radiographic density, the mAs must be cut in half (from 16.2 to 8.1) to compensate. Then, if 500 is the new milliamperage, we must determine what exposure time is required to achieve 8.1 mAs:

$$500x = 8.1$$
$$x = 0.016 \text{ second at 87 kVp and } 36 \text{ inches SID}$$

(*Selman, pp 214–215*)

114.   **(C)** If the imaging system speed is cut in half (from 400 to 200 speed), the result will be half of the original density on the radiograph. Therefore, to maintain the original density, the mAs must be doubled from the original 20 to 40 mAs. Grids are used to absorb scattered radiation from the remnant beam before it can contribute to the latent image. Because the grid removes scattered (and some primary) radiation from the beam, an increase in exposure factors is required. The amount of increase is dependent on the grid ratio: The higher the grid ratio, the higher the correction factor. The correction factor for an 8:1 grid is 4; therefore, the mAs (40) is multiplied by 4 to arrive at the new required mAs (160). Using

the mAs equation mA $\times$ s = mAs, it is determined that 0.4 second will be required at 400 mA:

$$400x = 160$$
$$x = 0.4 \text{ second}$$

(Fauber, pp 62, 148)

115. **(B)** The sensitometric, or characteristic, *curve* is used to illustrate the relationship between the exposure, given the film and the resulting film density. It can be used to predict a particular film *emulsion's* response (speed, sensitivity) by determining how long it takes to record a particular density. The sensitometric curve is used in *sensitometry* to monitor automatic processing efficiency and consistency. A film is given a series of predetermined exposures and processed. The resulting densities are plotted, and the resulting curve is compared with a known correct curve. Any deviation between the two may indicate processing difficulties. The sensitrometric curve illustrates the effects of exposure and processing on radiographic film emulsion; it is unrelated to film speed. *(Shephard, pp 104–108)*

116. **(A)** When the variable-kVp method is used, a particular mAs is assigned to each body part. As part thickness increases, the kVp (penetration) is also increased. The body part being radiographed must be carefully measured, and *for each centimeter of increase in thickness, 2 kVp is added* to the exposure. *(Shephard, pp 299–300)*

117. **(B)** DXA imaging is used to evaluate bone mineral density (BMD). Bone densitometry, DXA, can be used to *evaluate bone mineral content of the body, or part of it*, to *diagnosis osteoporosis* or to *evaluate the effectiveness of treatments for osteoporosis*. It is the most widely used method of *bone densitometry*—it is *low dose, preceise*, and *uncomplicated* to use/perform. DXA uses *two photon energies*—one for soft tissue and one for bone. Since bone is more dense and attenuates x-ray photons more readily, their *attenuation is calculated* to represent the degree of bone density. Soft tissue attenuation information is not used to measure bone density. *(Ballinger & Frank, vol 3, pp 488–489)*

118. **(D)** Factors that regulate the number of x-ray photons produced at the target can be used to control radiographic density, namely milliamperage and exposure time (mAs). Radiographic density is directly proportional to mAs; if the mAs is cut in half, the radiographic density will decrease by one half. Although kilovoltage is used primarily to regulate radiographic contrast, it may also be used to regulate radiographic density in variable—kVp techniques, according to the 15% rule. *(Selman, pp 213–214)*

119. **(B)** The illustrated radiograph demonstrates a 1.5-inch unexposed strip along the length of the film. This occurred because, although the patient was centered correctly to the collimator light and x-ray field, the x-ray tube was not centered to the grid. If the patient was off-center, the entire image would be exposed and the patient's spine would be off-center. Grid cutoff would not appear as such a sharply delineated line, but rather as a gradually decreasing density. *(Fauber, p 125)*

120. **(B)** If the safelight bulb is of a higher wattage than it should be, the safelight filter is incorrect for the film type, or the filter is cracked, film fog can occur. If film is not stored in a radiation-safe area, it can be fogged by background radiation. Screen lag is not caused by improper film storage conditions, but rather by aged or defective intensifying screens. *(Selman, pp 190–191)*

121. **(D)** The purpose of the thin layer of lead that is often located behind the rear intensifying screen in a cassette is to absorb x-rays that penetrate the screens, strike the rear of the cassette, and bounce back toward the film emulsion, resulting in scattered radiation fog. The thin layer of lead absorbs these x-ray photons and thus improves the radiographic image. *(Shephard, pp 41–42)*

122. **(B)** As films are developed, the developer solution becomes weaker and oxidation products are produced in the solution. If sufficient replenishment of new developer solution does not take place, the activity of the older solution decreases, and chemical fog is produced.

Films lack contrast and have a flat, gray appearance. *(Shephard, p 153)*

123. **(B)** Quantum mottle is a grainy appearance on a finished radiograph that is seen especially in fast-imaging systems. It is very similar in appearance to an enlarged photograph taken with fast film; it has a spotted or freckled appearance. *Fast imaging systems (fast film and fast screens, as well as CR/DR systems)* with *low mAs and high kVp factors* are most likely to be the cause of quantum mottle. *(Bushong, p 273)*

124. **(D)** *The shortest possible exposure time should be used to minimize motion unsharpness.* Motion causes unsharpness that destroys detail. Careful and accurate patient *instruction* is essential for minimizing voluntary motion. *Suspended respiration* eliminates respiratory motion. Using the shortest possible *exposure time* is essential for decreasing involuntary motion. Immobilization is also very useful in eliminating motion unsharpness. *(Carlton & Adler, p 410)*

125. **(D)** One of the biggest advantages of *CR* is the *dynamic range*, or *latitude*, it offers. The characteristic curve of x-ray film emulsion has a certain "range of correct exposure," limited by the toe and shoulder of the curve. In CR, there is a *linear relationship* between the exposure, given the PSP (*p*hotostimulable *p*hosphor, or *i*mage *p*late) and its resulting luminescence, as it is scanned by the laser. This affords much greater exposure latitude and technical inaccuracies can be effectively eliminated. Overexposure of up to 500% and underexposure of up to 80% are reported as recoverable, thus eliminating most retakes. This surely affords increased efficiency; *however, this does not mean that images can be exposed arbitrarily.* The radiographer must keep dose reduction in mind. The same exposure factors as screen–film systems, or less, are generally recommended for CR.

Intensifying screens used in screen–film x-ray imaging tend to produce high contrast. The faster the screens, the higher the contrast; higher contrast is often associated with decreased latitude. AEC refers to automatic exposure control and is unrelated to dynamic range or latitude. *(Ballinger & Frank, vol 3, p 234; Shepharnd, pp 336–338)*

126. **(A)** Soft tissue radiography requires the use of long-wavelength, low-energy x-ray photons. Very little filtration is used in mammography. Certainly, anything more than 1.0 mm of aluminum would remove the useful soft photons, and the desired high contrast could not be achieved. Dedicated mammographic units usually have molybdenum targets (for the production of soft radiation) and a small amount of molybdenum filtration. *(Carlton & Adler, p 581)*

127. **(C)** Quality control in mammography includes scrupulous testing of virtually all component parts of the mammographic imaging system. It includes processor checks, screen maintenance, accurate and consistent viewing conditions, and evaluation of phantom images, to name a few. The device pictured is the structures to be imaged within a mammography phantom. A mammographic phantom contains Mylar fibers, simulated masses, and specks of simulated calcifications. The American College of Radiology accreditation criteria state that a minimum of 10 objects (4 fibers, 3 specks, and 3 masses) must be visualized on test images. Changes in any part(s) of the imaging system (film, screens, image receptors, x-ray equipment, filtration, or viewbox) can result in unsuccessful results. *(Bushong, p 350)*

128. **(A)** The *characteristic (sensitometric) curve* is used to show the *relationship between the exposure given the film and the resulting film density.* It can therefore be used to evaluate a particular film emulsion's response (speed, sensitivity) by determining how long it takes to record a particular density. A *dose–response curve* is used in radiation protection and illustrates the quantity of dose required to produce a particular effect. The *reciprocity law* states that a particular mAs, regardless of the combination of milliamperage and time, should produce the same degree of blackening. The *inverse square law* illustrates the relationship between distance and radiation intensity. *(Fauber, pp 202–203)*

129. **(B)** A wire mesh supported between two rigid pieces of clear plastic is used to evaluate screen–film contact. The mesh is placed on an

image receptor and radiographed. Upon viewing, any areas that appear unsharp or blurry are indicative of poor screen–film contact. A screen lag test is performed by radiographing a phantom using an empty cassette–image receptor, then loading it with film and leaving for it a few minutes. If, after processing, there is any indication of an image, there is most probably screen lag. *(Shephard, p 54)*

130. **(A)** To calculate mAs, multiply milliamperage times exposure time. In this case, 300 mA × 0.017 s = 5.10 mAs. Careful attention to proper decimal placement will help avoid basic math errors. *(Shephard, p 170)*

131. **(C)** Externally, CR (computed radiography) cassettes appear very much like traditional film–screen cassettes. However, the main function of a CR cassette is to support and protect the IP that lies within the CR cassettes. CR cassettes do not contain intensifying screens or film and therefore do not need to be light tight. The photostimulable IP is not affected by light. *(Shephard, p 51)*

132. **(B)** Radiographic technique charts are highly recommended for use with every x-ray unit. A technique chart identifies the standardized factors that should be used with that particular x-ray unit, for various examinations/positions, of anatomic parts of different sizes. To be used effectively, these technique charts require that the anatomic part in question be measured correctly with a *caliper*.

A *fulcrum* is of importance in tomography; a *densitometer* is used in sensitometry and QA. *(Ballinger & Frank, vol 3, p 237)*

133. **(D)** As screen speed is increased, exposure factors must be decreased to maintain the original image density. A change from 100 to 200 speed usually requires that the mAs be reduced by one half. If screen speed were changed from 400 to 200 speed, twice the mAs would be required. *(Shephard, pp 67–68)*

134. **(B)** Rare earth phosphors have a greater *conversion efficiency* than do other phosphors. Lanthanum oxybromide is a blue-emitting

rare earth phosphor, and gadolinium oxysulfide is a green-emitting rare earth phosphor. Cesium iodide is the phosphor used on the input screen of image intensifiers; it is not a rare earth phosphor. *(Shephard, p 68)*

135. **(B)** The heel effect is characterized by a variation in beam intensity, which *gradually increases from anode to cathode*. This can be effectively put to use when performing radiographic examinations on large body parts with uneven tissue density. For example, the AP thoracic spine is thicker caudally than cranially, and so the thicker portion is best placed under the cathode. However, in the lateral projection of the thoracic spine, the upper portion is thicker because of superimposed shoulders, and therefore that portion is best placed under the cathode end of the beam. The femur is also uneven in density, particularly in the AP position, and can benefit from use of the heel effect. However, the sternum and its surrounding anatomy are fairly uniform in thickness and would not benefit from use of the anode heel effect. *The anode heel effect is most pronounced when using large-size IRs, at short SIDs, and with an anode having a steep (small) target angle. (Saia, p 298)*

136. **(D)** Because *pneumoperitoneum* is an abnormal accumulation of *air or gas* in the peritoneal cavity, it would require a *decrease* in exposure factors. *Obstructed bowel* usually involves distended, air- or gas-filled bowel loops, again requiring a *decrease* in exposure factors. With *ascites*, there is an abnormal accumulation of *fluid* in the abdominal cavity, necessitating an *increase* in exposure factors. *Renal colic* is the pain associated with the passage of renal calculi; no change from the normal exposure factors is usually required. *(Carlton & Adler, p 258)*

137. **(D)** The lead strips in a parallel grid are *parallel to one another*, and therefore are *not parallel to the x-ray beam*. The more divergent the x-ray beam, the more likely there is to be cutoff/decreased density at the lateral edges of the radiograph. This problem becomes more pronounced at short SIDs. If there was a centering or tube angle problem, there would be more likely to be a

noticeable density loss on one side *or* the other. *(Saia, p 324)*

138. **(B)** Locate density 1.5 on the vertical axis. Follow it across to where it intersects with image 1, then to where it intersects with image 2. At each intersection, follow the vertical line down and note the corresponding log relative exposure. Image 1 requires an exposure of about 1.6 to record a density of 1.5, while image 2 requires an exposure of about 1.8 to record the same density. Image 2 is the slower film and requires more exposure to record a density of 1.5. The faster film always occupies the position farthest to the left in a comparison of two or more films. *(Selman, p 221; Shephard, p 105)*

139. **(B)** Radiographic density is described as the *overall degree of blackening of a radiograph or a part of it.* The mAs regulates the number of x-ray photons produced at the target, and thus regulates radiographic density. If it is desired to double the radiographic density, one simply doubles the mAs; therefore, mAs and radiographic density are directly proportional. *(Selman, p 214)*

140. **(B)** As the distance from the object to the IR (OID) increases, so does magnification distortion thereby decreasing recorded detail. Some magnification is inevitable in radiography, as it is not possible to place anatomic structures directly on the image recorder. However, our understanding of how to minimize magnification distortion is an important part of our everyday work. *(Fauber, pp 90–91)*

141. **(A)** A *compensating filter* is used when the part to be radiographed is of uneven thickness or density (in the chest, mediastinum vs lungs). The filter (made of aluminum or lead acrylic) is constructed in such a way that it will absorb much of the primary radiation that would expose the low-tissue density area, while allowing the primary radiation to pass unaffected to the high-tissue density area. A *collimator* is used to decrease the production of scattered radiation by limiting the volume of tissue irradiated. The *grid* functions to trap scattered radiation before it reaches the IR, thus reducing scattered radiation fog. *(Selman, pp 254–255)*

142. **(D)** The advantages of automatic processors are quick, efficient operation and consistent results. Quick operation is attained with increased solution temperatures. The usual temperature of a 90-second processor is 90° to 95°. Excessively high developer temperature can cause chemical fog. *(Selman, p 200)*

143. **(A)** An increase in kilovoltage increases the overall average energy of the x-ray photons produced at the target, thus giving them greater penetrability. (This can increase the incidence of Compton interaction and therefore the production of scattered radiation.) Greater penetration of all tissues serves to lengthen the scale of contrast. However, excessive scattered radiation reaching the IR will cause a fog and carries no useful information. *(Selman, pp 127–128)*

144. **(C)** The FOV and matrix size are independent of one another, that is, either can be changed and the other will remain unaffected. However, *pixel size is affected by changes in either the FOV or matrix size.* For example, if the matrix size is increased, pixel size decreases. If FOV increases, pixel size increases. Pixel size is inversely related to resolution. As pixel size decreases, resolution increases. *(Fosbinder & Kelsey, p 285).*

145. **(A)** SID is *directly* related to recorded detail because as SID increases, so does recorded detail (because magnification is decreased). OID is *inversely* related to recorded detail because as OID increases, recorded detail decreases. As screen speed increases, recorded detail decreases, as a result of greater diffusion of light. Therefore, of the given choices, only SID is *directly* related to recorded detail. OID and screen speed are *inversely* related to recorded detail. *(Shephard, pp 221–224)*

146. **(A)** The single most important factor regulating radiographic contrast is kVp. The lower the kVp, the shorter the scale of contrast. All the mAs values in this problem have been adjusted for kVp changes to maintain density, but just a glance at each of the kilovoltages is often a good indicator of which will produce the longest scale or shortest scale contrast. *(Shephard, pp 306, 308)*

147. **(D)** *Grid ratio* is defined as *the ratio of the height of the lead strips to the width of the interspace material;* the higher the lead strips, the more scattered radiation they will trap and the greater the grid's efficiency. The greater the *number of lead strips per inch,* the thinner and less visible they will be on the finished radiograph. The function of a grid is to absorb scattered radiation in order to improve radiographic contrast. The *selectivity* of a grid is determined by the amount of primary radiation *transmitted* through the grid divided by the amount of scattered radiation *transmitted* through the grid. *(Selman, pp 236–237)*

148. **(A)** To test a film's response to processing, the film must first be given a predetermined exposure with a *sensitometer.* The film is then processed, and the densities are read using a *densitometer.* Any significant variation from the expected densities is further investigated. A *step wedge* is used to evaluate the effect of kVp on contrast, and a *spinning top* test is used to check timer accuracy. *(Shephard, pp 99–100)*

149. **(D)** The crescent-shaped *kink, or crinkle, marks* seen on the radiographic image are caused by acutely bending the x-ray film. The artifact will usually appear as a *plus-density* (dark) artifact if it is produced *before* exposure, and as a *minus-density* (light) artifact if it is produced *after* exposure. X-ray film emulsion is very sensitive to mishandling, particularly after exposure. *(Saia, pp 378, 406)*

150. **(B)** Many cassettes/image receptors have a thin lead foil layer behind the rear screen to absorb backscattered radiation that is energetic enough to exit the rear screen, strike the metal back, and bounce back to fog the image. When this happens, the image receptor's metal hinges or straps may be imaged in high-kVp radiography. The lead foil absorbs the backscatter before it can fog the film. *(Shephard, pp 41–42)*

151. **(B)** *Emphysema* is abnormal distention of the alveoli (or tissue spaces) with air. The presence of abnormal amounts of air makes it necessary to *decrease* from normal exposure factors. *Congestive heart failure* and *pleural effu-*sion involve abnormal amounts of fluid in the chest and thus require an *increase* in exposure factors. *(Carlton & Adler, p 258)*

152. **(D)** *Focusing distance* is the term used to specify the optimal SID used with a particular focused grid. It is usually expressed as *focal range,* indicating the minimum and maximum SID workable with that grid. Lesser or greater distances can result in grid cutoff. Although proper distance is important in computed tomography, chest, and magnification radiography, focusing distance is unrelated to them. *(Selman, pp 239–240)*

153. **(B)** The steepness of the characteristic curve is representative of image contrast. The steeper the curve, the greater the density *differences* and the *higher* the contrast. The speed of the film is determined by the curve's position on the log relative scale: When comparing two or more characteristic curves, the *faster* film lies farthest to the left. The faster the film speed, the less the exposure latitude. *(Shephard, p 105)*

154. **(A)** Grids are used in radiography to trap scattered radiation that would otherwise cause fog on the radiograph. *Grid ratio* is defined as the ratio of the height of the lead strips to the distance between them. *Grid frequency* refers to the number of lead strips per inch. *Focusing distance* and *grid radius* are terms denoting the distance range with which a focused grid may be used. *(Selman, p 236)*

155. **(B)** *The shortest possible exposure should be used as a matter of routine.* Parkinson's disease is characterized by uncontrollable tremors, and the resulting unsharpness can destroy image detail. It is therefore necessary to use as fast an imaging system as possible. High-speed (rare earth) intensifying screens will permit a considerable reduction in mAs (specifically, exposure time). Compensating filtration is unrelated to the problem and is not indicated here. *(Fauber, p 188)*

156. **(B)** Grid ratio compares the height of the lead strip to the distance between the lead strips. Focused grids have their lead strips angled so as to parallel the divergent x-ray beam. The

higher the grid ratio, the greater the grid's efficiency in absorbing scattered radiation before it reaches the image receptor—but the *more critical* the centering and distance specifications. Although higher ratio focused grids absorb more SR they have a narrower focal range (focusing distance) and grid/tube centering becomes much more critical. Focused grids must not be accidentally inverted—to do so would cause the lead strips to be placed exactly in the path of the lead strips (grid cutoff), everywhere but in the center of the grid. (*Ballinger & Frank, vol 3, p 235*)

157. **(D)** Every film emulsion has a characteristic curve representative of that film's speed, contrast, and latitude. A gentle curve (as opposed to a steep curve) usually indicates a film with slow speed, low contrast, and more latitude. (*Shephard, p 105*)

158. **(C)** The radiograph is an illustration of poor screen–film contact. Motion and scattered radiation fog can be ruled out because the blurriness is seen only in the apical region. Screen–film contact is evaluated using a wire mesh that is placed on the questionable image receptor and radiographed (see Fig. 4–31). Any areas of unsharpness represent poor contact, which can result from warped screens, a foreign body in the image receptor, or a damaged image receptor frame. (*Selman, pp 183–186*)

159. **(C)** There are two types of distortion: size and shape. *Shape distortion* relates to the alignment of the x-ray tube, the part to be radiographed, and the image recorder. There are two kinds of shape distortion: *elongation* and *foreshortening*. *Size distortion* is *magnification*, and it is related to the OID and the SID. Magnification can be reduced by either increasing the SID or decreasing the OID. However, an increase in SID must be accompanied by an increase in mAs to maintain density. It is therefore preferable, in the interest of exposure, to reduce OID whenever possible. (*Fauber, p 90*)

160. **(D)** Perfect contact between the intensifying screens and the film is essential to maintain image sharpness. Any separation between them allows diffusion of fluorescent light and

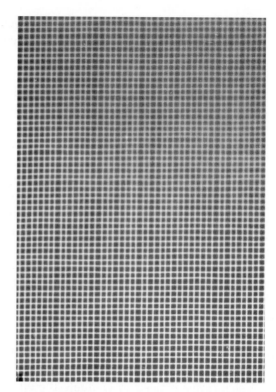

Figure 4–31. From the American College of Radiology Learning File. Courtesy of the ACR.

subsequent blurriness and loss of detail. Screen–film contact can be diminished if the image receptor frame is damaged and misshapen, if the front is warped, or if there is a foreign body between the screens, elevating them. (*Selman, p 185*)

161. **(D)** High-kilovoltage factors are frequently used to even out densities in anatomic parts with high tissue contrast (eg, the chest). However, as high kilovoltage produces added scattered radiation, it generally must be used with a grid. It would be inappropriate to perform an AP abdomen with high kilovoltage because it has such low subject contrast. Barium-filled structures are frequently radiographed using 120 kV or more to penetrate the barium—to see through to structures behind. (*Carlton & Adler, p 468*)

162. **(D)** Every film emulsion has a particular base-plus fog, which should not exceed 0.2. This base density is a result of the *manufacturing* process (environmental radiation) and the *blue tint* added to the base to reduce glare. The remaining fog density is a result of the *chemical*

development process, when exposed silver bromide grains are converted to black metallic silver. *(Carlton & Adler, p 318)*

163. **(B)** The original mAs (regulating radiographic density) was 200. The original kVp (regulating radiographic contrast) was 90. The mAs was cut in half, to 100, causing a decrease in density. The kVp was increased (by 15%) to *compensate for the density loss* and thereby *increase the scale of contrast*. *(Shephard, p 203)*

164. **(C)** Increased photon energy is caused by an increase in kVp, resulting in more penetration of the part and a *longer* scale of contrast. Increasing the grid ratio will result in a larger percentage of scattered radiation being absorbed and hence a *shorter* scale of contrast. *(Shephard, pp 203–204)*

165. **(C)** If the fixer fails to harden the gelatin emulsion sufficiently, water will remain within the still-swollen emulsion. The dryer mechanism will be unable to completely rid the emulsion of wash water, and the film will emerge from the processor damp and tacky. On the other hand, excessive hardening action may produce brittle radiographs. High air velocity usually encourages more complete drying. Unbalanced processing temperatures can result in blistering of the emulsion. Developer underreplenishment results in "light" images and can be the cause of transport problems as a result of insufficient hardener. *(Carlton & Adler, p 303)*

166. **(B)** The term *latitude* may refer to either *film emulsion latitude* or *exposure latitude*. Exposure latitude refers to the margin of error inherent in a particular group of exposure factors. Selection of high-kVp and low-mAs factors will allow greater exposure latitude than low-kVp and high-mAs factors. Film emulsion latitude is chemically built into the film emulsion and refers to the emulsion's ability to record a long range of densities from black to white (long-scale contrast). *(Bushong, p 185)*

167. **(C)** The *wider* dimension of the x-ray film is usually placed on the feed tray so that the film is fed into the processor in that direction. The *entrance roller* is the first roller of the transport system, located at the end of the feed tray; this is where the microswitch that determines the amount of replenishment is located. The *length* of the film (the shorter dimension) activates the microswitch, and replenisher is added according to the length of the film; a 10 × 12-inch film will receive less replenisher than will a 14 × 17-inch film. Crossover rollers are located between the different tanks. The receiving bin is where the films exit the processor. The replenishment pump is activated by the microswitch. *(Bushong, pp 212–213)*

168. **(D)** The illustrated shoulder radiograph looks dark and overexposed. On careful examination, especially of the clavicle and upper ribs areas, it is seen to be double-exposed. Two clavicles are seen separately, and there seems to be an abundance of superimposed first to third ribs. Two exposures were inadvertently made on different phases of respiration; thus, there is an overexposed double exposure. A high-contrast film would have more light/underexposed areas; chemical fog usually produces a very gray image; light fog generally results in a very black finished radiograph. *(Bushong, pp 373–374)*

169. **(D)** *Differential absorption* refers to the x-ray absorption characteristics of neighboring anatomic structures. The radiographic representation of these structures is referred to as *radiographic contrast*; it may be enhanced with high-contrast technical factors, especially using low kilovoltage levels. At low kilovoltage levels, the photoelectric effect predominates. *(Bushong, pp 181–184)*

170. **(B)** According to the inverse square law of radiation, as the distance between the radiation source and the IR decreases, the exposure rate increases. Therefore, a decrease in technical factors is indicated. The *density maintenance formula* is used to determine new mAs values when changing distance:

$$\frac{(\text{old mAs}) \ 18}{(\text{new mAs}) \ x} = \frac{(\text{old } D^2) \ 42^2}{(\text{new } D^2) \ 38^2}$$

$$\frac{18}{x} = \frac{1764}{1444}$$

$$1764x = 25{,}992$$

$$x = 14.7 \text{ mAs at 38 inches SID}$$

Then, to determine the new exposure time (mA × s = mAs),

$$300x = 14.7$$
$$x = 0.049 \text{ second at } 300 \text{ mA}$$

(Selman, p 214)

171. (B) If A and B are reduced to 5 mAs for mAs consistency, the kVp will increase to 85 kVp in both cases, thereby balancing radiographic densities. Thus, the greatest density is determined by the shortest SID (greatest exposure rate). *(Shephard, pp 306–307)*

172. (A) Only two pieces of apparatus are needed to construct a sensitometric curve (Fig. 4–32). First, a *penetrometer* (aluminum step wedge) is used to expose a film. Once the film is processed, a *densitometer* is needed to read the resulting densities. Log relative exposure is charted along the *x* (horizontal) axis; an increase in log relative exposure of 0.3 results from doubling the exposure. Optical density is plotted on the *y* (vertical) axis and represents the amount of light transmitted through a film compared to the amount of light striking the film (expressed as a logarithm). *(Bushong, p 274)*

173. (B) As the film emulsion is exposed to light or x-rays, latent image formation takes place. The exposed silver halide crystals are *reduced* to black metallic silver in the developer solution. Automatic processor developer agents are *hydroquinone* and *phenidone*. The preservative—sodium sulfite—helps prevent oxidation. The *activator* provides the necessary alkalinity for the developer solution, and *hardener* is added to the developer in automatic processing to keep emulsion swelling to a minimum. *(Fauber, p 164)*

174. (D) *X-rays produced at the target make up a heterogeneous primary beam.* There are many "soft," low-energy photons that, if not removed, would contribute only to greater patient (skin) dose. They do not have enough energy to penetrate the patient and expose the film; they just penetrate a small thickness of the patient's tissue and are absorbed. These photons are removed by aluminum filters. *(Fauber, pp 32–33)*

175. (C) Radiographers are usually able to stop voluntary motion, using suspended respiration, careful instruction, and immobilization. However, *involuntary* motion must also be considered. To have a "stop action" effect on the heart when radiographing the chest, it is essential to use a short exposure time. *(Fauber, pp 87–88)*

176. (C) Diagnostic x-ray photons interact with tissue in a number of ways, but mostly they are involved in the production of *Compton scatter* or in the *photoelectric effect*. *Compton scatter* is pictured; it occurs when a relatively *high-energy* (kV) photon uses *some* of its energy to eject an *outer*-shell electron. In doing so, the photon is deviated in direction and becomes a scattered photon. Compton scatter causes objectionable scattered radiation fog in large structures such as the abdomen and poses a radiation hazard to personnel during procedures such as fluoroscopy. In the *photoelectric effect*, a relatively *low*-energy x-ray photon uses *all* its energy to eject an *inner*-shell electron, leaving a "hole" in the K shell. An L-shell electron then drops down to fill the K vacancy, and in so doing emits a characteristic ray whose energy is equal to the difference between the binding energies of the K and L

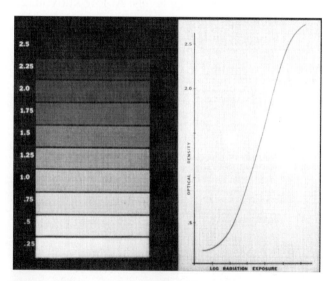

Figure 4–32. From the American College of Radiology Learning File. Courtesy of the ACR.

shells. The photoelectric effect occurs with *high-atomic-number* absorbers such as bone and positive contrast media, and is responsible for the production of radiographic contrast. It is helpful for the production of the radiographic image, but it contributes to the dose received by the patient (because it involves complete absorption of the incident photon). *(Saia, p 224)*

177. **(D)** The archival quality of a film refers to its ability to retain its image for a long period of time. Many states have laws governing how long a patient's medical records, including films, must be retained. Very importantly, they must be retained in their original condition. *Archival quality is poor if radiographic films begin to show evidence of stain after being stored for only a short time.* Probably the most common cause of stain, and hence of poor archival quality, is *retained fixer* within the emulsion. Fixer may be retained as a result of poor washing or because there was insufficient hardener *(underreplenishment)* in the developer, thus permitting fixer to be retained by the swollen emulsion. A test for quantity of retained fixer in film emulsion is often included as part of a quality control program. Stain may also be caused by poor *storage conditions.* Storage in a hot, humid place will cause even the smallest amount of retained fixer to react with silver, causing stain. *(Shephard, pp 110, 135, 137)*

178. **(B)** A review of the problem reveals that three changes are being made: an increase in SID, a change from a 400-speed system to a 200-speed system, and a change in exposure time (to be considered last). Because the original mAs was 9, cutting the speed of the system in half (from 400 to 200) will require a doubling of the mAs, to 18 mAs, in order to maintain density. Now we must deal with the distance change. Using the density maintenance formula (and remembering that 18 is now the *old* mAs), we find that the required new mAs at 42 inches is 22.

$$\frac{(\text{old mAs}) \, 18}{(\text{new mAs}) \, x} = \frac{(\text{Old } D^2) \, 38^2}{(\text{new } D^2) \, 42^2}$$

$$1444x = 31{,}752$$
$$x = 21.9 \text{ mAs at 42 inches SID}$$

Because we are not changing mA, we must determine the exposure time that, when used with 300 mA, will yield 22 mAs.

$$300 \, x = 22$$
$$x = 0.07\text{-second exposure}$$

(Selman, p 124)

179. **(D)** *High-kilovoltage* exposures produce large amounts of *scattered radiation*, and therefore high-ratio grids are used in an effort to trap more of this scattered radiation. However, *accurate centering and positioning* become more critical to *avoid grid cutoff. (Selman, p 243)*

180. **(B)** The *quantity* of x-ray photons produced at the target is the function of mAs. The *quality* (wavelength, penetration, energy) of x-ray photons produced at the target is the function of kVp. The kVp also has an effect on exposure rate, because an increase in kVp will increase the number of high-energy x-ray photons produced at the target. Exposure rate *decreases* with an increase in SID. *(Selman, p 117)*

181. **(A)** More scattered radiation is generated within a part as the kilovoltage is increased, the size of the field is increased, and the thickness and density of tissue increases. As the quantity of scattered radiation increases from any of these sources, more density is added to the radiographic image. *(Carlton & Adler, p 375)*

182. **(D)** *Luminescence* is the production of energy in the form of light. Two types of luminescence are fluorescence and phosphorescence. *Fluorescence* occurs when an intensifying (radiographic) screen absorbs x-ray photon energy, emits light, and ceases to emit light as soon as the energizing source ceases. Fluoroscopic screens continue to emit light for a short time after the exposure has terminated. This characteristic (phosphorescence) is a desirable quality in fluoroscopic screens. *Lag* occurs when an intensifying (radiographic) screen continues to fluoresce after the x-ray stimulation has terminated. This characteristic is undesirable and causes excessive density. Screen speed is identified by the amount of light emitted by the phosphors. *(Carlton & Adler, p 330)*

183. (D) The chest is composed of tissues with widely differing densities (bone and air). In an effort to "even out" these tissue densities and better visualize pulmonary vascular markings, high kilovoltage is generally used. This produces more uniform penetration and results in a *longer scale of contrast,* with visualization of the pulmonary vascular markings as well as bone (which is better penetrated) and air densities. The increased kilovoltage also affords the advantage of greater exposure latitude (an error of a few kV will make little if any difference). The fact that the kilovoltage is increased means that the mAs is accordingly reduced, and thus patient *dose is reduced* as well. A grid is usually used whenever high kilovoltage is required. (*Carlton & Adler, p 471*)

184. (C) The slower the screen speed, the smaller the quantity of fluorescent light emitted during x-ray exposure. Therefore, slow-speed screens *require more x-ray exposure* to provide adequate radiographic density and cannot be used when exposure reduction or fast exposure time is essential. However, because they are associated with less diffusion of fluorescent light, they *produce better recorded detail* and are used to image structures requiring excellent recorded detail. Pediatric radiography is likely to require fast screens to reduce exposure time and dose. (*Shephard, p 67*)

185. (C) Film base functions to support the silver halide emulsion. Today's film base is made of tough, nonflammable *polyester. Cellulose nitrate* was used in the past, but it was highly flammable. *Cellulose acetate,* also used in the past, was not flammable, but it was not as durable as polyester. The earliest supports for emulsion were plates of glass (hence the term *flat plate*). (*Selman, p 194*)

186. (D) *Collimators* restrict the size of the irradiated field, thereby limiting the volume of irradiated tissue, and hence less scattered radiation is produced. Once radiation has scattered and emerged from the body, it can be trapped by the grid's lead strips. *Grids* effectively remove much of the scattered radiation in the remnant beam before it reaches the x-ray IR. *Compression* can be applied to reduce the effect of

excessive fatty tissue (eg, in the abdomen), in effect reducing the thickness of the part to be radiographed. (*Selman, pp 234, 247, 289*)

187. (A) The scatterer between the target and the image recorder is the patient. After the radiation has scattered once, it has been significantly attenuated. The intensity of scattered radiation 1 m from the patient is approximately 0.1% of the intensity of the primary beam. (*Bushong, p 552*)

188. (A) DXA imaging is used to evaluate BMD (bone mass density). It is the most widely used method of *bone densitometry*—it is *low dose, preceise,* and *uncomplicated* to use/perform. DXA uses *two photon energies*—one for soft tissue and one for bone. Since bone is more dense and attenuates x-ray photons more readily, their *attenuation is calculated* to represent the degree of bone density. Soft tissue attenuation information is not used to measure bone density. Any images obtained in DXA/bone densitometry are strictly to evaluate the *accuracy of the ROI* (region of interest); they are not used for further diagnostic purposes—additional diagnostic examinations are done for any required further evaluation. Bone densitometry, DXA, can be used to evaluate bone mineral content of the body, or part of it, to diagnosis osteoporosis or to evaluate the effectiveness of treatments for osteoporosis. (*Ballinger & Frank, vol 3, pp 488–489*)

189. (D) Each of the three is included in a good QA program. *Beam alignment* must be accurate to within 2% of the SID. *Reproducibility* means that repeated exposures at a given technique must provide consistent intensity. *Linearity* means that a given mAs, using different mA stations with appropriate exposure time adjustments, will provide consistent intensity. (*Bushong, p 460*)

190. (A) If a radiograph lacks sufficient blackening, an increase in mAs is required. The mAs regulates the *number* of x-ray photons produced at the target. An increase or decrease in mAs of *at least 30%* is necessary to produce a perceptible effect. Increasing the kVp by 15%

will have about the same effect as *doubling* the mAs. (*Shephard, p 173*)

191. **(D)** Exposure rate is regulated by milliamperage. Distance significantly affects the exposure rate, according to the inverse square law of radiation. Kilovoltage also has an effect on exposure rate, because an increase in kVp will increase the number of high-energy photons produced at the target. The size of the x-ray field determines the volume of tissue irradiated, and hence the amount of scattered radiation generated, but is unrelated to the exposure rate. (*Selman, p 117*)

192. **(D)** *Static electricity* is a problem, especially in cool, dry weather. *Sliding* the film in and out of the cassette–image receptor can be the cause of a static electrical discharge. Removing one's sweater in the darkroom on a dry winter day can cause static electrical sparking. The film exposed by a large static discharge ("tree static") frequently exhibits black, branching artifacts such as those illustrated. *Poor screen–film contact* results in very blurry areas of the finished radiograph. A *foreign body* in the image receptor will be sharply imaged on the finished radiograph. An *inverted focused grid* will result in an area of exposure down the middle of the image and grid cutoff everywhere else. (*Saia, p 407*)

193. **(A)** Beam restrictors function to limit the size of the irradiated field. In doing so, they limit the volume of tissue irradiated (thereby decreasing the percentage of scattered radiation generated in the part) and help reduce patient dose. Beam restrictors do not affect the quality (energy) of the x-ray beam—that is the function of kVp and filtration. Beam restrictors do not absorb scattered radiation—that is a function of grids. (*Shephard, p 27*)

194. **(C)** The answer to this question conforms to the general rule that when two or more characteristic curves are being compared, the fastest film emulsion is the one furthest to the left. The one difference is that there are intersecting characteristic curves here. Simply see which curve is farther to the left *above the intersection* (number 1) and which is farther to the left *below the intersection* (number 2). As you can see, film 1 has more sensitivity (speed) above the point of intersection. (*Selman, p 221; Shephard, p 105*)

195. **(A)** Artifacts can be a result of *exposure, handling and storage,* or *processing.* Exposure artifacts include *motion,* double exposure, poor screen–film contact—the effects of these are seen as a result of the exposure. Handling and storage artifacts include *static* electricity discharge, crinkle marks, scratches, and light or radiation fog—these all occur as a result of improper usage or storage. Processing artifacts occur while the film is in the automatic processor and include *pi lines,* guide shoe marks, and chemical fog. (*Bushong, p 473*)

196. **(B)** If the exposure time is cut in half, one would normally double the milliamperage to maintain the same mAs and, consequently, the same radiographic density. However, increasing the kVp by 15% has a similar effect. For example, if the original kVp was 85, 15% of that is 13, and therefore the new kVp would be 98. The same percentage value would be used to cut the radiographic density in half (reduce kVp by 15%). (*Shephard, pp 178–181*)

197. **(D)** In the RAO position, the sternum must be visualized through the thorax and heart. Prominent pulmonary vascular markings can hinder good visualization. A method frequently used to overcome this problem is to use an mAs with a long exposure time. The patient is permitted to breathe normally during the (extended) exposure and, by doing so, blurs out the prominent vascularities. (*Ballinger & Frank, vol 1, p 474*)

198. **(C)** According to the density maintenance formula, if the SID is changed to 48 inches, 14.4 mAs is required tso maintain the original radiographic density.

$$\frac{(\text{old mAs}) \, 10}{(\text{new mAs}) \, x} = \frac{(\text{old } D^2) \, 40^2}{(\text{new } D^2) \, 48^2}$$

$$\frac{10}{x} = \frac{1600}{2304}$$

$$1600x = 23{,}040$$

$$x = 14.4 \text{ mAs at 48 inches SID}$$

Then, to compensate for changing from a 12:1 grid to an 8:1 grid, the mAs becomes 11.5:

$$\frac{\text{(old mAs) }14.4}{\text{(new mAs) }x} = \frac{\text{(old grid factor) }5}{\text{(new grid factor) }4}$$

$$5x = 57.6$$
$$x = 11.5 \text{ mAs with 8:1 grid at}$$
$$48 \text{ inches SID}$$

Thus, 11.5 mAs is required to produce a image density similar to that of the original radiograph.

The following are the factors used for mAs conversion from nongrid to grid:

No grid = 1 × the original mAs
5:1 grid = 2 × the original mAs
6:1 grid = 3 × the original mAs
8:1 grid = 4 × the original mAs
12:1 grid = 5 × the original mAs
16:1 grid = 6 × the original mAs

(Selman, pp 214, 243)

199. **(B)** Guide shoes are found at crossover and turnaround assemblies and function to direct the film around corners as it changes direction. If a guide shoe becomes misaligned, it will scratch the emulsion and leave the characteristic *guide shoe marks* running in the direction of film travel, as seen in the pictured radiograph. *Pi lines* appear as plus-density lines running perpendicular to the direction of film travel; they are sometimes seen in new processors or after a complete maintenance/overhaul. *Hesitation marks* are plus-density lines occurring as a result of pauses, or hesitations, in a faulty roller transport system. *(Shephard, pp 154, 156)*

200. **(B)** *Radiographic contrast* is defined as the degree of *difference between adjacent densities*. These density differences represent sometimes very subtle differences in the absorbing properties of adjacent body tissues. The type of *film emulsion* used also brings with it its own contrast characteristics. Different types of film emulsions have different degrees of contrast "built into" them chemically. The technical factor used to regulate contrast is kilovoltage. Radiographic contrast is unrelated to mAs. *(Selman, pp 218–220)*

201. **(D)** Attenuation (decreased intensity through scattering or absorption) of the x-ray beam is a result of its *original energy and its interactions with different types and thicknesses of tissue*. The greater the original energy/quality (the higher the kilovoltage) of the incident beam, the less the attenuation. The greater the effective *atomic number* of the tissues (tissue type determines absorbing properties), the greater the beam attenuation. The greater the *volume of tissue* (subject density and thickness), the greater the beam attenuation. *(Bushong, p 185)*

202. **(C)** Intensifying screens react to the presence of x-ray photons and change their energy to visible fluorescent light energy, which serves to expose the adjacent film emulsion. If an intensifying screen becomes stained, either partly or wholly, the stained area will not react to x-ray photons as completely and will emit less light. Therefore, the film emulsion adjacent to the stained area(s) will exhibit decreased density on the finished radiograph. *(Shephard, p 75)*

203. **(C)** The diffusion of fluorescent light from intensifying screens is responsible for a loss of recorded detail on double-emulsion film. Therefore, by changing the system to include only one intensifying screen and single-emulsion film, as in mammographic systems, light diffusion is reduced and better recorded detail results. Patient dose is somewhat greater than with a two-screen cassette system, but the advantage of significantly improved recorded detail greatly offsets this. *(Shephard, p 49)*

204. **(B)** X-ray film emulsion is sensitive and requires proper handling and storage. It should be stored in a cool (40° to 60°F), dry (40% to 60% humidity) place. Exposure to excessive temperatures or humidity can lead to film fog and loss of contrast. Static marks are a result of low humidity. *(Fauber, p 182)*

205. **(D)** The faster the imaging system, the greater the sacrifice of image clarity (recorded detail). As *intensifying-screen speed* increases, recorded detail decreases. Perfect *screen-film contact* is essential for good detail. Any areas of poor contact result in considerable blurriness in the

radiographic image. *Focal spot* blur is related to focal spot size; smaller focal spots produce less blur and thus better recorded detail. *(Selman, pp 206–210)*

206. **(C)** Film emulsion consists of *silver halide crystals suspended in gelatin.* Sodium sulfite is a film-processing preservative, and potassium bromide is a developer restrainer. Potassium and chrome alum are emulsion hardeners used in fixer solution. *(Selman, p 174)*

207. **(C)** Recorded detail is evaluated by how sharply tiny anatomic details are imaged on the radiograph. The area of blurriness that may be associated with small image details is termed *geometric blur.* The blurriness can be produced by using a large focal spot, or by diffused fluorescent light from intensifying screens. The image proper (ie, without blur) is termed the *umbra. Mottle* is a grainy appearance caused by fast imaging systems. *(Selman, pp 206–207)*

208. **(B)** A fractional focal spot of 0.3 mm or smaller is essential for reproducing fine detail without focal spot blurring in *magnification* radiography. As the object image is magnified, so will be any associated blur unless a fractional focal spot is used. Use of the fractional focal spot on a routine basis is unnecessary; it is not advised because it causes unnecessary wear on the x-ray tube and offers little radiographic advantage. *(Shephard, p 217)*

209. **(D)** The lateral skull radiograph pictured illustrates the result of great care taken by the radiographer to secure patient comfort. A skull examination was requested for this patient of advanced years. The radiographer positioned the patient, taking care to position and collimate accurately, all the while trying to ensure the patient's comfort by letting her keep her pillow! The foam stuffing of the pillow is nicely imaged. Although the artifacts somewhat resemble Paget's disease or osteoporosis, note that they extend outside the collimated field. Safelight fog would be shown as a more uniform "blanket" of fog. *(Saia, p 408)*

210. **(B)** Because lead content increases when grid ratio increases, a greater amount of scattered

radiation is trapped before reaching the IR. Fewer grays are therefore recorded, and a shorter scale of contrast results. *Radiographic density* would *decrease* with an increase in grid ratio. Grid ratio is unrelated to distortion. *(Carlton & Adler, p 396)*

211. **(B)** X-ray film emulsion becomes more sensitive to safelight fog *following exposure* to fluorescent light from intensifying screens. Care must be taken not to leave exposed film on the darkroom workbench for any length of time, as its sensitivity to safelight fog is now greatly heightened. *(Saia, p 405)*

212. **(B)** The distance between transport rollers in an automatic processor is extremely critical and allows for exact film thickness with minimum emulsion swelling. If the emulsion is allowed to swell excessively (as a result of excessive temperature or inadequate replenishment), the emulsion will stick to the rollers and cause a processor jam-up. *Glutaraldehyde is a hardener that is added to the developer to keep the emulsion swelling to a minimum.* Unexposed silver halide crystals are removed in the fixer solution. *(Shephard, p 135)*

213. **(D)** As OID is increased, recorded detail is diminished as a result of magnification distortion. If the OID cannot be minimized, an increase in SID is required to reduce the effect of magnification distortion. However, the relationship between OID and SID is not an equal relationship. In fact, to compensate for every 1 inch of OID, an increase of 7 inches of SID is required. Therefore, an OID of 6 inches requires an SID increase of 42 inches. That is why, a chest radiograph with a 6-inches air gap is usually performed at a 10-foot SID. *(Saia, p 290)*

214. **(D)** *Grid ratio* is defined as the ratio between the height of the lead strips and the width of the distance between them (ie, their height divided by the distance between them). If the height of the lead strips is 4.0 mm and the lead strips are 0.25 mm apart, the grid ratio must be 16:1 (4.0 divided by 0.25). The thickness of the lead strip is unrelated to grid ratio. *(Selman, p 236)*

215. **(D)** If developer *temperature* is too high, some of the less-exposed or unexposed silver halide crystals may be reduced, thus creating chemical fog. If the developer solution has become *oxidized* from exposure to air, chemical fog also results. If developer *replenishment* is excessive, too much new solution is replacing the deteriorated developer, and chemical fog is again the result. *(Carlton & Adler, p 296; Selman, p 197)*

216. **(C)** Radiographic density is greatly affected by changes in the *SID*, as expressed by the inverse square law of radiation. As distance from the radiation source increases, exposure rate decreases and radiographic density decreases. Exposure rate is inversely proportional to the square of the SID. *Aluminum filtration, kilovoltage,* and *scattered radiation* all have a significant effect on density, but they are not the primary controlling factors. *(Selman, p 214)*

217. **(D)** Shape distortion is caused by *misalignment of the x-ray tube, the part to be radiographed, and the image recorder/film.* An object can be falsely imaged (*foreshortened* or *elongated*) by incorrect placement of the tube, the body part, or the image recorder. Only one of the three need be misaligned for distortion to occur. *(Saia, p 293)*

218. **(C)** The radiograph illustrated in Figure 4–24 demonstrates adequate positioning, inspiration, and beam restriction. However, it has *too much background density* (too much mAs), *excessively high contrast* (too low kVp, too short a scale of contrast), and areas of *inadequate penetration.* This radiograph should be repeated at a lower mAs and appropriately higher kVp. *(Carlton & Adler, pp 367–369)*

219. **(D)** *Radiographic contrast is the sum of film emulsion contrast and subject contrast.* Subject contrast has by far the greatest influence on radiographic contrast. Several factors influence subject contrast, each as a result of beam attenuation differences in the irradiated tissues. As patient *thickness* and tissue *density* increase, attenuation increases and subject contrast is increased. As *kilovoltage* increases, higher energy photons are produced, beam attenuation is decreased, and subject contrast decreases. *(Carlton & Adler, pp 387–389)*

220. **(A)** If the SID is above or below the recommended focusing distance, the primary beam will not coincide with the angled lead strips at the lateral edges. Consequently, there will be absorption of the primary beam, termed grid cutoff. If the grid failed to move during the exposure, there would be grid lines throughout. Central ray angulation in the direction of the lead strips is appropriate and will not cause grid cutoff. If the central ray was off-center, there would be uniform loss of density. *(Carlton & Adler, p 274)*

221. **(B)** Review the groups of factors. First, because mAs has no effect on the scale of contrast produced, eliminate mAs from consideration by drawing a line through the column. Then, check the two entries in each column that are most likely to produce long-scale contrast. For example, in the kVp column, because higher kVp will produce longer-scale contrast, place check marks next to each 90 kVp. In the film–screen column, the slower screens (200) will produce lower (longer scale) contrast than the faster screens; place a check mark next to each. Because lower ratio grids permit a larger quantity of scattered radiation to reach the IR, the 5:1 and 8:1 grids will produce a longer scale of contrast than the higher ratio grids; check them. As the volume of irradiated tissue increases, so does the amount of scattered radiation produced and, consequently, the longer the scale of radiographic contrast; therefore, check the 14 × 17-inch field sizes. An overview shows that the factors in groups A and C have two check marks, whereas the factors in group B have four check marks, indicating that group B will produce the longest scale contrast. *(Shephard, pp 306–308)*

222. **(C)** Positive-contrast medium is *radiopaque*; negative-contrast material is *radioparent*. Barium sulfate (radiopaque, positive-contrast material) is most frequently used for examinations of the intestinal tract, and high-kVp exposure factors are used to penetrate (to see through and behind) the barium. Water-based iodinated

contrast media (Conray, Amipaque) are also positive-contrast agents. However, the K-edge binding energy of iodine prohibits the use of much greater than 70 kVp with these materials. Higher kVp values will obviate the effect of the contrast agent. Air is an example of a negative-contrast agent, and high-kVp factors are clearly not indicated. (*Shephard, pp 200–201*)

223. **(A)** Proper use of focal spot size is of paramount importance in magnification radiography. A magnified image that is diagnostic can be obtained only by using a *fractional focal spot of 0.3 mm or smaller*. The amount of blur or geometric unsharpness produced by focal spots that are larger in size render the radiograph undiagnostic. (*Selman, p 226*)

224. **(B)** The abdomen is a thick structure that contains many structures of similar density, and thus it requires increased exposure and a grid to absorb scattered radiation. The lumbar spine and hip are also dense structures requiring increased exposure and use of a grid. The knee, however, is frequently small enough to be radiographed without a grid. The general rule is that structures measuring more than 10 cm should be radiographed with a grid. (*Saia, p 322*)

225. **(A)** Grids are composed of alternate strips of lead and interspace material and are used to trap scattered radiation after it emerges from the patient and before it reaches the IR. Accurate centering of the x-ray tube is required. If the x-ray tube is off-center, but within the recommended focusing distance, there will usually be an overall loss of density. Over- or underexposure under the anode is usually the result of exceeding the focusing distance limits in addition to being off-center. (*Carlton & Adler, p 273*)

226. **(D)** As *photon energy* increases, more penetration and greater production of scattered radiation occur, producing a longer scale of contrast. As *grid ratio* increases, more scattered radiation is absorbed, producing a shorter scale of contrast. As OID increases, the distance between the part and the IR acts as a grid, and consequently less scattered radiation reaches the IR, producing a shorter scale

of contrast. Focal spot size is related only to recorded detail. (*Shephard, p 203*)

227. **(C)** First, evaluate the change(s): The kVp was decreased by about 15% [95–15% = 80.7]. A 15% decrease in kVp will cut the radiographic density in half; therefore, it is necessary to use *twice* the original mAs to maintain the original density. The original mAs was 21, and so we now need 42 mAs, using the 500-mA station. Because mA × s = mAs,

$$500x = 42$$
$$x = 0.084 \text{ second}$$

(*Fauber, pp 55, 59–60*)

228. **(D)** As the kilovoltage is decreased, x-ray beam energy (ie, penetration) is also decreased. Consequently, a *shorter scale of contrast* is obtained and, at lower kilovoltage levels, there is less *exposure latitude* (less margin for error in exposure). As kilovoltage is reduced, the mAs must be increased accordingly to maintain adequate density. This increase in mAs results in greater *patient dose*. (*Shephard, p 204*)

229. **(C)** *Image A* was made using 80 kVp at 75 mAs; *Image B* was made using 100 kVp at 18 mAs; all other exposure factors remained the same. As kVp is increased, the percentage of scattered radiation relative to primary radiation increases, hence the grayer appearance of image B. Use of optimal kilovoltage for each anatomic part is helpful in keeping scatter to a minimum. The production of scattered radiation will also be limited if the field size is as small as possible. A grid is the most effective way to remove scattered photons from those exiting the patient. Grids are designed to selectively absorb scattered radiation while absorbing as little of the primary radiation as possible. Images produced with higher ratio grids will possess fewer grays than those made with lower ratio grids. (*Saia, p 362*)

230. **(D)** Geometric unsharpness is affected by all three factors listed. As *OID* increases, so does magnification. OID is *directly* related to magnification. As *focal-object distance* and *SID* decrease, magnification increases. Focal-object distance and SID are *inversely* related to magnification. (*Carlton & Adler, pp 403–405*)

231. **(C)** *Kilovoltage* and the *HVL* affect both the quantity and the quality of the primary beam. The principal qualitative factor for the primary beam is kVp, but an increase in kVp will also create an increase in the *number* of photons produced at the target. *HVL* is defined as the amount of material necessary to decrease the intensity of the beam to one half of its original value, thereby effecting a change in both beam quality and quantity. The mAs value is adjusted to regulate the number of x-ray photons produced at the target. X-ray beam quality is unaffected by changes in mAs. *(Carlton & Adler, p 181)*

232. **(D)** A quality assurance program includes regular overseeing of all components of the imaging system: equipment calibration, film and cassettes, processor, x-ray equipment, and so on. With regular maintenance, testing, and repairs, equipment should operate efficiently and consistently. In turn, radiographic quality will be consistent and repeat exposures will be minimized, thereby reducing patient exposure. *(Carlton & Adler, pp 439–440)*

233. **(D)** The darkroom must be constructed in such a way as to be free from any white-light leaks. The film bin should be secure and should have a sign warning against opening in white light. Safelight bulbs must be of the correct wattage, and the filter should be appropriate for the type of film used. *(Fauber, p 183)*

234. **(C)** Every box of film comes with the *expiration date* noted. Film used after its expiration date will usually suffer a *loss of speed and contrast* and will exhibit fog. Film should be ordered in quantities that will ensure that it is used before it becomes outdated, and it should be rotated in storage so that the oldest is used first. *(Fauber, p 182)*

235. **(A)** The screen-film system and radiographic density are directly proportional; that is, if the system speed is doubled, the radiographic density is doubled. In this case, we started at 40 mAs with a 50-speed system. If the system speed is doubled to 100, we should decrease the mAs to 20. If the speed is again doubled to 200, we use half of the 20 mAs, or 10 mAs. Or,

mAs conversion factors and the following formula may be used:

$$\frac{\text{screen speed factor 1}}{\text{screen speed factor 2}} = \frac{\text{mAs 1}}{\text{mAs 2}}$$

$$\frac{2}{0.5} = \frac{40}{x}$$

$$2x = 20$$
$$x = 10 \text{ mAs with 200}$$
$$\text{screen-film system.}$$

(Saia, p 327)

236. **(B)** According to the *15% rule*, if the kVp is increased by 15%, radiographic density will be doubled. Therefore, to compensate for this change and to maintain radiographic density, the mAs should be reduced to 6 mAs. *(Saia, p 320)*

237. **(C)** *Motion*, voluntary or involuntary, is most detrimental to good recorded detail. Even if all other detail factors are adjusted to maximize detail, if motion occurs during exposure, detail is lost. The most important ways to reduce the possibility of motion are using the shortest possible exposure time, careful patient instruction (for suspended respiration), and adequate immobilization when necessary. Minimizing magnification through the use of *increased* SID and *decreased* OID functions to improve recorded detail. *(Carlton & Adler, p 403)*

238. **(D)** Compression of the breast tissue during mammographic imaging improves the technical quality of the image for several reasons. Compression brings breast structures into *closer contact* with the image recorder, thus reducing geometric blur and improving detail. As the breast tissue is compressed and essentially becomes thinner, less *scattered radiation* is produced. Compression serves as excellent *immobilization* as well. *(Peart, p 49)*

239. **(D)** Distortion is caused by *improper alignment of the tube, body part, and image recorder.* Anatomic structures within the body are rarely parallel to the IR in a simple recumbent position. In an attempt to overcome this distortion, we position the part to be parallel with the IR, or angle the central ray to "open up" the part. Examples of this technique are obliquing the pelvis to place the ilium parallel to the IR, or angling the central ray cephalad to "open up" the sigmoid colon. (*Shephard, pp 228–234*)

240. **(A)** Limiting the *size of the irradiated field* is a most effective method of decreasing the production of scattered radiation. The smaller the *volume of tissue* irradiated, the smaller the amount of scattered radiation generated; this can be accomplished using *compression* (prone position instead of supine or a compression band). Use of a grid does not affect the *production* of scattered radiation, but rather *removes it* once it has been produced. (*Saia, p 322*)

241. **(B)** *Rare earth* phosphors have a much higher conversion efficiency (and therefore speed) and have all but replaced the older calcium tungstate screens. The *larger* the phosphor and the *thicker the layer* of phosphors (active layer), the greater the light emission and therefore the speed. *Antihalation* backing is a component of single-emulsion film that prevents crossover of fluorescent light within an image receptor. (*Selman, pp 180–183*)

242. **(B)** The formula for mAs is mA × s = mAs. Substituting known values,

$$0.05x = 30$$
$$x = 600 \text{ mA}$$

(*Selman, p 214*)

243. **(C)** The rate of chemical replenishment in automatic processing is based on the *amount (length) of film processed*. Typically, a 14 × 17 film will require 60–70 mL of developer replenisher and 100–110 mL of fixer replenisher. Processor transport speed is constant. Solution temperature and agitation are unrelated to replenishment. (*Bushong, p 210; Shephard, p 146*)

244. **(C)** As kVp is reduced, the number of high-energy photons produced at the target is reduced; therefore, a decrease in radiographic density occurs. If a grid has been used improperly (off-centered or out of focal range), the lead strips will absorb excessive amounts of primary radiation, resulting in grid cutoff

and loss of radiographic density. If the SID is inadequate (too short), an *increase* in radiographic density will occur. (*Selman, pp 214, 240–242*)

245. **(C)** Radiographic density is directly proportional to mAs. If exposure time is *halved* from 0.04 (1/25) to 0.02 (1/50) second, radiographic density will be cut in half. Changing to 150 mA will also halve the mAs, effectively halving the radiographic density. If the kVp is decreased by 15%, from 85 to 72 kVp, radiographic density will be halved according to the *15% rule*. To cut the density in half, the mAs must be reduced to 6 (rather than 10). (*Selman, pp 213–214*)

246. **(B)** Magnification radiography is used to enlarge details to make them more perceptible. Hairline fractures, minute blood vessels, and microcalcifications are candidates for magnification radiography. The problem of magnification unsharpness is overcome by using a *fractional focal spot*; larger focal spot sizes will produce excessive blurring unsharpness. Grids are usually unnecessary in magnification radiography because of the air-gap effect produced by the OID. A direct-exposure technique would not be likely to be used because of the excessive exposure required. (*Selman, pp 226–228*)

247. **(C)** About half the silver in a film emulsion remains to form the image. The other half is removed from the film during the fixing process. Therefore, fixer solution has a high silver content. Silver is a *toxic metal* and cannot simply be disposed of into the public sewer system. As silver is also a precious metal, it becomes financially wise to recycle the silver removed from x-ray film. The three most commonly used silver recovery systems are the *electrolytic, metallic replacement,* and *chemical precipitation methods*. In *electrolytic* units, an electric current is passed through the fixer solution. Silver ions are attracted to, and become plated onto, the negative electrode of the unit. The plated silver is periodically scraped from the cathode and accurately measured so that the hospital can be appropriately reimbursed. The electrolytic method is a practical recovery system for moderate- and

high-use processors. The *metallic replacement* (or displacement) method of silver recovery uses a steel mesh/steel wool type of cartridge that traps silver as fixer is run through it. This system is useful for low-volume processors and is often also used as a backup to the electrolytic unit. *Chemical precipitation* adds chemicals that release electrons into the fixer solution. This causes the metallic silver to precipitate out, fall to the bottom of the tank, and form a recoverable sludge. This method is used principally by commercial silver dealers. *(Carlton & Adler, pp 308–310)*

248.   **(A)** A 15-min oblique image of an IVU is pictured. IV urography requires the use of iodinated contrast media. *Low kilovoltage* (about 70) is usually employed to enhance the photoelectric effect and, in turn, better visualize the renal collecting system. *High kilovoltage* will produce excessive scattered radiation and obviate the effect of the contrast agent. A higher milliamperage with a shorter exposure time is preferred to decrease the possibility of motion. *(Saia, p 347)*

249.   **(B)** As the kilovoltage is increased, a *greater number* of electrons are driven across to the anode with *greater force*. Therefore, as energy conversion takes place at the anode, *more high-energy* (short-wavelength) photons are produced. However, because they are higher energy photons, there will be less patient absorption. *(Selman, pp 117–118)*

250.   **(B)** The artifact seen in the figure has *sharply delineated edges*, indicating that it is located adjacent to the intensifying screens within the cassette. The *farther* the object is from the image receptor, the more *blurred* its edges will be as a result of magnification distortion. *(Saia, p 378)*

Subspecialty List

67. Image processing and quality assurance
68. Image processing and quality assurance
69. Selection of technical factors
70. Selection of technical factors
71. Selection of technical factors
72. Selection of technical factors
73. Selection of technical factors
74. Selection of technical factors
75. Selection of technical factors
76. Selection of technical factors
77. Selection of technical factors
78. Selection of technical factors
79. Selection of technical factors
80. Selection of technical factors
81. Selection of technical factors
82. Selection of technical factors
83. Selection of technical factors
84. Selection of technical factors
85. Selection of technical factors
86. Selection of technical factors
87. Selection of technical factors
88. Criteria for image evaluation
89. Selection of technical factors
90. Selection of technical factors
91. Image processing and quality assurance
92. Image processing and quality assurance
93. Selection of technical factors
94. Selection of technical factors
95. Selection of technical factors
96. Selection of technical factors
97. Selection of technical factors
98. Image processing and quality assurance
99. Selection of technical factors
100. Criteria for image evaluation
101. Selection of technical factors
102. Selection of technical factors
103. Selection of technical factors
104. Selection of technical factors
105. Selection of technical factors
106. Selection of technical factors
107. Criteria for image evaluation
108. Image processing and quality assurance
109. Image processing and quality assurance
110. Selection of technical factors
111. Selection of technical factors
112. Image processing and quality assurance
113. Selection of technical factors
114. Selection of technical factors
115. Image processing and quality assurance
116. Selection of technical factors
117. Computed/digital imaging
118. Selection of technical factors
119. Criteria for image evaluation
120. Image processing and quality assurance
121. Image processing and quality assurance
122. Image processing and quality assurance
123. Selection of technical factors
124. Selection of technical factors
125. Computed/digital imaging
126. Image processing and quality assurance
127. Image processing and quality assurance
128. Image processing and quality assurance
129. Image processing and quality assurance
130. Selection of technical factors
131. Computed/digital imaging
132. Selection of technical factors
133. Selection of technical factors
134. Selection of technical factors
135. Selection of technical factors
136. Selection of technical factors
137. Evaluation of radiographs
138. Image processing and quality assurance
139. Selection of technical factors
140. Selection of technical factors
141. Selection of technical factors
142. Selection of technical factors
143. Selection of technical factors
144. Computed/digital imaging
145. Selection of technical factors
146. Selection of technical factors
147. Selection of technical factors
148. Image processing and quality assurance
149. Criteria for image evaluation
150. Selection of technical factors
151. Selection of technical factors
152. Selection of technical factors
153. Image processing and quality assurance
154. Selection of technical factors
155. Selection of technical factors
156. Selection of technical factors
157. Image processing and quality assurance
158. Criteria for image evaluation
159. Selection of technical factors
160. Image processing and quality assurance
161. Selection of technical factors
162. Image processing and quality assurance
163. Criteria for image evaluation
164. Selection of technical factors
165. Image processing and quality assurance
166. Image processing and quality assurance
167. Image processing and quality assurance
168. Criteria for image evaluation

169. Selection of technical factors
170. Selection of technical factors
171. Selection of technical factors
172. Image processing and quality assurance
173. Image processing and quality assurance
174. Selection of technical factors
175. Selection of technical factors
176. Selection of technical factors
177. Image processing and quality assurance
178. Criteria for image evaluation
179. Selection of technical factors
180. Selection of technical factors
181. Selection of technical factors
182. Selection of technical factors
183. Selection of technical factors
184. Selection of technical factors
185. Image processing and quality assurance
186. Selection of technical factors
187. Selection of technical factors
188. Computed/digital imaging
189. Image processing and quality assurance
190. Selection of technical factors
191. Selection of technical factors
192. Criteria for image evaluation
193. Selection of technical factors
194. Selection of technical factors
195. Selection of technical factors
196. Selection of technical factors
197. Selection of technical factors
198. Selection of technical factors
199. Criteria for image evaluation
200. Selection of technical factors
201. Selection of technical factors
202. Criteria for image evaluation
203. Selection of technical factors
204. Image processing and quality assurance
205. Selection of technical factors
206. Image processing and quality assurance
207. Selection of technical factors
208. Selection of technical factors
209. Criteria for image evaluation
210. Selection of technical factors
211. Image processing and quality assurance
212. Image processing and quality assurance
213. Selection of technical factors
214. Selection of technical factors
215. Image processing and quality assurance
216. Selection of technical factors
217. Selection of technical factors
218. Criteria for image evaluation
219. Selection of technical factors
220. Criteria for image evaluation
221. Selection of technical factors
222. Selection of technical factors
223. Selection of technical factors
224. Selection of technical factors
225. Criteria for image evaluation
226. Selection of technical factors
227. Selection of technical factors
228. Selection of technical factors
229. Criteria for image evaluation
230. Selection of technical factors
231. Selection of technical factors
232. Image processing and quality assurance
233. Image processing and quality assurance
234. Image processing and quality assurance
235. Selection of technical factors
236. Selection of technical factors
237. Selection of technical factors
238. Selection of technical factors
239. Selection of technical factors
240. Selection of technical factors
241. Selection of technical factors
242. Selection of technical factors
243. Image processing and quality assurance
244. Criteria for image evaluation
245. Selection of technical factors
246. Selection of technical factors
247. Image processing and quality assurance
248. Criteria for image evaluation
249. Selection of technical factors
250. Criteria for image evaluation

CHAPTER 5

Equipment Operation and Maintenance
Questions

DIRECTIONS (Questions 1 through 120): Each of the numbered items or incomplete statements in this section is followed by answers or by completions of the statement. Select the *one* lettered answer or completion that is *best* in each case.

1. Moving the image intensifier closer to the patient during fluoroscopy

   1. decreases the source-image distance (SID).
   2. decreases patient dose.
   3. improves image quality.

   (A) 1 only
   (B) 1 and 2 only
   (C) 1 and 3 only
   (D) 1, 2, and 3

2. How is the thickness of the tomographic section related to the tomographic angle?

   (A) The greater the tomographic angle, the thicker the section.
   (B) The greater the tomographic angle, the thinner the section.
   (C) The less the tomographic angle, the thinner the section.
   (D) The tomographic angle is unrelated to section thickness.

3. Typical examples of digital imaging include

   1. magnetic resonance imaging (MRI).
   2. computed tomography (CT).
   3. pluridirectional tomography.

   (A) 1 only
   (B) 1 and 2 only
   (C) 1 and 3 only
   (D) 1, 2, and 3

4. The batteries in battery-operated mobile x-ray units provide power to

   1. the x-ray tube.
   2. machine locomotion.
   3. the braking mechanism.

   (A) 1 only
   (B) 2 only
   (C) 1 and 2 only
   (D) 1, 2, and 3

5. Radiographs from a particular three-phase, full-wave-rectified x-ray unit, made using known correct exposures, were underexposed. A synchronous spinning top test was performed using 200 mA, 1/12 second, and 70 kVp, and a 20° arc is observed on the test film. Which of the following is *most* likely the problem?

   (A) The 1/12-second time station is inaccurate.
   (B) The 200-mA station is inaccurate.
   (C) A rectifier is not functioning.
   (D) The processor needs servicing.

6. If exposure factors of 85 kVp, 400 mA, and 0.12 second yield an output exposure of 150 mR, what is the mR/mAs?

   (A) 0.32
   (B) 3.1
   (C) 17.6
   (D) 31

7. Which of the following will occur as a result of a decrease in the anode target angle?

1. Less pronounced anode heel effect
2. Decreased effective focal spot size
3. Greater photon intensity toward the cathode side of the x-ray tube

(A) 1 only
(B) 1 and 2 only
(C) 2 and 3 only
(D) 1, 2, and 3

8. Which of the waveforms illustrated in Figure 5–1 represents single-phase, full-wave rectified equipment?

(A) Figure 1
(B) Figure 2
(C) Figure 3
(D) Figure 4

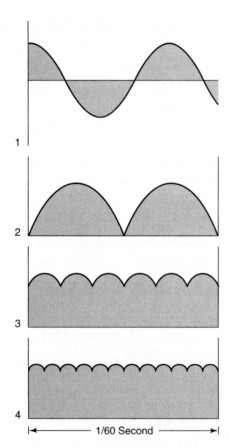

Figure 5–1. Reproduced with permission from Saia DA. *Radiography: Program Review and Examination Preparation*, 2nd ed. Stamford, CT: Appleton & Lange, 1999.

9. Components of digital imaging include

1. computer manipulation of the image.
2. formation of an electronic image on the radiation detector.
3. formation of an x-ray image directly on the image receptor.

(A) 1 only
(B) 1 and 2 only
(C) 2 and 3 only
(D) 1, 2, and 3

10. The minimum response time of an automatic exposure control (AEC)

(A) is the time required to energize the intensifying phosphors.
(B) is its shortest possible exposure time.
(C) functions to protect the patient from overexposure.
(D) functions to protect the tube from excessive heat.

11. The source of electrons within the x-ray tube is

(A) electrolysis.
(B) thermionic emission.
(C) rectification.
(D) induction.

12. Which of the following causes pitting, or many small surface melts, of the anode's focal track?

(A) Vaporized tungsten on the glass envelope
(B) Loss of anode rotation
(C) A large amount of heat to a cold anode
(D) Repeated, frequent overloading

13. In fluoroscopy, the automatic brightness control adjusts the

(A) kVp and mA.
(B) backup timer.
(C) mA and time.
(D) kVp and time.

14. A photostimulable phosphor plate is used with

    (A) computed radiography (CR).
    (B) radiographic intensifying screens.
    (C) fluoroscopic intensifying screens.
    (D) image intensified fluoroscopy.

15. Which of the following will serve to increase the effective energy of the x-ray beam?

    1. Increase in added filtration
    2. Increase in kilovoltage
    3. Increase in milliamperage

    (A) 1 only
    (B) 2 only
    (C) 1 and 2 only
    (D) 1, 2, and 3

16. Which of the following combinations would pose the *least* hazard to a particular anode?

    (A) 1.2-mm focal spot, 92 kVp, 1.5 mAs
    (B) 0.6-mm focal spot, 80 kVp, 3 mAs
    (C) 1.2-mm focal spot, 70 kVp, 6 mAs
    (D) 0.6-mm focal spot, 60 kVp, 12 mAs

17. Which of the following combinations will present the greatest heat-loading capability?

    (A) 17° target angle, 1.2-mm actual focal spot
    (B) 10° target angle, 1.2-mm actual focal spot
    (C) 17° target angle, 0.6-mm actual focal spot
    (D) 10° target angle, 0.6-mm actual focal spot

18. Congruence of the x-ray beam with the light field is tested using

    (A) a pinhole camera.
    (B) a star pattern.
    (C) radiopaque objects.
    (D) a slit camera.

19. Which of the following devices is (are) component(s) of a typical fluoroscopic video display system?

    1. Videotape recorder
    2. TV camera
    3. TV monitor

    (A) 1 only
    (B) 1 and 3 only
    (C) 2 and 3 only
    (D) 1, 2, and 3

20. If the primary coil of the high-voltage transformer is supplied by 220 V and has 200 turns, and the secondary coil has 100,000 turns, what is the voltage induced in the secondary coil?

    (A) 40 kV
    (B) 110 kV
    (C) 40 V
    (D) 110 V

21. What is the relationship between kilovoltage (kV) and the half-value layer (HVL)?

    (A) As kV increases, the HVL increases.
    (B) As kV decreases, the HVL decreases.
    (C) If the kV is doubled, the HVL doubles.
    (D) If the kV is doubled, the HVL is squared.

22. Exposures less than the minimum response time of an AEC may be required when

    1. using high mA.
    2. using fast film–screen combinations.
    3. examining large patients or body parts.

    (A) 1 only
    (B) 1 and 2 only
    (C) 2 and 3 only
    (D) 1, 2, and 3

23. In which of the following portions of the x-ray circuit is a step-down transformer located?

    (A) High-voltage side
    (B) Filament circuit
    (C) Rectification system
    (D) Secondary side

24. Patient dose during fluoroscopy is affected by the

    1. distance between the patient and the input phosphor.
    2. amount of magnification.
    3. tissue density.

    (A) 1 only
    (B) 3 only
    (C) 2 and 3 only
    (D) 1, 2, and 3

25. If 92 kV and 12 mAs were used for a particular abdominal exposure with single-phase equipment, what mAs would be required to produce a similar radiograph with three-phase, six-pulse equipment?

    (A) 36
    (B) 24
    (C) 8
    (D) 6

26. Which of the following devices converts electrical energy to mechanical energy?

    (A) Motor
    (B) Generator
    (C) Stator
    (D) Rotor

27. The essential function of the photomultiplier is to

    (A) provide a brighter fluoroscopic image.
    (B) automatically restrict the field size.
    (C) terminate the x-ray exposure once the image receptor is correctly exposed.
    (D) automatically increase or decrease incoming line voltages.

28. A slit camera is used to measure

    1. focal spot size.
    2. intensifying-screen resolution.
    3. SID resolution.

    (A) 1 only
    (B) 1 and 2 only
    (C) 1 and 3 only
    (D) 1, 2, and 3

29. A spinning top device can be used to evaluate

    1. timer accuracy.
    2. rectifier failure.
    3. the effect of kVp on contrast.

    (A) 1 only
    (B) 2 only
    (C) 1 and 2 only
    (D) 1, 2, and 3

30. Which of the following will improve the spatial resolution of image-intensified images?

    1. A very thin coating of cesium iodide on the input phosphor
    2. A smaller-diameter input screen
    3. Increased total brightness gain

    (A) 1 only
    (B) 1 and 2 only
    (C) 1 and 3 only
    (D) 1, 2, and 3

31. Circuit devices that will conduct electrons in only one direction are

    1. resistors.
    2. valve tubes.
    3. solid-state diodes.

    (A) 1 only
    (B) 1 and 3 only
    (C) 2 and 3 only
    (D) 1, 2, and 3

32. Which of the following occurs during Bremsstrahlung radiation production?

    (A) An electron makes a transition from an outer to an inner electron shell.
    (B) An electron approaching a positive nuclear charge changes direction and loses energy.
    (C) A high-energy photon ejects an outer-shell electron.
    (D) A low-energy photon ejects an inner-shell electron.

33. Tungsten alloy is the usual choice for the anode target material of radiographic equipment because it

1. has a high atomic number.
2. has a high melting point.
3. can readily dissipate heat.

(A) 1 only
(B) 1 and 2 only
(C) 2 and 3 only
(D) 1, 2, and 3

34. Which of the illustrations in Figure 5–2 depicts the ionization-chamber type of automatic exposure control?

(A) Figure A.
(B) Figure B.
(C) Both are ionization-chamber-type AEC.
(D) Neither is ionization-chamber-type AEC.

35. The voltage ripple associated with a three-phase, 12-pulse rectified generator is about

(A) 100%.
(B) 32%.
(C) 13%.
(D) 3%.

36. As the x-ray tube filament ages, it becomes progressively thinner because of evaporation. The vaporized tungsten is frequently deposited on the window of the glass envelope. This may

1. act as an additional filter.
2. reduce tube output.
3. result in arcing and tube puncture.

(A) 1 only
(B) 1 and 2 only
(C) 2 and 3 only
(D) 1, 2, and 3

37. Which of the following devices is used to control voltage by varying resistance?

(A) Autotransformer
(B) High-voltage transformer
(C) Rheostat
(D) Fuse

38. All of the following are components of the image intensifier, *except* the

(A) photocathode.
(B) focusing lenses.
(C) TV monitor.
(D) accelerating anode.

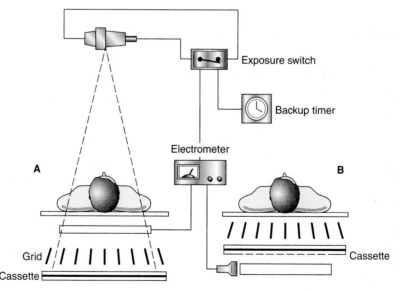

Figure 5–2. Reproduced with permission from Saia DA. *Radiography: Program Review and Examination Preparation,* 2nd ed. Stamford, CT: Appleton & Lange, 1999.

39. When using the smaller field in a dual-field image intensifier,

    1. a smaller patient area is viewed.
    2. the image is magnified.
    3. the image is less bright.

    (A) 1 only
    (B) 1 and 3 only
    (C) 2 and 3 only
    (D) 1, 2, and 3

40. A particular AP thoracic measurement is 25 cm. What tomographic sections are indicated if we desire one midline and one each anterior and posterior to midline?

    (A) 8, 9, and 10 cm
    (B) 10, 11, and 12 cm
    (C) 12, 13, and 14 cm
    (D) 14, 15, and 16 cm

41. Together, the filtering effect of the x-ray tube's glass envelope and its oil coolant are referred to as

    (A) inherent filtration.
    (B) added filtration.
    (C) compensating filtration.
    (D) port filtration.

42. In which type of equipment does kVp decrease during the actual length of the exposure?

    1. Condenser discharge mobile equipment
    2. Battery-operated mobile equipment
    3. Fixed x-ray equipment

    (A) 1 only
    (B) 1 and 2 only
    (C) 2 and 2 only
    (D) 1, 2, and 3

43. The procedure whose basic operation involves reciprocal motion of the x-ray tube and film is

    (A) cinefluorography.
    (B) spot filming.
    (C) tomography.
    (D) image intensification.

44. Which of the following is (are) characteristics of the x-ray tube?

    1. The target material should have a high atomic number and a high melting point.
    2. The useful beam emerges from the port window.
    3. The cathode assembly receives both low and high voltages.

    (A) 1 only
    (B) 2 only
    (C) 1 and 2 only
    (D) 1, 2, and 3

45. When the radiographer selects kilovoltage on the control panel, which device is adjusted?

    (A) Step-up transformer
    (B) Autotransformer
    (C) Filament circuit
    (D) Rectifier circuit

46. Dedicated radiographic units are available for

    1. chest radiography.
    2. head radiography.
    3. mammography.

    (A) 1 only
    (B) 2 only
    (C) 1 and 2 only
    (D) 1, 2, and 3

47. What is the device that directs the light emitted from the image intensifier to various viewing and imaging apparatus?

    (A) Output phosphor
    (B) Beam splitter
    (C) Spot film changer
    (D) Automatic brightness control

48. As electrons impinge on the target surface, less than 1% of their kinetic energy is changed to

    (A) x-rays.
    (B) heat.
    (C) gamma rays.
    (D) recoil electrons.

49. Which of the following contribute(s) to inherent filtration?

1. X-ray tube glass envelope
2. X-ray tube port window
3. Aluminum between the tube housing and the collimator

(A) 1 only
(B) 1 and 2 only
(C) 1 and 3 only
(D) 1, 2, and 3

50. A quality control program includes checks on which of the following radiographic equipment conditions?

1. Reproducibility
2. Linearity
3. Positive beam limitation/automatic collimation

(A) 1 only
(B) 1 and 2 only
(C) 1 and 3 only
(D) 1, 2, and 3

51. What x-ray tube component does the number 5 in Figure 5–3 indicate?

(A) Anode stem
(B) Rotor
(C) Stator
(D) Focal track

52. What x-ray tube component does the number 7 in Figure 5–3 indicate?

(A) Anode stem
(B) Rotor
(C) Stator
(D) Focal track

53. All of the following x-ray circuit devices are located between the incoming power supply and the primary coil of the high-voltage transformer *except* the

(A) timer.
(B) kV meter.
(C) mA meter.
(D) autotransformer.

54. Which of the following systems function(s) to compensate for changing patient/part thicknesses during fluoroscopic procedures?

(A) Automatic brightness control
(B) Minification gain
(C) Automatic resolution control
(D) flux gain

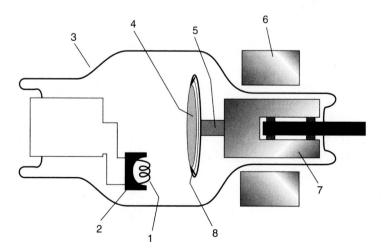

Figure 5–3. Reproduced with permission from Saia DA. *Radiography: Program Review and Examination Preparation,* 2nd ed. Stamford, CT: Appleton & Lange, 1999.

55. Disadvantages of moving grids over stationary grids include which of the following?

    1. They can prohibit the use of very short exposure times.
    2. They increase patient radiation dose.
    3. They can cause phantom images when anatomic parts parallel their motion.

    (A) 1 only
    (B) 1 and 2 only
    (C) 2 and 3 only
    (D) 1, 2, and 3

56. The functions of a picture archiving and communication system (PACS) include

    1. storage of analog images.
    2. acquisition of digital images.
    3. storage of digital images.

    (A) 1 only
    (B) 1 and 2 only
    (C) 2 and 3 only
    (D) 1, 2, and 3

57. How many half-value layers will it take to reduce an x-ray beam whose intensity is 78 R/min to an intensity of less than 10 R/min?

    (A) 2
    (B) 3
    (C) 4
    (D) 8

58. Double-focus x-ray tubes have two

    (A) port windows.
    (B) anodes.
    (C) filaments.
    (D) rectifiers.

59. An incorrect relationship between the primary beam and the center of a focused grid results in

    1. an increase in scattered radiation production.
    2. grid cutoff.
    3. insufficient radiographic density.

    (A) 1 only
    (B) 1 and 2 only
    (C) 2 and 3 only
    (D) 1, 2, and 3

60. Which of the following voltage ripples is (are) produced by single-phase equipment?

    1. 100% voltage ripple
    2. 13% voltage ripple
    3. 3.5% voltage ripple

    (A) 1 only
    (B) 2 only
    (C) 2 and 3 only
    (D) 1, 2, and 3

61. The radiograph illustrated in Figure 5–4 was made using a single-phase, full-wave-rectified unit with a timer and rectifiers that are known to be accurate and functioning correctly. What exposure time was used to produce this image?

    (A) 1/10 second
    (B) 0.05 second
    (C) 1/12 second
    (D) 0.025 second

62. Advantages of battery-powered mobile x-ray units include their

    1. ability to store a large quantity of energy.
    2. ability to store energy for extended periods of time.
    3. lightness and ease of maneuverability.

    (A) 1 only
    (B) 1 and 2 only
    (C) 2 and 3 only
    (D) 1, 2, and 3

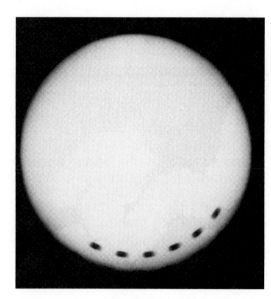

Figure 5–4.

63. The total brightness gain of an image intensifier is a result of

1. flux gain.
2. minification gain.
3. focusing gain.

(A) 1 only
(B) 2 only
(C) 1 and 2 only
(D) 1 and 3 only

64. Which of the following information is necessary to determine the maximum safe kVp, using the appropriate x-ray tube rating chart?

1. mA and exposure time
2. Focal spot size
3. Imaging-system speed

(A) 1 only
(B) 1 and 2 only
(C) 2 and 3 only
(D) 1, 2, and 3

65. In which of the following examinations would a cassette front with very low absorption properties be especially important?

(A) Abdominal radiography
(B) Extremity radiography
(C) Angiography
(D) Mammography

66. With three-phase equipment, the voltage across the x-ray tube

1. drops to zero every 180°.
2. is 87% to 96% of the maximum value.
3. is at nearly constant potential.

(A) 1 only
(B) 2 only
(C) 1 and 2 only
(D) 2 and 3 only

67. To be used more efficiently by the x-ray tube, alternating current is changed to unidirectional current by the

(A) filament transformer.
(B) autotransformer.
(C) high-voltage transformer.
(D) rectifiers.

68. If the distance from the focal spot to the center of the collimator's mirror is 6 inches, what distance should the illuminator's light bulb be from the center of the mirror?

(A) 3 inches
(B) 6 inches
(C) 9 inches
(D) 12 inches

69. To maintain image clarity in an image intensifier system, the path of electron flow from the photocathode to the output phosphor is controlled by

(A) the accelerating anode.
(B) electrostatic lenses.
(C) the vacuum glass envelope.
(D) the input phosphor.

70. The device used to test the accuracy of the x-ray timer is the

(A) densitometer.
(B) sensitometer.
(C) penetrometer.
(D) spinning top.

71. Which of the following equipment is mandatory for performance of a myelogram?

    (A) Cine camera
    (B) 105-mm spot film
    (C) Tilting x-ray table
    (D) Tomography

72. The device that receives the remnant beam, converts it into light, and then increases the brightness of that light is the

    (A) cine camera.
    (B) spot film camera.
    (C) image intensifier.
    (D) television monitor.

73. Features of x-ray tube targets that function to determine heat capacity include the

    1. rotation of the anode.
    2. diameter of the anode.
    3. size of the focal spot.

    (A) 1 only
    (B) 1 and 2 only
    (C) 1 and 3 only
    (D) 1, 2, and 3

74. Which of the following terms describes the amount of electric charge flowing per second?

    (A) Voltage
    (B) Current
    (C) Resistance
    (D) Capacitance

75. The brightness level of the fluoroscopic image can vary with

    1. milliamperage.
    2. kilovoltage.
    3. patient thickness.

    (A) 1 only
    (B) 1 and 2 only
    (C) 1 and 3 only
    (D) 1, 2, and 3

76. Which of the following techniques is used to evaluate the dynamics of a part?

    (A) Fluoroscopy
    (B) Stereoscopy
    (C) Tomography
    (D) Phototiming

77. Which of the following is the correct formula for determining heat units for a three-phase, 12-pulse x-ray machine?

    (A) $kVp \times mA \times time$
    (B) $mA \times kVp \times mAs$
    (C) $kVp \times mAs \times 1.35$
    (D) $mA \times time \times kVp \times 1.41$

78. If a high-voltage transformer has 100 primary turns and 35,000 secondary turns, and is supplied by 220 V and 75 A, what are the secondary voltage and current?

    (A) 200 A and 77 V
    (B) 200 mA and 77 kVp
    (C) 20 A and 77 V
    (D) 20 mA and 77 kVp

79. Rare earth phosphors that may be used in intensifying screens include

    1. cesium iodide.
    2. gadolinium oxysulfide.
    3. lanthanum oxybromide.

    (A) 1 only
    (B) 1 and 2 only
    (C) 2 and 3 only
    (D) 1, 2, and 3

80. Star and wye configurations are related to

    (A) autotransformers.
    (B) three-phase transformers.
    (C) rectification systems.
    (D) automatic exposure controls.

81. A technique chart should be prepared for each AEC x-ray unit and should contain the following information for each type of examination:

1. Photocell(s) used
2. Optimum kVp
3. Backup time

(A) 1 only
(B) 1 and 2 only
(C) 2 and 3 only
(D) 1, 2, and 3

82. A light-absorbing dye is frequently incorporated during the manufacture of screens to

(A) reduce the diffusion of fluorescent light.
(B) decrease film contrast.
(C) increase screen speed.
(D) increase the useful life of the screen.

83. All of the following are associated with the anode *except*

(A) the line focus principle.
(B) the heel effect.
(C) the focal track.
(D) thermionic emission.

84. Figure 5–5 illustrates the

(A) anode heel effect.
(B) reciprocity law.
(C) line focus principle.
(D) inverse square law.

85. The number 2 in Figure 5–5 indicates the

(A) effective focal spot.
(B) actual focal spot.
(C) focal track.
(D) thermionic emission.

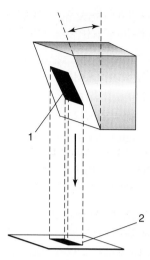

Figure 5–5. Reproduced with permission from Saia DA. *Radiography: Program Review and Examination Preparation,* 2nd ed. Stamford, CT: Appleton & Lange, 1999.

86. The advantages of capacitor discharge mobile x-ray equipment include

1. compact size.
2. light weight.
3. high kVp capability.

(A) 1 only
(B) 1 and 2 only
(C) 2 and 3 only
(D) 1, 2, and 3

87. Capacitor discharge mobile x-ray units

1. use a grid-controlled x-ray tube.
2. are typically charged before the day's work.
3. provide a direct current output.

(A) 1 only
(B) 2 only
(C) 1 and 3 only
(D) 1, 2, and 3

88. X-ray tube life may be extended by

1. using low-mAs/high-kVp exposure factors.
2. avoiding lengthy anode rotation.
3. avoiding exposures to a cold anode.

(A) 1 only
(B) 1 and 2 only
(C) 1 and 3 only
(D) 1, 2, and 3

89. Which of the following modes of a trifield image intensifier will result in the highest patient dose?

    (A) Its 25-inch mode.
    (B) Its 17-inch mode.
    (C) Its 12-inch mode.
    (D) Diameter does not affect patient dose.

90. Off-focus, or extrafocal, radiation may be minimized by

    (A) avoiding the use of very high kilovoltages.
    (B) restricting the x-ray beam as close to its source as possible.
    (C) using compression devices to reduce tissue thickness.
    (D) avoiding extreme collimation.

91. The advantage(s) of collimators over aperture diaphragms and flare cones include(s)

    1. the variety of field sizes available.
    2. more efficient beam restriction.
    3. better cleanup of scattered radiation.

    (A) 1 only
    (B) 1 and 2 only
    (C) 1 and 3 only
    (D) 2 and 3 only

92. An automatic exposure control device can operate on which of the following principles?

    1. A photomultiplier tube charged by a fluorescent screen
    2. A parallel-plate ionization chamber charged by x-ray photons
    3. Motion of magnetic fields inducing current in a conductor

    (A) 1 only
    (B) 2 only
    (C) 1 and 2 only
    (D) 1, 2, and 3

93. Which of the following functions to increase the mA?

    (A) Increase in charge of anode
    (B) Increase in heat of the filament
    (C) Increase in kVp
    (D) Increase in focal spot size

94. A backup timer for the AEC serves to

    1. protect the patient from overexposure.
    2. protect the x-ray tube from excessive heat.
    3. increase or decrease master density.

    (A) 1 only
    (B) 1 and 2 only
    (C) 2 and 3 only
    (D) 1, 2, and 3

95. Fractional-focus tubes, with a 0.3-mm focal spot or smaller, have special application in

    (A) magnification radiography.
    (B) fluoroscopy.
    (C) tomography.
    (D) image intensification.

96. In the radiographic rating charts shown in Figure 5–6, what is the maximum safe kVp that may be used with the 1-mm focal spot, single-phase x-ray tube, using 300 mA and 1/50-second exposure?

    (A) 80
    (B) 95
    (C) 105
    (D) 112

97. In Figure 5–6, which of the illustrated x-ray tubes permit(s) an exposure of 400 mA, 0.1 second, and 80 kVp?

    1. Tube A
    2. Tube B
    3. Tube C

    (A) 1 only
    (B) 1 and 2 only
    (C) 2 and 3 only
    (D) 1, 2, and 3

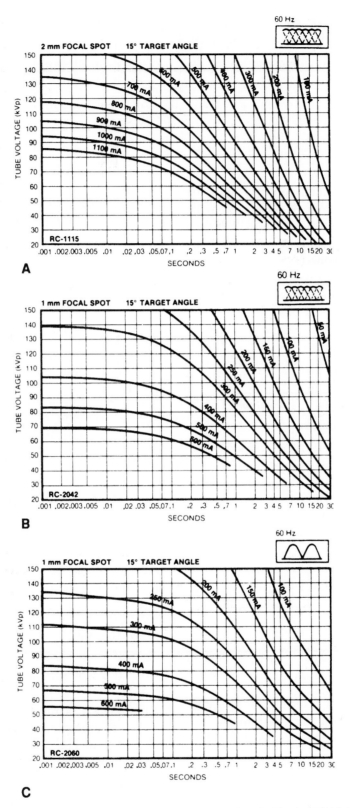

Figure 5–6. Reproduced with permission from Dunlee Tech Data Publication 50014, May 1988.

98. In Figure 5–6, what is the maximum safe mA that may be used with 0.1-second exposure and 120 kVp, using the three-phase, 2-mm focal spot x-ray tube?

(A) 400
(B) 500
(C) 600
(D) 700

99. Referring to the anode cooling chart in Figure 5–7, if the anode is saturated with 300,000 heat units (HU), how long will the anode need to cool before another 160,000 heat units can be safely applied?

(A) 3 minutes
(B) 4 minutes
(C) 5 minutes
(D) 7 minutes

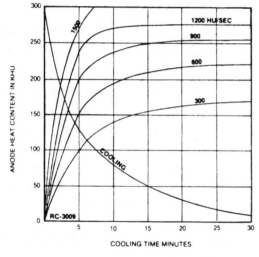

Figure 5–7. Reproduced with permission from Dunlee Tech Data Publication 50014, May 1988.

100. A high-speed electron entering the tungsten target is attracted to the positive nucleus of a tungsten atom and, in the process, is decelerated. This results in

(A) characteristic radiation.
(B) Bremsstrahlung radiation.
(C) Compton scatter.
(D) photoelectric effect.

101. Anode angle will have an effect on the

1. severity of the heel effect.
2. focal spot size.
3. heat load capacity.

(A) 1 only
(B) 2 only
(C) 1 and 2 only
(D) 1, 2, and 3

102. Light-sensitive automatic exposure control devices are known as

(A) phototimers.
(B) ionization chambers.
(C) sensors.
(D) backup timers.

103. Delivery of large exposures to a cold anode or the use of exposures exceeding tube limitation can result in

1. increased tube output.
2. cracking of the anode.
3. rotor bearing damage.

(A) 1 only
(B) 1 and 2 only
(C) 2 and 3 only
(D) 1, 2, and 3

104. To determine how quickly an x-ray tube will disperse its accumulated heat, the radiographer uses a(n)

(A) technique chart.
(B) radiographic rating chart.
(C) anode cooling curve.
(D) spinning top test.

105. Which of the following formulas would the radiographer use to determine the total number of HU produced with a given exposure using three-phase, six-pulse equipment?

(A) mA $\times$ time $\times$ kVp
(B) mA $\times$ time $\times$ kVp $\times$ 3.0
(C) mA $\times$ time $\times$ kVp $\times$ 1.35
(D) mA $\times$ time $\times$ kVp $\times$ 1.41

106. A device used to ensure reproducible radiographs, regardless of tissue density variations, is the

    (A) phototimer.
    (B) penetrometer.
    (C) grid.
    (D) rare earth screen.

107. Radiographs from a particular single-phase, full-wave–rectified x-ray unit were overexposed, using known correct exposures. A spinning top test was performed at 200 mA, 0.05-second, and 70 kVp, and eight dots were visualized on the finished film. Which of the following is indicated?

    (A) The 0.05-second time station is inaccurate.
    (B) The 200-mA station is inaccurate.
    (C) A rectifier is not functioning.
    (D) The processor needs servicing.

108. If a radiograph exposed using an AEC is overexposed because an exposure shorter than the minimum response time was required, the radiographer generally should

    (A) decrease the mA.
    (B) use the minus density.
    (C) use the plus density.
    (D) decrease the kVp.

109. Which of the following would be appropriate cassette front material(s)?

    1. Tungsten
    2. Magnesium
    3. Bakelite

    (A) 1 only
    (B) 1 and 2 only
    (C) 2 and 3 only
    (D) 1, 2, and 3

110. The most commonly used types of AEC devices are the

    1. ion chamber.
    2. photomultiplier tube.
    3. cathode ray tube.

    (A) 1 and 2 only
    (B) 1 and 3 only
    (C) 2 and 3 only
    (D) 1, 2, and 3

111. Capacitor discharge mobile x-ray units use capacitors to power the

    1. the x-ray tube.
    2. machine locomotion.
    3. the braking mechanism.

    (A) 1 only
    (B) 2 only
    (C) 1 and 2 only
    (D) 1, 2, and 3

112. A three-phase timer can be tested for accuracy using a synchronous spinning top. The resulting image looks like a

    (A) series of dots or dashes, each representative of a radiation pulse.
    (B) solid arc, with the angle (in degrees) representative of the exposure time.
    (C) series of gray tones, from white to black.
    (D) multitude of small, meshlike squares of uniform sharpness.

113. Accurate operation of the AEC device is dependent on

    1. the thickness and density of the object.
    2. positioning of the object with respect to the photocell.
    3. beam restriction.

    (A) 1 only
    (B) 1 and 2 only
    (C) 2 and 3 only
    (D) 1, 2, and 3

114. The image intensifier's input phosphor is generally composed of

(A) cesium iodide.
(B) zinc cadmium sulfide.
(C) gadolinium oxysulfide.
(D) calcium tungstate.

115. The total number of x-ray photons produced at the target is contingent on the

1. tube current.
2. target material.
3. square of the kilovoltage.

(A) 1 only
(B) 1 and 2 only
(C) 2 and 3 only
(D) 1, 2, and 3

116. A parallel-plate ionization chamber receives a particular charge as x-ray photons travel through it. This is the operating principle of which of the following devices?

(A) Automatic exposure control
(B) Image intensifier
(C) Cine film camera
(D) Spot film camera

117. Excessive anode heating can cause vaporized tungsten to be deposited on the port window. This can result in

1. decreased tube output.
2. tube failure.
3. electrical sparking.

(A) 1 only
(B) 2 only
(C) 1 and 2 only
(D) 1, 2, and 3

118. The input phosphor of the image intensifier tube functions to convert

(A) kinetic energy to light.
(B) x-rays to light.
(C) electrons to light.
(D) fluorescent light to electrons.

119. Which of the following circuit devices operate(s) on the principle of self-induction?

1. Autotransformer
2. Choke coil
3. High-voltage transformer

(A) 1 only
(B) 1 and 2 only
(C) 2 and 3 only
(D) 1, 2, and 3

120. Which of the following statement regarding dual x-ray absorptiometry are true?

1. It is a low-dose procedure.
2. Two x-ray photon energies are used.
3. Photon attenuation by bone is calculated.

(A) 1 only
(B) 1 and 2 only
(C) 1 and 3 only
(D) 1, 2, and 3

Answers and Explanations

1. **(D)** Moving the image intensifier *closer to the patient* during fluoroscopy *reduces* the distance between the x-ray tube (source) and the image intensifier (image receptor), that is, the *SID*. It follows that the distance between the part being imaged (object) and the image intensifier (image receptor), that is, the *OID*, is also reduced. The shorter OID produces *less magnification* and *better image quality*. As the SID is reduced, the intensity of the x-ray photons at the image intensifier's input phosphor increases, stimulating the automatic brightness control (ABC) to decrease the mA and thereby *decreasing patient dose* (see Fig. 5–8). *(Fosbinder & Kelsey, pp 265–267)*

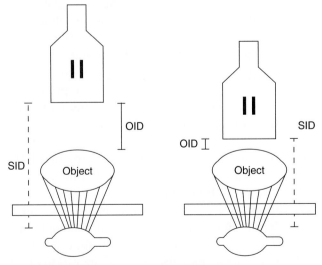

Figure 5–8. Bringing the image intensifier (II) closer to the patient *decreases SID* and *patient dose* (because the input phosphor receives more x-ray photons, the ABC automatically decreases the mA). Bringing the II closer to the patient *decreases OID* and *magnification*.

2. **(B)** Tomography is a procedure that uses reciprocal motion between the x-ray tube and the film to image structures at a particular level in the body, while blurring everything above and below that level. The thickness of the level visualized can be varied by changing the tube angle (amplitude). In general, the greater the tube angle, the thinner the section imaged. Thinner sections may be used for imaging small or intricate structures. *(Bushong, pp 317)*

3. **(B)** CT and MRI are two common examples of *digital imaging.* Special equipment is also available for digital radiography (DR) or CR: images produced by either a fan-shaped x-ray beam received by linearly arrayed radiation detectors or a traditional fan-shaped x-ray beam received by a light-stimulated phosphor plate. Digital images can also be obtained in digital subtraction angiography (DSA), nuclear medicine, and diagnostic sonography. *Analog* images are conventional images; they can be converted to digital images with a device called a digitizer. *Pluridirectional tomography* refers to conventional tomographic equipment that is capable of several x-ray tube movements. *(Shephard, p 367)*

4. **(D)** Mobile x-ray machines are smaller and more compact than their fixed counterparts in the radiology department. It is important that they be relatively easy to move, that their size allows entry into patient rooms, and that their locks enable securing of the x-ray tube into the

required positions. Mobile x-ray machines are cordless and are either the battery-operated type or the condenser discharge type. *Battery operated* is probably the most commonly used where consistent and high-energy output is required. Two sets of batteries are used in these mobile units: One set is used for operating the *motor* that drives the unit and operates the *braking* mechanism ("dead-man brake") and the other set is used for operating the *x-ray tube.* Periodic recharging of the batteries is required. *(Ballinger & Frank, vol 3, p 235)*

5. **(A)** A synchronous spinning top test is used to test timer accuracy or rectifier function in three-phase equipment. Because three-phase, full-wave–rectified current would expose a 360° arc each second, a 1/12-second exposure should expose a 30° arc. Anything more or less indicates timer inaccuracy. If exactly one half of the expected arc appears, one should suspect rectifier failure. *(Saia, p 434)*

6. **(B)** Determining mR/mAs output is often done to determine linearity among x-ray machines. However, all the equipment being compared must be of the same type (eg, all single-phase; all three-phase, six-pulse; etc). If there is linearity among these machines, then identical technique charts can be used. In the example given, 400 mA and 0.12 second were used, equaling *48 mAs.* If the output for 48 mAs was 150 mR, then 1 mAs is equal to 3.1 mR (150 mR ÷ 48 mAs = 3.1 mR/mAs). *(Bushong, pp 248–249)*

7. **(C)** Target angle has a pronounced geometric effect on the effective, or projected, focal spot size. As the target angle *decreases,* the effective (projected) focal spot becomes smaller. This is advantageous because it will improve radiographic detail without creating a heat-loading crisis at the anode (as would occur if the actual focal spot size were reduced to produce a similar detail improvement). There are disadvantages, however. With a smaller target angle, the anode heel effect increases; photons are more noticeably absorbed by the "heel" of the anode, resulting in a smaller percentage of x-ray photons at the anode end of the x-ray beam and a concentration of x-ray photons at

the cathode end of the radiograph. *(Shephard, p 221)*

8. **(B)** Four waveforms are illustrated. Number 1 represents unrectified *alternating current,* which has constantly changing amplitude and periodically changing polarity; only the positive half-cycle is useful. Number 2 represents *single-phase, full-wave–rectified* current; the negative half-cycle is rectified to a useful positive half-cycle. Numbers 3 and 4 represent *three-phase rectified* current; number 3 is 3-phase, 6-*pulse,* and number 4 is 3-phase, 12-*pulse. (Kelsey & Fosbinder, pp 74–75, 83–85)*

9. **(B)** *Traditional x-ray imaging* involves formation of the x-ray image directly on the image receptor (film). *In digital imaging,* x-rays form an electronic image on a special radiation detector. This electronic image can be manipulated by a computer and stored in the computer memory or displayed as a matrix of intensities. This final digital image is often viewed on a computer monitor and looks just like a traditional x-ray image, but the computer often has the capability of postprocessing image enhancement. *(Bushong, p 402)*

10. **(B)** *The minimum response time, or minimum reaction time,* is the length of the shortest exposure possible with a particular AEC. If less than the minimum response time is required for a particular exposure, the radiograph will exhibit excessive density. The problem may become apparent when using fast film–screen combinations or high milliamperage, or when imaging small or easily penetrated body parts. The *backup timer* functions to protect the patient from overexposure and the x-ray tube from overload. *(Saia, p 246)*

11. **(B)** The thoriated tungsten filament of the cathode is heated by its own filament circuit. The x-ray tube filament is made of thoriated tungsten and is part of the cathode assembly. Its circuit provides current and voltage to heat it to incandescence, at which time it undergoes *thermionic emission*—the liberation of valence electrons from the filament atoms. *Electrolysis* describes the chemical ionization effects of an electric current. *Rectification* is the

process of changing AC to unidirectional current. (*Bushong, p 118*)

12. **(D)** As the filament ages, vaporized tungsten may be deposited on the port window and act as an additional filter. Tungsten may also vaporize as a result of anode abuse. Exposures in excess of safe values deliver sufficient heat to cause surface melts, or pits, on the focal track. This results in roughening of the anode surface and decreased tube output. Delivery of a large amount of heat to a cold anode can cause cracking if the anode does not have sufficient time to disperse the heat. Loss of anode rotation would cause one large melt on the focal track, as the electrons would bombard only one small area. If the anode is not heard rotating, the radiographer should not make an exposure. (*Selman, pp 137–138*)

13. **(A)** As body areas of different thicknesses and densities are scanned with the image intensifier, image brightness and contrast require adjustment. The *ABC* functions to maintain constant brightness and contrast of the output screen image, correcting for fluctuations in x-ray beam attenuation with *adjustments in kVp and/or mA*. There are also brightness and contrast controls on the monitor that the radiographer can regulate. (*Bushong, p 358*)

14. **(A)** A *photostimulable* (light-stimulated) *phosphor plate*, or simply *image plate*, is used in CR. CR does not use traditional intensifying screens or film. Rather, the CR cassette contains a *photostimulable* IP that functions as the image receptor (rather than as film emulsion). Upon exposure, the IP stores information. The cassette is placed into a special scanner/processor where the IP is scanned with a laser light and the stored image is displayed on the computer monitor. (*Shephard, pp 321–329*)

15. **(C)** As *filtration* is added to the x-ray beam, the lower-energy photons are removed and the overall energy or wavelength of the beam is greater. As *kilovoltage* is increased, more high-energy photons are produced, and again the overall, or average, energy of the beam is greater. An increase in *milliamperage* serves to

increase the number of photons produced at the target, but is unrelated to their energy. (*Selman, p 171*)

16. **(A)** Radiographic rating charts enable the operator to determine the maximum safe mA, exposure time, and kVp for a particular exposure using a particular x-ray tube. An exposure that can be made safely with the large focal spot may not be safe for use with the small focal spot of the same x-ray tube. The total number of HU that an exposure generates also influences the amount of stress (in the form of heat) imparted to the anode. The product of mAs and kVp determines HU. Group A produces 138 HU, group B produces 240 HU, group C produces 420 HU, and group D produces 720 HU. The *least hazardous* group of technical factors is, therefore, group A. Group D is also delivering its heat load to the small focal spot, making this the *most hazardous* group of technical factors. (*Selman, pp 144–145*)

17. **(B)** The smaller the focal spot, the more limited the anode is with respect to the quantity of heat it can safely accept. As the target angle decreases, the actual focal spot can be increased while still maintaining a small effective focal spot. Therefore, group B offers the greatest heat-loading potential, with a steep target angle and a large actual focal spot. It must be remembered, however, *that a steep target angle increases the heel effect*, and film coverage may be compromised. (*Selman, pp 145–146*)

18. **(C)** Radiographic results should be consistent and predictable with respect to positioning accuracy, exposure factors, and equipment operation. X-ray equipment should be tested and calibrated periodically as part of an *ongoing quality assurance* program. The *focal spot* should be tested periodically to evaluate its size and its impact on recorded detail; this is accomplished using a slit camera, a pinhole camera, or a star pattern. To test the *congruence of the light and x-ray fields*, a radiopaque object such as a paper clip or a penny is placed at each corner of the light field before the test exposure is made. After processing, the corners of the x-ray field should be exactly delineated by the radiopaque objects. (*Carlton & Adler, p 443*)

19. **(C)** The image on the image intensifier's output phosphor may be displayed for viewing through the use of either a *series of lenses* or a *fiberoptic* link. The two devices needed to view the image are a *TV camera tube* and a *TV monitor*. The TV camera tube (usually a Plumbicon or Vidicon) converts the output phosphor image into an electrical signal. The TV monitor (a cathode-ray tube) then converts the electrical signal into a visible light image. *(Thompson et al, p 370)*

20. **(B)** The high-voltage, or step-up, transformer functions to *increase voltage* to the necessary kilovoltage. It *decreases the amperage* to milliamperage. The amount of increase or decrease *depends on the transformer ratio,* that is, the ratio of the number of turns in the primary coil to the number of turns in the secondary coil. The transformer law is as follows:

To determine secondary *V*,

$$\frac{V_s}{V_p} = \frac{N_s}{N_p}$$

To determine secondary *I*:

$$\frac{N_s}{N_p} = \frac{I_p}{I_s}$$

Substituting known values,

$$\frac{x}{220} = \frac{100,000}{200}$$
$$200x = 22,000,000$$
$$x = 110,000 \text{ V } (110 \text{ kVp})$$

(Selman, pp 84–85)

21. **(A)** The *HVL* of a particular beam is defined as that thickness of a material that will reduce the exposure rate to one half of its original value. The more energetic the beam (the higher the kV), the greater the HVL thickness required to cut its intensity in half. *Therefore, it may be stated that kV and HVL have a direct relationship: As kV increases, HVL increases. (Selman, pp 122–123)*

22. **(B)** The minimum response time, or minimum reaction time, is the length of the shortest expo-

sure possible with a particular AEC. If less than the minimum response time is required for a particular exposure, the radiograph will exhibit excessive density. This problem becomes apparent when making exposures that require very short exposure times, such as when using high milliamperage and fast film–screen combinations. To resolve this problem, the radiographer should decrease the mA rather than the kVp, in order to leave contrast unaffected. *(Saia, p 246)*

23. **(B)** Transformers are used to change the value of alternating current (AC). They operate on the principle of mutual induction. The secondary coil of the step-up transformer is located in the high-voltage (secondary) side of the x-ray circuit. The step-down transformer, or filament transformer, is located in the filament circuit and serves to regulate the voltage and current provided to heat the x-ray tube filament. The rectification system is also located on the high-voltage, or secondary, side of the x-ray circuit. *(Selman, pp 155–156)*

24. **(D)** Moving the image intensifier closer to the patient during fluoroscopy decreases the SID and patient dose (as SID is reduced, the intensity of the x-ray photons at the image intensifier's input phosphor increases; the automatic brightness control then automatically decreases the mA, and therefore patient dose). Moving the image intensifier closer to the patient during fluoroscopy also decreases the OID, and therefore magnification. As tissue density increases, a greater exposure dose is required. *(Fosbinder & Kelsey, pp 265–267)*

25. **(C)** Single-phase radiographic equipment is much less efficient than three-phase equipment because it has a 100% voltage ripple. *With three-phase equipment, voltage never drops to zero,* and x-ray intensity is significantly greater. To produce similar density, only *two thirds* of the original mAs would be used for three-phase, six-pulse equipment ($2/3 \times 12 = 8$ mAs). With 3-phase, 12-pulse equipment, the original mAs would be cut in *half. (Saia, p 333)*

26. **(A)** A *motor* is the device used to convert electrical energy to mechanical energy. The *stator*

and *rotor* are the two principal parts of an *induction motor*. A *generator* converts mechanical energy into electrical energy. *(Selman, p 78)*

27. (C) A *photomultiplier, or phototimer,* is a type of AEC that is used to automatically terminate the x-ray exposure once the film is correctly exposed. Another type of AEC is the *ionization chamber.* An image intensifier functions to provide a brighter fluoroscopic image, and positive beam limitation (PBL), or automatic collimation, serves to restrict the field size to the size of the cassette–image receptor used in the bucky tray. The line voltage compensator automatically adjusts the incoming line voltage to the x-ray machine to correct for any voltage drops or surges. *(Selman, pp 153–154)*

28. (A) A quality control program requires the use of a number of devices to test the effi-

ciency of various parts of the imaging system (Fig. 5–9). A *slit camera*, as well as a star pattern or pinhole camera, is used to test focal spot size. A parallel line–type resolution test pattern is used to test the resolution capability of intensifying screens. *(Bushong, p 462)*

29. (C) The spinning top test is used to evaluate *timer accuracy* or *rectifier failure*. With single-phase, full-wave–rectified equipment (120 pulses/sec); for example, 12 dots should be visualized when using the 1/10-second time station. A few dots more or less indicate timer inaccuracy. If the test demonstrated exactly six dots, rectifier failure is strongly suspected. With three-phase equipment, a special synchronous spinning top (or oscilloscope) is used and a solid black arc is obtained rather than dots. The length of this arc is measured and compared with the known correct arc. *(Selman, pp 105–106)*

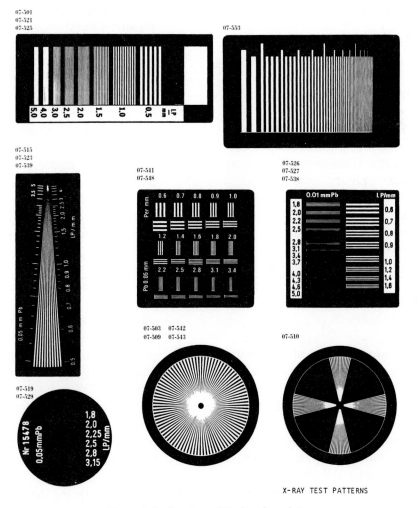

X-RAY TEST PATTERNS

Figure 5–9. Courtesy of Nuclear Associates.

30. **(B)** An image's *spatial resolution* refers to its recorded detail. The effect of the input screen's phosphor layer is similar to the effect of the phosphor layer thickness in intensifying screens; that is, as the phosphor layer can be made thinner, recorded detail increases. Also, the smaller the input phosphor diameter, the greater the spatial resolution. A brighter image is easier to see, but does not affect resolution. *(Bushong, pp 360–363)*

31. **(C)** *Rectifiers change AC into unidirectional current by allowing current to flow through them in only one direction. Valve tubes* are vacuum rectifier tubes found in older equipment. *Solid-state diodes* are the types of rectifiers used in today's x-ray equipment. Rectification systems are found between the secondary coil of the high-voltage transformer and the x-ray tube. *Resistors,* such as rheostats or choke coils, are circuit devices used to vary voltage or current. *(Selman, p 101)*

32. **(B)** Two types of interaction between high-speed incident electrons and the tungsten target atoms account for the production of x-rays within the x-ray tube. (1) In the production of brems ("braking") radiation, a high-speed electron is attracted to the positive nuclear charge of a tungsten atom. In doing so, it is "braked" and gives up energy in the form of an x-ray photon. Most of the primary beam is made up of brems radiation. (2) If the incident electron were to eject a K-shell electron, an L-shell electron would move in to fill the vacancy. It releases a photon (K characteristic ray) whose energy equals the difference between the K- and L-shell energy levels. This is characteristic radiation; it is responsible for only a small portion of the primary beam. *(Saia, p 224)*

33. **(D)** The x-ray anode may be a molybdenum disc coated with a tungsten–rhenium alloy. Because tungsten has a *high atomic number* (74), it produces high-energy x-rays more efficiently. Since a great deal of heat is produced at the target, tungsten's *high melting point* (3410°C) helps avoid damage to the target surface. Heat produced at the target should be dissipated readily, and tungsten's *conductivity is similar to that of copper.* Therefore, as heat is applied to the focus, it can be conducted throughout the disc to equalize the temperature and thus avoid pitting, or localized melting, of the focal track. *(Selman, p 138)*

34. **(A)** AEC devices are used in today's equipment and serve to produce consistent and comparable radiographic results. In one type of AEC, there is an *ionization chamber* just beneath the tabletop above the cassette–image receptor (A). The part to be examined is centered to it (the sensor) and radiographed. When a predetermined quantity of ionization has occurred (equal to the correct density), the exposure automatically terminates. In the other type of AEC, the *phototimer,* a small fluorescent screen is positioned beneath the cassette–image receptor (B). When remnant radiation emerging from the patient exposes the film and exits the image receptor, the fluorescent screen emits light. Once a predetermined amount of fluorescent light is "seen" by the photocell sensor, the exposure is terminated. A special cassette–image receptor, one without lead foil backing, is often required with this type of AEC. *In either case, the manual timer should be used as a backup timer.* In case of AEC malfunction, this would terminate the exposure, thus avoiding patient overexposure and tube overload. *(Saia, p 306)*

35. **(D)** Voltage ripple refers to the percentage drop from maximum voltage each pulse of current experiences. In single-phase rectified equipment, the entire pulse (half-cycle) is used; therefore, there is first an increase to the maximum (peak) voltage value and then a decrease to zero potential (90° past peak potential). The entire waveform is used; if 100 kV were selected, the actual average kilovoltage output would be approximately 70. Three-phase rectification produces almost constant potential, with just small ripples (drops) in maximum potential between pulses. Approximately a 13% voltage ripple (drop from maximum value) characterizes the operation of three-phase, six-pulse generators. Three-phase, 12-pulse generators have about a 3.5% voltage ripple. *(Selman, p 162)*

36. **(D)** Through the action of thermionic emission, as the tungsten filament continually

gives up electrons, it gradually becomes thinner with age. This evaporated tungsten is frequently deposited on the inner surface of the glass envelope at the tube window. When this happens, *it acts as an additional filter* of the x-ray beam, thereby *reducing tube output*. Also, the tungsten deposit may actually attract electrons from the filament, creating a tube current and causing *puncture of the glass envelope. (Selman, pp 137–138)*

37. **(C)** The *autotransformer* operates on the principle of *self-induction* and functions to select the correct voltage to be sent to the *high-voltage transformer* to be "stepped up" to kilovoltage. The high-voltage transformer increases the voltage and decreases the current. The *rheostat* is a type of *variable resistor* that is used to change voltage or current values. It is frequently found in the filament circuit. A *fuse* is a device used to protect the circuit elements from overload by opening the circuit in the event of a power surge. *(Selman, pp 90–91)*

38. **(C)** The *input phosphor* of an image intensifier receives remnant radiation emerging from the patient and converts it to a fluorescent light image. Directly adjacent to the input phosphor is the *photocathode,* which is made of a photoemissive alloy (usually a cesium and antimony compound). The fluorescent light image strikes the photocathode and is converted to an electron image. The electrons are carefully focused, to maintain image resolution, by the *electrostatic focusing lenses,* through the *accelerating anode* and to the *output phosphor* for conversion back to light. The *TV monitor* is not part of the image intensifier, but serves to display the image that is transmitted to it from the output phosphor. *(Bushong, pp 360–363)*

39. **(D)** When a dual-field image intensifier is switched to the smaller field, the electrostatic focusing lenses are given a greater charge to focus the electron image more tightly. The focal point, then, moves further from the output phosphor (the diameter of the electron image is therefore smaller as it reaches the output phosphor), and the brightness gain is somewhat diminished. Hence, the patient area viewed is somewhat smaller and is magnified.

However, the minification gain has been reduced and the image is somewhat less bright. *(Bushong, p 363)*

40. **(C)** Conventional x-ray images are two-dimensional and result in anatomic structures being superimposed on one another in the radiographic image. We use various methods to achieve the third dimension and to separate superimposed structures. Taking two projections at right angles to each other, using oblique positions, and using tube angulation are all ways of accomplishing this without special equipment. Tomographic equipment enables us to acquire images of particular *levels* of structures within the body, using the principles of reciprocal motion and a fulcrum. Exposing the image receptor with the fulcrum set at a particular level will clearly demonstrate that level, with all structures above and below it blurred by the motion of the x-ray tube and image receptor. If a part measures 25 cm, the midline is 13 cm (there are 12 cm anterior to the 13-cm level and 12 cm posterior to the 13-cm level), so the required series of cuts would be at 12, 13, and 14 cm. *(Selman, p 281)*

41. **(A)** The x-ray beam emitted from the target has a heterogeneous nature. The low-energy photons within it must be removed because they are not penetrating enough to contribute to the image, and because they *do* contribute to the patient's skin dose. The glass envelope and oil coolant provide approximately 0.5 to 1.0 mm Al equivalent filtration, which is referred to as *inherent* because it is a built-in, permanent part of the tube head. *(Selman, p 132)*

42. **(A)** Mobile x-ray machines are compact and cordless and are either the battery-operated type or the condenser discharge type. *Condenser discharge* mobile x-ray units do not use batteries; this type mobile unit requires that it be charged before each exposure. A condenser (or capacitor) is a device that stores electrical energy. The stored energy is used to operate the x-ray tube only. Because this machine does not carry many batteries, it is much lighter and does not need a motor to drive or brake it. The major disadvantage of the capacitor/condenser discharge unit is that, as the capacitor

discharges its electrical charge, the kVp gradually decreases throughout the length of the exposure—therefore limiting tube output and requiring recharging between exposures. (*Ballinger & Frank, vol 3, p 235*)

43. **(C)** Structures that we wish to visualize are frequently superimposed on other structures of lesser interest. Tomography uses reciprocal motion between the x-ray tube and the film to image structures at a particular level in the body, while blurring everything above and below that level. The thickness of the level visualized can be changed by changing the tube angle (amplitude). The greater the tube angle, the thinner the section imaged. (*Selman, pp 276–277*)

44. **(D)** Anode target material with a *high atomic number* produces higher energy x-rays more efficiently. Because a great deal of heat is produced at the target, the material should have a *high melting point* so as to avoid damage to the target surface. Most of the x-rays generated at the focal spot are directed downward and pass through the x-ray tube's *port window*. The cathode filament receives *low-voltage* current to heat it to the point of thermionic emission. Then *high voltage* is applied to drive the electrons across to the focal track. (*Selman, p 111*)

45. **(B)** Because the high-voltage transformer has a fixed ratio, there must be a means of changing the voltage sent to its primary coil; otherwise, there would be a fixed kVp. The autotransformer makes these changes possible. When kVp is selected on the control panel, the radiographer is actually adjusting the autotransformer and selecting the amount of voltage to send to the high-voltage transformer to be stepped up. The filament circuit supplies the proper current and voltage to the x-ray tube filament for proper thermionic emission. The rectifier circuit is responsible for changing AC to unidirectional current. (*Selman, pp 88–89*)

46. **(D)** Special units have been designed to accommodate examinations with high patient volume. Dedicated *chest* units are available that will transport a piece of unexposed film from the magazine into position between a pair

of intensifying screens, make a phototimed exposure, and transport the exposed film to the automatic processor. Dedicated head units are available for easy positioning of the skull, sinuses, mastoids, and so on. We are aware of the importance of high-quality mammographic examinations; dedicated *mammographic* units with molybdenum targets and other beneficial features are available. (*Saia, p 417*)

47. **(B)** The light image emitted from the output phosphor of the image intensifier is directed to the TV monitor for viewing and sometimes to recording devices such as a spot film camera or cine film. The light is directed to these places by a *beam splitter* or objective lens located between the output phosphor and the TV camera tube. The majority of the light will go to the recording device, while a small portion goes to the TV so that the procedure may continue to be monitored during filming. (*Selman, p 262*)

48. **(A)** The vast majority of target interactions involve the incident electrons and outer-shell tungsten electrons. No ionization occurs, and the energy loss is reflected in heat generation. The production of x-rays is an amazingly inefficient process: *More than 99% of the electrons'* kinetic energy is changed to *heat energy and less than 1% into x-ray* photon energy. This presents a serious heat buildup problem in the anode, as heat production is directly proportional to tube current. (*Selman, p 115*)

49. **(B)** *Inherent* filtration is that which is "built into" the construction of the x-ray tube. Before exiting the x-ray tube, x-ray photons must pass through the tube's glass envelope and port window; the photons are filtered somewhat as they do so. This inherent filtration is usually the equivalent of 0.5 mm Al. Aluminum filtration *placed* between the x-ray tube housing and the collimator is added to contribute to the total necessary requirement of 2.5 mm Al equivalent. The collimator itself is considered part of the *added filtration* (1.0 mm Al equivalent) because of the silver surface of the mirror within. It is important to remember that as aluminum filtration is added to the x-ray tube, the HVL increases. (*Selman, p 132*)

50. (D) The accuracy of all three is important to ensure adequate patient protection. *Reproducibility* means that repeated exposures at a given technique must provide consistent intensity. *Linearity* means that a given mAs, using different mA stations with appropriate exposure time adjustments, will provide consistent intensity. *PBL* is automatic collimation and must be accurate to 2% of the SID. Light-localized collimators must be available and must be accurate to within 2 percent. *(Bushong, p 462)*

51–52. (51, A; 52, B) Figure 5–3 illustrates the component parts of a rotating-anode x-ray tube enclosed within a glass envelope (number 3) to preserve the *vacuum* necessary for x-ray production. Number 8 is the rotating anode with its beveled focal track at the periphery and its *stem* (at number 5). Numbers 6 and 7 are the *stator* and *rotor*—the two components of an induction motor, whose function it is to rotate the anode. Number 1 is the filament of the cathode assembly, which is made of thoriated tungsten and functions to liberate electrons when heated to white hot. Number 2 is the molybdenum focusing cup, which functions to direct the filament electrons to the focal spot. *(Saia, p 424)*

53. (C) All circuit devices located before the primary coil of the high-voltage transformer are said to be on the primary or low-voltage side of the x-ray circuit. The timer, autotransformer, and (prereading) kV meter are all located in the low-voltage circuit. The mA meter, however, is connected at the midpoint of the secondary coil of the high-voltage transformer. When studying a diagram of the x-ray circuit, it will be noted that the mA meter is grounded at the midpoint of the secondary coil (where it is at zero potential). Therefore, it may be safely placed in the control panel. *(Selman, pp 150–151)*

54. (A) Parts being examined during fluoroscopic procedures change in thickness and density as the patient is required to change positions, and as the fluoroscope is moved to examine different regions of the body that have varying thickness and tissue densities. The *automatic*

brightness control functions to vary the required mAs and/or kVp as necessary. With this method, patient dose varies, and image quality is maintained. Minification and flux gain contribute to total brightness gain. *(Bushong, p 360)*

55. (B) One generally thinks in terms of moving grids being totally superior to stationary grids because moving grids function to blur the images of the lead strips on the radiographic image. Moving grids do, however, have several disadvantages. First, their complex mechanism is expensive and subject to malfunction. Second, today's sophisticated x-ray equipment makes possible the use of extremely short exposures, a valuable feature whenever motion may be a problem (as in pediatric radiography). However, grid mechanisms frequently are not able to oscillate rapidly enough for the short exposure times, and as a result the grid motion is "stopped" and the lead strips are imaged. Third, patient dose is increased with moving grids. Since the central ray is not always centered to the grid because it is in motion, lateral decentering occurs (resulting in diminished density), and consequently an increase in exposure is needed to compensate (either manually or via AEC). *(Shephard, p 249)*

56. (C) PACS refers to a picture archiving and communication system. *Analog* images (conventional images) can be digitized with a digitizer. *PACS* systems receive *digital* images and display them on monitors for interpretation. These systems also store images and allow their retrieval at a later time. PACS systems provide us with the option of a completely filmless radiology department. *(Shephard, pp 365–367)*

57. (B) HVL may be used to express the quality of an x-ray beam. *The HVL of a particular beam is that thickness of an absorber that will decrease the intensity of the beam to one half of its original value.* If the original intensity of the beam was 78 R/min, the first HVL will reduce it to 39 R/min, the second HVL will reduce it to 19.5 R/min, and the third HVL will reduce the intensity to 9.75 R/min. *(Bushong, p 52)*

58. (C) A double-focus tube has two focal spot sizes available. These focal spots are actually two *paths* available on the focal track. There are, however, two filaments. When the small focal spot is selected, the small filament is heated, and electrons are driven across to the smaller portion of the focal track. When the large focal spot is selected, the large filament is heated, and electrons are driven across to the larger portion of the focal track. *(Selman, p 137)*

59. **(C)** The lead strips of a focused grid are angled to correspond to the configuration of the divergent x-ray beam. Thus, any radiation that is changing direction, as is typical of scattered radiation, will be trapped by the lead foil strips. However, if the central ray and the grid center do not correspond, the lead strips will absorb primary radiation. The absorption of primary radiation is termed *cutoff* and results in diminished radiographic density. *(Carlton & Adler, pp 273–274)*

60. **(A)** With single-phase, full-wave–rectified equipment, the voltage drops to zero every 180° (of the AC waveform); that is, there is *100% voltage ripple.* With three-phase equipment, the voltage ripple is significantly smaller. Three-phase, 6-pulse equipment has a *13% voltage ripple,* and three-phase, 12-pulse equipment has only a *3.5% ripple.* Three-phase, 12-pulse equipment comes closest to constant potential, as the voltage never falls below 96.5% of maximum value. *(Selman, p 96)*

61. **(B)** When a spinning top is used to test the timer efficiency of full-wave–rectified single-phase equipment, the result is a *series of dots* or dashes, with each dot representing a pulse of radiation. With full-wave–rectified current and a possible 120 dots (pulses) available per second, one should visualize 12 dots at 1/10 second, 6 dots at 0.05 second, 10 dots at 1/12 second, and 3 dots at 0.025 second. Because three-phase equipment is at almost constant potential, a synchronous spinning top must be used for timer testing, and the result is a *solid arc* (rather than dots). The number of degrees covered by the arc is measured and equated to a particular exposure time. *(Saia, p 434)*

62. **(B)** There are two main types of mobile x-ray equipment: capacitor discharge and battery-powered. Although capacitor discharge units are light and therefore fairly easy to maneuver, the battery-powered mobile unit is very heavy (largely because it carries its heavy-duty power source). It is, however, capable of storing a large mAs capacity for extended periods of time. These units frequently have a capacity of 10,000 mAs, with 12 hours required for a full charge. *(Carlton & Adler, p 101)*

63. **(C)** The brightness gain of image intensifiers is 5000 to 20,000. This increase is accomplished in two ways. First, as the electron image is focused to the output phosphor, it is accelerated by high voltage (this is *flux gain*). Second, the output phosphor is only a fraction of the size of the input phosphor, and this decrease in image size represents another brightness gain, termed *minification gain. Total brightness gain is equal to the product of minification gain and flux gain. (Saia, p 244)*

64. **(B)** Given the milliamperage and exposure time, a radiographic rating chart enables the radiographer to determine the maximum safe kVp for a particular exposure. Because the heat load an anode will safely accept varies with the size of the focal spot and the type of rectification, these variables must be identified. Each x-ray tube has its own radiographic rating chart. The speed of the imaging system has no impact on the use of a radiographic rating chart. *(Selman, p 145)*

65. **(D)** Because mammography uses such low kVp levels, cassette–image receptor front material becomes especially important. Any attenuation of the beam by the image receptor front would be most undesirable. Low-attenuating carbon fibers or special plastics that resist impact and heat softening (eg, polystyrene and polycarbonate) are frequently used as image receptor front material. *(Carlton & Adler, p 585)*

66. **(D)** With *single-phase,* full-wave–rectified equipment, the voltage is constantly changing from 0% to 100% of its maximum value. It drops to 0 every 180° (of the AC waveform); that is, there is 100% voltage ripple. With *three-phase* equipment, the voltage ripple is significantly smaller. Three-phase, *six-pulse*

equipment has a 13% voltage ripple, and three-phase, *12-pulse* equipment has a 3.5% ripple. Therefore, *the voltage never falls below 87% to 96.5% of its maximum value with three-phase equipment,* and it closely approaches constant potential [direct current (DC)]. *(Carlton & Adler, pp 98–99)*

67. **(D)** Rectifiers (solid-state or the older valve tubes) permit the flow of current in only one direction. They serve to change AC, which is needed in the low-voltage side of the x-ray circuit, to unidirectional current. Unidirectional current is necessary for the efficient operation of the x-ray tube. *The rectification system is located between the secondary coil of the high-voltage transformer and the x-ray tube.* The *filament transformer* functions to adjust the voltage and current going to heat the x-ray tube filament. The *autotransformer* varies the amount of voltage being sent to the primary coil of the high-voltage transformer so that the appropriate kVp can be obtained. The *high-voltage transformer* "steps up" the voltage to the required kilovoltage and steps down the amperage to milliamperage. *(Carlton & Adler, p 78)*

68. **(B)** The collimator assembly includes a series of lead shutters, a mirror, and a light bulb. The mirror and light bulb function to project the size, location, and center of the irradiated field. The bulb's emitted beam of light is deflected by a mirror placed at an angle of 45° in the path of the light beam. *In order for the projected light beam to be the same size as the x-ray beam, the focal spot and the light bulb must be exactly the same distance from the center of the mirror. (Carlton & Adler, p 442)*

69. **(B)** The *input phosphor* of an image intensifier receives remnant radiation emerging from the patient and converts it to a fluorescent light image. Directly adjacent to the input phosphor is the *photocathode,* which is made of a photoemissive alloy (usually a cesium and antimony compound). The fluorescent light image strikes the photocathode and is converted to an electron image. The electrons are carefully focused, to maintain image resolution, by the *electrostatic focusing lenses,* through

the *accelerating anode* and to the *output phosphor* for conversion back to light. *(Carlton & Adler, p 537)*

70. **(D)** The spinning top test may be used to test timer accuracy in single-phase equipment. A spinning top is a metal disc with a small hole in its outer edge that is placed on a pedestal about 6 inches high. An exposure is made (eg, 0.1 second) while the top spins. Because a full-wave–rectified unit produces 120 x-ray photon impulses per second, in 0.1-second the film should record 12 dots (if the timer is accurate). Because three-phase equipment produces almost constant potential rather than pulsed radiation, the standard spinning top cannot be used. An oscilloscope or synchronous spinning top must be employed to test the timers of three-phase equipment. *(Selman, p 106)*

71. **(C)** Myelography requires that contrast media be instilled into the lumbar subarachnoid space and distributed via gravity to various levels of the subarachnoid space. This gravitational distribution is accomplished through the use of an x-ray table that is capable of angling or tilting during the procedure. *(Bontrager, p 734)*

72. **(C)** The visual apparatus that is responsible for visual acuity and contrast perception is the *cones* within the retina. Cones are also used for daylight vision. Therefore, the most desirable condition for fluoroscopic viewing is to have a bright enough image to permit cone (daylight) vision, for better detail perception. The image intensifier accomplishes this. The intensified image is then transferred to a TV monitor for viewing. Cine and spot film cameras record fluoroscopic events. *(Selman, pp 259–260)*

73. **(D)** Each time an x-ray exposure is made, less than 1% of the total energy is converted to x-rays, and the remainder (more than 99%!) of the energy is converted to heat. Thus, it is important to use target material with a high atomic number and high melting point. The larger the actual focal spot size, the larger the area over which the generated heat is spread and the more tolerant the x-ray tube is. Heat is particularly damaging to the target if it is

concentrated or limited to a small area. A target that rotates during the exposure is spreading the heat over a large area, the entire surface of the focal track. If the diameter of the anode is greater, the focal track will be longer and heat will be spread over an even larger area. (*Saia, p 225*)

74. **(B)** *Current* is defined as the amount of electric charge flowing per second. *Voltage* is the potential difference existing between two points. *Resistance* is the property of a circuit that opposes current flow. *Capacitance* describes a quantity of stored electricity. (*Selman, pp 46–47*)

75. **(D)** The thicker and more dense the anatomic part being studied, the less bright will be the fluoroscopic image. Both mA and kVp affect the fluoroscopic image in a way similar to the way in which they affect the radiographic image. For optimum contrast, especially taking patient dose into consideration, higher kVp and lower mA are generally preferred. (*Bushong, p 363*)

76. **(A)** The dynamics, or motion, of a part must be studied during a "real-time" examination such as *fluoroscopy* affords. *Stereoscopy* is a technique used to produce a radiographic third dimension. *Tomography* produces sectional images of body parts by blurring superimposed structures above and below the section, or level, of interest. A *phototimer* is one type of AEC device. (*Bushong, p 362*)

77. **(D)** Each time an x-ray exposure is made, heat is produced in the x-ray tube. Actually, of all the energy used to make an exposure, *99.8% is converted to heat* and only 0.2% is converted to x-ray photon energy. Since greater heat production leads to increased wear and tear on the x-ray tube, thereby decreasing its useful life, it behooves the radiographer to be able to calculate HU and to understand the means of keeping heat production to a minimum. HU for a *single-phase* x-ray unit are determined by using the formula HU = mA × kVp × time. HU for a *three-phase, six-pulse* x-ray unit are determined by using the formula: HU = mA × kVp × time × 1.35. HU for a *three-phase, 12-pulse* x-ray unit are determined by using the formula: HU =

mA × kVp × time × 1.41. High-mAs technical factors produce far more heat units than low-mAs technical factors. (*Carlton & Adler, p 125*)

78. **(B)** The high-voltage, or step-up, transformer functions to increase voltage to the necessary kilovoltage. It decreases the amperage to milliamperage. The amount of increase or decrease is dependent on the transformer ratio—the ratio of the number of turns in the primary coil to the number of turns in the secondary coil. The transformer law is as follows:

To determine secondary V,

$$\frac{V_s}{V_p} = \frac{N_s}{N_p}$$

To determine secondary I:

$$\frac{N_s}{N_p} = \frac{I_p}{I_s}$$

Substituting known factors,

$$\frac{x}{220} = \frac{35,000}{100}$$
$$100x = 7,700,000$$
$$x = 77,000 \text{ V (77 kVp)}$$

$$\frac{35,000}{100} = \frac{75}{x}$$
$$35,000x = 7500$$
$$x = 0.214 \text{ Amps (214 mA)}$$

(*Selman, pp 84–85*)

79. **(C)** Rare earth phosphors are not scarce; they are difficult to separate from other materials with which they are combined in the earth. Rare earth phosphors are much more efficient than calcium tungstate in absorbing x-ray photons and converting their energy into fluorescent light. Examples of rare earth phosphors are *gadolinium* oxysulfide and *lanthanum* oxybromide. *Cesium iodide* is the phosphor of preference for the input phosphor of an image intensifier. (*Selman, p 182*)

80. **(B)** The terms *star* and *wye* (or *delta*) refer to the configuration of transformer windings in three-phase equipment. Instead of having a

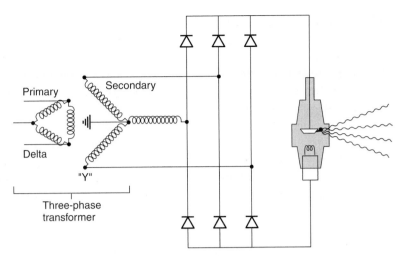

Figure 5–10. Reproduced with permission from Saia DA. *Radiography: Program Review and Examination Preparation,* 2nd ed. Stamford, CT: Appleton & Lange, 1999.

single primary coil and a single secondary coil, the high-voltage transformer has three primary and three secondary windings—one winding for each phase (see Fig. 5–10). Autotransformers operate on the principle of self-induction and have only one winding. Three-phase x-ray equipment often has three autotransformers. *(Selman, p 163)*

81. **(D)** The AEC automatically adjusts the exposure required for body parts that have different *thicknesses and densities.* Proper functioning of the phototimer depends on accurate positioning by the radiographer. The correct *photocell*(s) must be selected, and the anatomic part of interest must completely cover the photocell to achieve the desired density. If *collimation* is inadequate, and a field size larger than the part is used, excessive scattered radiation from the body or tabletop can cause the AEC to terminate the exposure prematurely, resulting in an underexposed radiograph. Backup time should always be selected on the manual timer to prevent patient overexposure and to protect the x-ray tube from excessive heat production should the AEC malfunction. Selection of the optimum kV for the part being radiographed is essential—no practical amount of mAs can make up for inadequate penetration (kV), and excessive kV can cause the AEC to terminate the exposure prematurely. *A technique chart is therefore strongly recommended for use with AEC; it should indicate the optimum kV*

for the part, the photocells that should be selected, and the backup time that should be set. (Carlton & Adler, p 508)

82. **(A)** Remnant radiation emerging from the patient causes fluorescence of the cassette's front intensifying screen. This fluorescent light not only exposes the adjacent film emulsion, but also can pass through the film base to the opposite emulsion. Because the fluorescent light diffuses as it travels to the opposite emulsion, there is a decrease in image sharpness. This occurrence, called crossover, is minimized by the incorporation of a light-absorbing dye in the active layer. *(Shephard, pp 73–74)*

83. **(D)** The rotating *anode* has a target (or focal spot) on its beveled edge, which forms the target angle. As the anode rotates, it constantly turns a new face to the incoming electrons; this is the focal track. That portion of the focal track that is bombarded by electrons is the actual focal spot, and because of the target's angle, the effective or projected focal spot is always smaller (line focus principle). The anode heel effect refers to decreased beam intensity at the anode end of the x-ray beam. The electrons impinging on the target have "boiled off" the *cathode* filament as a result of thermionic emission. *(Selman, pp 138–139)*

84–85. **(84, C; 85, A)** Figure 5–5 depicts the *line focus principle;* it illustrates that the *actual focal* *spot* (number 1) is always larger than the *effective*, or projected/apparent, focal spot (number 2). The actual focal spot is a finite area on the anode that is bombarded by electrons from the filament. Because of the anode's bevel, the effective focal spot is foreshortened and therefore is smaller than the actual focal spot. The anode heel effect has to do with the variation in intensity of the x-ray beam as it is emitted from the focus. The anode heel effect is more apparent with small anode angles. *(Selman, pp 138–139)*

86. **(B)** Mobile x-ray machines are compact and cordless and are either the battery-operated type or the condenser discharge type. *Condenser discharge* mobile x-ray units do not use batteries; this type mobile unit requires that it be charged before each exposure. A condenser (or capacitor) is a device that stores electrical energy. The stored energy is used to operate the x-ray tube only. Because this machine does not carry many batteries, it is much lighter and does not need a motor to drive or brake it. The major *disadvantage* of the capacitor/condenser discharge unit is that, as the capacitor discharges its electrical charge, the kVp gradually decreases throughout the length of the exposure—therefore limiting tube output and requiring recharging between exposures. *(Ballinger & Frank, vol 3, p 235)*

87. **(C)** There are two main types of mobile x-ray units: capacitor discharge and battery-powered. The capacitor discharge units consist of a capacitor, or condenser, which is given a charge and then stores energy until the x-ray tube uses it to produce x-rays. The charge may not be stored for extended periods, however, because it tends to "leak" away; the capacitor must be charged just before the exposure is made. Its x-ray tube is grid-controlled, permitting very fast (short) exposure times. Capacitors discharge a direct current (as opposed to single- or three-phase pulsating current) in which the kilovoltage decreases by a value of approximately 1 kV/mAs. Thus, although the value at the onset of the exposure may be 20 mAs and 80 kVp, at the end of the exposure the kV value will be approximately 60. In addition, capacitor discharge units permit only limited mAs values, usually 30 to 50 mAs per charge. *(Bushong, pp 123–124)*

88. **(D)** X-ray tube life may be extended by using exposure factors that produce a minimum of heat, that is, a lower mAs and higher kVp combination, whenever possible. When the rotor is activated, the filament current is increased to produce the required electron source (thermionic emission). Prolonged rotor time, then, can lead to shortened filament life as a result of early vaporization. Large exposures to a cold anode will heat the anode surface, and the big temperature difference can cause cracking of the anode. This can be avoided by proper warming of the anode prior to use, thereby allowing sufficient dispersion of heat through the anode. *(Selman, pp 143–145)*

89. **(C)** Most image intensifier tubes are either dual-field or trifield, indicating the diameter of the input phosphor. When a change to a smaller diameter mode is made, the voltage on the electrostatic focusing lenses is increased, and the result is a *magnified, but dimmer,* image. The milliamperage will automatically be increased to compensate for the loss in brightness with a magnified image, resulting in *higher patient dose in the smaller-diameter modes.* *(Bushong, p 363)*

90. **(B)** Off-focus, or extrafocal, radiation is produced as electrons strike metal surfaces other than the focal track and produce x-rays that emerge with the primary beam at a variety of angles. This radiation is responsible for indistinct images outside the collimated field. Mounting a pair of shutters as close to the source as possible minimizes off-focus radiation. *(Bushong, p 140)*

91. **(B)** There are three types of beam restrictors: aperture diaphragms, cones and cylinders, and collimators. The most practical and efficient type is the collimator. Its design makes available an infinite number of field size variations that are not available with the other types of beam restrictors. Because aperture diaphragms and flare cones have a fixed aperture size and shape, their beam restriction is not as efficient as that of the variable-size collimator. Aperture

diaphragms, cones, and cylinders may be placed on a collimator track so that the illuminated crosshairs are visualized. Although the collimator assembly contributes approximately 1.0 mm Al equivalent to the added filtration of the x-ray tube (because of the plastic exit portal and silver-coated reflective mirror), its functions are unrelated to the cleanup of scattered radiation. This is because the *patient* is the principal scatterer, and grids function to clean up scattered radiation generated by the patient. (*Bushong, pp 241–243*)

92. **(C)** A *phototimer* is one type of *AEC* that actually measures light. As x-ray photons penetrate and emerge from a part, a fluorescent screen beneath the image receptor glows, and the fluorescent light charges a photomultiplier tube. Once a predetermined charge has been reached, the exposure automatically terminates. A parallel-plate *ionization chamber* is another type of AEC. A radiolucent chamber is located beneath the patient (between the patient and the film). As photons emerge from the patient, they enter the chamber and ionize the air within it. Once a predetermined charge has been reached, the exposure is automatically terminated. Motion of magnetic fields inducing current in a conductor refers to the principle of mutual induction. (*Selman, pp 153–154*)

93. **(B)** The x-ray tube filament is made of thoriated tungsten. When heated to incandescence (white hot), the filament liberates electrons—a process called thermionic emission. It is these electrons that will become the tube current (mA). As heat is increased, more electrons are released and mA increases. (*Bushong, p 132*)

94. **(B)** When an AEC is installed in the x-ray circuit, it is calibrated to produce radiographic densities as required by the radiologist. Once the part being radiographed has been exposed to produce the correct film density, the AEC automatically terminates the exposure. The manual timer should be used as a backup timer; in case the AEC fails to terminate the exposure, the backup timer would protect the patient from overexposure and the x-ray tube from excessive heat load. The master density

is generally set on normal to produce the required densities. In special cases, when this produces excessive or insufficient density, the master density may be adjusted to plus or minus density. (*Selman, p 154*)

95. **(A)** *Magnification radiography* may be used to demonstrate small, delicate structures that are difficult to image with conventional radiography. Because object-image distance (OID) is an integral part of magnification radiography, the problem of magnification unsharpness arises. The use of a *fractional focal spot (0.3 mm or smaller)* is essential to the maintenance of image sharpness in magnification films. *Radiographic rating charts* should be consulted, as the heat load to the anode may be critical in magnification radiography. The long exposures typical of *image-intensified fluoroscopy* and *tomography* make the use of a fractional focal spot generally impractical and hazardous to the anode. (*Selman, p 226*)

96. **(C)** A radiographic rating chart enables the radiographer to determine the maximum safe mA, exposure time, and kVp for a given exposure using a particular x-ray tube. Because the heat load that an anode will safely accept varies with the size of the focal spot, type of rectification, and anode rotation, these variables must also be identified. Each x-ray tube has its own characteristics and its own rating chart. First, find the chart with the identifying single-phase sine wave in the upper right corner of the chart and the correct focal spot size in the upper left corner of the chart (chart C). Once the correct chart has been identified, locate 1/50 (0.02) second on the horizontal axis and follow its line up to where it intersects with the 300-mA curve. Then draw a line to where this point meets the vertical (kVp) axis; it meets at between 100 and 110 kVp, or approximately 107 kVp. This is the maximum permissible kVp exposure at the given mAs for this x-ray tube. The radiographer should always use somewhat less than the maximum exposure. This same procedure is followed to answer the next two questions. (*Selman, p 145*)

97. **(B)** Only x-ray tubes A and B, the three-phase-rectified x-ray tubes, will safely permit

this exposure. Locate 0.1 second on the horizontal axis and follow it up to where it intersects with the 400-mA curve. X-ray tube A will permit over 150 kVp safely, while x-ray tube B will safely permit only about 92 kVp. Notice the significant difference between the two, which is solely due to the difference in focal spot size! X-ray tube C will permit only about 75 kVp at the given mAs. (*Selman, p 145*)

98. **(C)** Find the correct chart for the three-phase, 2-mm focal spot x-ray tube. Locate 0.1 second on the horizontal (seconds) axis and follow it up to where it intersects with the 120-kVp line on the vertical (kVp) axis. They intersect midway between the 600- and 700-mA curves, at approximately 650 mA. Thus, 600 mA is the maximum safe milliamperage for this particular group of exposure factors and x-ray tube. (*Selman, p 145*)

99. **(B)** Each x-ray exposure made by the radiographer produces hundreds or thousands of heat units at the target. If the examination requires several consecutive exposures, the potential for extreme heat load is increased. Just as each x-ray tube has its own radiographic rating chart, each tube also has its own anode cooling curve to describe its unique heating and cooling characteristics. An x-ray tube generally cools most rapidly during the first 2 minutes of nonuse. First, note that the tube is saturated with heat at 300,000 HU. In order for another 160,000 HU to be safely applied, the x-ray tube must first release 160,000 HU, which means that it has to cool down at least to 140,000 HU. Find the 140,000 point on the vertical axis and follow across to where it intersects with the cooling curve. It intersects at about the 4-minute point. (*Selman, p 147*)

100. **(B)** The incident electron has a certain amount of energy as it approaches the tungsten target. If the positive nucleus of a tungsten atom attracts the electron, changing its course, a certain amount of energy is released during the "braking" action. This energy is given up in the form of an x-ray photon called *Bremsstrahlung ("braking") radiation. Characteristic radiation* is also produced at the target (less frequently) when an incident electron

ejects a K-shell electron, and an L-shell electron drops into its place. Energy is liberated in the form of a characteristic ray, and its energy is representative of the difference in energy levels. *Compton scatter* and the *photoelectric effect* are interactions between x-ray photons and tissue atoms. (*Selman, p 113*)

101. **(D)** As the anode angle is decreased (made steeper), a larger actual focal spot may be used, while still maintaining the same small effective focal spot. Because the actual focal spot is larger, it can accommodate a greater heat load. However, with steeper (smaller) anode angles, the anode heel effect is accentuated and can compromise film coverage. (*Selman, pp 138–139*)

102. **(A)** AECs are used in today's equipment and serve to produce consistent and comparable results. In one type of AEC, there is an ionization chamber beneath the tabletop above the image receptor. The part to be examined is centered to it (the sensor) and radiographed. When a predetermined quantity of ionization has occurred (equal to the correct density), the exposure automatically terminates. With the second type of AEC, the phototimer, a small fluorescent screen is positioned *beneath* the cassette. When remnant radiation emerging from the patient exposes the film and exits the cassette, the fluorescent screen emits light. Once a predetermined amount of fluorescent light has been "seen" by the photocell sensor, the exposure is automatically terminated. In either case, the manual timer should be used as a *backup timer;* in case of AEC malfunction, the exposure would terminate, thus avoiding patient overexposure and tube overload. (*Saia, p 244*)

103. **(C)** A large quantity of heat applied to a cold anode can cause enough surface heat to crack the anode. Excessive heat to the target can cause pitting or localized melting of the focal track. Localized melts can result in vaporized tungsten deposits on the glass envelope, which can cause a filtering effect, decreasing tube output. Excessive heat can also be conducted to the rotor bearings, causing increased friction and tube failure. (*Selman, p 146*)

104. (C) An *anode cooling curve* identifies how many HU the anode can accommodate and the length of time required for adequate cooling between exposures. A *radiographic rating chart* is used to determine if the selected mA, exposure time, and kVp are within safe tube limits. A *technique chart* is used to determine the correct exposure factors for a particular part of the body of a given thickness. A *spinning top test* is used to test for timer inaccuracy or rectifier failure. *(Selman, p 147)*

105. (C) The number of HU produced during a given exposure with single-phase equipment is determined by multiplying mA × time × kVp. Correction factors are required with three-phase equipment. Unless the equipment manufacturer specifies otherwise, HU for *three-phase, six-pulse* equipment are determined by multiplying mA × time × kVp × 1.35. HU for 3-phase, 12-pulse equipment are determined by multiplying mA × time × kVp × 1.41. *(Selman, pp 145–146)*

106. (A) Radiographic reproducibility is an important concept in producing high-quality diagnostic films. Radiographic results should be consistent and predictable, not only in terms of positioning accuracy, but with respect to exposure factors as well. AEC devices (phototimers and ionization chambers) automatically terminate the x-ray exposure once a predetermined quantity of x-rays has penetrated the patient, thus ensuring consistent results. *(Saia, p 443)*

107. (A) The spinning top test is used to test timer accuracy or rectifier operation. Because single-phase, full-wave–rectified current has 120 useful impulses per second, a 1-second exposure of the spinning top should demonstrate 120 dots. Therefore, a *0.05*-second exposure should demonstrate *six* dots. Anything more or less than that indicates that the time station needs calibration. If exactly *one half* of the expected number of dots appears, one should suspect *rectifier* failure. *(Saia, p 444)*

108. (A) Because using the master control's minus-density adjustment involves decreasing the exposure time (and this is not possible), this adjustment will be ineffective. Decreasing the kVp will produce a change in radiographic contrast. Because too long an exposure time results in excessive density, the best way to compensate is to decrease the milliamperage. *(Carlton & Adler, p 105; Shephard, p 286)*

109. (C) The cassette is used to support the intensifying screens and x-ray film. It should be strong and should provide good screen–film contact. The cassette front should be made of a sturdy material with a low atomic number, because attenuation of the remnant beam is undesirable. Bakelite (the forerunner of today's plastics) and magnesium (the lightest structural metal) are the materials most commonly used for cassette fronts. The high atomic number of tungsten makes it inappropriate as a cassette front material. *(Shephard, p 41)*

110. (A) AECs were originally developed to achieve more consistent and reproducible film densities. This consistency reduces the number of retakes, thereby reducing patient exposure dose. The two AECs that are most commonly used employ either a *photomultiplier* tube or an *ion* (or ionization) *chamber*. The ion chamber is positioned between the table and the cassette, whereas the photomultiplier is located below the cassette (Fig. 5–11). *(Shephard, pp 275–276)*

111. (A) Mobile x-ray machines are smaller and more compact than their fixed counterparts in the radiology department. It is important that they be relatively easy to move, that their size allows entry into patient rooms, and that their locks enable securing of the x-ray tube into the required positions. Mobile x-ray machines are cordless and are either the battery-operated type or the condenser discharge type. *Condenser discharge* mobile x-ray units do not use batteries; this type mobile unit requires that it be charged before each exposure. A condenser (or capacitor) is a device that stores electrical energy. The stored energy is used to operate the x-ray tube only. Because this machine does not carry many batteries, it is much lighter and does not need a motor to drive or brake it. The major disadvantage of the capacitor/condenser discharge unit is

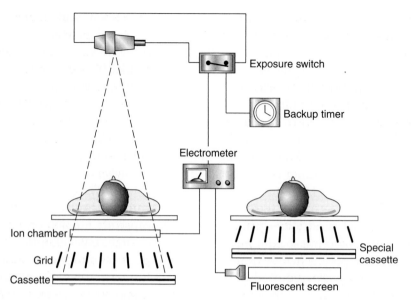

Figure 5–11. Reproduced with permission from Saia DA. *Radiography: Program Review and Examination Preparation,* 2nd ed. Stamford, CT: Appleton & Lange, 1999.

that, as the capacitor discharges its electrical charge, the kVp gradually decreases throughout the length of the exposure, hence, the need for recharging between exposures. (*Ballinger & Frank, vol 3, p 235*)

112. **(B)** When a spinning top is used to test the efficiency of a *single-phase* timer, the result is a *series of dots* or dashes, with each representing a pulse of radiation. With full-wave–rectified current and a possible 120 dots (pulses) available per second, one should visualize 12 dots at 1/10 second, 24 dots at 1/5 second, 6 dots at 1/20 second, and so on. However, because *three-phase* equipment is at almost constant potential, a synchronous spinning top must be used, and the result is a *solid arc* (rather than dots). The number of degrees taken up by the arc is measured and equated to a particular exposure time. A multitude of small, meshlike squares describes a screen contact test. An aluminum step wedge (penetrometer) may be used to demonstrate the effect of kVp on contrast (demonstrating a series of gray tones from white to black), with a greater number of grays demonstrated at higher kVp levels. (*Saia, p 434*)

113. **(C)** The AEC automatically terminates the exposure when the proper density has been recorded on the film. The important advan-

tage of the phototimer, then, is that it can accurately duplicate radiographic densities. It is very useful in providing accurate comparison in follow-up examinations, and in decreasing patient exposure dose by reducing the number of "retakes" needed because of improper exposure. The AEC automatically adjusts the exposure required for body parts with different *thicknesses and densities.* However, proper functioning of the phototimer depends on accurate positioning by the radiographer. The correct *photocell*(s) must be selected, and the anatomic part of interest must completely cover the photocell to achieve the desired density. If *collimation* is inadequate and a field size larger than the part is used, excessive scattered radiation from the body or tabletop can cause the AEC to terminate the exposure prematurely, resulting in an underexposed radiograph. (*Carlton & Adler, pp 503–506*)

114. **(A)** The image intensifier's input phosphor receives the remnant beam from the patient and converts it to a fluorescent light image. To maintain resolution, the input phosphor is made of cesium iodide crystals. *Cesium iodide* is much more efficient in this conversion process than was the phosphor previously used, zinc cadmium sulfide. Calcium tungstate was the phosphor used in cassette intensifying screens for many years prior to the development of rare earth phosphors such as gadolinium oxy-sulfide. *(Bushong, p 360)*

115. **(D)** The greater the *number of electrons* making up the electron stream and bombarding the target, the greater the number of x-ray photons produced. Although kV is usually associated with the energy of the x-ray photons, because *a greater number of more energetic electrons* will produce more x-ray photons, an increase in kV will also increase the *number* of photons produced. Specifically, the quantity of radiation produced increases as the *square* of the kilovoltage. The material composition of the tube target also plays an important role in the number of x-ray photons produced. The higher the *atomic number* of this material, the denser and more closely packed the atoms making up the material are, and therefore the greater the chance of an interaction between a high-speed electron and the target material. *(Bushong, p 132)*

116. **(A)** A *parallel-plate ionization chamber* is a type of AEC. A radiolucent chamber is beneath the patient (between the patient and the film). As photons emerge from the patient, they enter the chamber and ionize the air within it. Once a predetermined charge has been reached, the exposure is automatically terminated. *(Carlton & Adler, pp 503–506)*

117. **(D)** Vaporized tungsten may be deposited on the inner surface of the glass envelope at the tube (port) window. It acts as an *additional filter*, thereby *reducing tube output*. The tungsten deposit may also attract electrons from the filament, *creating sparking* and *causing puncture* of the glass envelope and subsequent tube failure. *(Selman, pp 137–138)*

118. **(B)** The image intensifier's input phosphor receives the remnant radiation emerging from the patient and converts it into a fluorescent light image. Very close to the input phosphor, separated by a thin transparent layer, is the photocathode. The photocathode is made of a photoemissive alloy, usually an antimony and cesium compound. The fluorescent light image strikes the photocathode and is converted to an electron image that is focused by the electrostatic lenses to the output phosphor. *(Bushong, p 360)*

119. **(B)** The principle of self-induction is an example of the second law of electromagnetics (Lenz's law), which states that an induced current within a conductive coil will oppose the direction of the current that induced it. It is important to note that self-induction is a characteristic of AC *only*. The fact that AC is constantly changing direction accounts for the opposing current set up in the coil. Two x-ray circuit devices operate on the principle of self-induction. The *autotransformer* operates on the principle of self-induction and enables the radiographer to vary the kilovoltage. The *choke coil* also operates on the principle of self-induction; it is a type of variable resistor that may be used to regulate filament current. The high-voltage transformer operates on the principle of mutual induction. *(Selman, p 89)*

120. **(D)** DXA imaging is used to evaluate bone mineral density (BMD). It is the most widely used method of *bone densitometry*—it is *low dose, preceise,* and *uncomplicated* to use/perform. DXA uses *two photon energies*—one for soft tissue and one for bone. Since bone is more dense and attenuates x-ray photons more readily, their *attenuation is calculated* to represent the degree of bone density. Bone densitometry, DXA, can be used to evaluate bone mineral content of the body, or part of it, to diagnosis osteoporosis or to evaluate the effectiveness of treatments for osteoporosis. *(Ballinger & Frank, vol 3, pp 488–489)*

Subspecialty List

56. Radiographic equipment
57. Principles of radiation physics
58. Radiographic equipment
59. Radiographic equipment
60. Radiographic equipment
61. Radiographic equipment
62. Radiographic equipment
63. Radiographic equipment
64. Quality control of radiographic equipment and accessories
65. Quality control of radiographic equipment and accessories
66. Radiographic equipment
67. Radiographic equipment
68. Quality control of radiographic equipment and accessories
69. Radiographic equipment
70. Fluoroscopic unit
71. Radiographic equipment
72. Radiographic equipment
73. Quality control of radiographic equipment and accessories
74. Principles of radiation physics
75. Radiographic equipment
76. Radiographic equipment
77. Radiographic equipment
78. Radiographic equipment
79. Radiographic equipment
80. Radiographic equipment
81. Radiographic equipment
82. Radiographic equipment
83. Principles of radiation physics
84. Radiographic equipment
85. Radiographic equipment
86. Radiographic equipment
87. Radiographic equipment
88. Radiographic equipment
89. Radiographic equipment
90. Principles of radiation physics
91. Radiographic equipment
92. Radiographic equipment
93. Radiographic equipment
94. Radiographic equipment
95. Radiographic equipment
96. Radiographic equipment
97. Radiographic equipment
98. Radiographic equipment
99. Radiographic equipment
100. Principles of radiation physics
101. Radiographic equipment
102. Radiographic equipment
103. Quality control of radiographic equipment and accessories
104. Quality control of radiographic equipment and accessories
105. Quality control of radiographic equipment and accessories
106. Radiographic equipment
107. Quality control of radiographic equipment and accessories
108. Radiographic equipment
109. Radiographic equipment
110. Radiographic equipment
111. Radiographic equipment
112. Quality control of radiographic equipment and accessories
113. Radiographic equipment
114. Radiographic equipment
115. Principles of radiation physics
116. Radiographic equipment
117. Radiographic equipment
118. Radiographic equipment
119. Radiographic equipment
120. Radiographic equipment

Practice Test 1
Questions

DIRECTIONS (Questions 1 through 200): Each of the numbered items or incomplete statements in this section is followed by answers or by completions of the statement. Select the *one* lettered answer or completion that is *best* in each case.

1. In the 15° medial oblique projection of the ankle, the

    1. tibiofibular joint is visualized.
    2. talotibial joint is visualized.
    3. plantar surface should be vertical.

    (A) 1 only
    (B) 1 and 2 only
    (C) 2 and 3 only
    (D) 1, 2, and 3

2. Techniques that function to reduce the spread of microbes are termed

    (A) surgical asepsis.
    (B) medical asepsis.
    (C) sterilization.
    (D) disinfection.

3. Which of the lines indicated in Figure 6–1 correctly demonstrates the relationship between the exposure received by the PSP and its resulting luminescence as it is laser scanned?

    (A) line A is representative of PSP exposure.
    (B) Line B is representative of PSP exposure.
    (C) neither line is representative of PSP exposure.
    (D) both lines are representative of PSP exposure.

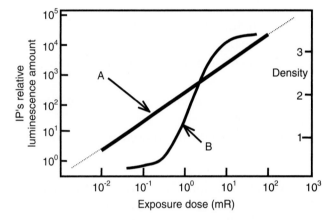

Figure 6–1. Courtesy FUJIFILM Medical Systems USA, Inc.

4. An automatic exposure control device can operate on which of the following principles?

    1. A photomultiplier tube charged by a fluorescent screen
    2. A parallel-plate ionization chamber charged by x-ray photons
    3. Motion of magnetic fields inducing current in a conductor

    (A) 1 only
    (B) 2 only
    (C) 1 and 2 only
    (D) 1, 2, and 3

5. As the CR laser scanner recognizes various tissue densities, it constructs a graphic representation of pixel value distribultion called a

    (A) processing algorithm
    (B) histogram
    (C) lookup table
    (D) exposure index

6. An accurately positioned oblique projection of the first through fourth lumbar vertebrae will demonstrate the classic "scotty dog." What bony structure does the scotty dog's neck represent?

   (A) Superior articular process
   (B) Pedicle
   (C) Transverse process
   (D) Pars interarticularis

7. The function of the developer solution chemicals is to

   (A) reduce the manifest image to a latent image.
   (B) increase production of silver halide crystals.
   (C) reduce the latent image to a manifest image.
   (D) remove the unexposed crystals from the film.

8. Which of the following barium-filled anatomic structures is best demonstrated in the left anterior oblique (LAO) position?

   (A) Hepatic flexure
   (B) Splenic flexure
   (C) Sigmoid colon
   (D) Iliocecal valve

9. The AP projection of the sacrum requires the central ray to be directed

   (A) perpendicular to the midline midway between the anterior superior iliac spine (ASIS) and the pubis.
   (B) to the midline approximately 2 inches superior to the pubis.
   (C) 15° cephalad to a point approximately 2 inches superior to the pubis.
   (D) 15° caudad to a point approximately 2 inches superior to the pubis.

10. Which of the following dose–response curve characteristics represent genetic and some somatic responses to radiation?

    1. Linear
    2. Nonthreshold
    3. Sigmoidal

    (A) 1 only
    (B) 1 and 2 only
    (C) 1 and 3 only
    (D) 1, 2, and 3

11. Which of the following procedures requires that contrast medium be injected into the ureters?

    (A) Cystogram
    (B) Urethrogram
    (C) Retrograde pyelogram
    (D) Cystourethrogram

12. The *rad* is the unit of

    (A) radiation dose.
    (B) exposure.
    (C) dose equivalent.
    (D) ionization in air.

13. Which of the following combinations would pose the *most* hazard to a particular anode?

    (A) 0.6 mm focal spot, 75 kVp, 30 mAs
    (B) 0.6 mm focal spot, 85 kVp, 15 mAs
    (C) 1.2 mm focal spot, 75 kVp, 30 mAs
    (D) 1.2 mm focal spot, 85 kVp, 15 mAs

14. Which of the following structures is best demonstrated in Figure 6–2?

    (A) Sigmoid colon
    (B) Splenic flexure
    (C) Hepatic flexure
    (D) Rectosigmoid

15. The radiograph seen in Figure 6–2 was made in which of the following positions?

    (A) Anatomical position (AP) recumbent
    (B) Right lateral decubitus
    (C) RPO
    (D) RAO

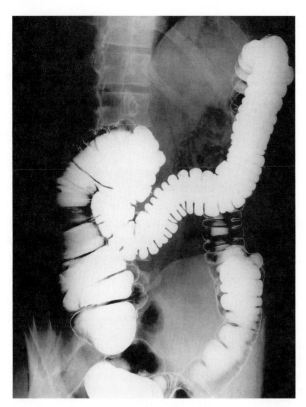

Figure 6–2. Courtesy of Stamford Hospital, Department of Radiology.

16. How can the radiographer reduce the amount of scattered radiation generated during a radiographic examination?

    1. Use optimum kVp.
    2. Collimate closely.
    3. Use a grid.

    (A) 1 only
    (B) 1 and 2 only
    (C) 1 and 3 only
    (D) 1, 2, and 3

17. Federal regulations regarding infection control in the workplace, as amended by the Occupational Safety and Health Administration (OSHA), make the following requirements:

    1. Hepatitis B immunizations must be made available to all hospital employees.
    2. puncture proof containers must be provided for all used needles.
    3. follow-up care must be provided to any staff accidentially exposed to blood splach/needle stick.

    (A) 1 only
    (B) 1 and 2 only
    (C) 2 and 3 only
    (D) 1, 2, and 3

18. A minor reaction to the intravenous (IV) administration of a contrast agent can include

    1. a few hives.
    2. nausea.
    3. flushed face.

    (A) 1 only
    (B) 1 and 2 only
    (C) 1 and 3 only
    (D) 1, 2, and 3

19. An emetic is used to

    (A) induce vomiting.
    (B) stimulate defecation.
    (C) promote elimination of urine.
    (D) inhibit coughing.

20. The presence of dust or scratches on intensifying screens will cause

    (A) decreased density in those areas of the image.
    (B) increased density in those areas of the image.
    (C) decreased density in all areas of the image.
    (D) increased density in all areas of the image.

21. Which of the following is (are) features of fluoroscopic equipment that are designed especially to eliminate unnecessary radiation to
patient and personnel?

1. Protective curtain
2. Filtration
3. Collimation

(A) 1 only
(B) 1 and 2 only
(C) 1 and 3 only
(D) 1, 2, and 3

22. Which of the following will best demonstrate
the lumbosacral junction in the AP position?

(A) CR perpendicular to L3
(B) CR perpendicular to L5–S1
(C) CR caudad 30° to 35°
(D) CR cephalad 30° to 35°

23. Which interaction between x-ray photons and
matter results in total absorption of the incident photon?

(A) Photoelectric effect
(B) Compton scattering
(C) Coherent scattering
(D) Pair production

24. During endoscopic retrograde cholangiopancreatography (ERCP) examination, contrast
medium is injected into the

(A) hepatic duct.
(B) cystic duct.
(C) pancreatic duct.
(D) common bile duct.

25. How can object-image distance (OID) be reduced for a posteroanterior (PA) projection of
the wrist?

(A) Extend the fingers.
(B) Flex the metacarpophalangeal joints.
(C) Extend the forearm.
(D) Oblique the metacarpals 45°.

26. A grid is usually employed

1. when radiographing a large or dense body
part.
2. when using high kilovoltage.
3. when less patient dose is required.

(A) 1 only
(B) 3 only
(C) 1 and 2 only
(D) 1, 2, and 3

27. Which of the following is the factor of choice
for the regulation of radiographic (optical)
density?

(A) kVp
(B) mAs
(C) SID
(D) Filtration

28. The image seen in Figure 6–3 exhibits

(A) adhesive tape artifact.
(B) quantum mottle.
(C) insufficient optical density.
(D) motion.

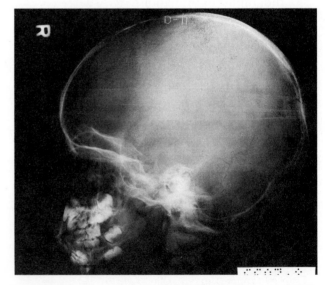

Figure 6–3. From the American College of Radiology Learning File.
Courtesy of the ACR.

29. Terms that refer to shape distortion include

    1. foreshortening.
    2. attenuation.
    3. elongation.

    (A) 1 only
    (B) 1 and 2 only
    (C) 1 and 3 only
    (D) 1, 2, and 3

30. The function of the 5-minute fluoroscopy timer is to

    (A) alert the fluoroscopist that 5 minutes has elapsed.
    (B) terminate the procedure.
    (C) alert the technologist to reload the camera.
    (D) signal completion of the examination.

31. The *control* dosimeter that comes from the monitoring company should be

    (A) stored in a radiation-free area.
    (B) kept in a designated control booth.
    (C) kept in the film processing area.
    (D) used as an extra badge for new personnel.

32. Which of the following is the preferred scheduling sequence?

    (A) Lower GI, abdomen ultrasound, upper GI
    (B) Abdomen ultrasound, lower GI, upper GI
    (C) Abdomen ultrasound, upper GI, lower GI
    (D) Upper GI, lower GI, abdomen ultrasound

33. The RAO position is used to project the sternum to the left of the thoracic vertebrae in order to take advantage of

    (A) pulmonary markings.
    (B) heart shadow.
    (C) posterior ribs.
    (D) costal cartilages.

34. How would the introduction of a 6-inch OID affect image contrast?

    (A) Contrast would be increased.
    (B) Contrast would be decreased.
    (C) Contrast would not change.
    (D) The scale of contrast would not change.

35. A patient is being positioned for a particular radiographic examination. The x-ray tube, image recorder, and grid are properly aligned, but the body part is angled. Which of the following will result?

    (A) Grid cutoff at the periphery of the image
    (B) Grid cutoff along the center of the image
    (C) Increased density at the periphery
    (D) Image distortion

36. Rapid onset of severe respiratory or cardio-vascular symptoms after ingestion or injection of a drug, vaccine, contrast agent, or food, or after an insect bite, *best* describes

    (A) asthma.
    (B) anaphylaxis.
    (C) myocardial infarct.
    (D) rhinitis.

37. If your patient is unable to stay erect for a paranasal sinus examination, which of the following alternatives should be chosen?

    (A) Recumbent AP
    (B) Lateral recumbent
    (C) Lateral cross-table recumbent
    (D) Recumbent Waters'

38. The right anterior oblique of the cervical spine requires which of the following combinations of tube angle and direction?

    (A) 15° to 20° caudad
    (B) 15° to 20° cephalad
    (C) 25° to 30° caudad
    (D) 25° to 30° cephalad

39. The patient is usually required to drink barium sulfate suspension in order to demonstrate which of the following structure(s)?

1. Cecum
2. Ilium
3. Stomach

(A) 1 and 2 only
(B) 1 and 3 only
(C) 2 and 3 only
(D) 3 only

40. All of the following have an effect on patient dose *except*

(A) inherent filtration.
(B) added filtration.
(C) SID.
(D) focal spot size.

41. Which of the following positions would *best* demonstrate the left apophyseal articulations of the lumbar vertebrae?

(A) LPO
(B) RPO
(C) Left lateral
(D) PA

42. The National Council on Radiation Protection and Measurements (NCRP) has recommended what total equivalent dose limit to the embryo/fetus?

(A) 0.05 rem
(B) 0.5 rem
(C) 50 mrem
(D) 5000 mrem

43. Fluids and medications are administered to patients intravenously for which of the following reasons?

1. To promote rapid response
2. To administer parenteral nutrition
3. To achieve a local effect

(A) 1 only
(B) 1 and 2 only
(C) 1 and 3 only
(D) 1, 2, and 3

44. Occupational exposure received by the radiographer is mostly from

(A) Compton scatter.
(B) the photoelectric effect.
(C) coherent scatter.
(D) pair production.

45. To maintain image clarity, the path of electron flow from photocathode to output phosphor is controlled by

(A) the accelerating anode.
(B) electrostatic lenses.
(C) the vacuum glass envelope.
(D) the input phosphor.

46. Which of the following positions will move the fundus of the gallbladder seen in Figure 6–4 away from the superimposed transverse process?

(A) RAO
(B) LAO
(C) LPO
(D) Left lateral decubitus

47. The processor rollers that are out of solution and function to transfer the film from one solution to another are the

(A) deflector plates.
(B) guide shoes.
(C) crossover rollers.
(D) turnaround assembly.

48. Examples of primary radiation barriers include

1. radiographic room walls.
2. lead aprons.
3. radiographic room floor.

(A) 1 only
(B) 1 and 2 only
(C) 1 and 3 only
(D) 1, 2, and 3

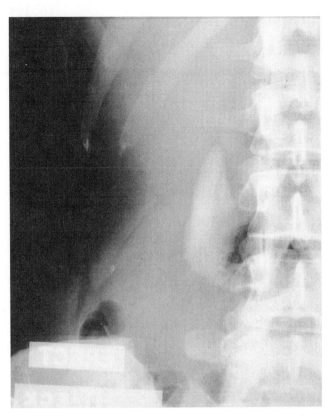

Figure 6–4. From the American College of Radiology Learning File. Courtesy of the ACR.

49. Which of the following can affect histogram appearance?

1. Centering accuracy
2. Positioning accuracy
3. Processing algorithm accuracy

(A) 1 only
(B) 1 and 2 only
(C) 2 and 3 only
(D) 1, 2, and 3

50. Bone densitometry is often performed to

1. measure degree of bone (de)-mineralization.
2. evaluate results of osteoporosis treatment/therapy.
3. evaluate condition of soft tissue adjacent to bone.

(A) 1 only
(B) 1 and 2 only
(C) 2 and 3 only
(D) 1, 2, and 3

51. Indirect modes of disease transmission include

1. airborne.
2. fomite.
3. vector.

(A) 1 only
(B) 1 and 2 only
(C) 1 and 3 only
(D) 1, 2, and 3

52. If a patient received 2000 mrad during a 10-minute fluoroscopic examination, what was the dose rate?

(A) 0.02 rad/min
(B) 0.2 rad/min
(C) 2.0 rad/min
(D) 20 rad/min

53. The legal doctrine *respondeat superior* relates to which of the following?

(A) Let the master answer.
(B) The thing speaks for itself.
(C) A thing or matter settled by justice.
(D) A matter settled by precedent.

54. The total number of x-ray photons produced at the target is contingent upon the

1. tube current.
2. target material.
3. square of the kilovoltage.

(A) 1 only
(B) 1 and 2 only
(C) 2 and 3 only
(D) 1, 2, and 3

55. Each of the following statements regarding respiratory structures is true *except*

(A) the left lung has two lobes.
(B) the lower portion of the lung is the base.
(C) each lung is enclosed in peritoneum.
(D) the mainstem bronchus enters the lung hilum.

56. In order for a phosphor to be suitable for use in intensifying screens, it should have which of the following characteristics?

    1. High conversion efficiency
    2. High x-ray absorption
    3. High atomic number

    (A) 1 only
    (B) 3 only
    (C) 1 and 2 only
    (D) 1, 2, and 3

57. An acute infection of the lungs is called

    (A) atelectasis.
    (B) pneumothorax.
    (C) pneumonia.
    (D) COPD.

58. If the exposure rate at 2.0 meters from a source of radiation is 18 R/min, what will be the exposure rate at 5 meters from the source?

    (A) 2.8 mR/min
    (B) 4.5 mR/min
    (C) 18 mR/min
    (D) 85 mR/min

59. Which of the following will reduce patient dose during fluoroscopy?

    1. Decreasing the source-skin distance (SSD)
    2. Using 2.5 mm Al filtration
    3. Restricting tabletop intensity to less than 10 R/min

    (A) 1 only
    (B) 1 and 2 only
    (C) 2 and 3 only
    (D) 1, 2, and 3

60. An axial projection of the clavicle is often helpful in demonstrating a fracture that is not visualized using a perpendicular central ray. When examining the clavicle in the AP position, how is the central ray directed for the axial projection?

    (A) Cephalad
    (B) Caudad
    (C) Medially
    (D) Laterally

61. An exposure was made using 600 mA, 0.04-second exposure, and 85 kVp. Each of the following changes will serve to decrease the radiographic density by one half *except* change to

    (A) 1/50-second exposure.
    (B) 72 kVp.
    (C) 18 mAs.
    (D) 300 mA.

62. The medical term used to describe the expectoration of blood is

    (A) hematemesis.
    (B) hemoptysis.
    (C) hematuria.
    (D) epistaxis.

63. Which of the following is (are) accurate positioning or evaluation criteria for an anteroposterior projection of the normal knee?

    1. Femorotibial interspaces equal bilaterally
    2. Patella superimposed on distal tibia
    3. CR enters 1/2 in distal to base of patella

    (A) 1 only
    (B) 1 and 2 only
    (C) 1 and 3 only
    (D) 1, 2, and 3

64. The focal spot–to–table distance in mobile fluoroscopy must

    (A) be at least 15 inches.
    (B) not exceed 15 inches.
    (C) be at least 12 inches.
    (D) not exceed 12 inches.

65. Which of the following structures will usually contain air, in the PA position on a sthenic patient, during a double-contrast upper GI (UGI) examination?

(A) Duodenal bulb
(B) Descending duodenum
(C) Pyloric vestibule
(D) Gastric fundus

66. If the quantity of black metallic silver on a particular radiograph is such that it allows 1% of the illuminator light to pass through the image, that image has a density of

(A) 0.01.
(B) 0.1.
(C) 1.0.
(D) 2.0.

67. The condition of below-normal blood pressure is termed

(A) hyperthermia.
(B) hypotension.
(C) hypoxia.
(D) bradycardia.

68. A "blowout fracture" usually occurs in which aspect of the orbital wall?

(A) Superior
(B) Inferior
(C) Medial
(D) Lateral

69. What is the name of the structure indicated as number 4 in Figure 6–5?

(A) Lunate
(B) Hamate
(C) Triquetrum
(D) Scaphoid

70. What position was required to obtain the image seen in Figure 6–5?

(A) Radial flexion/deviation
(B) Ulnar flexion/deviation
(C) Semipronation oblique
(D) Semisupination oblique

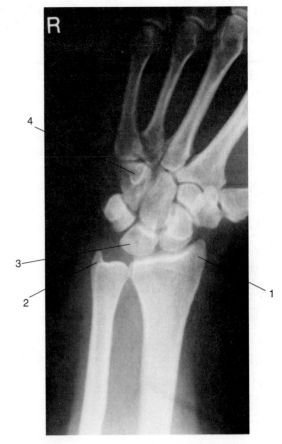

Figure 6–5. Courtesy of Stamford Hospital, Department of Radiology.

71. The condition in which pulmonary alveoli lose their elasticity and become permanently inflated, causing the patient to consciously exhale, is

(A) bronchial asthma.
(B) bronchitis.
(C) emphysema.
(D) tuberculosis.

72. Tungsten alloy is the usual choice of target material for radiographic equipment because it

1. has a high atomic number.
2. has a high melting point.
3. can readily dissipate heat.

(A) 1 only
(B) 1 and 2 only
(C) 2 and 3 only
(D) 1, 2, and 3

73. The portion of a hypodermic needle that attaches to the syringe is termed its

    (A) hub.
    (B) gauge.
    (C) length.
    (D) bevel.

74. If 92 kV and 12 mAs were used for a particular abdominal exposure with single-phase equipment, what mAs would be required to produce a similar radiograph with three-phase, six-pulse equipment?

    (A) 36
    (B) 24
    (C) 8
    (D) 6

75. Gonadal shielding should be provided for male patients in which of the following examinations?

    1. Femur
    2. Abdomen
    3. Pelvis

    (A) 1 only
    (B) 1 and 2 only
    (C) 2 and 3 only
    (D) 1, 2, and 3

76. The image intensifier's input phosphor differs from the output phosphor in that the input phosphor

    (A) is much larger than the output phosphor.
    (B) emits electrons whereas the output phosphor emits light photons.
    (C) absorbs electrons whereas the output phosphor absorbs light photons.
    (D) is a fixed size, and the size of the output phosphor can vary.

77. Which of the two sensitometric curves shown in Figure 6–6 requires more exposure to produce a density of 2.0 on the finished radiograph?

    (A) Image 1
    (B) Image 2

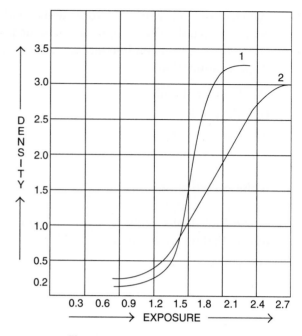

Figure 6–6. Courtesy of David Perri.

78. Which of the following pathologic conditions require(s) a decrease in exposure factors?

    1. Pneumothorax
    2. Emphysema
    3. Multiple myeloma

    (A) 1 only
    (B) 1 and 2 only
    (C) 2 and 3 only
    (D) 1, 2, and 3

79. Which of the following projections require(s) that the shoulder be placed in external rotation?

    1. AP humerus
    2. Lateral forearm
    3. Lateral humerus

    (A) 1 only
    (B) 1 and 2 only
    (C) 2 and 3 only
    (D) 1, 2, and 3

80. In which section of the automatic processor seen in Figure 6–7 are the exposed silver halide crystals changed to black metallic silver?

(A) Section 1

(B) Section 2

(C) Section 3

(D) Section 4

81. It is essential to question female patients of childbearing age regarding the

1. date of their last menstrual period.
2. possibility of their being pregnant.
3. number of x-ray examinations they have had in the past 12 months.

(A) 1 only

(B) 1 and 2 only

(C) 1 and 3 only

(D) 1, 2, and 3

82. Geometric unsharpness is influenced by which of the following?

1. Distance from object to image
2. Distance from focus to object
3. Distance from focus to image

(A) 1 only

(B) 1 and 2 only

(C) 1 and 3 only

(D) 1, 2, and 3

83. Which of the following adult radiographic examinations usually require(s) use of a grid?

1. Ribs
2. Vertebrae
3. Shoulder

(A) 1 only

(B) 1 and 2 only

(C) 1 and 3 only

(D) 1, 2, and 3

84. Which of the following radiologic examinations would deliver the greatest entrance skin exposure (ESE)?

(A) Chest

(B) Skull

(C) Abdomen

(D) Thoracic spine

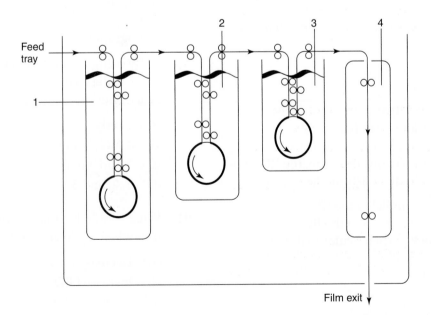

Figure 6–7. Reproduced with permission from Saia DA. *Radiography: Program Review and Examination Preparation,* 2nd ed. Stamford, CT: Appleton & Lange, 1999.

85. Combinations of milliamperage and exposure time that produce a particular mAs will produce identical radiographic density. This statement is an expression of the

    (A) inverse square law.
    (B) line focus principle.
    (C) reciprocity law.
    (D) *D* log E curve.

86. If single-emulsion film was loaded into its cassette with the emulsion facing away from the intensifying screen, the resulting image would demonstrate

    (A) decreased density.
    (B) increased density.
    (C) crossover.
    (D) fog.

87. Which of the following is (are) well demonstrated in the oblique position of the cervical vertebrae?

    1. Intervertebral foramina
    2. Disk spaces
    3. Apophyseal joints

    (A) 1 only
    (B) 1 and 2 only
    (C) 1 and 3 only
    (D) 1, 2, and 3

88. When medications are administered *parenterally*, they are given

    (A) orally.
    (B) orally or intravenously.
    (C) intravenously or intramuscularly.
    (D) by any route other than orally.

89. During an intravenous urogram, the RPO position is used to demonstrate the

    1. left kidney parallel to the IR.
    2. right kidney parallel to the IR.
    3. right kidney perpendicular to the IR.

    (A) 1 only
    (B) 2 only
    (C) 1 and 2 only
    (D) 1 and 3 only

90. A star pattern is used to measure

    1. focal spot resolution.
    2. intensifying-screen resolution.
    3. SID resolution.

    (A) 1 only
    (B) 1 and 2 only
    (C) 1 and 3 only
    (D) 1, 2, and 3

91. All other factors remaining the same, if a 14 × 17-inch field is collimated to a 4-inch square field, the radiographic image will demonstrate

    (A) more density.
    (B) less density.
    (C) more detail.
    (D) less detail.

92. Component part(s) of x-ray film include the following:

    1. Phosphor layer
    2. Gelatin emulsion
    3. Adhesive layer

    (A) 1 only
    (B) 1 and 3 only
    (C) 2 and 3 only
    (D) 1, 2, and 3

93. In which of the following ways can higher radiographic contrast be obtained in abdominal radiography?

    1. By using lower kilovoltage
    2. By using a contrast medium
    3. By limiting the field size

    (A) 1 only
    (B) 1 and 2 only
    (C) 1 and 3 only
    (D) 1, 2, and 3

94. What should be done to correct for magnification when using air-gap technique?

    (A) Decrease OID
    (B) Increase OID
    (C) Decrease SID
    (D) Increase SID

95. In the AP projection of an asthenic patient whose knee measures less than 19 cm from ASIS to tabletop, the central ray should be directed

(A) perpendicularly.
(B) 5° medially.
(C) 5° cephalad.
(D) 5° caudad.

96. Which of the following statements is (are) true regarding Figure 6–8?

1. Excessive kVp was used.
2. High contrast is demonstrated.
3. Insufficient penetration is evident.

(A) 1 only
(B) 1 and 2 only
(C) 2 and 3 only
(D) 1, 2, and 3

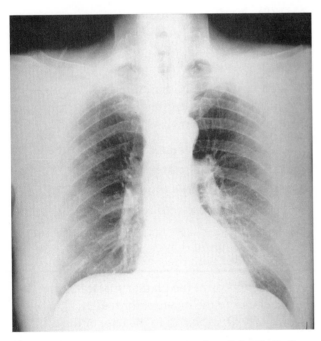

Figure 6–8. Reproduced with permission from Saia DA. *Radiography: Program Review and Examination Preparation*, 2nd ed. Stamford, CT: Appleton & Lange, 1999.

97. Most laser film must be handled

(A) under a Wratten 6B safelight.
(B) under a GBX safelight.
(C) in total darkness.
(D) with high-temperature processors.

98. During measurement of blood pressure, which of the following occurs as the radiographer controls arterial tension with the sphygmomanometer?

(A) The brachial vein is collapsed.
(B) The brachial artery is temporarily collapsed.
(C) The antecubital vein is monitored.
(D) Oxygen saturation of arterial blood is monitored.

99. Which of the following may be used as landmark(s) for an AP projection of the hip?

1. Two-inch medial to the anterior superior iliac spine (ASIS)
2. Prominence of the greater trochanter
3. Midway between the iliac crest and pubic symphysis

(A) 1 only
(B) 1 and 2 only
(C) 1 and 3 only
(D) 1, 2, and 3

100. Unlawful touching of a person without his or her consent is termed

(A) assault.
(B) battery.
(C) false imprisonment.
(D) invasion of privacy.

101. Exposure factors of 110 kVp and 12 mAs are used with an 8:1 grid for a particular exposure. What should be the new mAs if a 12:1 grid is substituted?

(A) 3
(B) 9
(C) 15
(D) 18

102. A diabetic patient who has not taken insulin while preparing for a fasting radiologic examination is susceptible to a hypoglycemic reaction. This is characterized by

1. fatigue.
2. cyanosis.
3. restlessness.

(A) 1 only
(B) 1 and 2 only
(C) 1 and 3 only
(D) 1, 2, and 3

103. Which of the following conditions will require an increase in x-ray photon energy/penetration?

(A) Fibrosarcoma
(B) Osteomalacia
(C) Paralytic ileus
(D) Ascites

104. Which of the following factors affect(s) both radiographic density and intensifying screen speed?

1. Thickness of phosphor layer
2. Type of phosphors used
3. Thickness of spongy screen support

(A) 1 only
(B) 1 and 2 only
(C) 1 and 3 only
(D) 1, 2, and 3

105. What is the name of the device that functions to expose a film with an optical step wedge having a number of densities ranging from white to black?

(A) Densitometer
(B) Sensitometer
(C) Penetrometer
(D) Potentiometer

106. A "controlled area" is one that is

(A) restricted to access by radiation workers only.
(B) monitored by survey meters.
(C) occupied by radiation workers.
(D) occupied by the general population.

107. The AP axial projection of the chest for pulmonary apices

1. requires 15° to 20° cephalad angulation.
2. projects the apices above the clavicles.
3. should demonstrate the medial ends of the clavicles equidistant from the vertebral column.

(A) 1 only
(B) 1 and 2 only
(C) 1 and 3 only
(D) 1, 2, and 3

108. Which of the following statements referring to Figure 6–9 is (are) correct?

1. Image A was performed AP.
2. Image B was performed AP.
3. The AP image was obtained using ureteral compression.

(A) 1 only
(B) 2 only
(C) 1 and 3 only
(D) 2 and 3 only

109. The process of radiation passing through tissue and depositing energy through ionization processes is known as

(A) the characteristic effect.
(B) Compton scatter.
(C) linear energy transfer.
(D) the photoelectric effect.

110. The radiograph seen in Figure 6–10 can be produced with the

1. long axis of the plantar surface perpendicular to the image recorder.
2. CR 40° cephalad to the base of the third metatarsal.
3. CR 20° cephalad to the talotibial joint.

(A) 1 only
(B) 2 only
(C) 1 and 2 only
(D) 1 and 3 only

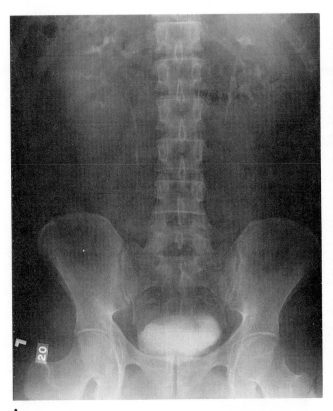 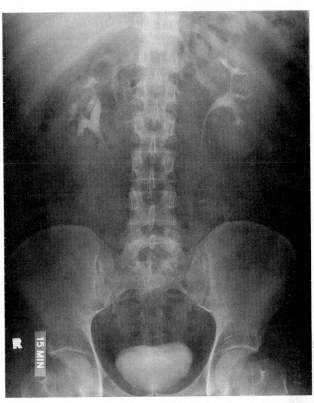

A   **B**

Figure 6–9A, B. Courtesy of Stamford Hospital, Department of Radiology.

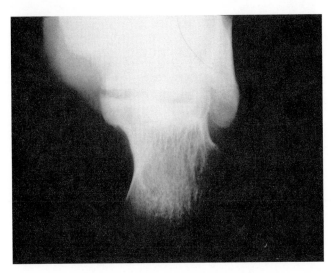

Figure 6–10. Courtesy of The Stamford Hospital, Department of Radiology.

111. Difficulty in breathing precipitated by stress and causing bronchospasm *best* describes

    (A) asthma.

    (B) anaphylaxis.

    (C) myocardial infarct.

    (D) rhinitis.

112. To within what percentage of the SID must the collimator light and actual irradiated area be accurate?

    (A) 2%

    (B) 5%

    (C) 10%

    (D) 15%

113. The brightness level of the fluoroscopic image can vary with

    1. milliamperage.
    2. kilovoltage.
    3. patient thickness.

    (A) 1 only

    (B) 1 and 2 only

    (C) 1 and 3 only

    (D) 1, 2, and 3

114. Which of the following methods can be effectively used to decrease differential absorption, providing a longer scale of contrast in the diagnostic range?

1. Using high kVp and low mAs factors
2. Using compensating filtration
3. Using factors that increase the photoelectric effect

(A) 1 only
(B) 1 and 2 only
(C) 2 and 3 only
(D) 1, 2, and 3

115. Which of the following pathologic conditions are considered *additive* conditions with respect to selection of exposure factors?

1. Osteoma
2. Bronchiectasis
3. Pneumonia

(A) 1 and 2 only
(B) 1 and 3 only
(C) 2 and 3 only
(D) 1, 2, and 3

116. Compared to that of the hyposthenic and asthenic habitus types, the gallbladder of a hypersthenic patient is most likely to be located

(A) higher and more medial.
(B) lower and more medial.
(C) higher and more lateral.
(D) lower and more lateral.

117. Which of the following correctly identifies the letter *T* in the radiograph seen in Figure 6–11?

(A) Gliding joint
(B) Pivot joint
(C) Diarthrotic joint
(D) Amphiarthrotic joint

118. Which of the following correctly identifies the letter *L* in the radiograph seen in Figure 6–11?

(A) Hamate
(B) Lunate
(C) Scaphoid
(D) Trapezium

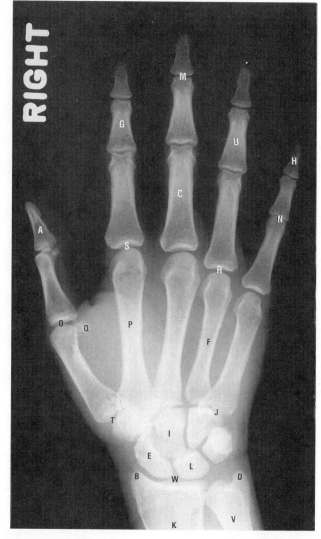

Figure 6–11. Courtesy of Bob Wong.

119. Which of the following can affect radiographic contrast?

1. Processing
2. Pathology
3. OID

(A) 1 only
(B) 1 and 2 only
(C) 1 and 3 only
(D) 1, 2, and 3

120. Crescent-shaped black marks on the finished radiograph are usually due to

   (A) bending the film acutely.
   (B) improper development.
   (C) improper film storage.
   (D) static electricity.

121. If 300 mA has been selected for a particular exposure, what exposure time should be selected to produce 18 mAs?

   (A) 0.04 second
   (B) 0.06 second
   (C) 0.4 second
   (D) 0.6 second

122. If the center photocell was selected for a lateral projection of the lumbar spine that was positioned with the spinous processes instead of the vertebral bodies centered to the grid, how would the resulting radiograph look?

   (A) The image would be underexposed.
   (B) The image would be overexposed.
   (C) The image would be correctly exposed.
   (D) An exposure could not be made.

123. What type of shock results from loss of blood?

   (A) Septic
   (B) Neurogenic
   (C) Cardiogenic
   (D) Hypovolemic

124. What is the most superior structure of the scapula?

   (A) Apex
   (B) Acromion process
   (C) Coracoid process
   (D) Superior angle

125. Which of the following contribute(s) to base-plus fog?

   1. Chemical fog
   2. Base tint
   3. Background radiation

   (A) 1 only
   (B) 1 and 2 only
   (C) 1 and 3 only
   (D) 1, 2, and 3

126. The roentgen, as a unit of measurement, expresses

   (A) absorbed dose.
   (B) exposure in air.
   (C) dose equivalent.
   (D) dose to biologic material.

127. Which reducing agent is responsible for producing the gray tones on the radiographic image?

   (A) Hydroquinone
   (B) Phenidone
   (C) Sodium sulfite
   (D) Ammonium thiosulfate

128. Which of the following cell types has the greatest radiosensitivity?

   (A) Nerve cells
   (B) Muscle cells
   (C) Spermatids
   (D) Lymphocytes

129. Which of the following radiologic examinations requires preparation consisting of a low-residue diet, cathartics, and enemas?

   (A) Upper GI series
   (B) Small-bowel series
   (C) Barium enema
   (D) IV cystogram

130. Although the stated focal spot size is measured directly under the actual focal spot, focal spot size in fact varies along the length of the x-ray beam. At which portion of the x-ray beam is the effective focal spot the largest?

(A) At its outer edge
(B) Along the path of the central ray
(C) At the cathode end
(D) At the anode end

131. Extravasation occurs when

(A) there is an absence of collateral circulation.
(B) there are a multitude of vessels supplying one area.
(C) excessive contrast medium is injected.
(D) contrast medium is injected into surrounding tissue.

132. A lesion with a stalk projecting from the intestinal mucosa into the lumen is a(n)

(A) fistula.
(B) polyp.
(C) diverticulum.
(D) abscess.

133. Both radiographic images seen in Figure 6–12 were made of the same subject using identical exposure factors. Which of the following statements correctly describes these images?

1. Image A demonstrates less optical density because a shorter SID was used.
2. Image A demonstrates more optical density because the subject was turned PA.
3. Image B demonstrates more optical density because a shorter SID was used.

(A) 1 only
(B) 2 only
(C) 3 only
(D) 1 and 2 only

134. What is the minimum requirement for lead aprons, according to CFR 20?

(A) 0.05 mm Pb
(B) 0.50 mm Pb
(C) 0.25 mm Pb
(D) 1.0 mm Pb

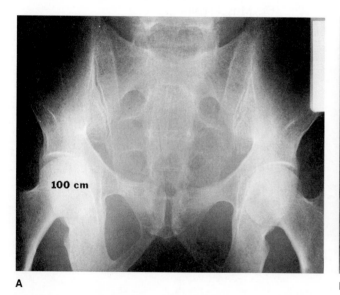

A

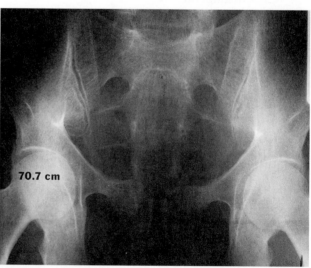

B

Figure 6–12. Reproduced with permission from Saia DA. *Radiography: Program Review and Examination Preparation*, 2nd ed. Stamford, CT: Appleton & Lange, 1999.

135. Which of the following would be *most* likely to cause the greatest skin dose (ESE)?

    (A) Short SID
    (B) High kVp
    (C) Increased filtration
    (D) Increased mA

136. Stochastic effects of radiation include

    (A) blood changes.
    (B) genetic alterations.
    (C) cataractogenesis.
    (D) reduced fertility.

137. The cycle of infection includes the following components:

    1. Reservoir of infection
    2. Pathogenic organism
    3. Means of transmission

    (A) 1 only
    (B) 1 and 2 only
    (C) 1 and 3 only
    (D) 1, 2, and 3

138. Which of the following is (are) located on the distal aspect of the humerus?

    1. Capitulum
    2. Intertubercular groove
    3. Coronoid fossa

    (A) 1 only
    (B) 1 and 2 only
    (C) 1 and 3 only
    (D) 1, 2, and 3

139. A cathartic is used to

    (A) induce vomiting.
    (B) stimulate defecation.
    (C) promote elimination of urine.
    (D) inhibit coughing.

140. Which of the following positions is *most* likely to offer the best visualization of the pulmonary apices?

    (A) Lateral decubitus
    (B) Dorsal decubitus
    (C) Erect lateral
    (D) AP axial lordotic

141. Which of the following is used to obtain a lateral projection of the upper humerus on patients who are unable to abduct their arm?

    (A) Bicipital groove projection
    (B) Superoinferior lateral
    (C) Inferosuperior axial
    (D) Transthoracic lateral

142. If 85 kV and 20 mAs were used for a particular abdominal exposure with single-phase equipment, what mAs would be required to produce a similar radiograph with 3-phase, 12-pulse equipment.

    (A) 40
    (B) 25
    (C) 20
    (D) 10

143. Which of the following is (are) demonstrated in the AP projection of the thoracic spine?

    1. Intervertebral spaces
    2. Apophyseal joints
    3. Intervertebral foramina

    (A) 1 only
    (B) 2 only
    (C) 1 and 3
    (D) 1, 2, and 3

144. Which of the following positions would demonstrate the right lumbar apophyseal articulations closest to the IR?

    (A) LAO
    (B) RAO
    (C) LPO
    (D) RPO

145. All of the following are related to recorded detail *except*

    (A) motion.
    (B) film–screen contact.
    (C) SID.
    (D) grid ratio.

146. Grid interspace material can be made of

    1. plastic.
    2. lead.
    3. aluminum.

    (A) 1 only
    (B) 1 and 2 only
    (C) 1 and 3 only
    (D) 1, 2, and 3

147. What is the annual TEDE limit for radiation workers?

    (A) 5000 rem
    (B) 500 rem
    (C) 5000 mrem
    (D) 50 mrem

148. If 0.05 second was selected for a particular exposure, what mA would be necessary to produce 15 mAs?

    (A) 900
    (B) 600
    (C) 500
    (D) 300

149. Body substances and fluids that are considered infectious, or potentially infectious, include

    1. sputum.
    2. synovial fluid.
    3. cerebrospinal fluid.

    (A) 1 only
    (B) 1 and 2 only
    (C) 2 and 3 only
    (D) 1, 2, and 3

150. A radiographer who discloses confidential information to unauthorized individuals may be found guilty of

    (A) invasion of privacy.
    (B) slander.
    (C) libel.
    (D) defamation.

151. Which of the following medications commonly found on emergency carts functions to raise blood pressure?

    (A) Heparin
    (B) Norepinephrine
    (C) Nitroglycerin
    (D) Lidocaine

152. Focal spot blur is greatest

    (A) toward the anode end of the x-ray beam.
    (B) toward the cathode end of the x-ray beam.
    (C) directly along the course of the central ray.
    (D) as the SID is increased.

153. The biggest advantage of coupling the image intensifier to the TV camera or CCD via a lens coupling device is its

    (A) compact size
    (B) durability
    (C) ability to accommodate cine and/or spot films
    (D) east maneuverability

154. Which of the following is (are) tested as part of a quality assurance (QA) program?

    1. Beam alignment
    2. Reproducibility
    3. Linearity

    (A) 1 only
    (B) 1 and 2 only
    (C) 1 and 3 only
    (D) 1, 2, and 3

155. The secondary center of ossification in long bones is the

   (A) periosteum.
   (B) endosteum.
   (C) epiphysis.
   (D) diaphysis.

156. Sternal compressions during cardiopulmonary resuscitation (CPR) are made with the heels of the hands located about

   (A) 1 ½ inches superior to the xiphoid tip.
   (B) 1 ½ inches inferior to the xiphoid tip.
   (C) 3 inches superior to the xiphoid tip.
   (D) 3 inches inferior to the xiphoid tip.

157. Which of the following effects does an antibiotic have on the body?

   (A) Decreases pain
   (B) Helps delay clotting
   (C) Increases urine output
   (D) Combats bacterial growth

158. Which of the following groups of organs/ structures are located in the left upper quadrant?

   (A) Left kidney, left suprarenal gland, and gastric fundus
   (B) Left suprarenal gland, pylorus, and duodenal bulb
   (C) Hepatic flexure, cecum, and pancreas
   (D) Gastric fundus, liver, and cecum

159. If 32 mAs and 50-speed screens were used to produce a particular radiographic density, what new mAs value would be required to produce the same density if the screen speed was changed to 400?

   (A) 4
   (B) 40
   (C) 175
   (D) 256

160. Recommended method(s) of minimizing motion unsharpness include

   1. suspended respiration.
   2. short exposure time.
   3. patient instruction.

   (A) 1 only
   (B) 1 and 2 only
   (C) 1 and 3 only
   (D) 1, 2, and 3

161. Which of the following is most useful for bone age evaluation?

   (A) Lateral skull
   (B) PA chest
   (C) AP pelvis
   (D) PA hand

162. How is SID related to exposure rate and radiographic density?

   (A) As SID increases, exposure rate increases and radiographic density increases.
   (B) As SID increases, exposure rate increases and radiographic density decreases.
   (C) As SID increases, exposure rate decreases and radiographic density increases.
   (D) As SID increases, exposure rate decreases and radiographic density decreases.

163. Which of the following contributes most to patient dose?

   (A) The photoelectric effect
   (B) Compton scatter
   (C) Classical scatter
   (D) Thompson scatter

164. An animal host of an infectious organism that transmits the infection via a bite or sting is a

   (A) vector.
   (B) fomite.
   (C) host.
   (D) reservoir.

165. In an AP abdomen taken at 105-cm SID during an IV urography series, one renal shadow measures 9 cm in width. If the OID is 18 cm, what is the actual width of the kidney?

(A) 5 cm
(B) 7.5 cm
(C) 11 cm
(D) 18 cm

166. Which of the following affect(s) both the quantity and quality of the primary beam?

1. Half-value layer (HVL)
2. kVp
3. mA

(A) 1 only
(B) 2 only
(C) 1 and 2 only
(D) 1, 2, and 3

167. What is the best position/projection to demonstrate the longitudinal arch of the foot?

(A) Mediolateral
(B) Lateromedial
(C) Mediolateral weight-bearing lateral
(D) Lateromedial weight-bearing lateral

168. Which of the x-ray circuit devices seen in Figure 6–13 operates on the principle of mutual induction?

1. Number 1
2. Number 2
3. Number 3

(A) 1 only
(B) 1 and 2 only
(C) 2 and 3 only
(D) 1, 2, and 3

169. Referring to the simplified x-ray circuit seen in Figure 6–13, what is indicated by the number 4?

(A) Step-up transformer
(B) kV meter
(C) Grounded mA meter
(D) Rectification system

170. The line focus principle expresses the relationship between

(A) actual and effective focal spot.
(B) SID used and resultant density.
(C) exposure given the IR and resultant density.
(D) kilovoltage used and the resulting contrast.

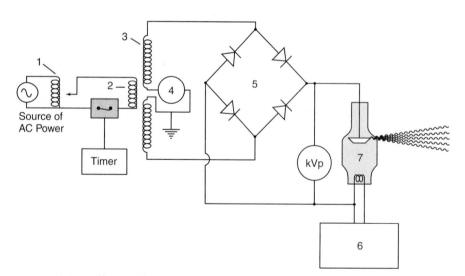

Figure 6–13.

171. The type of isolation practiced to prevent the spread of infectious agents in aerosol form is

    (A) respiratory isolation.
    (B) protective isolation.
    (C) contact isolation.
    (D) strict isolation.

172. Which of the following is (are) essential to high-quality mammographic examinations?

    1. Small focal spot x-ray tube
    2. Short-scale contrast
    3. Use of a compression device

    (A) 1 only
    (B) 1 and 2 only
    (C) 1 and 3 only
    (D) 1, 2, and 3

173. When green-sensitive rare earth screens are properly matched with the correct film, what type of safelight should be used in the darkroom?

    (A) Wratten 6B
    (B) GBX
    (C) Amber
    (D) None

174. X-ray tube life may be extended by

    1. using low-mAs/high-kVp exposure factors.
    2. avoiding lengthy anode rotation.
    3. avoiding exposures to a cold anode.

    (A) 1 only
    (B) 1 and 2 only
    (C) 1 and 3 only
    (D) 1, 2, and 3

175. A focal spot size of 0.3 mm or smaller is essential for which of the following procedures?

    (A) Bone radiography
    (B) Magnification radiography
    (C) Tomography
    (D) Fluoroscopy

176. What determines the amount of fluorescent light emitted from a fluorescent screen?

    1. Thickness of the active layer
    2. Type of phosphor used
    3. kV range used for exposure

    (A) 1 only
    (B) 1 and 2 only
    (C) 2 and 3 only
    (D) 1, 2, and 3

177. The term used to describe the gradual decrease in exposure rate as an x-ray beam passes through matter is

    (A) attenuation.
    (B) absorption.
    (C) scattered radiation.
    (D) secondary radiation.

178. The principal function of filtration in the x-ray tube is to reduce

    (A) patient skin dose.
    (B) operator exposure.
    (C) scattered radiation.
    (D) image noise.

179. The effects of radiation on biologic material are dependent on several factors. If a quantity of radiation is delivered to a body over a long period of time, the effect

    (A) will be greater than if it is delivered all at one time.
    (B) will be less than if it is delivered all at one time.
    (C) has no relation to how it is delivered in time.
    (D) is solely dependent on the radiation quality.

180. Which of the following shoulder projections can be used to evaluate the lesser tubercle in profile?

    (A) External rotation position
    (B) Internal rotation position
    (C) Neutral rotation position
    (D) Inferosuperior axial

181. The x-ray beam and collimator light field must coincide to within

(A) 10% of the OID.
(B) 2% of the OID.
(C) 10% of the SID.
(D) 2% of the SID.

182. The use of which of the following is (are) essential in magnification radiography?

1. High-ratio grid
2. Fractional focal spot
3. Direct exposure technique

(A) 1 only
(B) 2 only
(C) 1 and 3 only
(D) 1, 2, and 3

183. A minimum total amount of aluminum filtration (inherent plus added) of 2.5 mm is required in equipment operated

(A) above 50 kVp.
(B) above 60 kVp.
(C) above 70 kVp.
(D) above 80 kVp.

184. Which type of error results in grid cutoff at the periphery of the radiographic image?

(A) Off-focus
(B) Off-center
(C) Off-level
(D) Off-angle

185. Major effects of irradiation of macromolecules include

1. point lesions.
2. cross-linking.
3. main-chain scission.

(A) 1 only
(B) 1 and 2 only
(C) 1 and 3 only
(D) 1, 2, and 3

186. Which of the following will have an effect on radiographic contrast?

1. Beam restriction
2. Grids
3. Focal spot size

(A) 1 only
(B) 1 and 2 only
(C) 2 and 3 only
(D) 1, 2, and 3

187. Which of the following techniques might have been employed in the production of Figure 6–14?

1. Motion
2. Anode heel effect
3. Compression

(A) 1 only
(B) 1 and 2 only
(C) 1 and 3 only
(D) 1, 2, and 3

188. Which of the following statements is (are) true with respect to the differences between the male and female bony pelvis?

1. The female pelvic outlet is wider.
2. The pubic angle is 90° or less in the male.
3. The male pelvis is more shallow.

(A) 1 only
(B) 1 and 2 only
(C) 2 and 3 only
(D) 1, 2, and 3

189. All of the following are rules of good body mechanics except

(A) provide a wide base of support.
(B) keep back straight, avoid twisting.
(C) pull, do not push the load.
(D) keep the load close to the body.

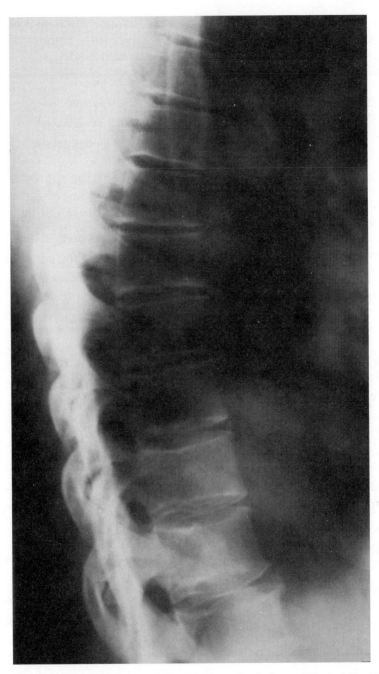

Figure 6–14. Reproduced with permission from Shephard. *Radiographic Image Production and Manipulation.* New York: McGraw-Hill, 2003.

190. The advantages of large format spot film cameras, such as 100 mm and 105 mm, over smaller format cameras, such as 70 mm and 90 mm, include

1. improved image quality.
2. decreased patient dose.
3. decreased x-ray tube heat load.

(A) 1 only
(B) 1 and 2 only
(C) 2 and 3 only
(D) 1, 2, and 3

191. Periodic equipment care includes evaluation of the

1. intensifying screens.
2. milliamperage.
3. timer.

(A) 1 only
(B) 1 and 3 only
(C) 2 and 3 only
(D) 1, 2, and 3

192. Which of the following formulas would the radiographer use to determine the total number of heat units (HU) produced with a given exposure using 3-phase, 12-pulse equipment?

(A) mA × time × kVp
(B) mA × time × kVp × 3.0
(C) mA × time × kVp × 1.35
(D) mA × time × kVp × 1.41

193. An increase in exposure factors is usually required in which of the following circumstances?

1. Edema
2. Ascites
3. Acromegaly

(A) 1 only
(B) 1 and 2 only
(C) 1 and 3 only
(D) 1, 2, and 3

194. Biologic material is most sensitive to radiation exposure under which of the following conditions?

(A) Anoxic
(B) Hypoxic
(C) Oxygenated
(D) Deoxygenated

195. What is the appropriate action if a patient has signed consent for a procedure but, once on the radiographic table, refuses the procedure?

(A) Proceed—the consent form is signed.
(B) Send the patient back to his or her room.
(C) Honor the patient's request and proceed with the next patient.
(D) Immediately stop the procedure and inform the radiologist and the referring physician of the patient's request.

196. The line focus principle refers to the fact that

(A) the actual focal spot is larger than the effective focal spot.
(B) the effective focal spot is larger than the actual focal spot.
(C) x-rays travel in straight lines.
(D) x-rays cannot be focused.

197. Impingement on the wrist's median nerve causing pain and disability of the affected hand and wrist is known as

(A) carpal boss syndrome.
(B) carpal tunnel syndrome.
(C) carpopedal syndrome.
(D) radioulnar syndrome.

198. What is the function of x-ray tube component number 2 in Figure 6–15?

(A) To release electrons when heated
(B) To release light when heated
(C) To direct electrons to the focal track
(D) To direct light to the focal track

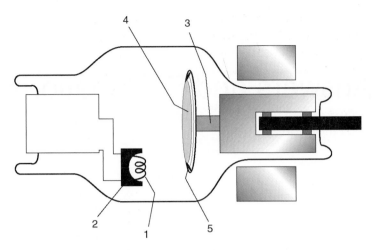

Figure 6–15.

199. Of what material is x-ray tube component number 5 in Figure 6–15 made?

(A) Cesium

(B) Copper

(C) Molybdenum

(D) Tungsten

200. Of what material is x-ray tube component number 2 in Figure 6–15 made?

(A) Cesium

(B) Copper

(C) Molybdenum

(D) tungsten

Answers and Explanations

1. **(C)** The medial oblique projection of the ankle can be performed either as a 15° to 20° oblique or as a 45° oblique. The 15° to 20° oblique demonstrates the ankle mortise, that is, the articulations between the talus, tibia, and fibula. The 45° oblique opens the distal tibiofibular joint. In all three cases, the plantar surface must be vertical. *(Ballinger & Frank, vol 1, p 280)*

2. **(B)** *Medical asepsis* refers to practices that reduce the spread of microbes, and therefore the chance of spreading disease or infection. Washing your hands is an example of medical asepsis. It reduces the spread of infection, but it does not eliminate all microorganisms. *Disinfection* involves the use of chemicals to either inactivate or inhibit the growth of microbes. The complete killing of all microorganisms is termed *sterilization*. *Surgical asepsis* refers to the technique used when performing procedures to prevent contamination. *(Adler & Carlton, p 211)*

3. **(A)** One of the biggest advantages of CR/DR is the *latitude* it offers. The characteristic curve of typical film emulsion has a "range of correct exposure," limited by the toe and shoulder of the curve. In CR/DR, there is a *linear* relationship between the exposure given the photostimulable phosphor (PSP) and its resulting luminescence as it is scanned by the laser, as illustrated in the figure shown. This affords much *greater exposure latitude*; technical inaccuracies can be effectively eliminated. Overexposure of up to 500% and underexposure of up to 80% are reported as recoverable, thus eliminating most retakes. *This surely affords increased efficiency; however, this does not mean that images can be exposed arbitrarily.* The professional radiographer has a responsibility to keep dose reduction to a minimum. The same exposure factors as screen–film systems, or less, are generally recommended for CR/DR. *(Shephard, p 332)*

4. **(C)** A *phototimer* is one type of *automatic exposure control (AEC)* that actually measures light. As x-ray photons penetrate and emerge from a part, a fluorescent screen beneath the cassette glows, and the fluorescent light charges a photomultiplier tube. Once a predetermined charge has been reached, the exposure automatically terminates. A parallel-plate *ionization chamber* is another type of AEC. A radiolucent chamber is beneath the patient (between the patient and the IR). As photons emerge from the patient, they enter the chamber and ionize the air within it. Once a predetermined charge has been reached, the exposure is automatically terminated. Motion of magnetic fields inducing a current in a conductor refers to the principle of mutual induction. *(Fauber, pp 232–233)*

5. **(B)** The CR laser scanner recognizes the various tissue density values (eg, bone, muscle, fat, air/gas, metal, contrast media, pathologic processes, etc) and constructs a gray-scale *histogram* of the values represented in the imaged part. A histogram is a *graphic representation*

showing the distribution of pixel values. The radiographer has selected a *processing algorithm* by selecting the anatomical part and particular projection on the computer. The CR unit matches that information with a particular *Lookup Table (LUT)*—a characteristic curve that best matches the anatomical part being imaged. Hence, *histogram analysis* and use of the appropriate *LUT* together function to produce predictable image quality in CR.

Histogram appearance can be affected by a number of things. Degree of accuracy in positioning and centering can have a significant effect on histogram appearance (as well as patient dose). Change is affected in average exposure level and exposure's latitude; these changes will be reflected in the images informational numbers ("S number," "Exposure Index," etc). Other factors affecting histogram appearance and, therefore, these informational numbers, include selection of the *correct processing algorithm* (eg, chest vs femur vs cervical spine), changes in scatter, SID, OID, and collimation. In short, anything that affects scatter and/or dose. (*Saia, PREP*)

6. **(D)** The 45° oblique position of the lumbar spine is generally performed for demonstration of the *apophyseal joints*. In a correctly positioned oblique lumbar spine, *"scotty dog"* images are demonstrated. The scotty's *ear* corresponds to the superior articular process, his *nose* to the transverse process, his *eye* to the pedicle, his *neck* to the pars interarticularis, his *body* to the lamina, and his *front foot* to the inferior articular process. (*Ballinger & Frank, vol 1, p 434*)

7. **(C)** The *latent image* is the invisible image produced within the film emulsion as a result of exposure to radiation. The developer solution converts this to a visible, manifest image. The exposed silver halide grains in the emulsion undergo chemical change in the develop1er solution, and the *unexposed* crystals are removed from the film during the fixing process. (*Fauber, p 163*)

8. **(B)** In the prone oblique positions (RAO, LAO), the flexure disclosed is the one closer to the image receptor. Therefore, the LAO posi-

tion will "open up" the splenic flexure; the RAO position will demonstrate the hepatic flexure. The AP oblique positions (RPO, LPO) demonstrate the side farther from the image receptor. (*Ballinger & Frank, vol 2, p 142*)

9. **(C)** For the AP projection of the sacrum, the patient is AP supine with the MSP perpendicular to the x-ray tabletop. The central ray is directed 15° cephalad to a point 2 inches superior to the pubis (approximately midway between the ASIS and the pubic symphysis). In this projection, the central ray angulation parallels the sacral curve and provides less distorted visualization of the sacrum and its foramina. (*Saia, p 133*)

10. **(B)** Genetic effects of radiation and some somatic effects, like leukemia, are plotted on a *linear* dose–response curve. The linear dose-response curve has *no threshold,* that is, *there is no dose below which radiation is absolutely safe.* The sigmoidal dose–response curve has a threshold and is thought to be generally correct for most somatic effects. (*Bushong, p 498*)

11. **(C)** Contrast injection into the ureters can be achieved only by first catheterizing the bladder, locating the ureteral orifices, then injecting the contrast agent into the ureters. This procedure is called a *retrograde* (because contrast is being introduced against the normal direction of flow) *pyelogram*. A *cystogram* is an examination of the bladder. A *cystourethrogram* is an examination of the bladder and urethra. (*Ballinger & Frank, vol 2, p 167*)

12. **(A)** There are several radiation units that are used to express quantity and effects of radiation. *Rad* (radiation *a*bsorbed *d*ose) expresses energy deposited (as a result of ionizations) in any kind of absorber. The unit of exposure, the *roentgen,* is used to express the quantity of ionization in air. The unit of dose equivalent is the *rem* (radiation *e*quivalent *m*an), which expresses dose to biologic material. (*Selman, p 131*)

13. **(A)** Radiographic rating charts enable the operator to determine the maximum safe mA,

exposure time, and kVp for a particular exposure using a particular x-ray tube. An exposure that can be made safely with the large focal spot may not be safe for use with the small focal spot of the same x-ray tube. The total number of HU that an exposure generates also influences the amount of stress (in the form of heat) imparted to the anode. The product of mAs and kVp determines HU. Groups A and C produce 2250 HU; groups B and D produce 1275 HU. Groups B and D deliver less heat load, but group D delivers it to a *larger* area (actual focal spot) making this the *least hazardous* group of technical factors. The *most* hazardous group of technical factors is group A. *(Selman, p 145)*

14–15. (14, C; 15, D) The radiograph illustrates an air-contrast barium enema examination. The intent of this examination is to coat the intestinal mucosa with barium, then fill the lumen with air. Typically, some structures will be imaged filled with barium, and others will be imaged as double-contrast (barium and air); how structures are filled depends to a large extent on the position employed. Radiographic examinations of the large bowel generally include the AP or PA axial position to "open" the S-shaped *sigmoid* colon, the lateral position especially for the *rectum*, and the LAO and RAO (or LPO and RPO) to "open" the colic *flexures*. Left and right decubitus positions are usually employed only in double-contrast barium enemas to better demonstrate double contrast of the *medial and lateral walls* of the ascending and descending colon. An *LPO* position is illustrated. The *LPO* and *RAO* positions demonstrate the hepatic *flexure and adjacent ascending colon*. The *LAO* and *RPO* positions demonstrate the *splenic flexure and descending colon. (Ballinger & Frank, vol 2, p 141)*

16. (B) *The amount of scattered radiation generated in a given exposure increases as three factors increase:* the *kVp*, the *field size*, and the *thickness and density of the tissues*. Therefore, using optimum kVp and collimating as closely as possible are two ways to reduce the amount of scattered radiation produced. The use of a grid reduces the amount of scattered radiation *reaching the IR*; grids are unrelated to the *production of* scattered radiation. *(Selman, pp 233–234)*

17. (C) Federal regulations regarding infection control in the workplace, as amended by OSHA, require development of policies conforming to OSHA guidelines and instruction in their application/use. These regulations also require provision of Hepatitis B immunization (free of charge) for all staff who might be exposed to blood/body sybstances; follow-up care for any staff accidentally exposed to blood/body fluids/needle stick injuries; readily accessible personal protective equipment (PPE) and impermeable puncture-proof containers for used needles/syringes. It also requires that all health-care workers and their employers follow/enforce Standard Precautions, Transmission-Based Precautions, and these OSHA guidelines under penalty of law. *(Torres et al, p 63)*

18. (D) Adverse reactions to the intravascular administration of iodinated contrast media are not uncommon, but although the risk of a life-threatening reaction is relatively rare, the radiographer must be alert to recognize and deal effectively with a serious reaction should it occur. *Flushed* appearance and *nausea*, occasionally vomiting, and a few *hives* characterize a *minor* reaction. Early symptoms of a possible *anaphylactic* reaction include constriction of the throat, possibly due to laryngeal edema, dysphagia (difficulty swallowing), and itching of the palms and soles. The radiographer must maintain the patient's airway, summon the radiologist, and call a "code." *(Ehrlich, McCloskey, & Daly, p 234)*

19. (A) Emetics, such as ipecac, function to induce vomiting. Cathartics are used to stimulate defecation (bowel movements). Diuretics are used to promote urine elimination in individuals whose tissues are retaining excessive fluid, and antitussives are used to inhibit coughing. *(Ehrlich, McCloskey, & Daly, p 188)*

20. (A) If intensifying-screen phosphors are covered with dust, either they will not fluoresce or their fluorescence will not reach the IR emulsion. Similarly, if the screen is scratched and phosphors are removed, there will be no fluorescence to expose the IR. In both cases, then, those areas will exhibit little or no density. *(Shephard, p 75)*

21. **(D)** The *protective curtain,* usually made of leaded vinyl with at least 0.25 mm Pb equivalent, must be positioned between the patient and the fluoroscopist to greatly reduce exposure of the fluoroscopist to energetic scatter from the patient. As with overhead equipment, fluoroscopic total *filtration* must be at least 2.5 mm Al equivalent to reduce excessive exposure to soft radiation. *Collimator*/beam alignment must be accurate to within 2%. *(Bushong, p 569)*

22. **(D)** In the AP projection of the lumbar spine, the disk spaces of L1–4 are perpendicular to the IR and well visualized, but the L5–S1 disk space is angled 30° to 35° cephalad to the perpendicular. If the central ray is directed 30° to 35° *cephalad* midway between the ASIS and the symphysis pubis, the L5–S1 interspace will be well demonstrated. *(Saia, p 130)*

23. **(A)** *The photoelectric* effect and *Compton scattering* are the two predominant interactions between x-ray photons and matter in diagnostic x-ray. In the photoelectric effect, the low-energy incident photon *uses all its energy* to eject an atom's inner-shell electron. That photon ceases to exist—it has used all its energy to ionize the atom. The part has absorbed the x-ray photon. This interaction contributes to patient dose and produces short-scale contrast. In Compton scatter, the high-energy incident photon uses only part of its energy to eject an outer-shell electron. It retains most of its energy in the form of a scattered x-ray. *(Bushong, pp 176–177)*

24. **(D)** Endoscopic retrograde cholangiopancreatography is performed to diagnose disease of the *biliary* and/or *pancreatic* organs. Fluoroscopic control is used to introduce the *fiberoptic endoscope* through the mouth and into the duodenum. The hepatopancreatic ampulla (of Vater) is then located and cannulated, and contrast medium is injected into the *common bile duct.* *(Ballinger & Frank, vol 2, p 80)*

25. **(B)** When the hand is pronated and the fingers are extended for a PA projection of the wrist, the wrist arches and an OID is introduced between the wrist and the cassette. To reduce this OID, *the metacarpophalangeal joints should be flexed slightly.* This maneuver will bring the anterior surface of the wrist into contact with the cassette. *(Ballinger & Frank, vol 1, p 112)*

26. **(C)** Significant scattered radiation is produced when radiographing large or dense body parts and when using high kilovoltage. A radiographic grid is made of alternating lead strips and interspace material; it is placed between the patient and the IR to absorb energetic scatter emerging from the patient. Although a grid prevents much scattered radiation fog from reaching the radiograph, its use does necessitate a significant increase in patient exposure. *(Shephard, pp 244–245)*

27. **(B)** The principal quantitative factor regulating radiographic (or optical) density is *mAs.* The mAs selected is directly proportional to radiographic density (ie, if the mAs is cut in half, radiographic density will be halved). Although *SID* affects exposure rate (according to the inverse square law of radiation), and therefore affects density (according to the density maintenance formula), it is not used to regulate radiographic density. According to the 15% rule, *kVp* may be used to change radiographic density, but kVp is not a major quantitative factor. The principal use of *filtration* is to decrease patient skin dose; filtration of that sort will not affect the radiographic image. *(Shephard, p 170)*

28. **(A)** The pediatric lateral skull seen in Figure 6–3 demonstrates no *motion* and somewhat *excessive* optical density. However, an adhesive tape *artifact* can still be clearly identified across the skull from frontal bone to occiput. Tape used for immobilization is imaged easily and can make image details difficult to see. *(Saia, pp 404–409)*

29. **(C)** *Distortion* is misrepresentation of the actual size or shape of the object being imaged. Size distortion is *magnification.* Shape distortion is a result of improper alignment of the x-ray

tube, the part being radiographed, and the image recorder; the two types of shape distortion are *foreshortening* and *elongation*. The shape of various structures can be radiographically misrepresented as a result of their position in the body, when the part is out of the central axis of the x-ray beam, or when the central ray is angled (see Fig. 6–16). Parts are sometimes intentionally elongated for better visualization (eg, the sigmoid colon). Some body parts, because of their position in the body, are foreshortened, such as the carpal scaphoid. Attenuation refers to decreasing beam intensity and is unrelated to distortion. *(Shephard, pp 228–231)*

30. **(A)** The fluoroscopic unit is required to have a 5-minute cumulative timer. It is set to zero at the beginning of the examination and allowed to run continuously to indicate the amount of fluoroscopic exposure in minutes. After 5 minutes of fluoroscopy, a buzzer will sound, indicating to the fluoroscopist (who may be somewhat unaware of the passing time while studying the x-ray image) that 5 minutes of fluoroscopy has been used. The technologist will then reset the timer for another 5 minutes. The timer is there for radiation protection measures, to alert the fluoroscopist of the passing time. The technologist should not reset the timer until it has sounded, alerting the fluoroscopist. *(Bushong, p 569)*

31. **(A)** The control badge that comes with the month's supply of dosimeters is used as a standard for comparison with the used personnel badges. The control badge should be stored in a radiation-free area, away from the radiographic rooms. When it has been processed, its density is compared with the densities of the monitors worn in radiation areas. Densities greater than the density of the radiation-free monitor are reported in mrem units. *(Bushong, p 596)*

32. **(B)** Diagnostic imaging examinations must be scheduled appropriately. Retained barium sulfate contrast medium can obscure necessary anatomic details in x-ray studies or ultrasound studies that are scheduled later. Therefore, the ultrasound examination should come first, followed by the lower GI (barium enema), and finally the upper GI. Retained barium from the lower GI will probably not obscure upper GI structures. *(Torres et al, p 233–234)*

33. **(B)** The heart superimposes a homogeneous density over the sternum in the RAO position, thus providing clearer radiographic visualization of its bony structure. If the LAO position were used to project the sternum to the right of the thoracic vertebrae, the posterior ribs and pulmonary markings would cast confusing shadows over the sternum because of their differing densities. Prominent pulmonary

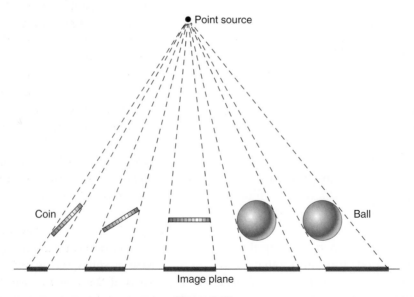

Figure 6–16.

markings can be obliterated using a "breath-ing technique," that is, using an exposure time long enough (with appropriately low mA) to equal at least a few respirations. *(Ballinger & Frank, vol 1, p 464)*

34. **(A)** *OID* can affect contrast when it is used as an air gap. If a 6-inch air gap (OID) is intro-duced between the part and IR, much of the scattered radiation emitted from the body will not reach the IR, as seen in Figure 6–17. The OID is thus acting as a low-ratio grid and in-creasing image contrast. *(Shephard, p 205)*

35. **(D)** Proper *alignment* of the x-ray tube, body part, and image recorder is required to avoid

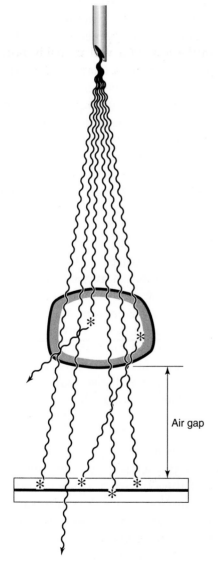

Air gap

Figure 6–17.

image *distortion* in the form of *foreshortening* or *elongation*. *Foreshortening* will usually re-sult when the *part* is out of alignment. *Elon-gation* is often a result of *angulation of the x-ray tube.* Grid lines or *grid cutoff* will occur when the *grid* itself is off-center or not in alignment with the x-ray tube. *(Shephard, pp 228–231)*

36. **(B)** Anaphylaxis is an acute reaction charac-terized by sudden onset of urticaria, respira-tory distress, vascular collapse, or systemic shock; it sometimes leads to death. It is caused by ingestion or injection of a sensitizing agent such as a drug, vaccine, contrast agent, or food, or by an insect bite. Asthma and rhinitis are examples of allergic reactions. Myocardi-cal infarction results from a blocked coronary artery. *(Jones et al, p 165)*

37. **(C)** Radiography of the paranasal sinuses should be performed in the erect position whenever possible to demonstrate the pres-ence of a *air–fluid level.* The only way air–fluid levels can be demonstrated is to have the *central ray parallel the floor,* as in erect, decubitus, and cross-table projections. Therefore, of the choices provided, the *cross-table lateral* is the only one that will demon-strate air–fluid levels. *(Ballinger & Frank, vol 2, p 362)*

38. **(A)** The cervical intervertebral foramina lie 45° to the midsagittal plane (MSP) and 15° to 20° to a transverse plane. When the *posterior oblique* position (LPO, RPO) is used, the cen-tral ray is directed 15° to 20° cephalad and the cervical intervertebral foramina demonstrated are those *farther* from the image recorder. There is therefore some magnification of the foramina (because of the OID). In the *anterior oblique* position (LAO, RAO), the central ray is directed 15° to 20° caudad, and the foramina disclosed are those *closer* to the image recorder. *(Ballinger & Frank, vol 1, p 402)*

39. **(D)** Oral administration of barium sulfate is used to demonstrate the upper digestive sys-tem, esophagus, fundus, and body and py-lorus of the *stomach,* and barium progression through the small bowel. The large bowel, in-

cluding the *cecum*, is usually demonstrated via rectal administration of barium. The *ilium* refers to the bony pelvis, whereas the ileum refers to the small bowel—which would be demonstrated by oral administration of barium. *(Jones et al, p 165)*

40. **(D)** *Inherent filtration* is composed of materials that are a permanent part of the tube housing: the x-ray tube's glass envelope and the oil coolant. *Added filtration*, usually thin sheets of aluminum, is included to make a total of 2.5 mm Al equivalent for equipment operated at 70 kVp and higher. *Filtration* is used to decrease patient dose by removing the low-energy photons that do not contribute to image formation but simply contribute to skin dose. According to the inverse square law of radiation, exposure dose increases as *distance* from the source decreases and vice versa. The effect of *focal spot size* is principally on recorded detail; it has no effect on patient dose. *(Shephard, pp 17–18)*

41. **(A)** The posterior oblique positions (LPO, RPO) of the lumbar vertebrae demonstrate the apophyseal articulations closer to the image receptor. The left apophyseal articulations are demonstrated in the LPO position, while the right apophyseal articulations are demonstrated in the RPO position. The lateral position is useful to demonstrate the intervertebral disk spaces, intervertebral foramina, and spinous processes. *(Saia, p 131)*

42. **(B)** The NCRP recommends a total equivalent dose limit to the embryo/fetus of *500 mrem (0.5 rem)*. That dose limit is the total for the entire gestational period. The dose limit for 1 month during pregnancy is 50 mrem (0.05 rem). *(Bushong, p 557)*

43. **(B)** Fluids and medications are administered to patients intravenously to achieve a more rapid response to the medication than if it were delivered orally or intramuscularly. The IV route is also often used to deliver parenteral nutrition to patients who cannot take their meals by mouth. Medications that are administered topically, such as calamine lotion, achieve a local effect. *(Ehrlich et al, p 192)*

44. **(A)** The photoelectric effect and Compton scattering are the two predominant interactions between x-ray photons and matter in diagnostic radiology. In the photoelectric effect, the low-energy incident photon is absorbed by the tissues being radiographed. In Compton scatter, the high-energy incident photon uses only part of its energy to eject an outer-shell electron. *It retains much of its original energy in the form of a scattered x-ray.* Radiologic personnel can be exposed to that high-energy scattered radiation, especially in fluoroscopy and mobile radiography. Lead aprons are used to protect us from exposure to scattered radiation during these procedures. *(Bushong, p 174)*

45. **(B)** The *input phosphor* of an image intensifier receives remnant radiation emerging from the patient and converts it to a fluorescent light image. Directly adjacent to the input phosphor is the *photocathode*, which is made of a photoemissive alloy (usually a cesium and antimony compound). The fluorescent light image strikes the photocathode and is converted to an electron image. The electrons are carefully focused, to maintain image resolution, by the *electrostatic focusing lenses*, through the *accelerating anode* and to the *output phosphor* for conversion back to light. *(Bushong, p 361)*

46. **(B)** The image displayed is an erect PA projection on a patient of hyposthenic body habitus. Note the low position of the gallbladder: It is a result of body habitus and position (viscera assume a lower position in the erect position). The gallbladder may be moved *away* from the spine by using the *LAO* position. The *right* lateral decubitus will also move the gallbladder away from the spine. *(Ballinger & Frank, vol 2, pp 68–71)*

47. **(C)** *Turnaround* assemblies are located at the bottom of each solution tank and function to direct the film from a downward to an upward motion. *Guide shoes*, also called *deflector plates*, serve to keep the film on its proper course by directing or guiding it around corners. The *crossover* rollers are located at the top of the processor, out of the solution, and

direct the film from one solution tank to the next. These are the racks that need daily cleaning to avoid chemical or emulsion buildup on their surface. Chemical or emulsion buildup on roller surfaces can cause film artifacts. *(Shephard, pp 141–143)*

48. **(C)** Primary radiation barriers are those barriers that protect from the primary, or useful, x-ray beam. Secondary radiation barriers are those that protect from secondary or scattered radiation. Examples of *primary* barriers are the radiographic room walls, doors, and floors, because the primary beam can often be directed toward them. *Secondary* radiation barriers include lead aprons, gloves, thyroid shields, and the radiographic room ceiling. These will protect from exposure to scattered radiation only. Secondary radiation barriers will not protect from the useful beam. *(Bushong, p 553)*

49. **(D)** The CR laser scanner recognizes the various tissue density values and constructs a representative gray-scale histogram. A histogram is a graphic representation showing the distribution of pixel values. Histogram analysis and use of the appropriate LUT together function to produce predictable image quality in CR. Histogram appearance can be affected by a number of things. Degree of accuracy in positioning and centering can have a significant effect on histogram appearance (as well as patient dose). Change is affected in average exposure level and exposure's latitude; these changes will be reflected in the images informational numbers ("S number," "Exposure Index," etc). Other factors affecting histogram appearance and, therefore, these informational numbers, include selection of the correct processing algorithm (eg, chest vs femur vs cervical spine), changes in scatter, SID, OID, and collimation. Figure 6–18 illustrates the effect of incorrect collimation on histogram appearance. In short, anything that affects scatter and/or dose. (Saia, PREP)

50. **(B)** Dual x-ray absorptiometry (DXA) imaging is used to evaluate bone mineral density (BMD). Bone densitometry, DXA, can be used to *evaluate bone mineral content of the body, or*

Example A	Example B
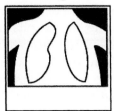	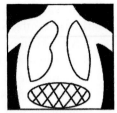
Properly collimated	Non-collimated beam
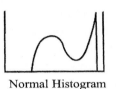	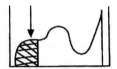
Normal Histogram	Wider Histogram

Figure 6–18. Courtesy FUJIFILM Medical Systems USA, Inc.

part of it, to *diagnosis osteoporosis* or to *evaluate the effectiveness of treatments for osteoporosis*. It is the most widely used method of *bone densitometry*—it is *low dose, preceise,* and *uncomplicated* to use/perform. DXA uses *two photon energies*—one for soft tissue and one for bone. Since bone is more dense and attenuates x-ray photons more readily, their *attenuation is calculated* to represent the degree of bone density. Soft tissue attenuation information is not used to measure bone density. *(Ballinger & Frank, vol 3, pp 488–489)*

51. **(D)** Airborne, fomite, and vector are all indirect modes of transmitting microorganisms. Direct contact involves actual touching of the infected person. A *fomite* is an inanimate object that has been in contact with an infectious microorganism (eg, doorknobs or x-ray tables). Although an inanimate object may serve as a temporary host for microbes, microbes flourish on and in the human host, where plenty of body fluids and tissues nourish and feed them. A *vector* is an animal host of an infectious organism that transmits the infection via a bite or sting, such as the mosquito or deer tick. *Airborne* contamination occurs via droplets (sneeze) or dust. *(Saia, p 34)*

52. **(B)** Two thousand *mrad* is equal to 2 *rad*. If 2 rad were delivered in 10 minutes, then the dose rate is 2 ÷ 10, or 0.2 rad/min. *(Selman, p 528)*

53. **(A)** The legal doctrine *res ipsa locquitur* relates to a matter that speaks for itself. For instance, if a patient was admitted to the hospital to have a kidney stone removed and incorrectly was given an appendectomy, that speaks for itself and negligence could be proven. *Respondeat superior* is the phrase meaning "let the master answer" or "the one ruling is responsible." If a radiographer is negligent, there may be an attempt to prove that the radiologist was responsible, because the radiologist oversees the radiographer. *Res judicata* means a thing or matter settled by justice. *Stare decisis* refers to a matter settled by precedent. *(Adler & Carlton, p 366)*

54. **(D)** The greater the number of electrons making up the *electron stream* and bombarding the target, the greater the number of x-ray photons produced. Although kilovoltage is usually associated with the energy of the x-ray photons, because *a greater number of more energetic electrons* will produce more x-ray photons, an increase in kilovoltage will also increase the *number* of photons produced. Specifically, the quantity of radiation produced increases as the *square of the kilovoltage*. The *material composition* of the tube target also plays an important role in the number of x-ray photons produced. The higher the atomic number, the denser and more closely packed the atoms making up the material, and therefore the greater the chance of an interaction between a high-speed electron and the target material. *(Selman, pp 112–115)*

55. **(C)** The trachea (windpipe) bifurcates into left and right *mainstem bronchi,* each of which enters its respective lung hilum. The *left* bronchus divides into *two* portions, one for each lobe of the left lung. The *right* bronchus divides into *three* portions, one for each lobe of the right lung. The lungs are conical in shape, consisting of upper pointed portions, termed the *apices* (plural of apex), and the broad lower portions (or *bases*). The lungs are enclosed in a double-walled serous membrane called the *pleura*. *(Tortora & Derrickson, p 857)*

56. **(D)** Intensifying-screen phosphors that have a *high atomic number* are more likely to *absorb* a high percentage of the incident x-ray photons and *convert* x-ray photon energy to fluorescent light energy. How efficiently the phosphors detect and interact with the x-ray photons is termed *quantum detection efficiency.* How effectively the phosphors make this energy conversion is termed *conversion efficiency.* *(Shephard, p 65)*

57. **(C)** *Pneumonia* is an acute infection of the lung parenchyma characterized by productive cough, chest pain, fever, and chills and frequently accompanied by rales. *Atelectasis* is partial or complete collapse of a lung or lobe of a lung. *Pneumothorax* is the condition of air or gas in the pleural space. *COPD (chronic obstructive pulmonary disease),* is the name given to a number of disease processes that decrease the lung's ability to perform its function of ventilation. *(Tortora & Derrickson, p 888)*

58. **(A)** The relationship between x-ray intensity and distance from the source is expressed in the inverse square law of radiation. The formula is

$$\frac{I_1}{I_2} = \frac{D_2^2}{D_1^2}$$

Substituting known values,

$$\frac{18}{x} = \frac{25\,(5^2)}{4\,(2^2)}$$

$$25x = 72$$

$$x = 2.88 \text{ mR/min at 5 meters}$$

Distance has a profound effect on dose received and therefore is one of the cardinal factors con-sidered in radiation protection. As distance from the source increases, dose received decreases. (Bushong, pp 68–70)

59. **(C)** Patient dose during fluoroscopy can be considerable because the x-ray tube is in close proximity to the patient. We can therefore decrease patient dose by *increasing* the SSD as much as possible. The law states that the SSD must be at least 15 inches with *fixed* fluoroscopic equipment and at least 12 inches with *mobile* fluoroscopic equipment. The use of 2.5 mm Al equivalent filtration in equipment operated above 70 kVp is also required by law to reduce patient skin dose. Another requirement

of fluoroscopic equipment is that the tabletop intensity not exceed 10 R/min. *(Bushong, p 569)*

60. **(A)** With the patient in the AP position, the central ray is directed cephalad 25° to 30°. This serves to project the clavicle away from the pulmonary apices and ribs, projecting most of the clavicle above the thorax. The reverse is true when the patient is examined in the PA position. *(Bontrager, p 188)*

61. **(C)** Radiographic density is directly proportional to mAs. If exposure time is *halved* from 0.04 (1/25) second to 0.02 (1/50) second, radiographic density will be cut in half. Changing to 300 mA will also halve the mAs, effectively halving the radiographic density. If the kVp is decreased by 15%, from 85 to 72 kVp, radiographic density will be halved according to the 15% rule. To cut the density in half, the mAs must be reduced to 12 (rather than to 18). *(Selman, p 214)*

62. **(B)** Expectoration (coughing or spitting up) of blood is called *hemoptysis*. Blood is originating from the mouth, larynx, or respiratory structure. *Hematemesis* refers to vomiting blood. If the blood is dark in color, it is probably gastric in origin; if it is bright red, it is most likely pharyngeal in origin. *Hematuria* is the condition of blood in the urine. *Epistaxis* is the medical term for nosebleed. *(Bontrager, p 80)*

63. **(C)** In the AP projection of the normal knee, the space between the tibial plateau and the femoral condyles is equal bilaterally. It is therefore important that there be no pelvic rotation that could change the appearance of an otherwise-normal relationship. The AP projection of the knee superimposes the patella and femur. The central ray should enter at the knee joint, located 1/2 inch distal to the patellar *apex*. *(Ballinger & Frank, vol 1, p 290)*

64. **(C)** Lead and distance are the two most important ways to protect from radiation exposure. Fluoroscopy can be particularly hazardous because the SID is so much shorter than in overhead radiography. Therefore, it

has been established that *mobile* fluoroscopic equipment must provide at least 12-inch source-to-tabletop/skin distance for the protection of the patient. *(Bushong, p 569)*

65. **(D)** The stomach is normally angled with the fundus lying posteriorly and the body, pylorus, and duodenum inferior to the fundus and angling anteriorly. Therefore, when the patient ingests barium and lies *AP* recumbent, the heavy barium gravitates easily to the fundus and fills it. With the patient *PA* recumbent, barium gravitates inferiorly to the body, pylorus, and duodenum, *displacing air into the fundus. (Ballinger, vol 2, pp 110–111)*

66. **(D)** If an x-ray image is placed on an illuminator and 100% of the illuminator's light is transmitted through the image, that image must have a density of 0. According to the equation

$$\text{Density} = \frac{\log_{10} \text{ incident light intensity}}{\text{transmitted light intesity}}$$

If 10% of the illuminator's light passes through the image, that image has a density of 1. If 1% of the light passes through the image, that image has a density of 2. *(Selman, p 213)*

67. **(B)** *Hypotension* occurs if the blood pressure drops below the normal ranges (110 to 140/60 to 90 mm Hg). It can occur in shock, hemorrhage, infection, and anemia. The condition in which a patient's heart rate slows below 60 beats per minute is *bradycardia. Hyperthermia* is the condition in which the patient's temperature is well above the normal average range (97.7 to 99.5°F). *Hypoxia* is a condition in which there is a decrease in the oxygen supplied to the tissues in the body. *(Adler & Carlton, pp 181–182)*

68. **(B)** The bony walls of the orbit are thin, fragile, and subject to fracture. A direct blow to the eye results in a pressure that can cause fracture. That fracture is usually to the *orbital floor* (the inferior aspect of the bony orbit). Because the fracture results from increased pressure within the eye, it is referred to as a "blowout" fracture. *(Ballinger, vol 2, p 289)*

69–70. (69, B; 70, A) The image seen in Figure 6–5 demonstrates a *radial flexion* deviation maneuver of the left wrist. To position, the hand and wrist are placed PA, and the elbow is moved toward the body without moving the hand and wrist. Or, the hand can be turned medialward in extreme radial flexion (deviation). This position is used to better demonstrate the *medial carpals* (pisiform, triangular, hamate, and medial aspect of capitate and lunate) and their interspaces. In the proximal carpal row, the *lunate* (number 3) is seen particularly well. Just medial to the lunate, the superimposed triquetrum and pisiform are seen. In the distal carpal row, the most lateral carpal, the *hamate* (number 4), is well seen. Just medial to it is the capitate. The self-superimposed and foreshortened scaphoid is seen distal to the radius and lateral to the lunate. The *radial styloid process* is number 1, and the *ulnar styloid* is number 2. *(Ballinger & Frank, vol 1, pp 117–118)*

71. (C) Emphysema is a progressive disorder caused by long-term irritation of the bronchial passages, such as by air pollution or cigarette smoking. Emphysema patients are unable to exhale normally because of the loss of elasticity of the alveolar walls. If emphysema patients receive oxygen, it is usually administered at a very slow rate, because their respirations are controlled by the level of carbon dioxide in the blood. *(Tortora & Derrickson, p 887)*

72. (D) The x-ray anode may be a molybdenum disc coated with a tungsten–rhenium alloy. Tungsten, with a *high atomic number* (74), produces high-energy x-rays quite efficiently. Since a great deal of heat is produced at the target, its *high melting point* (3410°C) helps avoid damage to the target surface. Heat produced at the target should be dissipated readily, and tungsten's *conductivity is similar to that of copper*. Therefore, as heat is applied to the focus, it can be conducted throughout the disc to equalize the temperature and thus avoid pitting, or localized melting, of the focal track. *(Selman, p 138)*

73. (A) The diameter of a needle is the needle *gauge*. The higher the gauge number, the thinner the diameter. For example, a very tiny-gauge needle such as 25 gauge may be used on a pediatric patient for IV injection, whereas a large-gauge needle such as 16 gauge may be used for donating blood. The *hub* of the needle is the portion of the needle that attaches to a syringe. The *length* of the needle varies depending on its use. A longer needle is needed for intramuscular injections, a shorter needle for a subcutaneous injection. The *bevel* of the needle is the slanted tip of the needle. For IV injections, the bevel should always face up. *(Adler & Carlton, p 294)*

74. (C) Single-phase radiographic equipment is much less efficient than three-phase equipment because it has a 100% voltage ripple. *With three-phase equipment, voltage never drops to zero*, and x-ray intensity is significantly greater. To produce similar density, only two thirds of the original mAs would be used for three-phase, six-pulse equipment ($2/3 \times 12 = 8$ mAs). With 3-phase, 12-pulse equipment, the original mAs would be cut in half. *(Saia, pp 329, 330)*

75. (D) Gonadal shielding should be used when the gonads lie within 5 cm of the collimated primary beam, when the patient has reasonable reproductive potential, and when clinical objectives permit. Because their reproductive organs lie outside the abdominal cavity, male patients are more easily and effectively shielded than are female patients, whose reproductive organs lie within the abdominal cavity. Therefore, radiographic examinations of the male abdomen and pelvic structures should include evidence of gonadal shielding. *(Bontrager, pp 209, 257)*

76. (A) The image intensifier's input phosphor is six to nine times larger than the output phosphor. It receives the remnant radiation emerging from the patient and converts it into a fluorescent light image. Very close to the input phosphor, separated only by a thin transparent layer, is the photocathode. The photocathode is made of a photoemissive alloy, usually a cesium and antimony compound. The fluorescent light image strikes the photocathode and is converted to an electron image, which is focused by the electrostatic lenses to the small output phosphor. *(Bushong, pp 360–363)*

77. **(B)** Locate density 2.0 on the vertical axis. Follow it across to where it intersects with image 1, and then to where it intersects with image 2. At each intersection, follow the vertical line down and note the corresponding log relative exposure. Image 1 requires an exposure of about 1.7 to record a density of 2.0, while image 2 requires an exposure of about 2.0 to record the same density. Image 2 is clearly the slower film. The faster film always occupies the position farthest to the left in a comparison of two or more films. *(Shephard, pp 104–107)*

78. **(D)** All three pathologic conditions involve processes that render tissues more easily penetrated by the x-ray beam. *Pneumothorax* is a collection of air or gas in the pleural cavity. *Emphysema* is a chronic pulmonary disease characterized by an increase in the size of the air-containing terminal bronchioles. These two conditions add air to the tissues, making them more easily penetrated. *Multiple myeloma* is a condition characterized by infiltration and destruction of bone and marrow. Each of these conditions requires that factors be decreased from the normal to avoid overexposure. *(Carlton & Adler, p 257)*

79. **(A)** When the arm is placed in the *AP* position, the *epicondyles are parallel* to the plane of the cassette and the shoulder is placed in *external rotation*. In this position, an AP projection of the humerus, elbow, and forearm can be obtained. For the lateral projection of the humerus, elbow, or forearm, the epicondyles must be perpendicular to the plane of the cassette. *(Ballinger & Frank, vol 1, p 144)*

80. **(A)** As the exposed film enters the processor from the feed tray, it first enters the *developer* section (1), where the emulsion's *exposed* silver bromide crystals are reduced to black metallic silver. The film then enters the *fixer* (2), where the *unexposed* silver grains are removed from the film by the clearing agent (hypo). The film then enters the wash section (3), where chemicals are removed from the film to preserve the image. From the wash section, the film enters the dryer section (4). *(Fauber, p 163)*

81. **(B)** It is the radiographer's responsibility to keep radiation exposure to patients and to him- or herself to a minimum. The embryo/fetus is particularly radiosensitive. One way to avoid irradiating a newly fertilized ovum is to inquire about the possibility of a female patient's being pregnant, or to ask her for the date of her last menstrual period. The safest time for a woman of childbearing age to have elective radiographic examinations is during the first 10 days following the onset of menstruation. *(Bushong, p 559)*

82. **(D)** Geometric unsharpness is affected by all three factors listed. As OID increases, so does magnification. As focal-object distance and SID decrease, so does magnification. OID may be said to be directly proportional to magnification. Focal-object distance and SID are inversely proportional to magnification. *(Shephard, pp 214–217)*

83. **(D)** Generally speaking, anatomic parts measuring in excess of 10 cm require a grid. The major exception to this rule is the chest. The larger the part, the more scattered radiation is generated. To avoid degradation of the image as a result of scattered radiation fog, a grid is used to absorb scatter. Parts generally requiring the use of a grid include the skull, spine, ribs, pelvis, shoulder, and femur. *(Carlton & Adler, p 266)*

84. **(C)** The quantity of radiation absorbed by the skin from the primary beam is referred to as the ESE. Although the primary x-ray beam is filtered, it is still quite heterogeneous, containing x-ray photons of low energy that do not contribute to image formation but do contribute to patient skin dose. Thus, the greater the intensity of the initial primary beam, the greater the ESE will be. Therefore, the chest delivers the lowest ESE (12 to 26 mR); the next is the skull (105 to 240 mR); then the thoracic spine (290 to 485 mR); and the examination delivering the greatest ESE is the abdomen (375 to 698 mR). *(Ballinger & Frank, vol 1, p 43)*

85. **(C)** A variety of milliamperage and exposure time settings can produce the same mAs. Each of the following milliamperage and time combinations produces 10 mAs: 100 mA and 0.1 second, 200 mA and 0.05 second, 300 mA and 1/30 second, and 400 mA and 0.025 second. These milliamperage and exposure time combinations should produce identical radiographic density. This is known as the *reciprocity law*. The radiographer can make good use of the reciprocity law when manipulating exposure factors to decrease exposure time and decrease motion unsharpness. *(Selman, p 214)*

86. **(A)** Single-emulsion film is used for particular examinations, such as mammography. It is used with a cassette that has a single intensifying screen and provides better detail than typical double-emulsion film and two-screen cassettes. It is essential that the light-sensitive emulsion be placed against the light-emitting screen. Single-emulsion film has an antihalation backing that efficiently absorbs reflected (crossover) light. Therefore, if the film were loaded with the antihalation side against the light-emitting screen, the film emulsion would receive very little exposure. *(Carlton & Adler, pp 281–282)*

87. **(A)** The cervical *intervertebral foramina* form a 45° angle with the MSP, and therefore are well visualized in a 45° oblique position. *Apophyseal* joints are formed by articulating surfaces of the inferior articular facet of one vertebra with the superior articular facet of the vertebra below; they are well demonstrated in the lateral position of the cervical spine. The *intervertebral disk spaces* are best demonstrated in the lateral position. *(Bontrager, p 294)*

88. **(D)** Some medications cannot be taken orally. They may be destroyed by the GI juices or may irritate the GI tract. Medications that are administered by any route other than orally are said to be given *parenterally*. This can include intravenously, intramuscularly, topically, intrathecally, or subcutaneously. *(Torres et al, p 270)*

89. **(D)** Since the kidneys do not lie parallel to the IR in the AP, the oblique positions are used during IV urography to visualize them better. With the AP oblique projections (RPO and LPO positions), the kidney that is *farther* away is placed *parallel* to the IR, and the kidney that is *closer* is placed *perpendicular* to the IR. Therefore, in the RPO position, the *right kidney*, being closer, is *perpendicular* to the IR. The *left kidney*, the one farther away, is placed *parallel* to the IR. *(Ballinger & Frank, vol 2, p 180)*

90. **(A)** A quality control program requires the use of a number of devices to test the efficiency of various components of the imaging system. A star pattern is a resolution testing device that is used to test the effect of focal spot size. A parallel-line–type resolution test pattern is used to test the resolving capability of intensifying screens. *(Selman, p 210)*

91. **(B)** As field size decreases, the volume of tissue being irradiated decreases, and consequently the production of scattered radiation decreases. When less scattered radiation contributes to the image, the result is *higher contrast* and *lower density*. Restriction of field size is an important way to reduce patient dose and improve image quality. Field size and scattered radiation are unrelated to recorded detail. *(Shephard, p 185)*

92. **(C)** The manufacture of x-ray film starts with a clear polyester *base* that serves as support for the emulsion. Applied next is an *adhesive* layer that functions to hold the *emulsion* to the base. Next is the emulsion, consisting of silver halide grains suspended in gelatin. Finally, a *supercoat* of clear hard gelatin is applied as an antiabrasive layer. A phosphor layer is used in the construction of intensifying screens. *(Shephard, pp 85–88)*

93. **(D)** Higher contrast is shorter scale contrast; it is present in an image that has few shades of gray between white and black. High radiographic contrast is, in part, a result of *lower energy photons* (lower kVp). High radiographic contrast also results when radiographing anatomic parts that have high subject contrast, such as the chest. The abdomen has low subject contrast, and therefore abdominal radiographs will tend to have very

low contrast unless technical factors are selected to increase contrast. To produce high radiographic contrast in abdominal radiography, lower kVp should be used. To better demonstrate high contrast within a viscus, a *contrast medium* such as barium, iodine, or air can be used. Restricting the *size of the field* will also function to increase contrast because less scattered radiation will be generated. *(Carlton & Adler, p 397)*

94. **(D)** OID is used to effect an increase in contrast in the absence of a grid, usually in chest radiography. If a 6-inch air gap (OID) is introduced between the part and the IR, much of the scattered radiation emitted from the body will not reach the IR; thus, the OID acts as a low-ratio grid and increases image contrast. However, the 6-inch OID air gap will make a very noticeable increase in magnification. To correct for this, the SID must be increased. Generally speaking, the SID needs to be increased 7 inches for every 1 inch of OID. With a 6-inch OID, the SID is usually increased from 6 feet to 10 feet (120 inches). *(Shephard, pp 263, 264)*

95. **(D)** In the AP projection of the knee, the position of the joint space is significantly affected by the patient's overall body habitus and the distance between the ASIS and the tabletop. When the patient is of sthenic habitus with a distance of 19 to 24 cm between ASIS and tabletop, the central ray is directed perpendicularly. When the patient is of asthenic habitus with a distance of less than 19 cm between ASIS and tabletop, the central ray is directed 5° caudad. With a patient with a hypersthenic habitus and an ASIS-to-table measurement greater than 24 cm, the central ray is directed 5° cephalad. *(Ballinger & Frank, vol 1, p 290)*

96. **(C)** The radiograph shows evidence of very few grays; this is short-scale, or high, contrast. There is inadequate penetration of the denser structures: the heart and the lung bases and apices. Penetration and contrast are a function of kilovoltage. Inadequate penetration and high contrast are a result of insufficient kVp. *(Saia, p 345)*

97. **(C)** Most laser film is panchromatic film and sensitive to all light, including both the Wratten 6B and the GBX safelight filters. Laser film will fog if it is handled under these safelight conditions. Most laser film is loaded into a film magazine in total darkness. Other processing conditions and temperatures are the same for laser film as for regular x-ray film. *(Shephard, p 92)*

98. **(B)** A *stethoscope and a sphygmomanometer* are used together to measure blood pressure. The sphygmomanometer's cuff is placed around the midportion of the upper arm. The cuff is inflated to a value higher than the patient's systolic pressure to *temporarily collapse the brachial artery.* As the inflation is gradually released, the first sound heard is the systolic pressure; the normal range is 110 to 140 mm Hg. When no more sound is heard, the dia-stolic pressure is recorded. The normal dia-stolic range is 60 to 90 mm Hg. Elevated blood pressure is called *hypertension. Hypotension,* low blood pressure, is not of concern unless it is caused by injury or disease; in that case, it can result in shock. *(Adler & Carlton, p 181)*

99. **(B)** For an AP projection of the hip, two bony landmarks are used. The central ray is directed perpendicular to a point located 2 inches medial to the *ASIS* at the level of the *greater trochanter.* A point midway between the iliac crest and the pubic symphysis is too superior and medial to coincide with the hip articulation. *(Ballinger & Frank, vol 1, p 329)*

100. **(B)** *Battery* refers to the unlawful laying of hands on a patient. Battery could be charged if a patient were moved about roughly or touched in a manner that is inappropriate or without the patient's consent. *Assault* is the threat of touching or laying hands on. If a patient feels threatened by a health-care provider, either because of the provider's tone or pitch of voice or because of words that are threatening, an assault charge may be made. *False imprisonment* may be considered if a patient states that he or she no longer wishes to continue with a procedure and is ignored, or if restraining devices are improperly used or used

without a physician's order. *Invasion of privacy issues arise when there has been a disclosure of confidential information. (Adler & Carlton, p 326)*

101. **(C)** To change nongrid to grid exposure, or to adjust exposure when changing from one grid ratio to another, recall the factor for each grid ratio:

No grid = 1 × the original mAs
5:1 grid = 2 × the original mAs
6:1 grid = 3 × the original mAs
8:1 grid = 4 × the original mAs
12:1 grid = 5 × the original mAs
16:1 grid = 6 × the original mAs

The grid conversion formula is

$$\frac{mAs_1}{mAs_1} = \frac{grid\ factor_1}{grid\ factor_1}$$

Substituting known quantities:

$$\frac{12}{x} = \frac{4}{5}$$
$$4x = 60$$
$$x = 15\ mAs\ with\ a\ 12{:}1\ grid$$

(Saia, p 328)

102. **(C)** Hypoglycemic reactions can be very severe and should be treated with an immediate dose of sugar in the form of juice or candy. Symptoms of hypoglycemia include fatigue, restlessness, irritability, and weakness. Diabetic patients who have not taken their insulin prior to a fasting examination should be given priority, and their examinations should be expedited as quickly as possible. *(Torres et al, pp 169–170)*

103. **(D)** The ability of x-ray photons to penetrate a body part has a great deal to do with the composition of that part (eg, bone vs soft tissue vs air) and the presence of any pathologic condition. Pathologic conditions can alter the normal nature of the anatomic part. Some conditions, such as *osteomalacia, fibrosarcoma,* and *paralytic ileus* (obstruction), result in a *decrease* in body tissue density. When body tissue density *decreases*, x-rays will *penetrate the tissues more readily*, that is, there is more x-ray penetrability. In conditions such as *ascites*, where body tissue density *increases* as a result

of the accumulation of fluid, x-rays *will not readily penetrate the body tissues*, that is, there is *less x-ray penetrability. (Carlton & Adler, p 258)*

104. **(B)** Factors that affect screen speed will also affect radiographic density. *Rare earth–type* phosphors absorb x-rays more efficiently and convert their energy into fluorescent light; they therefore affect both screen speed and radiographic density. The *thickness* of the phosphor layer affects speed and density similarly: As the thickness of the phosphor layer increases, speed and density increase. The *spongy layer* behind each intensifying screen helps ensure good screen–film contact and therefore good recorded detail. The spongy layer is unrelated to radiographic density. *(Shephard, p 68)*

105. **(B)** Two devices that are required for quality assurance evaluation purposes are a sensitometer and a densitometer. A *sensitometer* is a device that functions to *expose* a film; when developed, that film will illustrate an optical step wedge with a number of optical densities ranging from white through several shades of gray to black. A *densitometer* is a device that *reads* the various densities on the film. A *penetrometer*, or (usually aluminum) step wedge, can be used to demonstrate the effect of kVp on radiographic contrast. A *potentiometer* is another name for a variable resistor. *(Carlton & Adler, pp 317–318)*

106. **(C)** A "controlled area" is one that is occupied by radiation workers; the exposure rate in a controlled area must not exceed 100 mR/week. An uncontrolled area is one that is occupied by the general population; the exposure rate must not exceed 10 mR/week. Shielding requirements vary according to several factors, one of them being occupancy factor. *(Bushong, p 573)*

107. **(C)** The AP axial projection is used to project the clavicles from superimposition on the pulmonary apices. A 15° to 20° cephalad angle projects the clavicles above the apices. The radiograph is evaluated for rotation by checking the distance between the medial ends of the clavicles and the lateral border of

the vertebral column. *(Ballinger & Frank, vol 1, pp 544–545)*

108. **(B)** Radiograph A was performed *PA* and radiograph B performed *AP*, as evidenced by the bony pelvis anatomy. The PA projection (image A) shows the ilia more foreshortened, giving the pelvis a "closed" appearance, while in the AP projection the ilia and bladder area appears more "open." There was an appropriate selection of exposure factors, for the required anatomic structures are well visualized: renal shadows, psoas muscle, lumbar transverse processes, and inferior margin of the liver. There is no evidence of ureteral compression, which would be seen as air-filled bladders, or some other type of compression device, placed over the distal ureters. *(Ballinger & Frank, vol 2, p 124)*

109. **(C)** As radiation passes through tissue, different types of ionization processes can take place, depending on the photon energy and the type of material being irradiated. The photoelectric effect (whose end products include a characteristic ray) and Compton scatter are the two major interactions that take place in the diagnostic x-ray kVp range. The *rate* at which energy is deposited in (or transferred to) tissue during these interactions is termed *linear energy transfer* (LET). The greater the LET, the greater the potential biologic effect. Diagnostic x-ray is considered low-LET radiation. *(Bushong, p 495)*

110. **(C)** The radiograph illustrates a plantodorsal projection of the calcaneus. The patient is usually positioned with the leg extended and the long axis of the plantar surface perpendicular to the tabletop/image recorder. The central ray is directed 40° cephalad to the base of the third metatarsal. Structures that should be visualized include the sustentaculum tali, trochlear process, and calcaneal tuberosity. *(Bontrager, p 222)*

111. **(A)** *Asthma* is characterized by difficulty in breathing, causing bronchospasm. It is often precipitated by stress, and although dyspnea is a symptom, oxygen is not administered. Asthmatics carry a nebulizer that contains a medication to relieve the bronchospasm, thereby relieving their breathing distress. Anaphylaxis is an acute reaction characterized by sudden onset of urticaria, respiratory distress, vascular collapse, or systemic shock; it sometimes leads to death. It is caused by ingestion or injection of a sensitizing agent such as a drug, vaccine, contrast agent, or food, or by an insect bite. Asthma and rhinitis are examples of allergic reactions. *(Bontrager, p 636)*

112. **(A)** Restriction of field size is one important method of patient protection. However, the accuracy of the light field must be evaluated periodically as part of a QA program. Guidelines set forth for patient protection state that the collimator light and actual irradiated area must be accurate to within 2% of the SID. *(Thompson et al, p 403)*

113. **(D)** The thicker and more dense the anatomic part being studied, the less bright will be the fluoroscopic image. Both mA and kVp affect the fluoroscopic image in a way similar to the way they affect the radiographic image. For optimal contrast, especially taking patient dose into consideration, higher kVp and lower mA are generally preferred. *(Carlton & Adler, p 607)*

114. **(B)** When differences in absorption characteristics are decreased, body tissues absorb radiation more uniformly, and, as a result, more grays are seen on the radiographic image. A longer scale of contrast is produced. High-kVp and low-mAs factors achieve this. Compensating filtration is also used to "even out" densities in uneven anatomic parts, such as the thoracic spine. The photoelectric effect is the interaction between x-ray photons and matter that occurs at low kVp levels—levels that tend to produce short-scale contrast. *(Shephard, pp 193, 197, 199)*

115. **(D)** All these conditions are considered technically *additive* because they all involve an *increase in tissue density*. Osteoma, or exostosis, is a (usually benign) bony tumor that can develop on bone. *Bronchiectasis* is a chronic dilatation of the bronchi with accumulation of

fluid. *Pneumonia* is inflammation of the lung(s) with accumulation of fluid. Additional bony tissues and the pathological presence of fluid are additive pathological conditions and require an increase in exposure factors. *Destructive* conditions such as osteoporosis require a *decrease* in exposure factors. *(Carlton & Adler, p 258)*

116. **(C)** The four types of body habitus describe differences in visceral shape, position, tone, and motility. One body type is *hypersthenic*, the very large individual with short, wide heart and lungs; high transverse stomach and gallbladder; and peripheral colon. The *sthenic* individual is the average, athletic, most predominant type. The *hyposthenic* patient is somewhat thinner and a little more frail, with organs positioned somewhat lower. The *asthenic* type is smaller in the extreme, with a long thorax; a very long, almost pelvic stomach; and a *low medial gallbladder*. The colon is medial and redundant. *(Saia, p 167)*

117. **(C)** The radiograph is a PA projection of the hand and wrist; an oblique projection of the thumb is obtained. The letter *T* is pointing out the first carpometacarpal joint, formed by the base of the first metacarpal and the trapezium. This is classified as a *saddle*-type *diarthrotic* joint. Diarthrotic joints are *freely movable* joints and the most plentiful type joint in the human body. Amphiarthrotic joints are partially movable; synarthrotic joints are immovable. *(Ballinger & Frank, vol 1, p 91)*

118. **(B)** The eight carpal bones are well visualized in this PA projection of the hand and wrist. The letters *E* (scaphoid) and *L* (lunate) are in the proximal carpal row. The capitate *(I)* is seen in the distal carpal row; just lateral to the capitate is the carpal trapezium, seen articulating with the base of the first metacarpal. The PA projection of the hand provides an oblique projection of the first finger (thumb). *(Ballinger & Frank, vol 1, p 91)*

119. **(D)** All three factors can affect radiographic contrast. The type of chemistry used in the automatic *processor* and especially the temperature of the solution can have a big impact on the resulting image contrast. As temperature increases, contrast decreases. Since pathology can alter the degree of attenuation of the x-ray beam, it can affect contrast. The type of pathology will determine how contrast is affected. An *additive* pathology such as Paget's disease will increase contrast, while a *destructive* disease such as osteoporosis will decrease contrast. *OID* can affect contrast when it is used as an air gap. If a 6-inch air gap (OID) is introduced between the part and the IR, much of the scattered radiation emitted from the body will not reach the IR; the air gap thus acts as a grid and increases image contrast. *(Carlton & Adler, pp 397–398)*

120. **(A)** X-ray film is sensitive and requires proper handling and storage. Careless handling during production of the radiographic image can produce several kinds of artifacts. Crescent-shaped artifacts (crinkle marks) are a result of bending the film acutely over the fingertip while loading or unloading the cassette. A black crescent usually results from bending after exposure, whereas a white crescent occurs if the film is bent before exposure. Treelike, branching black marks on a radiograph are usually due to static electrical discharge. Problems with static electricity are especially prevalent during cold, dry weather and can be produced by simply removing a sweater in the darkroom. *(Selman, p 197)*

121. **(B)** The exposure factor that regulates radiographic density is *mAs*. The equation used to determine mAs is $mA \times s = mAs$. Substituting known factors,

$$300x = 18 \text{ mAs}$$
$$x = 0.06 \text{ second}$$

(Selman, p 214)

122. **(A)** If the photocell was centered more posteriorly to a thinner and less dense structure, then the exposure received would be correct for that less dense structure. The spinous processes would be well visualized, *but the denser vertebral bodies and surrounding structures* (pedicles and lamina) *would be underexposed*. Accurate selection of photocells and precise positioning is critical with the use of

automatic exposure devices. *(Carlton & Adler, pp 503–506)*

123. **(D)** Shock caused by an abnormally low volume of blood in the body is termed *hypovolemic* shock. *Neurogenic* shock can be caused by some kind of trauma to the nervous system, that is, spinal cord injury or extreme psychological stress. *Cardiogenic* shock is related to the heart and caused by failure of the heart to pump adequate blood to the body's vital organs. *Septic* shock can result when the body is invaded by bacteria; there are signs of acute septicemia and hypotension. *(Torres et al, p 163)*

124. **(B)** It is easy to determine the highest point of the scapula when it is viewed laterally. The coracoid process projects anteriorly and is quite superior. However, the acromion process, which is an anterior extension of the scapular spine, projects considerably more superior than the coracoid. *(Ballinger & Frank, vol 1, p 162)*

125. **(D)** Base-plus fog is the small amount of measurable density on unexposed and processed x-ray film. This fog is a result of environmental, background radiation that is present during film manufacture, transportation, and storage. The (usually blue) tint, given the base to enhance contrast, adds more density. Finally, the emulsion receives further fog as the film is chemically processed. Base-plus fog should not exceed 0.2D. *(Carlton & Adler, p 314)*

126. **(B)** There are several radiation units that are used to express quantity and effects of radiation. Radiation ionizes air, and the unit of measurement used to describe the amount of ionization (and therefore the quantity of radiation present) is the *roentgen*. The *rad* is the unit of absorbed dose. The *rem* is the unit of dose equivalent, which expresses radiation dose to biologic material. *(Bontrager, p 53)*

127. **(B)** The developer's reducing agents function to change exposed silver halide grains to black metallic silver. *Hydroquinone* builds up the blacks, whereas *phenidone* controls the subtle gray tones. *Sodium sulfite* is used in the

developer and fixer solutions and acts as a preservative. In the developer, it retards rapid oxidation of the solution. *Ammonium thiosulfate* (hypo) is the fixer's clearing agent, which functions to clear from the film unexposed silver grains that would otherwise darken on exposure to light. *(Carlton & Adler, p 319)*

128. **(D)** *Lymphocytes*, a type of white blood cell concerned with the immune system, have the greatest radiosensitivity of all body cells. *Spermatids* are also highly radiosensitive, though not to the same degree as lymphocytes. *Muscle* cells have a fairly low radiosensitivity, and *nerve* cells are the least radiosensitive in the body (in fetal life, however, nerve cells are highly radiosensitive). *(Dowd & Tilson, p 135)*

129. **(C)** To have high diagnostic quality, a *barium enema* examination requires rigorous and complete patient preparation. This usually consists of a modified low-residue diet for a few days before the examination, cathartics the day before, and cleansing enemas the morning of the examination. Instructions for a UGI, small bowel series, and IV cystogram are usually to be npo after midnight. *(Ballinger & Frank, vol 2, p 129)*

130. **(C)** X-ray tube targets are constructed according to the *line focus principle*—the focal spot is angled (usually 12° to 17°) to the vertical. As the actual focal spot is projected downward, it is foreshortened; thus, the effective focal spot is smaller than the actual focal spot. As the focal spot is projected toward the cathode end of the x-ray beam, it becomes larger and approaches its actual size. Figure 6–19 illustrates the variation of the effective focal spot size along the longitudinal tube axis. As the effective focal spot becomes larger toward the cathode end, the images of the phalanges illustrate gradual loss of re-corded detail. *(Bushong, p 140)*

131. **(D)** Extravasation occurs when medication or contrast medium is injected into the tissues surrounding a vein rather than into the vein itself. It can happen when the patient's veins are particularly deep and/or small. If this

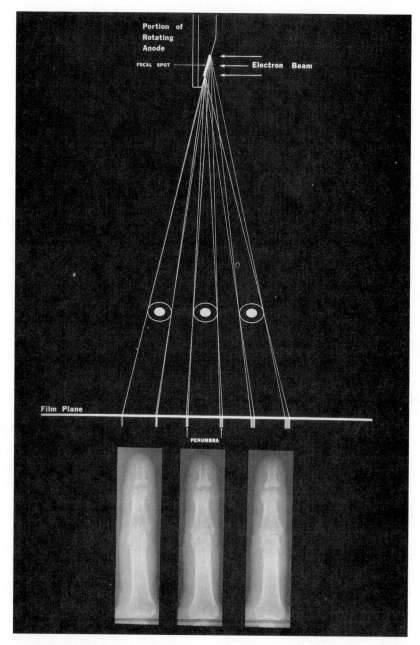

Figure 6–19. From the American College of Radiology Learning File. Courtesy of the ACR.

happens, the needle should be removed, pressure applied to prevent formation of a hematoma, and then hot packs applied to relieve pain. *(Torres et al, p 324)*

132. **(B)** A *polyp* is a tumor with a pedicle (stalk) that is commonly found in vascular organs projecting inward from its mucosal wall. Polyps are usually removed surgically because, although usually benign, they can become malignant. A *diverticulum* is an out-

pouching from the wall of an organ, such as the colon. A *fistula* is an abnormal tubelike passageway between organs or between an organ and the surface. An *abscess* is a localized collection of pus as a result of inflammation. *(Bontrager, p 426)*

133. **(C)** In Figure 6–12, image B is darker and therefore has more optical (radiographic) density. Radiographic density is significantly affected by mAs, SID, and exposure rate. In

this case, there is a difference in SID between the two images. As SID decreases, exposure rate increases and radiographic density increases. Image B is darker (has more optical density) than image A because image B was exposed at a shorter SID (and therefore a higher exposure rate). (*Bushong, pp 300–303*)

134. **(C)** Lead aprons are secondary radiation barriers and must *contain at least 0.25 (1/4) mm Pb* equivalent, usually in the form of lead-impregnated vinyl (according to CFR 20). Many radiology departments routinely use lead aprons containing 0.5 mm Pb (the NCRP recommends 0.5 mm Pb equiv. minimum). These aprons are heavier, but they attenuate a higher percentage of scattered radiation. (*Bushong, p 560*)

135. **(A)** The shorter the SID, the greater the skin dose (ESE). That is why there are specific SSD restrictions in fluoroscopy. X-ray beam quality has a significant effect on patient skin dose. The use of high kVp produces more high-energy penetrating photons, thereby decreasing skin dose. Filtration is used to remove the low-energy photons that contribute to skin dose from the primary beam. Although mA regulates the number of x-ray photons produced, it does not affect photon quality. (*Bushong, p 300–303*)

136. **(B)** *Stochastic* effects of radiation are non-threshold and randomly occurring. Examples of stochastic effects include carcinogenesis and genetic effects. The chance of occurrence of stochastic effects is directly related to the radiation dose; that is, as radiation dose increases, there is a greater likelihood of genetic alterations or development of cancer. *Nonstochastic* effects are predictable, threshold responses; that is, a certain quantity of radiation must be received before the effect will occur, and the greater the dose, the more severe the effect. (*Bushong, p 532*)

137. **(D)** The cycle of infection includes four components: a susceptible host, a reservoir of infection, a pathogenic organism, and a means of transmission. *Pathogenic organisms* are microscopic and include bacteria, fungi, and viruses.

The *reservoir of infection* is the environment in which the microorganism thrives; this can be the human body. A *susceptible host* may have reduced resistance to infection. The means of transmission is either direct (touch) or indirect (vector, fomite, airborne). (*Torres et al, p 53*)

138. **(C)** The distal humerus articulates with the radius and ulna to form the elbow joint. The lateral aspect of the distal humerus presents a raised, smooth, rounded surface, the *capitulum*, that articulates with the superior surface of the *radial head*. The *trochlea* is on the medial aspect of the distal humerus and articulates with the semilunar notch of the ulna. Just proximal to the capitulum and the trochlea are the *lateral* and *medial epicondyles*; the medial is more prominent and palpable. The *coronoid fossa* is found on the anterior distal humerus and functions to accommodate the coronoid process with the elbow in flexion. The *intertubercular (bicipital) groove* is located on the proximal humerus. (*Saia, pp 89*)

139. **(B)** *Cathartics* are used to stimulate defecation (bowel movements). *Diuretics* are used to promote urine elimination in individuals whose tissues are retaining excessive fluid. *Emetics* function to induce vomiting, and *antitussives* are used to inhibit coughing. (*Torres et al, p 288*)

140. **(D)** The *pulmonary apices* are often at least partially obscured by the clavicles. To visualize the entire *lung apex* and any suspicious areas, the clavicles must be "removed." This can be accomplished with the *AP axial lordotic position*. Through the arching of the patient's back and the cephalad angulation, the clavicles are projected upward and out of the pulmonary apices. *Decubitus* positions are used primarily to see *air–fluid levels*. Lateral and dorsal decubitus positions show fluid in the side that is down, and air in the side that is up. (*Ballinger & Frank, vol 1, p 544*)

141. **(D)** A *transthoracic* projection is used to obtain a lateral projection of the upper half to two thirds of the humerus when the arm cannot be abducted. The affected arm is placed next to the upright Bucky, the unaffected arm rests on the head, and the central ray is

directed horizontally through the thorax, exiting the upper humerus. The *superoinferior* and *inferosuperior* projections of the shoulder both require abduction of the arm. *(Saia, p 98)*

142. **(D)** Single-phase radiographic equipment is much less efficient than three-phase equipment because it has a 100% voltage ripple. *With three-phase equipment, voltage never drops to zero,* and x-ray intensity is significantly greater. To produce similar density, only *two thirds* of the original mAs would be used for three-phase, *six-pulse* equipment (2/3 × 20 = 13 mAs). With 3-phase, *12-pulse* equipment, the original mAs would be cut in *half;* thus, 10 mAs should be used. *(Saia, pp 329, 330)*

143. **(A)** The thoracic intervertebral (disk) spaces are demonstrated in the AP and lateral projections, although they are probably best demonstrated in the lateral. The thoracic apophyseal joints are 70° to the MSP and are demonstrated in a steep (70°) oblique position. The thoracic intervertebral foramina, formed by the vertebral notches of the pedicles, are 90° to the MSP. They are therefore well demonstrated in the lateral position. *(Bontrager, p 283)*

144. **(D)** The *posterior oblique positions* (LPO and RPO) of the lumbar vertebrae demonstrate the apophyseal joints *closer* to the IR. The left apophyseal joints are demonstrated in the LPO position, while the *right* apophyseal joints are demonstrated in the *RPO* position. The lateral position is useful to demonstrate the intervertebral disk spaces, intervertebral foramina, and spinous processes. *(Saia, p 131)*

145. **(D)** *Motion* is said to be the greatest enemy of recorded detail because it completely obliterates image sharpness. Poor *screen–film contact* reduces recorded detail because of the degree of light diffusion in the areas of poor contact. Areas of poor contact appear blurry. A decrease in *source–image distance* causes magnification and blurriness of recorded detail. Grid ratio is related to scattered radiation cleanup; it is unrelated to recorded detail. *(Shephard, pp 213–217)*

146. **(C)** A grid is a thin wafer placed between the patient and the IR to collect scattered radiation. It is made of alternating strips of lead and a radiolucent material such as *plastic* or *aluminum.* If the interspace material were also made of lead, little or no radiation would reach the IR, and no image would be formed. *(Shephard, pp 244–245)*

147. **(C)** Whenever a radiation worker could receive 10% or more of the annual TEDE (total effective dose equivalent) limit, that person must be provided with a radiation monitor. The annual TEDE limit for radiation workers is 5 rem (5000 mrem), but it is the responsibility of the radiographer to practice the ALARA principle, that is, to keep radiation dose as low as reasonably achievable. *(Sherer et al, p 228)*

148. **(D)** The formula for mAs is mA × s = mAs. Substituting known values,

$$0.05x = 15$$
$$x = 300 \text{ mA}$$

(Selman, p 214)

149. **(D)** Body substance precaution procedures identify various body fluids as infectious or potentially infectious. These body substances include pleural, pericardial, peritoneal, and amniotic fluids, synovial fluid, CSF, breast milk, and vaginal secretions. Also nasal secretions, tears, saliva, sputum, feces, urine, and wound drainage. *(Torres et al, p 63)*

150. **(A)** A radiographer who discloses confidential information to unauthorized individuals may be found guilty of *invasion of privacy.* If the disclosure is in some way detrimental or otherwise harmful to the patient, the radiographer may be accused of *defamation.* Spoken defamation is *slander;* written defamation is *libel. Assault* is to threaten harm; *battery* is to carry out the threat. *(Torres et al, p 11)*

151. **(B)** All four medications are routinely found on the typical emergency cart. *Heparin* is used to decrease coagulation and often used in the cardiovascular imaging suite to inhibit coagulation on catheters. *Norepinephrine* functions to raise the blood pressure, while *nitroglycerin* functions as a vasodilator, relaxing the walls of blood vessels and increasing

circulation. *Lidocaine* is used as a local anesthetic or antidysrhythmic. *(Adler & Carlton, p 257)*

152. **(B)** Focal spot blur, or geometric blur, is caused by photons emerging from a large focal spot. Because the projected focal spot is greatest at the cathode end of the x-ray tube, geometric blur is also greatest at the corresponding part (cathode end) of the radiograph. The projected focal spot size becomes progressively smaller toward the anode end of the x-ray tube. *(Bushong, p 140)*

153. **(C)** The image intensifier can be coupled to the TV camera via *a fiber optic bundle* or via a *lens coupling* device. The fiber optic connection offers less fragility, more compactness, and ease of manuverability. The big advantage of the objective lens is that it *allows the use of auxiliary imaging devices* such as a *cine camera or spot film camera. (Bushong, p 366)*

154. **(D)** Each of the three is included in a good QA program. *Beam alignment* must be accurate to 2% of the SID. *Reproducibility* means that repeated exposures at a given technique must provide consistent intensity. *Linearity* means that a given mAs, using different mA stations with appropriate exposure time adjustments, will provide consistent intensity. *(Bushong, pp 460–464)*

155. **(C)** Bones are classified as long, short, flat, and irregular. Many of the bones making up the extremities are long bones. Long bones have a *shaft* and two extremities (ends). The shaft (or *diaphysis*) of long bones is the *primary ossification center* during bone development. It is composed of compact tissue and covered with a membrane called *periosteum*. Within the shaft is the medullary cavity, which contains bone marrow and is lined by the membrane called *endosteum*. In the adult, yellow marrow occupies the shaft, and red marrow is found within the proximal and distal extremities of long bones. The *secondary ossification center*, the *epiphysis*, is separated from the diaphysis in early life by a layer of cartilage, the *epiphyseal plate*. As bone growth takes place, the epiphysis becomes part of the larger portion of bone and the epiphyseal plate disappears, but a characteristic line remains and is thereafter recognizable as the *epiphyseal line*. *(Saia, p 85)*

156. **(A)** Location of the heels of the hands is of great importance during CPR. They should be placed about $1\frac{1}{2}$ *inches superior to the xiphoid tip*. In this way, the heart will receive the compressions it requires without causing internal injuries. Rib fractures can depress and cause injury to the lung tissues within the rib cage. *(Torres et al, pp 172–176)*

157. **(D)** An *analgesic* is any drug, such as aspirin, that functions to relieve pain. An *anticoagulant* (eg, heparin) is used to prevent clotting of blood. A *diuretic* is used to increase urine output, and an *antibiotic* (eg, penicillin) fights the growth of bacterial microorganisms. *(Torres et al, p 291)*

158. **(A)** The abdomen is divided anatomically into *nine regions* and *four quadrants*. The *region* designation is usually used for anatomic studies, while the *quadrant* designation is most often used to describe the location of a lesion, pain, tumor, or other abnormality. Some of the structures found in the left upper quadrant (LUQ) are the fundus of the stomach, the left kidney and suprarenal gland, and the splenic flexure. *(Tortora & Derrickson, p 20)*

159. **(A)** With all other factors remaining the same, as intensifying-screen speed increases, radiographic density increases. Radiographic density is directly proportional to intensifying-screen speed; that is, if screen speed doubles, density doubles. The formula to determine how mAs should be corrected with screen speed changes is

Screen speed and mAs conversion factors are as follows:

Screen Speed	mAs Conversion Factor
50	4
100	2
200	1
400	0.5
800	0.25

Substituting known quantities,

$$\frac{4}{0.5} = \frac{32 \text{ mAs}}{x \text{ mAs}}$$

$$4x = 16$$

$$x = 4 \text{ mAs with 400 speed screens}$$

(Saia, p 361)

160. **(D)** *The shortest possible exposure time should be used to minimize motion unsharpness.* Motion causes unsharpness that destroys detail. Careful and accurate patient instruction is essential for minimizing voluntary motion. Suspended respiration eliminates respiratory motion. Using the shortest possible exposure time is essential to decreasing *involuntary* motion. Immobilization can also be useful in eliminating motion unsharpness. *(Selman, p 210)*

161. **(D)** A PA projection of the left hand and wrist is most often obtained to evaluate skeletal maturation. These images are compared to standard normal images for the age and sex of the child. Additional supplemental images may be requested. *(Bontrager, p 634)*

162. **(D)** According to the inverse square law of radiation, the intensity or exposure rate of radiation from its source is inversely proportional to the square of the distance. Thus, as distance from the source of radiation increases, exposure rate decreases. Because exposure rate and radiographic density are directly proportional, if the exposure rate of a beam directed to the image recorder is decreased, the resultant radiographic density would be decreased proportionally. *(Selman, p 117)*

163. **(A)** As radiation passes through tissue, different types of ionization processes can take place, depending on the photon energy and the type of material being irradiated. In the *photoelectric effect*, a relatively low-energy photon uses all its energy to eject an inner-shell electron from the target atom, leaving a vacancy in that shell. An electron from the shell beyond drops down to fill the vacancy and, in doing so, emits a characteristic ray. This type of interaction contributes most to

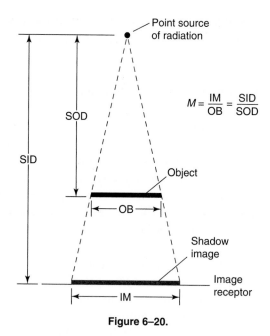

$$M = \frac{IM}{OB} = \frac{SID}{SOD}$$

Figure 6–20.

patient dose, because all the x-ray photon energy is being transferred to tissue. In *Compton scatter*, a high-energy incident photon uses some of its energy to eject an outer-shell electron. In doing so, the incident photon is deflected with reduced energy, but usually retains most of its original energy and exits the body as an energetic scattered photon. In Compton scatter, the scattered radiation will either contribute to image fog or pose a radiation hazard to personnel, depending on its direction of exit. In *classical scatter*, a low-energy photon interacts with an atom but causes no ionization; the incident photon disappears in the atom, then immediately reappears and is released as a photon of identical energy but changed direction. *Thompson scatter* is another name for classical scatter. *(Selman, pp 125–128)*

164. **(A)** A *vector* is an animal host of an infectious organism that transmits the infection via a bite or sting, such as the mosquito (malaria) and the deer tick (Lyme disease). A *fomite* is an inanimate object that has been in contact with an infectious microorganism. A *reservoir* is a site where an infectious organism can remain alive and from which transmission can occur. Although an inanimate object can be a reservoir for infection, living objects (such as humans) can also be reservoirs. For infection to spread, there must be a *host* environment.

Although an inanimate object may serve as a temporary host for microbes to grow, microbes flourish on and in the human host, where plenty of body fluids and tissue nourish and feed the microbes. (*Adler & Carlton, p 201*)

165. **(B)** As OID increases, magnification increases. Viscera and structures within the body will be varying distances from the image receptor, depending on their location within the body and the position used for the exposure. The size of a particular structure or image can be calculated using the following formula:

$$\frac{\text{Image size}}{\text{Object size}} = \frac{\text{SID}}{\text{SOD (SOD = SID–OID)}}$$

Substituting known quantities,

$$\frac{9 \text{ cm}}{x \text{ cm}} = \frac{105 \text{ cm}}{87 \text{ cm}}$$
$$105x = 83$$
$$x = 7.45 \text{ cm (approximate } actual \text{ } size\text{)}$$

The relationship between SID, SOD, and OID and the equation for determining image or object size is illustrated in Figure 6–20. (*Bushong, p 284*)

166. **(C)** Kilovoltage (kVp) and half-value layer (HVL) change *both* the quantity and quality of the primary beam. The principal qualitative factor of the primary beam is kVp, but an increase in kVp will also effect an increase in the *number* of photons produced at the target. HVL is defined as the amount of material necessary to decrease the intensity of the beam to one half of its original value, thereby effecting a change in both beam quality and quantity. The mAs value is adjusted to regulate the number of x-ray photons produced at the target. X-ray beam quality is unaffected by changes in mAs. (*Bushong, p 165*)

167. **(D)** Weight-bearing lateral projections of the foot are often requested to evaluate the longitudinal arch structure of the foot. The patient stands on a small platform. The x-ray cassette is placed between the feet, in a slot provided on the platform, with the top of the cassette against the medial aspect of the foot. The central ray is directed to enter the *lateral* aspect of the foot perpendicular to the base of the fifth metatarsal and to exit the *medial* side of the foot. (*Ballinger & Frank, vol 1, pp 254–255*)

168. **(C)** The *autotransformer* (number 1) controls/selects the amount of voltage sent to the primary winding of the high-voltage transformer and operates on the principle of *self*-induction. The *step-up* (high-voltage) *transformer* (primary coil is number 2, secondary coil is number 3) operates on the principle of *mutual* induction. The *step-up transformer* functions to change low voltage to the high voltage necessary to produce x-ray photons. The x-ray tube is identified as number 7. (*Selman, pp 83–84*)

169. **(C)** In the simplified x-ray circuit shown, the *autotransformer* is labeled number 1, the primary coil of the *high-voltage transformer* is number 2, and the *secondary coil* is labeled number 3. The autotransformer selects the voltage that will be sent to the high-voltage transformer to be stepped up to the thousands of volts required for x-ray production. At the midpoint of the secondary coil is *the grounded mA meter* (number 4). Since the mA meter is in the control panel and is associated with high voltage, it must be grounded. The *rectification system*, which is used to change alternating current to unidirectional current, is indicated by the number 5. The rectification system is located between the secondary coil of the high-voltage transformer (number 3) and the x-ray tube (number 7). (*Selman, pp 159, 161*)

170. **(A)** The line focus principle is a geometric principle illustrating that the *actual focal spot is larger than the effective (projected) focal spot*. The actual focal spot (target) is larger, to accommodate heat over a larger area, and angled so as to *project* a smaller focal spot, thus maintaining recorded detail by reducing blur. The relationship between the exposure given the IR and the resulting density is expressed in the inverse square law. The relationship between the kVp used and the resulting contrast may be illustrated using an aluminum step wedge. (*Selman, pp 138–139*)

171. **(A)** The type of isolation practiced to prevent the spread of infectious agents in aerosol form is *respiratory isolation*. A mask is sufficient protection from aerosol transmission of pathogens. *Protective isolation,* also referred to as reverse isolation, is used to protect patients whose immune systems are compromised. Patients receiving chemotherapy, burn patients, or patients who are human immunodeficiency virus– (HIV) positive may all have compromised immune systems. *Contact isolation* is used when there is a chance that infection may be spread by contact with body fluids. Gloves and a gown are used, and goggles and masks may be necessary if there is a chance of fluids spraying, such as in biopsy or drainage. *Strict isolation* is practiced with highly contagious diseases or viruses that may be spread by air and/or contact. *(Adler & Carlton, p 215)*

172. **(D)** Breast tissue has very low subject contrast, but it is imperative to visualize microcalcifications and subtle density differences. Fine detail is necessary to visualize any microcalcifications; therefore, a *small focal spot* tube is essential. *High,* short-scale contrast (and therefore low kilovoltage) is needed to accentuate minute differences in tissue density. A *compression device* serves to even out differences in tissue thickness (thicker at chest wall, thinner at nipple) and decrease OID, and helps decrease the production of scattered radiation. *(Selman, pp 288–289)*

173. **(B)** It is essential that the darkroom safelight filter color is correctly matched with the type/sensitivity of film emulsion being used. The GBX is a red filter that is safe with greensensitive film emulsion. The amber-colored Wratten 6B filter is safe for blue-sensitive film only. Although using no safelight is possible, it is not a practical way to function. *(Selman, p 191)*

174. **(D)** X-ray tube life may be extended by using exposure factors that produce a minimum of heat, that is, a lower mAs and higher kVp combination, whenever possible. When the rotor is activated, the filament current is increased to produce the required electron source (thermionic emission). Prolonged rotor time, then, can lead to shortened filament life as a result of early vaporization. Large exposures to a cold anode will heat the anode surface, and the big temperature difference can cause cracking of the anode. This can be avoided by proper warming of the anode prior to use, thereby allowing sufficient dispersion of heat through the anode. *(Selman, pp 143–145)*

175. **(B)** A fractional focal spot of 0.3 mm or smaller is essential for reproducing fine detail without focal spot blurring in magnification radiography. As the object image is magnified, so will be the associated blur unless the fractional focal spot is used. Fluoroscopic procedures would probably cause great wear on a fractional focal spot. Use of the fractional focal spot is not essential in bone radiography, although *magnification* of bony structures is often helpful in locating hairline fractures. *(Selman, pp 226–228)*

176. **(D)** The thicker the active layer of phosphors, the more fluorescent light is emitted from the screen. Different types of phosphors have different *conversion efficiencies;* rare earth phosphors emit more light during a given exposure than do calcium tungstate phosphors. As the kVp level is increased, so is the amount of fluoroscopic light emitted by intensifying screen phosphors. *(Selman, pp 177–182)*

177. **(A)** The gradual decrease in exposure rate as radiation passes through matter is called *attenuation*. Attenuation is attributed to the two major types of interactions that occur in tissue between x-ray photons and matter in the diagnostic x-ray range. In the photoelectric effect, absorption and secondary radiation occur. In the Compton effect, scattered radiation is produced. With each of these occurrences, there is a decrease in the exposure rate that is referred to as attenuation. *(Bushong, p 185)*

178. **(A)** X-rays produced in the x-ray tube make up a heterogeneous beam. There are many low-energy, or "soft," photons that do not contribute to the radiographic image because they never reach the IR. Instead, they stay in the patient, contributing to skin dose. It is

these photons that are removed by (aluminum) filtration. *(Bushong, p 12)*

179. **(B)** The effects of a quantity of radiation delivered to a body are dependent on several factors: the amount of radiation received, the size of the irradiated area, and how the radiation is delivered in time. If the radiation is delivered in *portions* over a period of time, it is said to be *fractionated* and has a *less harmful* effect than if the radiation were delivered all at once. With fractionation, cells have an opportunity to repair, and so some recovery occurs between doses. *(Bushong, p 496)*

180. **(B)** The *internal rotation* position places the humeral epicondyles perpendicular to the IR, the humerus in a true lateral position, and the lesser tubercle in profile. The *external rotation* position places the humeral epicondyles parallel to the IR, the humerus in a true AP position, and the greater tubercle in profile. The *neutral* position is often used for the evaluation of calcium deposits in the shoulder joint. *(Ballinger & Frank, vol 1, pp 164–165)*

181. **(D)** There are many radiation protection devices and laws associated with today's x-ray equipment. For example, the collimator light must accurately indicate the size and location of the x-ray beam *to within 2% of the SID*. Equipment that does not function properly contributes to excessive patient exposure, in the form of repeat examinations, and to poor image quality. *(Bushong, p 568)*

182. **(B)** Magnification radiography is used to enlarge details to a more perceptible degree. Hairline fractures and minute blood vessels are candidates for magnification radiography. The problem of magnification unsharpness is overcome by using a *fractional focal spot;* larger focal spot sizes will produce excessive blurring unsharpness. *Grids* are usually unnecessary in magnification radiography because of the air-gap effect produced by the OID. *Direct-exposure* technique would probably not be used because of the excessive exposure required. *(Selman, pp 226–228)*

183. **(C)** The x-ray tube's glass envelope and oil coolant are considered inherent ("built-in") filtration. Thin sheets of aluminum are added to make *a total of at least 2.5 mm Al equivalent filtration in equipment operated above 70 kVp.* The function of the filtration is to remove the low-energy photons that serve only to contribute to skin dose. *(Bushong, p 568)*

184. **(A)** The lead strips in a focused grid are made to parallel the x-ray beam. Therefore, scattered radiation, which radiates in directions other than that of the primary beam, will be absorbed by the grid. When the x-ray beam does not parallel the lead strips, some type of grid cutoff occurs. If the x-ray beam is not *centered* to the grid, or if the x-ray tube and grid surface are not parallel *(level)*, there will be a fairly uniform decrease in radiographic density across the entire image. However, if the grid is not used within its recommended SID *(focus)* range (ie, if the SID is too great or too little), there will be a decrease in density at the periphery of the image. *(Carlton & Adler, pp 272–274)*

185. **(D)** A *point lesion* is a disturbance of a single chemical bond, which can result in malfunction within the affected cell. Following irradiation, a small extension-type molecule can develop, extending from the main chain. This molecule can attach to a neighboring molecule or to another portion of the same molecule; this is referred to as *cross-linking*. Main-chain scission is breakage of the molecule's principal connection, so that the molecule is broken into smaller molecules. Each of these radiation effects on macromolecules is repairable. *(Bushong, p 505)*

186. **(B)** Radiographic contrast is described as the difference between densities, or scale of grays, in the radiographic image. Since the function of *grids* is to collect scattered radiation, they serve to shorten the scale of contrast. *Beam restrictors* function to limit the x-ray field size, thereby reducing the production of scattered radiation and shortening the scale of contrast. *Focal spot size* is one of the geometric factors affecting recorded detail; it has no effect on the scale of contrast. It is the function of radiographic contrast to make details visible.

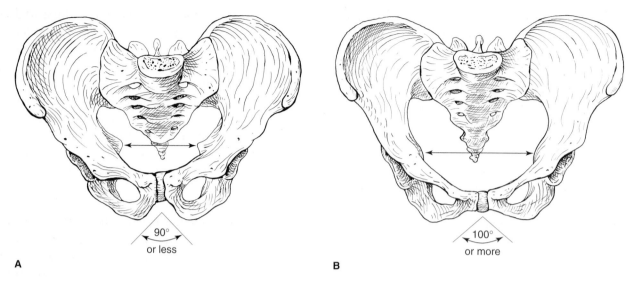

A   B

Figure 6–21. Reproduced with permission from Saia DA. *Radiography: Program Review and Examination Preparation,* 2nd ed. Stamford, CT: Appleton & Lange, 1999.

The sum of subject contrast and film contrast equals radiographic contrast. *(Carlton & Adler, p 397)*

187. **(B)** Figure 6–14 illustrates a lateral thoracic spine. *Motion* from "breathing technique" has been employed to blur out the superimposed pulmonary vascular markings and bony rib details in order to better demonstrate the bony structure of the thoracic spine. This is often referred to as autotomography, that is, the part moves itself rather than actual tomographic apparatus being employed. Since the shoulder area of the upper thoracic spine is so much thicker and more dense than the lower thoracic area, employment of the *anode heel effect* is also a valuable tool here. The thicker shoulder area is placed under the more intense cathode end of the x-ray beam, and the thinner anatomic part is placed under the anode end of the x-ray beam. *(Ballinger & Frank, vol 1, pp 418, 420)*

188. **(B)** The female pelvis differs from the male pelvis in that it is more shallow and its bones are generally lighter and more delicate (see Fig. 6–21). The pelvic outlet is wider and more circular in the female, and the ischial tuberosities and acetabula are farther apart; the angle formed by the pubic arch is also greater (more than 100°) in the female. All these bony char-

acteristics facilitate childbearing and birth. *(Ballinger & Frank, vol 1, p 328)*

189. **(C)** Proper body mechanics can help prevent painful back injuries by making proficient use of the muscles in the arms and legs. Proper body mechanics includes a *wide base of support*. The base of support is the part of the body in touch with the floor or other horizontal plane. The back should always be kept *straight;* twisting increases the chance of injury. When lifting a load, keep it as *close to the body* as possible to avoid back strain. Always *push* a load (like a mobile x-ray machine) rather than pull it. *(Torres et al, pp 82–83)*

190. **(A)** Spot film cameras have replaced conventional spot film cassettes. A significant advantage of spot film cameras is the big reduction in patient dose that their use permits. However, as the film format increases (from 70 mm to 100 mm), so do image quality, patient dose, and heat production. Patient dose, however, is so much smaller than the dose with conventional spot film cassettes that it is almost insignificant given the small improvement in image quality afforded by cassette spot films. *(Bushong, p 369)*

191. **(D)** Radiographic results should be consistent and predictable, not only with regard to positioning accuracy, but with respect to exposure

factors and image clarity as well. X-ray equipment and accessories must be calibrated periodically as part of an ongoing QA program. Intensifying screens should be cleaned regularly and screen–film contact evaluated annually. The quantity (mAs) and quality (kVp) of the primary beam have a big impact on the quality of the finished radiograph, and their accuracy, along with that of the x-ray timer, should be assessed regularly. The focal spot should be tested periodically to evaluate its impact on image sharpness. *(Bushong, pp 460–464)*

192. **(D)** The number of *heat units* produced during a given exposure with single-phase equipment is determined by multiplying mA × time × kVp. Correction factors are required with three-phase equipment. Unless the equipment manufacturer specifies otherwise, three-phase, *six*-pulse HU are determined by multiplying mA × time × kVp × 1.35. Three-phase, *12*-pulse HU are determined by multiplying mA × time × kVp × 1.41. *(Selman, p 145)*

193. **(D)** An increase in exposure factors will be required when imaging pathological conditions that cause greater attenuation of the x-ray beam. The x-ray beam suffers more attenuation as the thickness and/or density of the tissues increases. Examples include conditions involving an increase in part size as a result of fluid accumulation *(edema)* following trauma, an accumulation of fluid in the abdomen *(ascites)*, or an increase in bone size and density *(acromegaly)* as a result of an endocrine disorder. The radiographer needs a good working knowledge of pathological conditions, their effect on the body, and the resulting modifications in technical factors required. *(Carlton & Adler, p 258)*

194. **(C)** Tissue is most sensitive to radiation exposure when it is in an *oxygenated* condition. *Anoxic* refers to a general lack of oxygen in tissue; *hypoxic* refers to tissue with little oxygen. Anoxic and hypoxic tumors are typically avascular (with little or no blood supply) and therefore more radioresistant. *(Bushong, p 496)*

195. **(D)** According to the patient's bill of rights, the patient's verbal request supersedes any prior written consent. It is not appropriate to dismiss the patient without notifying the referring physician and the radiologist. The patient may very well need a particular radiographic examination to make a proper diagnosis or for presurgical planning, and the radiographer must inform the physician of the patient's decision immediately. *(Ehrlich et al, pp 54–55)*

196. **(A)** A distinction is made between the actual focal spot and the effective, or projected, focal spot. The *actual focal spot* is the finite area on the tungsten target that is actually bombarded by electrons from the filament. The *effective focal spot* is the foreshortened size of the focus as it is projected down toward the image receptor. This is called line focusing or the *line focus principle*. The quoted focal spot size is the effective focal spot size. *(Carlton & Adler, pp 117–119)*

197. **(B)** *Carpal tunnel syndrome* involves pain and numbness to some parts of the median nerve distribution (ie, palmar surface of thumb, index finger, and radial half of fourth finger and palm). Carpal tunnel syndrome frequently occurs in those who continually use vibrating tools or machinery. *Carpopedal spasm* is spasm of the hands and feet, commonly encountered during hyperventilation. *Carpal boss* is a bony growth on the dorsal surface of the third metacarpophalangeal joint. *(Bontrager, p 129)*

198–200. **(198, C; 199, D; 200, C)** The figure illustrates the x-ray tube component parts. Number 1 indicates the thoriated tungsten filament, which functions to release electrons when heated. Number 2 is the molybdenum focusing cup, which directs these electrons toward the anode's focal track. Number 4 is the rotating anode, and number 5 is the anode's focal track. The focal track is made of thoriated (for extra protection from heat) tungsten. When high-speed electrons are suddenly decelerated at the target, their kinetic energy is changed to x-ray photon energy. *(Bushong, pp 132–135)*

Subspecialty List

67. Patient care and education
68. Radiographic procedures
69. Radiographic procedures
70. Radiographic procedures
71. Equipment operation and maintenance
72. Equipment operation and quality control
73. Patient care and education
74. Image production and evaluation
75. Radiation protection
76. Equipment operation and quality control
77. Image production and evaluation
78. Image production and evaluation
79. Radiographic procedures
80. Image production and evaluation
81. Radiation protection
82. Image production and evaluation
83. Image production and evaluation
84. Radiation protection
85. Image production and evaluation
86. Image production and evaluation
87. Radiographic procedures
88. Patient care and education
89. Radiographic procedures
90. Equipment operation and quality control
91. Image production and evaluation
92. Image production and evaluation
93. Image production and evaluation
94. Image production and evaluation
95. Radiographic procedures
96. Image production and evaluation
97. Image production and evaluation
98. Patient care and education
99. Radiographic procedures
100. Patient care and education
101. Image production and evaluation
102. Patient care and education
103. Image production and evaluation
104. Image production and evaluation
105. Image production and evaluation
106. Radiation protection
107. Radiographic procedures
108. Radiographic procedures
109. Radiation protection
110. Radiographic procedures
111. Patient care and education
112. Radiation protection
113. Equipment operation and quality control
114. Image production and evaluation
115. Image production and evaluation
116. Radiographic procedures
117. Radiographic procedures
118. Radiographic procedures
119. Image production and evaluation
120. Image production and evaluation
121. Image production and evaluation
122. Equipment operation and quality control
123. Patient care and education
124. Radiographic procedures
125. Radiographic procedures
126. Radiation protection
127. Image production and evaluation
128. Radiation protection
129. Radiographic procedures
130. Image production and evaluation
131. Patient care and education
132. Patient care and education
133. Image production and evaluation
134. Radiation protection
135. Radiation protection
136. Radiation protection
137. Patient care and education
138. Radiographic procedures
139. Patient care and education
140. Radiographic procedures
141. Radiographic procedures
142. Equipment operation and quality control
143. Radiographic procedures
144. Radiographic procedures
145. Image production and evaluation
146. Image production and evaluation
147. Radiation protection
148. Image production and evaluation
149. Patient care and education
150. Patient care and education
151. Patient care and education
152. Equipment operation and quality control
153. Equipment operation and quality control
154. Equipment operation and quality control
155. Radiographic procedures
156. Patient care and education
157. Patient care and education
158. Radiographic procedures
159. Image production and evaluation
160. Image production and evaluation
161. Radiographic procedures
162. Image production and evaluation
163. Radiation protection
164. Patient care and education
165. Radiographic procedures
166. Radiation protection
167. Radiographic procedures
168. Equipment operation and quality control

169. Equipment operation and quality control
170. Equipment operation and quality control
171. Patient care and education
172. Radiographic procedures
173. Image production and evaluation
174. Equipment operation and quality control
175. Equipment operation and quality control
176. Image production and evaluation
177. Radiation protection
178. Radiation protection
179. Radiation protection
180. Radiographic procedures
181. Equipment operation and quality control
182. Image production and evaluation
183. Radiation protection
184. Image production and evaluation
185. Radiation protection
186. Image production and evaluation
187. Radiographic procedures
188. Radiographic procedures
189. Patient care and education
190. Equipment operation and quality control
191. Equipment operation and quality control
192. Equipment operation and quality control
193. Image production and evaluation
194. Radiation protection
195. Patient care and education
196. Equipment operation and quality control
197. Radiographic procedures
198. Equipment operation and quality control
199. Equipment operation and quality control
200. Equipment operation and quality control

CHAPTER 7

Practice Test 2
Questions

DIRECTIONS (Questions 1 through 200): Each of the numbered items or incomplete statements in this section is followed by answers or by completions of the statement. Select the *one* lettered answer or completion that is *best* in each case.

1. Ipecac is a medication used to induce vomiting and is classified as a(n)

   (A) diuretic.
   (B) antipyretic.
   (C) antihistamine.
   (D) emetic.

2. In which type of equipment does kVp decrease during the actual length of the exposure?

   1. Condenser discharge mobile equipment
   2. Battery operated mobile equipment
   3. Fixed x-ray equipment

   A. 1 only
   B. 1 and 2 only
   C. 2 and 3 only
   D. 1, 2, and 3

3. Which of the following is (are) characteristic of anemia?

   1. Decreased number of circulating red blood cells
   2. Decreased hemoglobin
   3. Hematuria

   (A) 1 only
   (B) 1 and 2 only
   (C) 1 and 3 only
   (D) 1, 2, and 3

4. The decision as to whether to deliver ionic or nonionic contrast media should include a preliminary patient history including, but not limited to,

   1. patient age.
   2. history of respiratory disease.
   3. history of cardiac disease.

   (A) 1 and 2
   (B) 1 and 3
   (C) 2 and 3
   (D) 1, 2, and 3

5. An exposure was made using 600 mA and 18 ms. If the mA is changed to 400, which of the following exposure times would *most* closely approximate the original radiographic density?

   (A) 16 ms
   (B) 0.16 second
   (C) 27 ms
   (D) 0.27 second

6. To demonstrate the glenoid fossa in profile, the patient is positioned

   (A) 45° oblique, affected side up.
   (B) 45° oblique, affected side down.
   (C) 25° oblique, affected side up.
   (D) 25° oblique, affected side down.

7. Which of the following involve(s) intentional misconduct?

1. Invasion of privacy
2. False imprisonment
3. Patient sustaining injury from a fall while left unattended

(A) 1 only
(B) 3 only
(C) 1 and 2 only
(D) 2 and 3 only

8. Which of the following types of adult tissues is (are) relatively insensitive to radiation exposure?

1. Muscle tissue
2. Nerve tissue
3. Epithelial tissue

(A) 1 only
(B) 1 and 2 only
(C) 2 and 3 only
(D) 1, 2, and 3

9. If the exposure rate to a body standing 3 feet from a radiation source is 12 mR/min, what will be the exposure rate to that body at a distance of 7 feet from the source?

(A) 2.2 mR/min
(B) 5.1 mR/min
(C) 28 mR/min
(D) 36 mR/min

10. Which of the dose–response curves pictured in Figure 7–1 illustrate(s) a linear threshold dose effect?

1. Curve number 1
2. Curve number 2
3. Curve number 3

(A) 1 only
(B) 3 only
(C) 2 and 3 only
(D) 1, 2, and 3

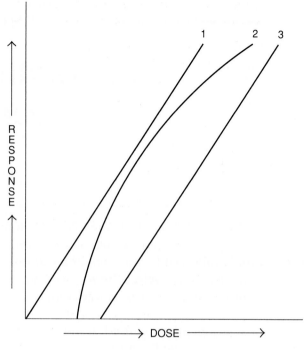

Figure 7–1.

11. The carpal scaphoid may be demonstrated in the following projection(s) of the wrist:

1. PA oblique
2. PA with radial flexion
3. PA with forearm elevated 20°

(A) 1 only
(B) 1 and 2 only
(C) 1 and 3 only
(D) 1, 2, and 3

12. Linear energy transfer (LET) may be *best* described as

(A) the amount of energy delivered per distance traveled in tissue.
(B) the unit of absorbed dose.
(C) radiation equivalent man.
(D) radiation absorbed dose.

13. A dorsal decubitus projection of the chest may be used to evaluate small amounts of

1. fluid in the posterior chest.
2. air in the posterior chest.
3. fluid in the anterior chest.

(A) 1 only
(B) 1 and 2 only
(C) 2 and 3 only
(D) 1, 2, and 3

14. Which of the following is (are) evaluation criteria for a PA chest for heart and lungs?

1. Ten posterior ribs should be seen above the diaphragm.
2. The medial ends of the clavicles should be equidistant from the vertebral column.
3. The scapulae should be seen through the upper lung fields.

(A) 1 only
(B) 1 and 2 only
(C) 2 and 3 only
(D) 1, 2, and 3

15. To eject a K shell electron from a tungsten atom, the incoming electron must have an energy of at least

(A) 60 keV.
(B) 70 keV.
(C) 80 keV.
(D) 90 keV.

16. Body substances and fluids that are considered infectious, or potentially infectious, include

1. feces.
2. breast milk.
3. wound drainage.

A. 1 only
B. 1 and 2 only
C. 2 and 3 only
D. 1, 2, and 3

17. The effective energy of the x-ray beam is increased by increasing the

1. added filtration.
2. kilovoltage.
3. milliamperage.

(A) 1 only
(B) 2 only
(C) 1 and 2 only
(D) 1, 2, and 3

18. The radiograph in Figure 7–2 could be improved in which of the following ways?

(A) The midsagittal plane (MSP) should be placed 45° with the plane of the cassette.
(B) The MSP should be placed 90° to the plane of the cassette.
(C) The chin should be elevated slightly.
(D) The head should be flexed slightly.

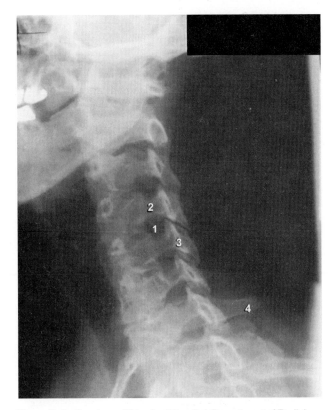

Figure 7–2. Courtesy of Stamford Hospital, Department of Radiology.

19. What is the anatomic structure indicated by the number 3 in the radiograph in Figure 7–2?

   (A) Spinous process
   (B) Transverse process
   (C) Pedicle
   (D) Intervertebral foramen

20. While measuring blood pressure, the first pulse that is heard is recorded as the

   (A) diastolic pressure.
   (B) systolic pressure.
   (C) venous pressure.
   (D) valvular pressure.

21. Characteristics of the patient with pulmonary emphysema include

   1. shoulder girdle elevation.
   2. increased AP diameter of chest.
   3. hyperventilation.

   (A) 1 only
   (B) 1 and 2 only
   (C) 2 and 3 only
   (D) 1, 2, and 3

22. Free air in the abdominal cavity is *best* demonstrated in which of the following?

   1. Lateral recumbent abdomen
   2. Erect AP abdomen
   3. Left lateral decubitus abdomen

   (A) 1 only
   (B) 2 only
   (C) 1 and 2 only
   (D) 2 and 3 only

23. Which of the following is (are) included in whole-body dose equivalents?

   1. Gonads
   2. Lens
   3. Extremities

   (A) 1 only
   (B) 1 and 2 only
   (C) 2 and 3 only
   (D) 1, 2, and 3

24. The late effects of radiation are considered to

   1. have no threshold dose.
   2. be directly related to dose.
   3. occur within hours of exposure.

   (A) 1 only
   (B) 1 and 2 only
   (C) 2 and 3 only
   (D) 1, 2, and 3

25. To radiograph an infant for suspected free air within the abdominal cavity, which of the following projections of the abdomen will demonstrate the condition with the *least* patient exposure?

   (A) PA erect with grid
   (B) Right lateral decubitus with grid
   (C) Right lateral decubitus without grid
   (D) Recumbent AP without grid

26. The AP oblique projection (medial rotation) of the elbow demonstrates which of the following?

   1. Radial head free of superimposition
   2. Olecranon process within the olecranon fossa
   3. Coronoid process free of superimposition

   (A) 1 only
   (B) 1 and 2 only
   (C) 2 and 3 only
   (D) 1, 2, and 3

27. What percentage of x-ray attenuation does a 0.5-mm lead equivalent apron at 100 kVp provide?

   (A) 51%
   (B) 66%
   (C) 75%
   (D) 94%

28. Which portion of the characteristic curve would *most* likely represent a density of 1.0?

   (A) Toe
   (B) Straight-line portion
   (C) Shoulder
   (D) D_{max}

29. The risk of inoculation with human immun-odeficiency virus (HIV) is considered high for the following entry sites:

1. Broken skin
2. Shared needles
3. Conjunctiva

(A) 1 only
(B) 1 and 2 only
(C) 2 and 3 only
(D) 1, 2, and 3

30. The term *parenteral* refers to which of the following medication routes?

(A) Oral
(B) Sublingual
(C) Mucosal
(D) Any, other than alimentary

31. The position illustrated in Figure 7–3 can be successfully used to demonstrate

1. PA oblique sternum
2. barium filled esophagus
3. right anterior ribs

(A) 1 only
(B) 1 and 2 only
(C) 2 and 3 only
(D) 1, 2, and 3

32. Which of the following positions may be used to effectively demonstrate the hepatic flexure during radiographic examination of the large bowel?

1. RAO
2. LAO
3. LPO

(A) 1 only
(B) 1 and 2 only
(C) 1 and 3 only
(D) 2 and 3 only

33. Which of the following is an acceptable approximate entrance skin exposure (ESE) for a PA chest?

(A) 6 mR
(B) 20 mR
(C) 38 mR
(D) 0.6 R

34. Hemovac or Penrose drains are used for

(A) bile duct drainage.
(B) tissue drainage of wounds or postoperative drainage.
(C) decompression of the gastrointestinal tract.
(D) feeding patients who are unable to swallow food.

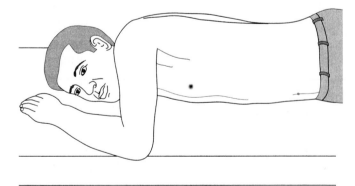

Figure 7–3.

35. Differences between body habitus types are likely to affect all of the following except the

   (A) size and shape of an organ.
   (B) position of an organ.
   (C) position of the diaphragm.
   (D) degree of bone porosity.

36. Geometric unsharpness is most likely to be greater

   (A) at long SIDs.
   (B) at the anode end of the image.
   (C) with small focal spots.
   (D) at the cathode end of the image.

37. Which of the x-ray circuit devices seen in Figure 7–4 operates on the principle of self-induction?

   (A) Number 1
   (B) Number 2
   (C) Number 3
   (D) Number 7

38. Referring to the simplified x-ray circuit seen in Figure 7–4, what is indicated by the number 5?

   (A) Step-up transformer
   (B) Autotransformer
   (C) Filament circuit
   (D) Rectification system

39. Which of the following is another name for an intermittent injection port?

   (A) Hypodermic needle
   (B) Butterfly needle
   (C) Heparin lock
   (D) Intravenous (IV) infusion

40. A light-absorbing dye is frequently incorporated during the manufacture of screens to

   (A) reduce the diffusion of fluorescent light.
   (B) increase image contrast.
   (C) increase screen speed.
   (D) increase the useful life of the screen.

41. The advantages of capacitor discharge mobile x-ray equipment include

   1. compact size.
   2. light weight.
   3. high kVp capability.

   A. 1 only
   B. 1 and 2 only
   C. 2 and 3 only
   D. 1, 2, and 3

42. A radiograph exposed using a 12:1 ratio grid may exhibit a loss of density at its lateral edges because the

   (A) SID was too great.
   (B) grid failed to move during the exposure.
   (C) x-ray tube was angled in the direction of the lead strips.
   (D) central ray was off-center.

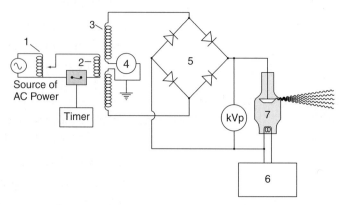

Figure 7–4.

43. Routine excretory urography usually includes a postmicturition radiograph of the bladder. This is done to demonstrate

1. tumor masses.
2. residual urine.
3. prostatic enlargement.

(A) 2 only
(B) 1 and 3 only
(C) 2 and 3 only
(D) 1, 2, and 3

44. The *best* projection to demonstrate the articular surfaces of the femoropatellar articulation is the

(A) AP knee.
(B) PA knee.
(C) tangential ("sunrise") projection.
(D) "tunnel" view.

45. Which of the following is (are) valid evaluation criteria for a lateral projection of the forearm?

1. The radius and the ulna should be superimposed distally.
2. The coronoid process and the radial head should be partially superimposed.
3. The humeral epicondyles should be superimposed.

(A) 1 only
(B) 1 and 2 only
(C) 2 and 3 only
(D) 1, 2, and 3

46. Very low humidity in the darkroom can lead to

(A) crinkle marks.
(B) static electrical discharge.
(C) excessive emulsion swelling.
(D) chemical fog.

47. The collimator light and actual irradiated area must be accurate to within

(A) 2% of the SID.
(B) 5% of the SID.
(C) 10% of the SID.
(D) 15% of the SID.

48. The radiographic image in Figure 7–5 was obtained while testing

(A) rectifier operation in a single-phase x-ray machine.
(B) rectifier operation in a three-phase x-ray machine.
(C) timer accuracy in a single-phase x-ray machine.
(D) timer accuracy in a three-phase x-ray machine.

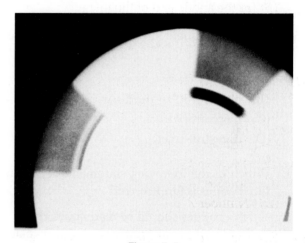

Figure 7–5

49. All of the following procedures demonstrate renal function, *except*

(A) IVP.
(B) descending urography.
(C) retrograde urography.
(D) infusion nephrotomography.

50. Which of the following waveforms has the lowest percentage voltage ripple?

(A) Single-phase
(B) Three-phase, 6-pulse
(C) Three-phase, 12-pulse
(D) High-frequency

51. The sternoclavicular joints will be *best* demonstrated in which of the following positions?

(A) Apical lordotic
(B) Anterior oblique
(C) Lateral
(D) Weight-bearing

52. What are the advantages of photospot camera imaging over cassette spot imaging during fluoroscopy?

    1. Lower patient dose
    2. Less interruption of the fluoroscopic examination
    3. Improved spatial resolution

    (A) 1 only
    (B) 1 and 2 only
    (C) 2 and 3 only
    (D) 1, 2, and 3

53. The *most* frequent site of nosocomial infection is the

    (A) urinary tract.
    (B) blood.
    (C) respiratory tract.
    (D) digestive tract.

54. Which of the following statements regarding film badges is (are) correct?

    1. Film badges should be read quarterly.
    2. Film badges must not leave the workplace.
    3. Film badges measure quantity and quality of radiation exposure.

    (A) 1 only
    (B) 1 and 2 only
    (C) 2 and 3 only
    (D) 1, 2, and 3

55. Which of the following radiographic accessories functions to produce uniform density on a radiograph?

    (A) Grid
    (B) Intensifying screens
    (C) Compensating filter
    (D) Penetrometer

56. The radiation dose to an individual is dependent on which of the following?

    1. Type of tissue interaction(s)
    2. Quantity of radiation
    3. Biologic differences

    (A) 1 only
    (B) 1 and 2 only
    (C) 1 and 3 only
    (D) 1, 2, and 3

57. A satisfactory radiograph was made without a grid, using a 72-inch SID and 8 mAs. If the distance is changed to 40 inches and an 8:1 ratio grid is added, what should be the new mAs?

    (A) 10 mAs
    (B) 18 mAs
    (C) 20 mAs
    (D) 32 mAs

58. The thoracic cavity is lined by

    (A) parietal pleura.
    (B) visceral pleura.
    (C) parietal peritoneum.
    (D) visceral peritoneum.

59. All of the following statements regarding three-phase current are true *except*

    (A) Three-phase current is constant-potential direct current.
    (B) Three-phase equipment produces more x-rays per mAs.
    (C) Three-phase produces higher-average-energy x-rays than single-phase.
    (D) The three-phase waveform has less ripple than the single-phase.

60. Which of the following contribute to the radiographic contrast present on the finished radiograph?

1. Tissue density
2. Pathology
3. Muscle development

(A) 1 and 2 only
(B) 1 and 3 only
(C) 2 and 3 only
(D) 1, 2, and 3

61. In 1906, Bergonié and Tribondeau theorized that undifferentiated cells are highly radiosensitive. Which of the following is (are) characteristic(s) of undifferentiated cells?

1. Young cells
2. Highly mitotic cells
3. Precursor cells

(A) 1 only
(B) 1 and 2 only
(C) 1 and 3 only
(D) 1, 2, and 3

62. When the collimated field must extend past the edge of the body, allowing primary radiation to strike the tabletop, as in a lateral lumbar spine, what may be done to prevent excessive radiographic density due to undercutting?

(A) Reduce the mAs
(B) Reduce the kVp
(C) Use a shorter SID
(D) Use lead rubber to absorb tabletop primary radiation

63. The radiograph of the pelvis seen in Figure 7–6 is unacceptable because of:

(A) motion.
(B) inadequate penetration.
(C) scattered radiation fog.
(D) excessive density.

64. The effect that differential absorption has on radiographic contrast of a high subject contrast part can be minimized by

1. using a compensating filter.
2. using high-kVp exposure factors.
3. increased collimation.

(A) 1 only
(B) 1 and 2 only
(C) 2 and 3 only
(D) 1, 2, and 3

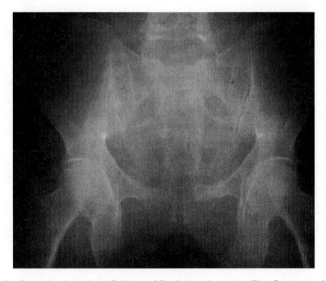

Figure 7–6. From the American College of Radiology Learning File. Courtesy of the ACR.

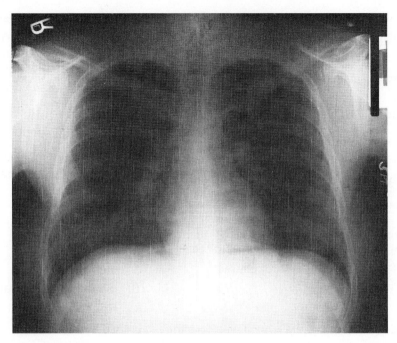

Figure 7–7. Courtesy FUJIFILM Medical Systems USA, Inc.

65. The vertical lines present on the radiograph in Figure 7–7 represent which of the following?

(A) Improperly placed guide shoes
(B) Sediment on processor rollers
(C) Pi lines
(D) Grid lines

66. Which of the following groups of exposure factors would be *most* appropriate for an adult intravenous pyelogram (IVP)?

(A) 300 mA, 0.02 second, 72 kVp
(B) 300 mA, 0.01 second, 82 kVp
(C) 150 mA, 0.01 second, 94 kVp
(D) 100 mA, 0.03 second, 82 kVp

67. Which of the following is (are) correct regarding care of protective leaded apparel?

1. Lead aprons should be fluoroscoped yearly to check for cracks.
2. Lead gloves should be fluoroscoped yearly to check for cracks.
3. Lead aprons should be hung on appropriate racks when not in use.

(A) 1 only
(B) 1 and 2 only
(C) 1 and 3 only
(D) 1, 2, and 3

68. An exposure was made at a 36-inch SID using 12 mAs and 75 kVp with a 400-speed imaging system and an 8:1 grid. A second radiograph is requested with improved recorded detail. Which of the following groups of technical factors will *best* accomplish this task?

(A) 15 mAs, 12:1 grid, 75 kVp, 400-speed system, 36 inches SID
(B) 15 mAs, 12:1 grid, 75 kVp, 400-speed system, 40 inches SID
(C) 30 mAs, 12:1 grid, 75 kVp, 200-speed system, 40 inches SID
(D) 12 mAs, 8:1 grid, 86 kVp, 200-speed system, 36 inches SID

69. Which of the following is the approximate skin dose for 5 minutes of fluoroscopy performed at 1.5 mA?

(A) 3.7 rad
(B) 7.5 rad
(C) 15 rad
(D) 21 rad

70. Which of the following will produce the greatest distortion?

    (A) AP projection of the skull
    (B) PA projection of the skull
    (C) 37° AP axial of the skull
    (D) 20° PA axial of the skull

71. The National Council on Radiation Protection and Measurements (NCRP) recommends an annual occupational effective (stochastic) dose equivalent limit of

    (A) 50 mSv (5 rem).
    (B) 100 mSv (10 rem).
    (C) 25 mSv (2.5 rem).
    (D) 200 mSv (20 rem).

72. All of the following statements regarding the bony thorax are true, *except*

    (A) the first seven pairs of ribs are referred to as vertebrosternal, or true ribs.
    (B) the only articulation between the thorax and the upper extremity is the sternoclavicular joint.
    (C) the gladiolus is the upper part of the sternum and is quadrilateral in shape.
    (D) the anterior ends of the ribs are about 4 inches below the level of the vertebral ends.

73. TV camera tubes used in image intensification, such as the Plumbicon and Vidicon, function to

    (A) increase the brightness of the input phosphor image.
    (B) transfer the output phosphor image to the TV monitor.
    (C) focus and accelerate electrons toward the output phosphor.
    (D) record the output phosphor image on 16- or 35- film.

74. The device that is used for the direct measurement of optical density is the

    (A) sensitometer.
    (B) densitometer.
    (C) penetrometer.
    (D) H&D curve.

75. The greater tubercle should be visualized in profile in which of the following?

    (A) AP shoulder, external rotation
    (B) AP shoulder, internal rotation
    (C) AP elbow
    (D) Lateral elbow

76. Which of the following may be used to control the production of scattered radiation?

    1. Restricted field size
    2. Use of optimal kVp
    3. Use of grids

    (A) 1 only
    (B) 1 and 2 only
    (C) 2 and 3 only
    (D) 1, 2, and 3

77. Improper spectral matching between rare earth intensifying screens and film emulsion results in

    (A) longer-scale contrast.
    (B) insufficient density.
    (C) decreased recorded detail.
    (D) excessive density.

78. An increase in the kilovoltage applied to the x-ray tube increases the

    1. percentage of high-energy photons produced.
    2. exposure rate.
    3. patient absorption.

    (A) 1 only
    (B) 1 and 2 only
    (C) 2 and 3 only
    (D) 1, 2, and 3

79. Silver reclamation may be accomplished in which of the following ways?

    1. Metallic replacement cartridge
    2. Electrolytic plating unit
    3. Removal from used film

    (A) 1 only
    (B) 2 only
    (C) 1 and 2 only
    (D) 1, 2, and 3

80. Acceptable method(s) of minimizing motion unsharpness is (are)

    1. suspended respiration.
    2. short exposure time.
    3. patient instruction.

    (A) 1 only
    (B) 1 and 2 only
    (C) 1 and 3 only
    (D) 1, 2, and 3

81. If a quantity of radiation is delivered to a body in a short period of time, its effect

    (A) will be greater than if it were delivered over a long period of time.
    (B) will be less than if it were delivered over a long period of time.
    (C) has no relation to how it is delivered in time.
    (D) is solely dependent on the radiation quality.

82. Shape distortion is influenced by the relationship between the

    1. x-ray tube and the part to be imaged.
    2. body part to be imaged and the IR.
    3. IR and the x-ray tube.

    (A) 1 and 2 only
    (B) 1 and 3 only
    (C) 2 and 3 only
    (D) 1, 2, and 3

83. In which section of the automatic processor seen in Figure 7–8 are the unexposed silver halide crystals removed from the emulsion?

    (A) Section 1
    (B) Section 2
    (C) Section 3
    (D) Section 4

84. Which of the following defines the *gonadal dose* that, if received by every member of the population, would be expected to produce the same total genetic effect on that population as the actual doses received by each of the individuals?

    (A) Genetically significant dose
    (B) Somatically significant dose
    (C) Maximum permissible dose
    (D) Lethal dose

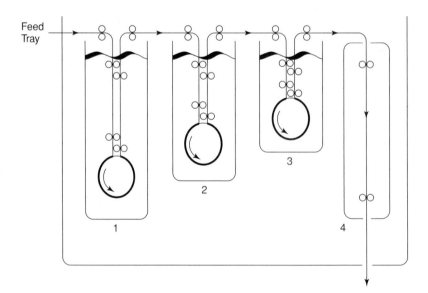

Figure 7–8. Reproduced with permission from Saia DA. *Radiography: Program Review and Examination Preparation*, 2nd ed. Stamford, CT: Appleton & Lange, 1999.

85. A patient with an upper respiratory tract infection is transported to the radiology department for a chest examination. Who should be masked?

1. Technologist
2. Transporter
3. Patient

(A) 1 only
(B) 1 and 2 only
(C) 3 only
(D) 1, 2, and 3

86. Phosphors suitable for use in intensifying screens should have which of the following characteristics?

1. High conversion efficiency
2. High x-ray absorption
3. Afterglow

(A) 1 only
(B) 1 and 2 only
(C) 3 only
(D) 1, 2, and 3

87. The radiograph in Figure 7–9 exhibits a loss of radiographic density as a result of

(A) x-ray tube angulation across grid lines.
(B) exceeding the focusing distance.
(C) incorrect grid placement.
(D) insufficient SID.

88. The housing surrounding an x-ray tube functions to

1. retain heat within the glass envelope.
2. protect from electric shock.
3. keep leakage radiation to a minimum.

(A) 1 and 2 only
(B) 1 and 3 only
(C) 2 and 3 only
(D) 1, 2, and 3

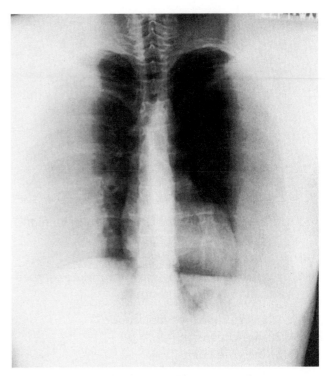

Figure 7–9. Courtesy of Stamford Hospital, Department of Radiology.

89. The reduction in x-ray photon intensity as the photon passes through a material is termed

(A) absorption.
(B) scattering.
(C) attenuation.
(D) divergence.

90. It is usually recommended that a thermoluminescent dosimeter (TLD) or film badge be worn

(A) under the lead apron at waist level.
(B) outside the lead apron at waist level.
(C) under the lead apron at collar level.
(D) outside the lead apron at collar level.

91. Which of the following groups of exposure factors will produce the longest scale of contrast?

(A) 200 mA, 0.25 second, 70 kVp, 12:1 grid
(B) 500 mA, 0.10 second, 90 kVp, 8:1 grid
(C) 400 mA, 0.125 second, 80 kVp, 12:1 grid
(D) 300 mA, 0.16 second, 70 kVp, 8:1 grid

92. Which of the following is the most likely site for a lumbar puncture?

    (A) S1–2
    (B) L3–4
    (C) L1–2
    (D) C6–7

93. How are LET and biologic response related?

    (A) They are inversely related.
    (B) They are directly related.
    (C) They are related in a reciprocal fashion.
    (D) They are unrelated.

94. An increase in kVp with appropriate compensation of mAs will result in

    1. increased exposure latitude.
    2. higher contrast.
    3. increased density.

    (A) 1 only
    (B) 1 and 2 only
    (C) 2 and 3 only
    (D) 1 and 3 only

95. If the quantity of black metallic silver on a particular radiograph is such that it allows 1% of the illuminator light to pass through the x-ray image, that image has a density of

    (A) 0.01.
    (B) 0.1.
    (C) 1.0.
    (D) 2.0.

96. Substituting intensifying screens having a speed of 200 in place of a 100-speed system will

    1. require one half of the exposure of 100-speed screens.
    2. increase the production of scattered radiation.
    3. enable the radiographer to decrease the exposure time.

    (A) 1 only
    (B) 1 and 2 only
    (C) 1 and 3 only
    (D) 1, 2, and 3

97. If the primary coil of the high-voltage transformer is supplied by 110 V and has 100 turns, and the secondary coil has 80,000 turns, what is the voltage induced in the secondary coil?

    (A) 135 kV
    (B) 88 kV
    (C) 135 V
    (D) 88 V

98. Figure 7–10 is an example of a

    (A) bar pattern test.
    (B) Wisconsin test tool.
    (C) star resolution test.
    (D) screen–film contact test.

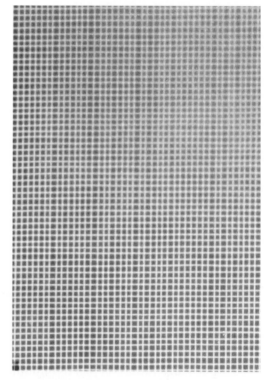

Figure 7–10. From the American College of Radiology Learning File. Courtesy of the ACR.

99. The fact that x-ray intensity across the primary beam can vary as much as 45% describes the

    (A) line focus principle.
    (B) transformer law.
    (C) anode heel effect.
    (D) inverse square law.

100. Which of the following conditions require(s) a decrease in technical factors?

1. Emphysema
2. Osteomalacia
3. Atelectasis

(A) 1 only
(B) 1 and 2 only
(C) 2 and 3 only
(D) 1, 2, and 3

101. Inherent and added filtration in the x-ray tube functions to

(A) reduce patient skin dose.
(B) shorten the scale of contrast.
(C) reduce scattered radiation.
(D) soften the x-ray beam.

102. Which of the following is (are) characteristics of a 16:1 grid?

1. It absorbs more primary radiation than an 8:1 grid.
2. It has more centering latitude than an 8:1 grid.
3. It is used with higher kVp exposures than an 8:1 grid.

(A) 1 only
(B) 1 and 3 only
(C) 2 and 3 only
(D) 1, 2, and 3

103. An exposure was made at 40-inch SID, using 5 mAs and 105 kVp with an 8:1 grid. In an effort to improve radiographic contrast, the image is repeated using a 12:1 grid and 90 kVp. Which of the following exposure times will be *most* appropriate, using 400 mA, to maintain the original density?

(A) 0.01 second
(B) 0.03 second
(C) 0.1 second
(D) 0.3 second

104. The brightness level of the fluoroscopic image is dependent on

1. milliamperage.
2. kilovoltage.
3. patient thickness.

(A) 1 only
(B) 1 and 2 only
(C) 1 and 3 only
(D) 1, 2, and 3

105. The pyloric canal and duodenal bulb are *best* demonstrated during an upper GI series in which of the following positions?

(A) RAO
(B) Left lateral
(C) Recumbent PA
(D) Recumbent AP

106. The functions of the automatic processor's roller system include

1. film transport.
2. agitation.
3. squeegee action.

(A) 1 only
(B) 1 and 2 only
(C) 1 and 3 only
(D) 1, 2, and 3

107. If a radiograph were made of an average-size knee using automatic exposure control (AEC) and all three photocells were selected, the resulting radiograph would demonstrate

(A) excessive density.
(B) insufficient density.
(C) poor detail.
(D) adequate exposure.

108. With mAs adjusted to produce equal exposures, all of the following statements are true *except*

   (A) A single-phase examination done at 10 mAs can be duplicated with 3-phase, 12-pulse at 5 mAs.

   (B) There is greater patient dose with three-phase equipment than with single-phase equipment.

   (C) Three-phase equipment can produce comparable radiographs with less heat unit (HU) buildup.

   (D) Three-phase equipment produces lower-contrast radiographs than single-phase equipment.

109. In which of the following examinations would a cassette front with very low absorption properties be especially desirable?

   (A) Extremity radiography
   (B) Abdominal radiography
   (C) Mammography
   (D) Angiography

110. Which of the following function(s) to reduce the amount of scattered radiation reaching the IR?

   1. Grid devices
   2. Restricted focal spot size
   3. Beam restrictors

   (A) 1 only
   (B) 1 and 2 only
   (C) 1 and 3 only
   (D) 1, 2, and 3

111. Which of the following statements is true with regard to the two radiographs in Figure 7–11?

   (A) Image 1 was exposed on expiration.
   (B) Image 2 was exposed on expiration.
   (C) Image 1 is a lordotic position.
   (D) Image 2 is a ventral decubitus position.

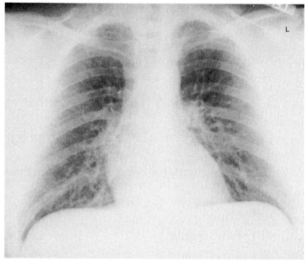

1

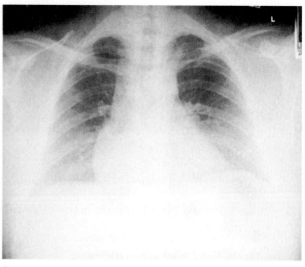

2

Figure 7–11. Courtesy of Stamford Hospital, Department of Radiology.

112. The amount of replenisher solution added as a film enters the automatic processor is related to the

   1. size of the film.
   2. temperature of the solution.
   3. number of films processed.

   (A) 1 only
   (B) 1 and 3 only
   (C) 2 and 3 only
   (D) 1, 2, and 3

113. With the patient positioned as illustrated in Figure 7–12, how should the central ray be directed to *best* demonstrate the intercondyloid fossa?

(A) Perpendicular to the popliteal depression

(B) 40° caudad to the popliteal depression

(C) Perpendicular to the long axis of the femur

(D) 40° cephalad to the popliteal depression

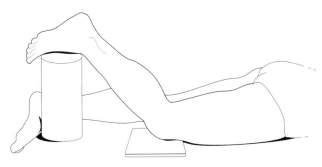

Figure 7–12.

114. CPR procedure for infants differs from that of adults with respect to

1. hand placement.
2. number of compressions.
3. volume of air delivered.

(A) 1 and 2 only

(B) 1 and 3 only

(C) 2 and 3 only

(D) 1, 2, and 3

115. A radiolucent contrast agent

1. absorbs a high number of x-ray photons.
2. causes anatomy to appear dark on the radiograph.
3. is composed of elements with low atomic numbers.

(A) 1 and 2 only

(B) 1 and 3 only

(C) 2 and 3 only

(D) 1, 2, and 3

116. Which of the following is a functional study used to demonstrate the degree of AP motion present in the cervical spine?

(A) Moving mandible position

(B) AP open-mouth projection

(C) Flexion and extension laterals

(D) AP right and left bending

117. The functions of the automatic processor's recirculation system include

1. keeping the solution in contact with the film emulsion.
2. maintaining uniform temperatures.
3. mixing and agitating solutions.

(A) 1 only

(B) 1 and 3 only

(C) 2 and 3 only

(D) 1, 2, and 3

118. Which of the labeled bones in Figure 7–13 identifies the tarsal navicular?

(A) Number 2

(B) Number 3

(C) Number 6

(D) Number 7

119. What does the number 8 in Figure 7–13 identify?

(A) Medial malleolus

(B) Lateral malleolus

(C) Medial cuneiform

(D) Talus

120. In what order should the following examinations be performed?

1. Upper GI
2. IVP
3. Barium enema

(A) 3, 1, 2

(B) 1, 3, 2

(C) 2, 1, 3

(D) 2, 3, 1

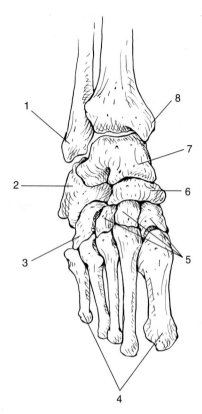

Figure 7–13. Reproduced with permission from Saia DA. *Radiography: Program Review and Examination Preparation,* 2nd ed. Stamford, CT: Appleton & Lange, 1999.

121. Several types of exposure timers may be found on x-ray equipment. Which of the following types of timers functions to accurately duplicate radiographic densities?

(A) Synchronous
(B) Impulse
(C) Electronic
(D) Phototimer

122. Sterile technique is required when contrast agents are administered

(A) through a nasogastric tube.
(B) intrathecally.
(C) rectally.
(D) orally.

123. Which of the following is *most* likely to occur as a result of using a 30-inch SID with a 14 × 17-inch IR to radiograph a fairly homogeneous structure?

(A) Production of quantum mottle
(B) Density variation between opposite ends of the IR
(C) Production of scatter radiation fog
(D) Excessively short-scale contrast

124. Which of the four baselines illustrated in Figure 7–14 should be used for a lateral projection of facial bones?

(A) Baseline 1
(B) Baseline 2
(C) Baseline 3
(D) Baseline 4

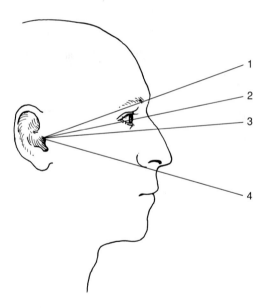

Figure 7–14. Reproduced with permission from Saia DA. *Radiography: Program Review and Examination Preparation,* 2nd ed. Stamford, CT: Appleton & Lange, 1999.

125. Which of the following statements is (are) true regarding the radiograph in Figure 7–15?

1. The part is rotated.
2. The patient is not shielded correctly.
3. There is excessive density.

(A) 1 only
(B) 2 only
(C) 1 and 2 only
(D) 1, 2, and 3

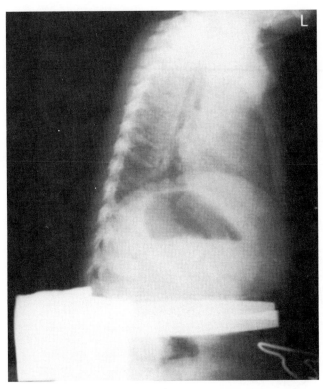

Figure 7–15. Courtesy of Stamford Hospital, Department of Radiology.

126. Which of the following is (are) considered long-term somatic effect(s) of exposure to ionizing radiation?

1. Life-span shortening
2. Carcinogenesis
3. Cataractogenesis

(A) 1 only
(B) 1 and 2 only
(C) 2 and 3 only
(D) 1, 2, and 3

127. Drugs that may be used to prolong blood clotting time include

1. heparin.
2. diphenhydramine (Benadryl).
3. lidocaine.

(A) 1 only
(B) 1 and 2 only
(C) 1 and 3 only
(D) 1, 2, and 3

128. The instrument that is frequently used in quality control programs to measure varying degrees of x-ray exposure is the

(A) aluminum step wedge.
(B) spinning top.
(C) densitometer.
(D) sensitometer.

129. Exposure factors of 80 kVp and 8 mAs are used for a particular nongrid exposure. What should be the new mAs if an 8:1 grid is added?

(A) 16 mAs
(B) 24 mAs
(C) 32 mAs
(D) 40 mAs

130. What is the name of the plane indicated by the number 2 in Figure 7–16?

(A) Midcoronal plane
(B) Midsagittal plane
(C) Transverse plane
(D) Horizontal plane

131. In which of the following procedures is quiet, shallow breathing recommended during the exposure to obliterate prominent pulmonary vascular markings?

1. RAO sternum
2. Lateral thoracic spine
3. AP scapula

(A) 1 only
(B) 1 and 2 only
(C) 2 and 3 only
(D) 1, 2, and 3

132. The infection streptococcal pharyngitis (strep throat) is caused by a

(A) virus.
(B) fungus.
(C) protozoon.
(D) bacterium.

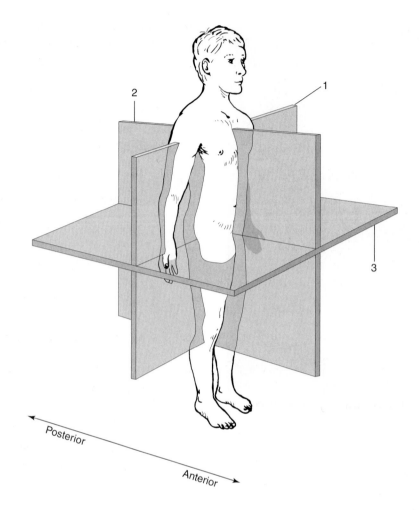

Figure 7–16. Reproduced with permission from Saia DA. *Radiography: Program Review and Examination Preparation,* 2nd ed. Stamford, CT: Appleton & Lange, 1999.

133. Which surface of the forearm must be adjacent to the IR to obtain a lateral projection of the fourth finger with optimal recorded detail?

(A) Anterior

(B) Posterior

(C) Medial

(D) Lateral

134. The submentovertical (SMV) oblique axial projection of the zygomatic arches requires that the skull be rotated

(A) 15° toward the affected side.

(B) 15° away from the affected side.

(C) 45° toward the affected side.

(D) 45° away from the affected side.

135. The radiographic position illustrated in Figure 7–17 is used to demonstrate

(A) ethmoidal and frontal sinuses.

(B) maxillary sinuses.

(C) sphenoidal sinuses through the open mouth.

(D) mastoid sinuses.

136. Which of the following functions to protect the x-ray tube and the patient from overexposure in the event that the phototimer fails to terminate an exposure?

(A) Circuit breaker

(B) Fuse

(C) Backup timer

(D) Rheostat

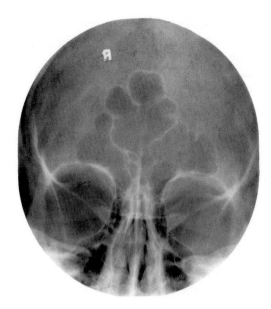

Figure 7–17. Courtesy of Stamford Hospital, Department of Radiology.

137. The AP axial projection of the pulmonary apices requires the central ray to be directed

(A) 15° cephalad.
(B) 15° caudad.
(C) 30° cephalad.
(D) 30° caudad.

138. Which cholangiographic procedure uses an indwelling drainage tube for contrast medium administration?

(A) Endoscopic retrograde cholangiographic pancreatography (ERCP)
(B) Operative cholangiography
(C) T-tube cholangiography
(D) Percutaneous transhepatic cholangiography

139. The radiographic accessory used to measure the thickness of body parts in order to determine optimum selection of exposure factors is the

A. fulcrum.
B. caliper.
C. densitometer.
D. ruler.

140. Which of the following combinations would deliver the least amount of heat to the anode of a 3-phase, 12- pulse x-ray unit?

(A) 400 mA, 0.12 second, 90 kVp
(B) 300 mA, 1/2 second, 70 kVp
(C) 500 mA, 1/30 second, 85 kVp
(D) 700 mA, 0.06 second, 120 kVp

141. Which of the following is *most* likely to result in the greatest increase in patient exposure?

(A) Changing from a 400 speed system to a 200 speed system
(B) Increasing kVp 15% and cutting mAs in half
(C) Using two tomographic cuts instead of two plain images
(D) From nongrid technique to 8:1 grid

142. Which of the following statements is (are) correct regarding the chest radiograph in Figure 7–18?

1. Rotation of the chest is demonstrated.
2. The pulmonary apices are not visualized.
3. The costophrenic angles are demonstrated.

(A) 1 only
(B) 1 and 3 only
(C) 2 and 3 only
(D) 1, 2, and 3

143. Which of the following positions may be used to effectively demonstrate the right posterior axillary ribs?

(A) LAO
(B) RAO
(C) RPO
(D) LPO

144. In myelography, the contrast medium is generally injected into the

(A) cisterna magna.
(B) individual intervertebral disks.
(C) subarachnoid space between the first and second vertebrae.
(D) subarachnoid space between the third and fourth lumbar vertebrae.

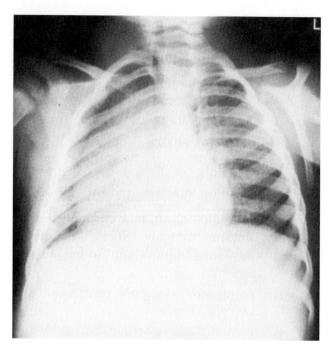

Figure 7–18. Courtesy of Stamford Hospital, Department of Radiology.

145. Improper support of a patient's fractured lower leg (tibia/fibula) while performing radiography could result in

    1. movement of fracture fragments.
    2. tearing of soft tissue, nerves, and blood vessels.
    3. initiation of muscle spasm.

    (A) 1 and 2 only
    (B) 1 and 3 only
    (C) 2 and 3 only
    (D) 1, 2 and 3

146. Which of the following is (are) demonstrated in the lateral projection of the cervical spine?

    1. Intervertebral joints
    2. Apophyseal joints
    3. Intervertebral foramina

    (A) 1 only
    (B) 1 and 2 only
    (C) 2 and 3 only
    (D) 1, 2, and 3

147. Which of the following statements is (are) correct with respect to postoperative cholangiography?

    1. A T-tube is in place in the common bile duct.
    2. Water-soluble contrast material is injected.
    3. The patency of biliary ducts is evaluated.

    (A) 1 only
    (B) 1 and 2 only
    (C) 2 and 3 only
    (D) 1, 2, and 3

148. If the entrance dose for a particular radiograph is 320 mR, the radiation exposure at 1 m from the patient will be approximately

    (A) 32 mR.
    (B) 3.2 mR.
    (C) 0.32 mR.
    (D) 0.032 mR.

149. Which of the following groups of exposure factors would deliver the *lowest* patient dose?

    (A) 2.5 mAs, 100 kVp, 400-speed screens
    (B) 10 mAs, 90 kVp, 200-speed screens
    (C) 10 mAs, 70 kVp, 800-speed screens
    (D) 10 mAs, 80 kVp, 400-speed screens

150. Which of the following would be the safest interval of time for a fertile woman to undergo abdominal radiography without significant concern for irradiating a recently fertilized ovum?

    (A) The first 10 days following the cessation of menstruation
    (B) The first 10 days following the onset of menstruation
    (C) The 10 days preceding the onset of menstruation
    (D) About 14 days before menstruation

151. What is the anatomic structure indicated by number 2 in the radiograph in Figure 7–19?

    (A) Mandibular angle
    (B) Coronoid process
    (C) Zygomatic arch
    (D) Maxillary sinus

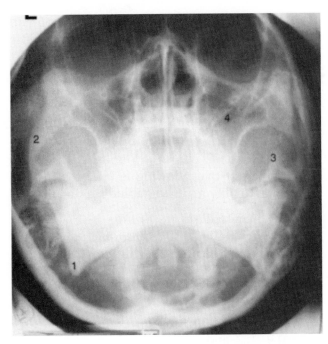

Figure 7–19. Courtesy of Stamford Hospital, Department of Radiology.

152. What is the anatomic structure indicated by number 4 in the radiograph in Figure 7–19?

(A) Mandibular angle
(B) Coronoid process
(C) Zygomatic arch
(D) Maxillary sinus

153. Esophageal varices are best demonstrated in which of the following positions?

(A) Erect
(B) Recumbent
(C) Fowler's
(D) Sims'

154. Greater latitude is available to the radiographer when using

1. high kVp factors.
2. a slow film–screen combination.
3. a high-ratio grid.

(A) 1 only
(B) 1 and 2 only
(C) 2 and 3 only
(D) 1, 2, and 3

155. Recorded detail is directly related to

1. source-image distance (SID).
2. tube current.
3. focal spot size.

(A) 1 only
(B) 1 and 2 only
(C) 2 and 3 only
(D) 1, 2, and 3

156. With the patient supine, the left side of the pelvis elevated 25°, and the central ray entering 1 inch medial to the left anterior superior iliac spine (ASIS), which of the following is demonstrated?

(A) Left sacroiliac joint
(B) Left ilium
(C) Right sacroiliac joint
(D) Right ilium

157. Double-focus x-ray tubes have two

1. focal spots.
2. filaments.
3. anodes.

(A) 1 only
(B) 1 and 2 only
(C) 1 and 3 only
(D) 2 and 3 only

158. What is the anatomic structure indicated by number 2 in the radiograph in Figure 7–20?

(A) Superior articular process
(B) Inferior articular process
(C) Transverse process
(D) Lamina

159. What is the anatomic structure indicated by number 4 in the radiograph in Figure 7–20?

(A) Superior articular process
(B) Inferior articular process
(C) Pedicle
(D) Lamina

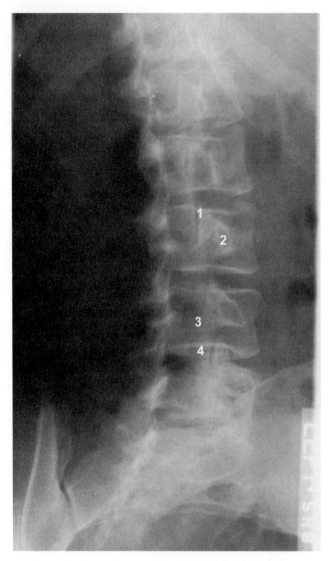

Figure 7–20. Courtesy of Stamford Hospital, Department of Radiology.

160. Which of the following statements is (are) true regarding the lateral projection of the lumbar spine?

 1. The MSP is parallel to the tabletop.
 2. The vertebral foramina are well visualized.
 3. The pedicles are well visualized.

 (A) 1 only
 (B) 1 and 2 only
 (C) 1 and 3 only
 (D) 1, 2, and 3

161. If a patient received 4500 mrad during a 6-min fluoroscopic examination, what was the dose rate?

 (A) 0.75 rad/min
 (B) 2.7 rad/min
 (C) 7.5 rad/min
 (D) 27 rad/hr

162. Which of the following is (are) essential to high-quality mammographic examinations?

 1. Small focal spot x-ray tube
 2. High radiographic contrast
 3. Use of a compression device

 (A) 1 only
 (B) 1 and 2 only
 (C) 1 and 3 only
 (D) 1, 2, and 3

163. The primary function of filtration is to reduce

 (A) patient skin dose.
 (B) operator dose.
 (C) image noise.
 (D) scattered radiation.

164. What is the anatomic structure indicated by the number 6 in Figure 7–21?

 (A) Coracoid process
 (B) Coronoid process
 (C) Trochlear notch
 (D) Radial notch

165. Which of the following correctly identifies the radial styloid process in the illustration in Figure 7–21?

 (A) Number 1
 (B) Number 4
 (C) Number 10
 (D) Number 11

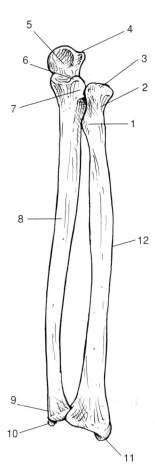

Figure 7–21. Reproduced with permission from Saia DA. *Radiography: Program Review and Examination Preparation*, 2nd ed. Stamford, CT: Appleton & Lange, 1999.

166. Which of the following statements is true regarding the PA axial projection of the paranasal sinuses?

1. The central ray is directed caudally to the orbitomeatal line (OML).
2. The petrous pyramids are projected into the lower one third of the orbits.
3. The frontal sinuses are visualized.

(A) 1 only
(B) 1 and 2 only
(C) 1 and 3 only
(D) 1, 2, and 3

167. Which of the following x-ray circuit devices operate(s) on the principle of mutual induction?

1. High-voltage transformer
2. Filament transformer
3. Autotransformer

(A) 1 only
(B) 1 and 2 only
(C) 1 and 3 only
(D) 1, 2, and 3

168. According to the line focus principle, an anode with a small angle provides

1. improved recorded detail.
2. improved heat capacity.
3. less heel effect.

(A) 1 and 2 only
(B) 1 and 3 only
(C) 2 and 3 only
(D) 1, 2, and 3

169. To better demonstrate the interphalangeal joints of the toes, which of the following procedures may be employed?

1. Angle the CR 15° caudad.
2. Angle the CR 15° cephalad.
3. Place a sponge wedge under the foot with toes elevated 15°.

(A) 1 only
(B) 1 and 2 only
(C) 1 and 3 only
(D) 2 and 3 only

170. The most commonly used method of low-flow oxygen delivery is the

(A) oxygen mask.
(B) nasal cannula.
(C) respirator.
(D) oxyhood.

171. All of the following statements regarding the RAO position of the sternum are true, *except*

(A) the sternum is generally projected to the left of the vertebral column.

(B) shallow breathing during the exposure can obliterate prominent pulmonary markings.

(C) it is helpful to project the sternum over the heart.

(D) a thin thorax requires a lesser degree of obliquity than a thicker thorax.

172. A signed consent form is necessary prior to performing all of the following procedures, *except*

(A) myelogram.

(B) cardiac catheterization.

(C) upper GI series.

(D) interventional vascular procedure.

173. When interviewing a patient, what is it that the health-care professional can observe?

(A) Symptoms

(B) History

(C) Objective signs

(D) Chief complaint

174. Which of the following statements is (are) true regarding the control badge that accompanies each shipment of personnel monitors?

1. It should be stored away from all radiation sources.

2. It should be stored in the main work area.

3. It should be used to replace an employee's lost monitor.

(A) 1 only

(B) 2 only

(C) 1 and 3 only

(D) 2 and 3 only

175. Patients' rights include which of the following?

1. The right to refuse treatment

2. The right to confidentiality

3. The right to possess his or her radiographs

(A) 1 only

(B) 1 and 2 only

(C) 1 and 3 only

(D) 1, 2, and 3

176. The ethical principle that aspires never to, above all, do harm describes:

(A) fidelity

(B) veracity

(C) nonmalficence

(D) beneficence

177. A radiographer would be in violation of the American Registry of Radiologic Technologists (ARRT) Code of Ethics for the Profession of Radiologic Technology for all of the following *except*

(A) failing to wear a lead apron when performing mobile radiography.

(B) failing to participate in continuing education.

(C) communicating information regarding suspected child abuse to the referring physician.

(D) refusing to participate in new and innovative technical procedures.

178. Hospitals and other health-care providers must ensure patient confidentiality, in compliance with which of the following legislations? Which of the following legislations is in place to ensure patient confidentiality?

A. MQSA

B. MRSA

C. HIPAA

D. HIPPA

179. Which of the following statements are true regarding radiographic examination of the acromioclavicular joints?

    1. The procedure is performed in the erect position.
    2. The use of weights helps demonstrate small joint changes.
    3. Weights are avoided if dislocation or separation is suspected.

    (A) 1 and 2 only
    (B) 1 and 3 only
    (C) 2 and 3 only
    (D) 1, 2, and 3

180. The ethical principle that refers to bringing about good, or benefiting others, is called

    (A) fidelity.
    (B) veracity.
    (C) nonmalficence.
    (D) beneficence.

181. Which of the following radiographic examinations require the patient to be npo 8 to 10 hours prior to examination for proper patient preparation?

    1. Abdominal survey
    2. Upper GI series
    3. BE

    (A) 1 and 2 only
    (B) 1 and 3 only
    (C) 2 and 3 only
    (D) 1, 2, and 3

182. What is the established fetal dose-limit guideline for pregnant radiographers during the entire gestation period?

    (A) 0.1 rem
    (B) 0.5 rem
    (C) 5.0 rem
    (D) 10 rem

183. The acquired immune deficiency syndrome (AIDS) virus may be transmitted

    1. by sharing contaminated needles.
    2. from mother to child during birth.
    3. by intimate contact with body fluids.

    (A) 1 only
    (B) 1 and 2 only
    (C) 1 and 3 only
    (D) 1, 2, and 3

184. An autoclave is used for

    (A) dry heat sterilization.
    (B) chemical sterilization.
    (C) gas sterilization.
    (D) steam sterilization.

185. Which of the following are considered *most* radiosensitive?

    (A) Lymphocytes
    (B) Ova
    (C) Neurons
    (D) Myocytes

186. Proper body mechanics includes a wide base of support. The base of support is the portion of the body

    (A) in contact with the floor or other horizontal surface.
    (B) in the midportion of the pelvis or lower abdomen.
    (C) passing through the center of gravity.
    (D) none of the above.

187. Which of the following is (are) classified as a rare earth phosphor?

    1. Lanthanum oxybromide
    2. Gadolinium oxysulfide
    3. Cesium iodide

    (A) 1 only
    (B) 1 and 2 only
    (C) 2 and 3 only
    (D) 1, 2, and 3

188. Double-contrast examinations of the stomach or large bowel are performed to better visualize

    (A) the position of the organ.
    (B) the size and shape of the organ.
    (C) diverticula.
    (D) the gastric or bowel mucosa.

189. A patient who has been recumbent for some time and gets up quickly may suffer from lightheadedness or feel faint. This is referred to as

    (A) dyspnea.
    (B) orthopnea.
    (C) hypertension.
    (D) orthostatic hypotension.

190. Contaminated needles are disposed of in special containers in which of the following ways?

    (A) Recap the needle, remove syringe, dispose of
    (B) Do not recap needle, remove from syringe, dispose of
    (C) Recap the needle, dispose of entire syringe
    (D) Do not recap needle, dispose of entire syringe

191. Which of the following is a fast-acting vasodilator used to lower blood pressure and relieve the pain of angina pectoris?

    (A) Digitalis
    (B) Dilantin
    (C) Nitroglycerin
    (D) Cimetidine (Tagamet)

192. An overall image density arising from factors other than the light or radiation used to expose the image is called

    (A) fog.
    (B) log relative exposure.
    (C) optical density.
    (D) artifact.

193. The annual dose limit for occupationally exposed individuals is valid for

    (A) alpha, beta, and x-radiations.
    (B) x- and gamma radiations only.
    (C) beta, x-, and gamma radiations.
    (D) all ionizing radiations.

194. If 85 kVp, 400 mA, and 1/8 second was used for a particular exposure using single-phase equipment, which of the following milliamperage or time values would be required, all other factors being constant, to produce a similar density using 3-phase, 12-pulse equipment?

    (A) 200 mA
    (B) 600 mA
    (C) 0.125 second
    (D) 0.25 second

195. In the parieto-orbital projection (Rhese method) of the optic canal, the median sagittal plane and central ray form what angle?

    (A) 90°
    (B) 37°
    (C) 53°
    (D) 45°

196. Which of the following should be used to evaluate glenohumeral joint dislocation?

    1. Inferosuperior axial
    2. Transthoracic lateral
    3. Scapular Y projection

    (A) 1 only
    (B) 1 and 2 only
    (C) 2 and 3 only
    (D) 1, 2, and 3

197. The Centers for Disease Control and Prevention (CDC) suggests that health-care workers protect themselves and their patients from blood and body fluid contamination by using

    (A) strict isolation precautions.
    (B) standard precautions.
    (C) respiratory precautions.
    (D) sterilization.

198. X-ray tube life may be extended by

1. using high-mAs, low-kVp exposure factors.
2. avoiding lengthy anode rotation.
3. avoiding exposures to a cold anode.

(A) 1 only
(B) 1 and 2 only
(C) 2 and 3 only
(D) 1, 2, and 3

199. Which of the following functions to increase the mA?

(A) Increasing the speed of anode rotation
(B) Increasing the transformer turns ratio
(C) Using three-phase rectification
(D) Increasing the heat of the filament

200. A technique chart should include which of the following information?

1. Recommended SID
2. Grid ratio
3. Screen–film combination

(A) 1 only
(B) 1 and 2 only
(C) 1 and 3 only
(D) 1, 2, and 3

Answers and Explanations

1. **(D)** Ipecac is a medication used to induce vomiting and is classified as an *emetic*. This is easy to remember if you think of what an emesis basin is for. A *diuretic* is a medication that stimulates the *production of urine*. Lasix (furosemide) is an example of a diuretic. An *antipyretic* is used to reduce fever. Tylenol (acetaminophen) is an example of an antipyretic. An *antihistamine* is used to relieve allergic effects. Benadryl (diphenhydramine hydrochloride) is an example of an antihistamine that is often on hand in radiology departments in the event of a minor reaction to contrast media. (*Adler & Carlton, p 265*)

2. **A.** Mobile x-ray machines are compact and cordless and are either the battery-operated type or the condenser discharge type. *Condenser discharge* mobile x-ray units do not use batteries; this type mobile unit requires that it be charged before each exposure. A condenser (or capacitor) is a device that stores electrical energy. The stored energy is used to operate the x-ray tube only. Because this machine does not carry many batteries, it is much lighter and does not need a motor to drive or brake it. The major *disadvantage* of the capacitor discharge unit is that, as the capacitor discharges its electrical charge, the kVp gradually decreases throughout the length of the exposure, therefore limiting tube output and requiring recharging between exposures. (*Ballinger & Frank, vol 3, p 235*)

3. **(B)** Anemia is a blood condition characterized by a decreased number of circulating red blood cells and decreased hemoglobin; it has many causes. Adequate hemoglobin is required to provide oxygen to the body. Anemia is treated according to its cause. Hematuria is the term used to describe blood in the urine and is unrelated to anemia. (*Tortora & Derrickson, p 689*)

4. **(D)** All of the choices listed in the question should be part of a preliminary patient history before deciding to inject ionic or nonionic contrast media. As patients age, their general health decreases, and they are therefore more likely to suffer from adverse reactions. Patients with a history of respiratory disease, such as asthma or emphysema and chronic obstructive pulmonary disease (COPD), are more likely to have a reaction, and to suffer greater distress in the event of a reaction. Patients with cardiac disease run an increased risk of changes in heart rate and myocardial infarction. Patients should also be screened for decreased renal or hepatic function, sickle-cell disease, diabetes, and pregnancy. (*Adler & Carlton, pp 314–317*)

5. **(C)** Since 18 ms is equal to 0.018 s, and since mA × time = mAs, the original mAs was 10.8. Now it is only necessary to determine what exposure time must be used with 400 mA to provide the same 10.8 mAs (and thus the same radiographic density). Because mA × time = mAs,

   $$400x = 10.8$$
   $$x = 0.027 \text{ second (27 milliseconds)}$$

   (*Selman, p 214*)

6. **(B)** When viewing the glenoid fossa from the anterior, it is seen to angle posteriorly and laterally approximately 45°. To view it in profile, then, it must be placed so that its surface is perpendicular to the image recorder. The patient is positioned in a 45° oblique, affected side down, which places the glenoid fossa approximately perpendicular to the image recorder. The arm is abducted slightly, the elbow flexed, and the hand and forearm placed over the abdomen. The CR is directed perpendicular to the glenohumeral joint. *(Ballinger & Frank, vol 1, pp 182–183)*

7. **(C)** Invasion of privacy—that is, public discussion of privileged and confidential information—is intentional misconduct. False imprisonment, such as unnecessarily restraining a patient, is also intentional misconduct. However, if a radiographer left a weak patient standing while leaving the room to check images or get supplies, and the patient fell and sustained an injury, that would be considered unintentional misconduct or negligence. *(Gurley & Callaway, p 187)*

8. **(B)** Because *muscle* and *nerve* tissues perform specific functions and do not divide, they are relatively *insensitive* to radiation exposure. *Epithelial* cells cover the outer surface of the body; they also line body cavities and tubes and passageways leading to the exterior. They contain very little intercellular substance and are devoid of blood vessels. Because *epithelial* cells constantly regenerate through mitosis, they are very *radiosensitive*. *(Dowd & Tilson, pp 121–122)*

9. **(A)** The relationship between x-ray intensity and distance from the source is expressed in the inverse square law of radiation. The formula is

$$\frac{I_1}{I_2} = \frac{D_2^2}{D_1^2}$$

Substituting known values,:

$$\frac{12 \text{ R/min}}{x} = \frac{49 \, (7^2)}{9 \, (3^2)}$$
$$49x = 108$$
$$x = 2.2 \text{ R/min at 7 feet}$$

Note the *inverse relationship* between distance and dose. As distance from the source of radiation increases, dose rate decreases significantly. *(Bushong, p 67)*

10. **(B)** Three dose–response (dose effect) curves are illustrated, representing the body's response to irradiation. *Dose* is indicated by the horizontal axis (increasing to the right); *response* is indicated by the vertical axis (increasing upward). Two of the curves (numbers 1 and 3) are *linear*, that is, a straight line. Curve 2 is not a straight line and is therefore *nonlinear*. Curves 2 and 3 show that a particular dose (*threshold* quantity) of radiation is required before any effect will occur; therefore, curve 2 is *nonlinear threshold* and curve 3 is *linear threshold*. Curve 1, however, shows that any dose of radiation (theoretically, even a single x-ray photon, ie, there is no threshold) can result in a particular biologic effect; therefore, it is *linear nonthreshold*. *(Bushong, p 498)*

11. **(D)** Lateral carpals, especially the scaphoid, are demonstrated in the *PA oblique* projection and the *ulnar flexion* maneuver. The scaphoid may also be demonstrated with the wrist *PA and elevated 20°*. The central ray is directed perpendicular to the carpal scaphoid. The medial carpals, especially the pisiform, are well demonstrated in the AP oblique projection and with the radial flexion maneuver. *(Saia, pp 96–97)*

12. **(A)** The velocity and charge of particulate radiation determines the amount of energy transferred (and, therefore, the number of ionizations) to the *tissue traversed*. A greater LET (number of ionizations) is delivered by particles with a slower velocity and greater charge. The greater the LET and the number of ionizations, the greater the biologic effect. The unit of absorbed dose is the rad (*radiation absorbed dose*). *Rem* is the acronym for *radiation equivalent man*—the unit of dose equivalent. *(Bushong, p 495)*

13. **(A)** The dorsal decubitus position is obtained with the patient *supine* and the x-ray beam directed *horizontally*. The finished radiograph

looks similar to a routine lateral projection of the chest. However, small amounts of *fluid* will gravitate posteriorly, and small amounts of *air* will rise anteriorly. *(Ballinger & Frank, vol 1, p 78)*

14. **(B)** Sufficient inspiration is demonstrated by the visualization of 10 posterior ribs projected above the diaphragm. Rotation of the chest is detected by asymmetry in the distance between the medial ends of the clavicles and the vertebral column. The scapulae should be free of superimposition with the lung fields; this is accomplished by rolling the shoulders forward while positioning for the PA. *(Ballinger & Frank, vol 1, p 527)*

15. **(B)** X-ray photons are produced in two ways as high-speed electrons interact with target tungsten atoms. First, if the high-speed electron is attracted by the nucleus of a tungsten atom and changes its course, as the electron is "braked," energy is given up *in the form of an x-ray photon*. This is called bremsstrahlung (braking) radiation, and it is responsible for the majority of the x-ray photons produced at the conventional tungsten target. Second, a high-speed electron *having an energy of at least 70 keV* may eject a tungsten K-shell electron, leaving a vacancy in the shell. An electron from the next energy level, the L shell, drops down to fill the vacancy, *emitting the difference in energy as a K characteristic ray.* Characteristic radiation makes up only about 15% of the primary beam. *(Bushong, p 176)*

16. **(D)** Body substance precaution procedures identify various body fluids as infectious or potentially infectious. These body substances include pleural, pericardial, peritoneal, and amniotic fluids, synovial fluid, CSF, breast milk, and vaginal secretions. Also, nasal secretions, tears, saliva, sputum, feces, urine, and wound drainage. *(Torres et al, p 63)*

17. **(C)** As *filtration* is added to the x-ray beam, the lower-energy photons are removed and the overall energy or wavelength of the beam is greater. As *kilovoltage* is increased, more high-energy photons are produced and, again, the overall or average energy of the beam is greater. *An increase in mA serves to increase the number of photons produced at the target, but is unrelated to their energy. (Bushong, pp 165, 166)*

18. **(C)** An oblique projection of the cervical spine is pictured. The first two cervical vertebrae are not well visualized because of superimposition of the mandible. The chin should be elevated somewhat to avoid this problem. Otherwise, the positioning is satisfactory, with good demonstration of the remainder of the cervical intervertebral foramina. The patient has been accurately rotated 45° with a 15 to 20° cephalic tube angle. *(Bontragen, p 294)*

19. **(B)** An oblique projection of the cervical spine is pictured. The patient has been accurately positioned RAO with the MSP 45° to the IR and the central ray angled 15° to 20° caudad. The chin should be elevated to better visualize the first two cervical vertebrae. This position offers excellent delineation of the *intervertebral foramina* (number 1) formed by the adjacent vertebral notches of *pedicles* (2). This projection gives an "on-end" view of the *transverse processes* (3). A portion of the *spinous processes* (4) may be seen, especially in the lower cervical vertebrae. *(Ballinger & Frank, vol 1, p 400)*

20. **(B)** With the blood pressure cuff wrapped snugly around the patient's brachial artery and the pump inflated to approximately 180 mm Hg, the valve is opened only slightly to release pressure very slowly. With the stethoscope over the brachial artery, listen for the pulse while watching the Hg column (gauge). Note the point at which the first pulse is heard as the *systolic* pressure. As the valve is opened further, the sound is louder; the point at which it suddenly becomes softer is recorded as the *diastolic pressure. (Torres et al, p 149)*

21. **(B)** Emphysema is a COPD characterized by pathologic distention of the pulmonary alveoli with (destructive) changes in their walls, resulting in a loss of elasticity. Emphysema is occasionally seen following asthma or tuberculosis, but it is most frequently caused by cigarette smoking. Because the emphysematous patient's greatest difficulty is exhalation, it becomes a conscious, forced effort. Breathing is

shallow and rapid. Forced and ineffective breathing results in *expansion of the AP diameter* of the chest and *elevated shoulder girdle* in established emphysema.

Hyperventilation results from too frequent deep breaths in the anxious or tense individual. This results in a feeling of dizziness and tingling of the extremities. *(Tortora & Derrickson, p 887)*

22. **(D)** When air–fluid levels are to be demonstrated, it is important to direct the central ray horizontally. If the central ray is angled or directed vertically, the air or fluid level will be distorted or entirely obliterated. Free air in the abdominal cavity is best visualized when the patient is left lateral decubitus or erect AP. The decubitus allows the air to accumulate around the homogeneous liver. *(Ballinger & Frank, vol 2, p 41)*

23. **(B)** Whole-body dose is calculated to include all the *especially radiosensitive* organs. The *gonads*, the *lens* of the eye, and the *blood-forming organs* are particularly radiosensitive. The annual dose limit for the skin, hands, and feet (extremities) is 50 rem per year. *(Bushong, p 557)*

24. **(B)** Exposure to high doses of radiation results in *early* effects. Examples of early effects are blood changes and erythema. If the exposed individual survives, then *late* or long-term effects must be considered. Individuals who receive *small* amounts of *low-level* radiation (such as those who are occupationally exposed) are concerned with the late effects of radiation exposure—those effects that can occur many years after the initial exposure. *Late effects* of radiation exposure, such as carcinogenesis, are considered to be related to the *linear nonthreshold* dose–response curve. That is, there is *no safe dose*; theoretically, even one x-ray photon can induce a later response. *(Bushong, pp 532, 537)*

25. **(C)** *Air–fluid levels* are demonstrated in the *erect* or *decubitus* position. *Grid* radiography requires about a three to four times greater dose than nongrid radiography. A right lateral decubitus without a grid, then, would demonstrate fluid levels with a considerably smaller

dose to the infant. A recumbent AP would not demonstrate air–fluid levels. *(Saia, p 322)*

26. **(C)** The AP oblique projection (medial rotation) of the elbow superimposes the radial head and neck on the proximal ulna. It demonstrates the *olecranon process within the olecranon fossa,* and it projects the *coronoid process free of superimposition.* The radial head is projected free of superimposition in the AP oblique projection (lateral rotation) of the elbow. *(Saia, p 10)*

27. **(C)** Lead aprons are worn by occupationally exposed individuals during fluoroscopic and mobile x-ray procedures. Lead aprons are available with various lead equivalents; 0.5 and 1.0 mm are the most common. The 1.0-mm lead equivalent apron will provide close to 100% protection at most kVp levels, but it is rarely used because it weighs anywhere from 12 to 24 lb! A *0.25-mm* lead equivalent apron will attenuate about 97% of a 50-kVp x-ray beam, 66% of a 75-kVp beam, and 51% of a 100-kVp beam. A *0.5-mm lead* equivalent apron will attenuate about 99.9% of a 50-kVp beam, 88% of a 75-kVp beam, and 75% of a 100-kVp beam. *(Bushong, p 597)*

28. **(B)** A *characteristic curve* is used to predict the speed, contrast, and exposure latitude of a particular film emulsion. It compares the exposure, given the film with the resultant density. It has *three portions:* the toe, the straight-line portion (region of correct exposure), and the shoulder. The *toe* occurs immediately after base-plus fog, whose density must not exceed 0.2. The ascending straight-line portion follows the toe; the *straight-line portion is the portion of correct exposure* and extends from about 0.25 to 2.5. The curve then bends and levels off at the *shoulder* (Dmax) portion of the curve. *(Bushong, p 277)*

29. **(B)** The overall chance that a person will become infected with HIV is high with entry sites such as the anus, broken skin, shared needles, infected blood products, and perinatal exposure. *Low-risk* entry methods include oral and nasal, conjunctiva, and accidental needle stick. *(Ehlrich et al, p 150)*

30. **(D)** The term *parenteral* denotes any medication route other than the alimentary canal (by mouth). Examples of parenteral routes are subcutaneous, intravenous, intramuscular, and intracardiac. The speed of absorption varies with the route used. *(Torres et al, p 270)*

31. **(B)** The RAO position is pictured. The barium-filled *esophagus* can be projected between the vertebrae and heart in this position. This RAO position is also used to superimpose the *sternum* onto the heart shadow, to provide uniform density throughout the sternum. The degree of obliquity depends on the patient's body habitus—greater obliquity required for thinner chests. The RAO position is also used to see axillary portions of *left anterior ribs*; in the anterior oblique positions, the affected side is away from the IR. *(Ballinger & Frank, vol 1, pp 500, 515)*

32. **(C)** The hepatic and splenic flexures are not generally well demonstrated in the AP and PA projections. To "open" the flexures, oblique projections are required. The *hepatic* flexure is usually well demonstrated in the RAO (right PA oblique) and LPO (left AP oblique) positions. The LAO and RPO positions are used to demonstrate the *splenic* flexure. *(Bontrager, p 509)*

33. **(B)** If it is desired to determine entrance skin exposure, a small ionization chamber (pocket dosimeter) can be placed on the skin and the approximate ESE read immediately. These devices are readily imaged, however, and are awkward to position. For these reasons, TLDs or OSLs are more easily used; they are precise and will not interfere with the radiographic image. The acceptable ESE for a PA chest is approximately 20 mR (12 to 26 mR is the acceptable range). An image taken with an ESE of 6 mR would be underexposed and require repeating. Similarly, ESEs of 38 mR and 0.6 R (600 mR) would lead to overexposed images that would need to be repeated. *(Ballinger & Frank, vol 1, p 43)*

34. **(B)** Hemovac or Penrose drains are used for tissue drainage of wounds or in postoperative drainage. Drainage tubes help prevent the formation of infection or fistulas in wounds and postoperative sites with large amounts of drainage. Bile duct drainage, when necessary, is performed with a T-tube, and radiographers often perform radiographic examinations of the T-tube to verify patency. Nasogastric and nasoenteric tubes may be used either for decompression of the gastrointestinal tract or to feed patients who are unable to swallow food normally. In addition, radiographic examination of the gastrointestinal tract may be performed by introducing a contrast agent into a nasogastric or nasoenteric tube. *(Torres et al, pp 255–256)*

35. **(D)** The four types of body habitus are (from upper extreme to lower extreme) hypersthenic, sthenic, hyposthenic, and asthenic. The gallbladder and stomach are higher and more lateral and the large bowel more peripheral in the hypersthenic. The diaphragm is in a higher position in the hypersthenic individual. Recognition of a patient's body habitus and its characteristics is an important part of accurate radiography. Bone porosity is generally unrelated to body habitus type. *(Ballinger & Frank, vol 1, p 59)*

36. **(D)** The x-ray tube anode is designed according to the *line focus principle,* that is, with the focal track beveled (Fig. 7–22). This allows a larger *actual* focal spot to project a smaller *effective* focal spot, resulting in improved recorded detail with less blur. However, because of the target angle, penumbral *blur varies along the longitudinal tube axis,* being greater at the cathode end of the image and less at the anode end of the image. *(Bushong, p 287)*

37. **(A)** The *autotransformer* controls/selects the amount of voltage sent to the primary winding of the high-voltage transformer and operates on the principle of *self*-induction. The *step-up* (high-voltage) *transformer* (the primary coil is number 2; the secondary coil is number 3) operates on the principle of *mutual* induction. The x-ray tube is identified as number 7. *(Selman, pp 88, 159)*

38. **(D)** The *rectification system,* which is used to change alternating current to unidirectional current, is indicated by number 5. The rectification system is located between the secondary

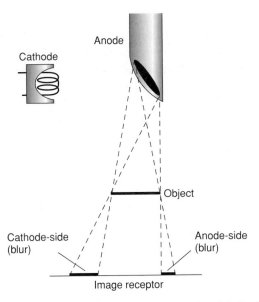

Cathode

Anode

Object

Cathode-side
(blur)

Anode-side
(blur)

Image receptor

Figure 7–22. Reproduced with permission from Saia DA. *Radiography: Program Review and Examination Preparation*, 2nd ed. Stamford, CT: Appleton & Lange, 1999.

coil of the high-voltage transformer (3) and the x-ray tube (7). The autotransformer is labeled 1, the primary coil of the high-voltage transformer is 2, the grounded mA meter is 4, and the filament circuit is 6. *(Selman, pp 98, 159)*

39. **(C)** Another name for an intermittent injection port is a *heparin lock*. As the name suggests, heparin locks are used for patients who will require sporadic injections. An intravenous catheter is placed in the vein, and an external adapter with a diaphragm allows for repeated injections. Heparin locks provide more freedom than an *IV infusion*, which also allows for repeated access. *Hypodermic needles* are usually used for drawing blood or drawing up fluids, whereas a *butterfly needle* is usually used for venipuncture. *(Torres et al, p 318)*

40. **(A)** Remnant radiation emerging from the patient causes fluorescence of the cassette's intensifying screens. When activated by x-ray photons, the individual phosphors emit light isotropically. Fluorescent light that is not perpendicular produces a blur, resulting in geometric unsharpness and decreased resolution. During manufacture, special dyes can be added to the active layer that will absorb much of the diffused fluorescence and allow a greater percentage of the image density to be created by

more perpendicular fluorescent light. These dyes improve resolution but result in a small loss of screen speed. *(Shephard, pp 73–74)*

41. **B.** Mobile x-ray machines are compact and cordless and are either the battery operated type or the condenser discharge type. *Condenser discharge* mobile x-ray units do not use batteries; this type mobile unit requires that it be charged before each exposure. A condenser (or capacitor) is a device that stores electrical energy. The stored energy is used to operate the x-ray tube only. Because this machine does not carry many batteries, it is much lighter and does not need a motor to drive or brake it. The major *disadvantage* of the capacitor discharge unit is that, as the capacitor discharges its electrical charge, the kVp gradually decreases throughout the length of the exposure, therefore limiting tube output and requiring recharging between exposures. *(Ballinger & Frank, vol 3, p 235)*

42. **(A)** If the SID is above or below the recommended focusing distance, the primary beam at the lateral edges will not coincide with the angled lead strips. Consequently, there will be absorption of the primary beam, termed *grid cutoff*. If the grid failed to move during the exposure, there would be grid lines throughout. Central ray angulation in the direction of the lead strips is appropriate and will not cause grid cutoff. If the central ray was off-center, there would be uniform loss of density. *(Selman, p 240)*

43. **(D)** Variance from the normal bladder contour will be noted while the bladder is full of contrast medium. However, a postmicturition (postvoiding) radiograph is also an essential part of an IVU/IVP. The presence of residual urine may be an indication of small tumor masses or, in male patients, enlargement of the prostate gland. *(Ballinger & Frank, vol 2, p 177)*

44. **(C)** The tangential ("sunrise") projection is used to demonstrate the *articular surfaces* of the femur and patella. It is also used to demonstrate *vertical fractures* of the patella. The AP, PA, and oblique projections of the knee are used primarily to evaluate the joint space and

articulating structures. The "tunnel" view is used to demonstrate the intercondyloid fossa. (Bontrager, p 241)

45. **(D)** To accurately position a lateral forearm, the elbow must form a 90° angle with the humeral epicondyles superimposed. The radius and ulna are superimposed distally. Proximally, the coronoid process and radial head are partially superimposed. Failure of the elbow to form a 90° angle, or the hand to be lateral, results in a less-than-satisfactory lateral projection of the forearm. (Ballinger & Frank, vol 1, p 130)

46. **(B)** X-ray film emulsion is sensitive and requires proper handling and storage. Careless handling can produce several kinds of artifacts. Treelike black branching marks are usually caused by static electrical discharge, which is especially prevalent during cold, dry weather. Acute bending of the film produces crinkle marks. Excessive emulsion swelling and chemical fog can be caused by increased solution temperature or insufficient replenishment. (Shephard, pp 110–111)

47. **(A)** Restriction of field size is one important method of patient protection. However, the accuracy of the light field must be evaluated periodically as part of a QA program. Guidelines set forth for patient protection state that the collimator light and actual irradiated area must be accurate to within 2% of the SID employed. (Bushong, p 568)

48. **(D)** A *spinning top* test may be performed to evaluate timer accuracy or rectifier efficiency in single-phase equipment. The number of dots or dashes imaged on the IR is counted and should equal the number of radiation "pulses" occurring during that exposure time. Because three-phase equipment does not emit pulsed radiation, but rather almost constant potential, a *synchronous spinning top* must be used to evaluate timer accuracy. The resulting image is a solid black arc. The angle of the arc is measured and should correspond to the known correct angle. (Selman, pp 105–106)

49. **(C)** *Retrograde urography* is not considered a functional study of the urinary system. *IVP,*

descending urography, and *infusion nephrotomography* are all considered functional urinary tract studies because the contrast medium is introduced intravenously and *excreted* by the kidneys. *Retrograde urography* involves introduction of contrast medium into the kidneys via catheter, thereby demonstrating their *structure,* but not their *function.* (Ballinger & Frank, vol 2, p 167)

50. **(D)** *Single-phase* current has a 100% voltage drop between peak voltages. Three-phase current decreases this voltage drop considerably. *Three-phase, six-pulse* current has about a 13% voltage drop between peak voltages, and *3-phase, 12-pulse* current has only about a 4% drop between peak voltages. However, *high-frequency* current is almost constant potential, having less than 1% voltage ripple. (Bushong, pp 122, 123)

51. **(B)** The (diarthrotic) sternoclavicular joints are formed by the medial (sternal) extremities of the clavicles and the clavicular notches of the manubrium (of the sternum). They can be demonstrated in the *LAO* and *RAO* positions. The LAO demonstrates the left sternoclavicular joint, while the RAO demonstrates the joint on the right. The patient is obliqued about 15° with the *side of interest adjacent* to the image recorder. (Ballinger & Frank, vol 1, p 485)

52. **(B)** Photospot camera film comes in 90- and 105-mm sizes. Comparing these two sizes, the larger size provides better resolution but more patient dose. However, when compared to cassette-loaded spot films, photospot camera film produces *less resolution* than cassette-loaded film, but requires *half the exposure.* The poorer resolution is insignificant when compared to all the advantages of photospot camera use. Additionally, photospot camera use involves *less interruption* of the procedure because frame after frame can be exposed without the interruption of changing cassette-loaded spot films. (Bushong, p 369)

53. **(A)** Nosocomial infections are infections acquired in hospitals. Despite the efforts of infectious disease departments, nosocomial infections continue to be a problem in hospitals

today. This is at least partly due to there being a greater number of older, more vulnerable patients and an increase in the number of invasive procedures performed today (needles, catheters, and so on). The most frequent site of nosocomial infection is the *urinary tract*, followed by *wounds*, the *respiratory tract*, and *blood*. (*Torres et al, p 47*)

54. **(C)** Film badges are supplied by a dosimetry service. They contain pieces of dental film held within a holder containing filters. When used properly, film badges measure the quantity and quality of radiation exposure. Film within the badges is usually changed *monthly*. The sensitive film emulsion is susceptible to deterioration and false readings if the badges are worn for longer periods, or if they are damaged by water, heat, light, and so on. To avoid the possibility of damage or exposure, film badges should not leave the workplace. (*Ballinger & Frank, vol 1, p 49*)

55. **(C)** When the anatomic part contains greatly differing densities, a *compensating filter* is frequently helpful. Compensating filters can be accommodated by tracks in the tube head. They can be wedge-shaped (with the thicker part of the wedge paralleling the thinner body part), thus compensating for greater or lesser tissue densities (as in a large decubitus abdomen). A *grid* is used to absorb scattered radiation before it reaches the IR; *intensifying screens* amplify the action of x-rays; and a *penetrometer* (aluminum step wedge) is used to illustrate the effect of kVp on contrast. (*Bushong, pp 69–170*)

56. **(D)** Photoelectric interaction in tissue involves complete absorption of the incident photon, whereas Compton interactions involve only partial transfer of energy. The larger the quantity of radiation and the greater the number of photoelectric interactions, the greater the patient dose. Radiation dose to more radiosensitive tissues, such as gonadal tissue or blood-forming organs, is more harmful than the same dose to muscle tissue. (*Bushong, p 197*)

57. **(A)** According to the inverse square law of radiation, as the distance between the radiation source and the IR decreases, the exposure rate increases. Therefore, a decrease in technical factors is first indicated to compensate for the distance change. The following formula (*density maintenance formula*) is used to determine new mAs values, when changing distance:

$$\frac{mAs_1}{mAs_2} = \frac{D_1^2}{D_2^2}$$

Substituting known values,

$$\frac{8}{x} = \frac{5184\,(72^2)}{1600\,(40^2)}$$
$$5184x = 12{,}800$$
$$x = 2.46 \text{ mAs at 40 inches SID}$$

To then compensate for adding an 8:1 grid, you must multiply the 2.4 mAs by a factor of 4. Thus, *9.6 mAs is required* to produce a image density similar to the original radiograph. The following are the factors used for mAs conversion from nongrid to grid:

No grid= 1 × original mAs
5:1 grid = 2 × original mAs
6:1 grid = 3 × original mAs
8:1 grid = 4 × original mAs
12:1 grid = 5 × original mAs
16:1 grid = 6 × original mAs

(*Bushong, pp 69, 252*)

58. **(A)** The thoracic and abdominal cavities are associated with serous membranes: the thoracic cavity with the *pleura* and the abdominal cavity with the *peritoneum*. The pleura and peritoneum each have two walls, a parietal (outer) wall and a visceral (inner) wall. The *parietal pleura* lines the thoracic cavity, while the *visceral pleura* is reflected over the surface of the lungs and projects between the fissures. The *parietal peritoneum* lines the abdominal cavity, and the *visceral peritoneum* invests the abdominal viscera. (*Tortora & Derrickson, p 857*)

59. **(A)** Three-phase current is obtained from three individual alternating currents superimposed on, but out of step with, one another by 120°. The result is an *almost* constant potential current, with only a very small voltage ripple

(4% to 13%), producing more x-rays per mAs. *(Saia, p 422)*

60. **(D)** The radiographic subject (the patient) is composed of many different tissue types of varying densities, resulting in varying degrees of photon attenuation and absorption. This *differential absorption* contributes to the various shades of gray (scale of radiographic contrast) on the finished radiograph. Normal tissue density may be significantly altered in the presence of pathology. For example, destructive bone disease can cause a dramatic decrease in tissue density. Abnormal accumulation of fluid (as in ascites) will cause a significant increase in tissue density. Muscle atrophy or highly developed muscles will similarly decrease or increase tissue density. *(Shephard, p 203)*

61. **(D)** Cells that are termed undifferentiated are *immature* or young. They have no specific function and/or structure. They are usually precursor cells; their most important function is to divide. Mitosis is the most radiosensitive portion of the cell cycle. *(Bushong, p 495)*

62. **(D)** When the primary beam is restricted to an area near the periphery of the body, sometimes part of the illuminated area overhangs the edge of the body. If the exposure is then made, scattered radiation from the tabletop (where there is no absorber) will undercut the part, causing excessive image density. If, however, a *lead rubber mat* is placed on the overhanging illuminated area, most of this scatter will be absorbed. This is frequently helpful in lateral lumbar spines and AP shoulders. *(Carlton & Adler, p 507)*

63. **(C)** Radiographic contrast is greatly affected by changes in kilovoltage (Fig. 7–23). As kVp increases, a greater number of high-energy photons are produced at the target. These photons are more penetrating, but they also produce more scattered radiation, contributing to *lower* radiographic contrast as a result of *scattered radiation fog*. Radiograph B was made using 100 kVp and 18 mAs. Radiograph A was made of the same part using 80 kVp and 75 mAs, all other factors constant. The image details in radiograph A are far more perceptible as a result of the production of less scattered radiation. *(Saia, p 344)*

64. **(B)** *Differential absorption* refers to the different attenuation, or absorption, properties of adjacent body tissues. Two parts with widely differing absorption characteristics will produce a high radiographic contrast. Frequently, exposure factors that would properly expose one part will severely overexpose or underexpose the neighboring part (as with lungs vs thoracic

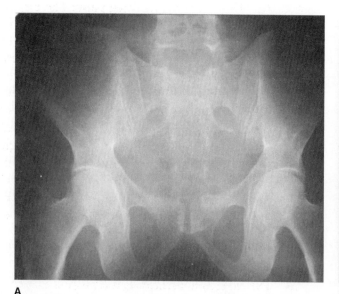
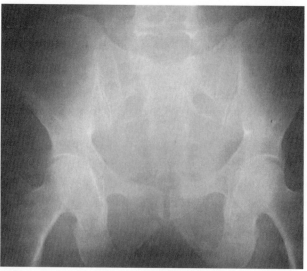

A   B

Figure 7–23. From the American College of Radiology Learning File. Courtesy of the ACR.

spine). This effect can be minimized by the use of a *compensating filter* or by the use of high kilovoltage (for more uniform penetration). Increased collimation is important in the control of patient dose and scattered radiation, not differential absorption. *(Bushong, pp 169, 170)*

65. **(A)** A misaligned *guide shoe* in the turnaround assembly will create evenly spaced minus-density lines as a result of emulsion scratching. *Dirty rollers* cause multiple black specks on the finished radiograph; these are present on the pictured radiograph as well. A *pi line* is a plus-density artifact found 3/4 inch from the leading edge of the film. *Grid lines* appear as minus-density lines resulting from improper positioning or centering of the grid or x-ray tube. *(Shephard, p 155)*

66. **(A)** Intravenous urography requires the use of iodinated contrast media. Low kilovoltage (about 70) is usually employed to enhance the photoelectric effect, and in turn to better visualize the renal collecting system. High kilovoltage will produce excessive scattered radiation and obviate the effect of the contrast agent. A higher milliamperage with a short exposure time is generally preferable. *(Fauber, p 264)*

67. **(D)** Proper care of leaded protective apparel is required to ensure its continued usefulness. If lead aprons and gloves are folded, cracks will develop, and this will decrease their effectiveness. Both items should be fluoroscoped annually to check for the formation of cracks. *(Bushong, pp 596, 597)*

68. **(C)** Look over the choices again, keeping in mind the factors that affect recorded detail. Looking first at SID, the options may be reduced to B and C because the increase to a 40-inch SID will certainly improve recorded detail. There is one other factor that will affect detail: the speed of the system (intensifying screens). Because a slower system will render better recorded detail, the best answer is C. The technical factors mAs, kVp, and grid ratio have no effect on recorded detail. *(Shephard, pp 247, 310)*

69. **(C)** Fluoroscopic skin dose is greater than radiographic skin dose because the x-ray source

is much closer to the patient. The generally accepted rule is that the skin receives 2 rad/min/mA. Therefore, 2 rad/min for 5 min equals 10 rad/mA. At 1.5 mA, the patient dose is 15 rad (2 rad/5 min/1.5 mA). *(Bushong, p 584)*

70. **(C)** Distortion is the result of *misalignment* of the x-ray tube, the anatomic part, and the IR. If these three parts are not parallel with one another, shape distortion occurs. The greater the misalignment, the greater the distortion. In the example cited, the image made with the *greatest tube angle* will produce the greatest distortion. Distortion is often introduced intentionally to visualize some structure to better advantage. The 37° (caudad) AP axial projection of the skull, for example, projects the facial bones inferiorly so that the occipital bone can be visualized to better advantage. *(Shephard, pp 231–234)*

71. **(A)** A 1984 review of radiation exposure data revealed that the average annual dose equivalent for monitored radiation workers was approximately 0.23 rem (2.3 mSv). The fact that this is approximately one tenth of the recommended limit indicates that the limit is adequate for radiation protection purposes. Therefore, the NCRP reiterates its 1971 recommended annual limit of 5 rem (50 mSv). *(Bushong, p 557)*

72. **(C)** The sternum has three parts: The uppermost portion is the *manubrium* (and is quadrilateral in shape), the midportion is the *body* or *gladiolus*, and the distal portion is the *ensiform* or *xiphoid* process. The sternum supports the clavicles superiorly and provides attachment for the ribs laterally. The first seven pairs of ribs are true or *vertebrosternal* ribs, as they attach directly to the sternum. The ribs angle obliquely *anteriorly and inferiorly* so that their anterior portions are 3 to 5 inches inferior to their posterior attachment. The *sternoclavicular* joints afford the only bony attachment between the thorax and the upper extremity. *(Bontrager, p 336)*

73. **(B)** Image intensification is a process that converts the dim fluoroscopic image into a much brighter image, much like normal daylight. As

x-ray photons emerge from the patient and enter the image intensifier, they first encounter the *input phosphor*, which is generally composed of cesium iodide phosphors. At the input phosphor, x-ray photons are converted to light photons, which in turn strike the photocathode. The *photocathode* is a photoemissive metal (usually antimony and cesium compounds); when struck by light, it emits electrons in proportion to the intensity of the light striking it. The electrons are then directed to the *output phosphor* via the *electrostatic focusing lenses*, speeded up in the neck of the tube by the *accelerating anode*, and directed to the output phosphor for further amplification. Most image intensifiers offer brightness gains of 5000 to 20,000. *From the output phosphor, the image is taken by the TV camera, most often a Plumbicon or Vidicon tube, and transferred to the TV monitor.* A cine camera is required to record images on 16- or 35-mm film. *(Thompson et al, p 370)*

74. **(B)** A *densitometer* indicates optical density by providing a digital readout of the quantity of light transmitted through an x-ray image. A *sensitometer* is a device used to produce a consistent gray scale exposure on film, usually in conjunction with processor sensitometry. A *penetrometer* is an aluminum step wedge that may be radiographed to produce a gray scale. H&D (Hurter & Driffield) curves are sensitometric curves of a film emulsion's response to light and radiation. *(Shephard, p 102)*

75. **(A)** The greater and lesser tubercles are prominences on the proximal humerus, separated by the bicipital groove. The AP projection of the humerus in *external rotation* demonstrates the *greater tubercle* in profile. With the arm placed in *internal rotation*, the humerus is placed in a true lateral position and the *lesser tubercle* is demonstrated. *(Bontrager, p 177)*

76. **(B)** As kVp is increased, x-ray photons begin to interact with atoms of tissue via the Compton scattered interaction. Scattered x-ray photons result, which serve only to add unwanted, undiagnostic densities (scattered radiation fog) to the radiologic image. (While Compton scatter reduces patient dose, compared to photo-

electric interactions, it can pose a significant radiation hazard to personnel during fluoroscopic procedures.) Therefore, the use of *optimal kVp* is recommended to reduce the production of scattered radiation. Scattered radiation is also a function of the *size* and content of the irradiated field. The greater the volume and atomic number of the tissue, the greater the production of scattered radiation. Although there is little that can be done about the atomic number of the structure to be radiographed, every effort can be made to keep the field size restricted to the essential area of interest in an effort to decrease production of scattered radiation. *Grids* have no effect on the *production* of scattered radiation, but they are very effective in removing scattered radiation from the beam before it strikes the IR. *(Fauber, pp 71, 103)*

77. **(B)** Calcium tungstate intensifying screens had a broad range of emitted light, and it was more likely that somewhat different film emulsions could still be compatible with them. However, rare earth phosphors emit light over a relatively short range, usually in the green portion of the spectrum. The film emulsion must be sensitive and responsive to that particular color, or the expected results will not occur. If, for example, a blue-sensitive emulsion were matched with green-emitting screens, the resulting radiograph would be underexposed because the blue-sensitive film emulsion was not responsive to the green-emitting phosphors. *(Shephard, pp 65–66)*

78. **(B)** As the kilovoltage is increased, a greater number of electrons are driven across to the anode with greater force. Therefore, as energy conversion takes place at the anode, *more high-energy photons are produced*. However, because they are *higher energy* photons, there will be less patient absorption. *(Fauber, p 58)*

79. **(D)** Unexposed, undeveloped silver is removed from film emulsion in the fixer solution. It is recovered (reclaimed) from the solution and sold. The silver may be reclaimed electrolytically or with a metallic replacement cartridge. Silver may also be reclaimed from

processed radiographs or unexposed film. (*Selman, p 203; Shephard, pp 155–160*)

80. **(D)** Motion causes unsharpness that destroys detail. Careful and accurate patient instruction is essential for minimizing voluntary motion. Suspended respiration eliminates respiratory motion. Using the shortest possible exposure time is essential to decrease involuntary motion. Immobilization can also be very useful in eliminating motion unsharpness. (*Fauber, pp 87–88*)

81. **(A)** The effects of a quantity of radiation delivered to a body are dependent on several factors: the amount of radiation received, the size of the irradiated area, and how the radiation is delivered in time. If the radiation is delivered in portions over a period of time, it is said to be *fractionated* and has a *less harmful* effect than if the radiation were delivered all at once. With fractionation, cells have an opportunity to repair, and so some recovery occurs between doses. (*Bushong, p 496*)

82. **(D)** Shape distortion is caused by misalignment of the x-ray tube, the body part to be radiographed, and the IR. An object can be falsely imaged (foreshortened or elongated) as a result of incorrect placement of the tube, the part, or the IR. Only one of the three need be misaligned for distortion to occur. (*Selman, pp 225–226*)

83. **(B)** As the exposed film enters the processor from the feed tray, it first enters the *developer* section (1), where *exposed* silver bromide crystals are reduced to black metallic silver. The film then enters the *fixer* (2), where the *unexposed* silver grains are removed from the film by the clearing agent. The film then enters the wash section (3), where chemicals are removed from the film to preserve the image. From the wash, the film enters the dryer section (4). (*Selman, p 194*)

84. **(A)** The genetically significant dose (GSD) illustrates that large exposures to a few people are cause for little concern when diluted by the total population. On the other hand, we all share the burden of that radiation that is received by the total population; and especially as the use of medical radiation increases, each individual's share of the total exposure increases. (*Bushong, p 589*)

85. **(C)** A patient with a respiratory disease can transmit infectious organisms via airborne contamination (if the patient sneezes or coughs). Therefore, patients with upper respiratory tract infection should be transported wearing a mask, to prevent the possibility of airborne contamination. It is not necessary for the radiographer to be masked. (*Torres et al, p 69*)

86. **(B)** Phosphors used in intensifying screens must *absorb* a high percentage of the incident x-ray photons and convert x-ray photon energy to fluorescent light energy. Afterglow is an undesirable characteristic of phosphors, as continued fluorescence causes unpredictable and increased density. (*Shephard, p 65*)

87. **(C)** If the x-ray tube is angled significantly *across the lead strips* of a focused grid, there is uniform loss of density (grid cutoff). Insufficient or excessive *distance* with focused grids causes loss of density (grid cutoff) along the periphery of the image. Figure 7–9 demonstrates grid cutoff everywhere except along a central vertical strip of the image. This density loss is due to the focused grid's being placed *upside down*. Thus, the middle vertical lead strips allow x-rays to pass, but because the lead strips cant laterally, they are directly opposite to the direction of the x-ray photons (rather than parallel to them), and severe grid cutoff results. (*Fauber, pp 123–124*)

88. **(C)** When high-speed electrons strike surfaces other than the tungsten target, x-rays may be produced and emitted in all directions. X-ray tubes therefore have a lead-lined metal protective housing to absorb much of this "leakage radiation." Leakage radiation must not exceed 100 mR/hr at a distance of 1 m from the tube. Because the production of x-radiation requires the use of exceedingly high voltage, the tube housing also serves to protect from electric shock. The production of x-rays involves the production of large quantities of heat, which can be damaging to the x-ray tube. Therefore,

an oil coolant surrounds the x-ray tube to further insulate it and to absorb heat from the x-ray tube structures. *(Bushong, p 131)*

89. **(C)** *Absorption* occurs when an x-ray photon interacts with matter and disappears, as in the photoelectric effect. *Scattering* (change in direction) occurs when there is *partial* transfer of energy to matter, as in the Compton effect. The *reduction in the intensity* of an x-ray beam as it passes through matter is called *attenuation. (Bushong, pp 185–186)*

90. **(D)** Most of the occupational exposure received by radiographers is received during fluoroscopy and mobile radiography, and the use of lead aprons is required during both of these procedures. The position of the personnel monitor relative to the lead apron therefore becomes important. It is recommended that the badge be worn outside the lead apron at collar level. In this position, the badge will record the maximum possible exposure received by the radiographer and will provide a realistic estimate of thyroid and lens exposure. *(Bushong, p 594)*

91. **(B)** Of the given factors, kilovoltage and grid ratio will have a significant effect on the scale of radiographic contrast. The mAs values are almost identical. Because an increased kilovoltage and low-ratio grid combination would allow the greatest amount of scattered radiation to reach the IR, thereby producing more gray tones, B is the best answer. Group D also uses a low-ratio grid, but the kilovoltage is too low to produce as many gray tones as B. *(Shephard, p 308)*

92. **(B)** The spinal cord is a column of nervous tissue about 17 inches (44 cm) in length. It is somewhat flattened anteroposteriorly and extends from the medulla oblongata of the brain to the level of L2 within the spinal canal. Because the adult spinal cord ends at the level of L2, a lumbar puncture is usually performed below that level—generally at the level of L3–4. A lumbar puncture may be performed for the removal of spinal fluid for diagnostic purposes or for the injection of medications. *(Tortora & Derrickson, p 440)*

93. **(B)** LET expresses the rate at which photon or particulate energy is transferred to (absorbed by) biologic material (through ionization processes); it is dependent on the type of radiation and absorber characteristics. Relative Biological Effectiveness describes the degree of response or amount of biologic change that one can expect of the irradiated material. As the amount of transferred energy (LET) increases (from interactions occurring between radiation and biologic material), the amount of biologic effect/damage will also increase; that is, the two are directly related. *(Bushong, p 495)*

94. **(A)** As the kilovoltage is increased, more penetration will occur and a greater range of densities (grays) will be apparent in the image. This is termed *long scale or low contrast*. In addition, as the kVp and scale of grays increase, the *exposure latitude increases*; the "margin for error" in technical factors becomes greater. As the mAs is decreased to compensate for the increased kVp, density should remain the same. *(Shephard, p 204)*

95. **(D)** If an x-ray image was placed on an illuminator and 100% of the illuminator's light was transmitted through the image, that image must have a density of 0. According to the equation,

$$\text{Density} = \log_{10} \frac{\text{incident light intensity}}{\text{transmitted light intensity}}$$

if 10% of the illuminator's light passes through the image, that image has a density of 1. If 1% of the light passes through the image, that image has a density of 2. *(Fauber, p 197)*

96. **(C)** At a given exposure, higher speed intensifying screens will emit more fluorescent light, thereby increasing radiographic density. Faster intensifying screens allow a considerable reduction in mAs, and therefore in patient dose and motion unsharpness. Intensifying-screen speed is unrelated to scattered radiation. *(Shephard, p 68)*

97. **(B)** The high-voltage, or step-up, transformer functions to *increase voltage* to the necessary

kilovoltage. It *decreases* the *amperage to milliamperage.* The amount of increase or decrease depends on the transformer ratio, that is, the ratio of the number of turns in the primary coil to the number of turns in the secondary coil. The transformer law is as follows: To determine secondary kV,

$$\frac{V_s}{V_p} = \frac{N_s}{N_p}$$

To determine secondary *I*,

$$\frac{N_s}{N_p} = \frac{I_p}{I_s}$$

Substituting known values,

$$\frac{x}{110} = \frac{80,000}{100}$$
$$100x = 8,800,000$$
$$x = 88,000 \text{ V (88 kVp)}$$

(Saia, p 420)

98. **(D)** The figure illustrates a *wire mesh* test for *screen–film contact.* If the intensifying screens and the film do not make perfect contact, recorded detail can be seriously compromised. In this test, a wire mesh supported between two rigid pieces of clear plastic is used to evaluate screen–film contact. The mesh is placed on a cassette and radiographed. Upon viewing, any areas that appear unsharp or blurry are indicative of poor screen–film contact. A *bar pattern* is used to evaluate screen resolution, a *star pattern* is used to evaluate the focal spot, and a *Wisconsin cassette* can be used to evaluate kVp calibration. *(Shephard, p 54)*

99. **(C)** A beveled focal track extends around the periphery of the anode disc; when a small angle is used, the beveled edge allows for a smaller effective focal spot and better detail. The disadvantage, however, is that photons are noticeably absorbed by the "heel" of the anode, resulting in a smaller percentage of x-ray photons at the anode end of the x-ray beam and a concentration of x-ray photons at the cathode end of the beam. This is known as the anode heel effect and can cause a primary beam variation of up to 45%. The anode heel

effect becomes more pronounced as the SID decreases, as IR size increases, and as target angle decreases. *(Bushong, pp 138–140)*

100. **(B)** *Subcutaneous emphysema* is a pathologic distention of tissues with air; *pulmonary emphysema* is a chronic disease characterized by overdistention of the alveoli with air. *Osteomalacia* is a softening of bone so that it becomes flexible, brittle, and deformed. Both of these conditions involve a *decrease in tissue density,* and therefore require a *decrease in exposure factors. Atelectasis* is a collapsed or airless lung; it requires an *increase* in exposure factors. *(Carlton & Adler, p 257)*

101. **(A)** The x-ray tube's glass envelope and oil coolant are considered *inherent* filtration. Thin sheets of aluminum are *added* to make a total of 2.5 mm Al equivalent filtration in equipment operated above 70 kVp. The function of aluminum filtration is to remove from the x-ray beam the soft (long-wavelength) x-ray photons that do not contribute to image formation but simply contribute to patient dose. These soft x-rays penetrate only a small thickness of tissue before being absorbed. *(Selman, p 411)*

102. **(B)** High-kilovoltage exposures produce large amounts of scattered radiation, and high-ratio grids are often used with high-kV techniques in an effort to absorb more of this scattered radiation. However, as more scattered radiation is absorbed, more primary radiation is absorbed as well. This accounts for the increase in mAs required when changing from an 8:1 to a 16:1 grid. In addition, precise centering and positioning become more critical; a small degree of inaccuracy is more likely to cause grid cutoff in a high-ratio grid. *(Bushong, pp 252–255)*

103. **(B)** The use of high kVp with a fairly low-ratio grid will be ineffective in ridding the remnant beam of scattered radiation. To improve contrast in this example, it has been decided to *decrease the kilovoltage by 15%,* thus making it necessary to *increase* the mAs from 5 to *10 mAs.* Because an increase in the grid ratio to 12:1 is also desired, another change in mAs will

be required (remember, 10 mAs is now the *old* mAs):

$$\frac{10 \text{ (old mAs)}}{x \text{ (new mAs)}} = \frac{4 \text{ (8:1 grid factor)}}{5 \text{ (12:1 grid factor)}}$$

$$4x = 50$$

$$x = 12.5 \text{ mAs at 90 kVp}$$

Now determine the *exposure time* required with 400 mA to produce 12.5 mAs:

$$400x = 12.5$$

$$x = 0.03 \text{ second exposure}$$

(Selman, p 214)

104. **(D)** The thicker and more dense the anatomic part being studied, the less bright will be the fluoroscopic image. Both mA and kVp affect the fluoroscopic image in a way similar to the way they affect the radiographic image. For optimum contrast, especially taking into consideration the patient dose, higher kVp and lower mA are generally preferred. *(Carlton & Adler, p 540)*

105. **(A)** The *RAO* position affords a good view of the pyloric canal and duodenal bulb. It is also a good position for the barium-filled esophagus, projecting it between the vertebrae and the heart. The *left lateral* projection of the stomach demonstrates the left retrogastric space; the *recumbent PA* is used as a general survey of the gastric surfaces; and the *recumbent AP* with slight left oblique affords a double contrast of the pylorus and duodenum. *(Bontrager, p 474)*

106. **(D)** The automatic processor's roller system consists of a series of rollers, propelled by gears, that transport the film from one solution to another and through the dryer section. As the film is being transported, solution is agitated along the film surface. Rollers coming into very close contact with the film provide a squeegee action to remove excess solution from the emulsion surface. *(Carlton & Adler, p 302)*

107. **(B)** Proper functioning of the phototimer depends on accurate positioning by the radiographer. The correct *photocell*(s) must be selected and the anatomic part of interest must com-

pletely cover the photocell(s) to achieve the desired density. If a photocell is left uncovered, scattered radiation from the part being examined will cause premature termination of exposure and an underexposed radiograph. *(Carlton & Adler, pp 505, 508)*

108. **(B)** If the same kilovoltage is used with single-phase and three-phase equipment, the three-phase unit will require about 50% less mAs to produce similar radiographs. Because three-phase equipment has much higher effective voltage than single-phase equipment, the three-phase radiograph will have lower contrast. Lower mAs can be used with three-phase equipment, and so heat units are not built up as quickly. *When technical factors are adjusted to obtain the same density and contrast, there is no difference in patient dose. (Selman, pp 162–164)*

109. **(C)** Because mammographic techniques operate at very low kVp levels, the cassette front material becomes especially important. The use of soft, low-energy x-ray photons is the underlying principle of mammography; any attenuation of the beam would be most undesirable. Special plastics that resist impact and heat softening, such as polystyrene and polycarbonate, are frequently used as cassette front material. *(Shephard, p 49)*

110. **(C)** There are several ways to reduce the amount of scattered radiation reaching the IR. First, the use of *optimum kVp* is essential; excessive kVp will increase the production of scattered radiation. Second, conscientious use of the *beam restrictor* (collimator) will reduce scattered radiation; the smaller the volume of irradiated tissue, the less scattered radiation is produced. The use of *grids* helps clean up scattered radiation before it reaches the IR. The size of the tube *focus* has an impact on image geometry and recorded detail, but it has no effect on scattered radiation. *(Shephard, p 203)*

111. **(A)** Inspiration and expiration images are frequently requested when examining patients for *pneumothorax*, or to demonstrate degree of *diaphragm excursion* or the presence of a *foreign body*. The *expiration* radiograph (image 1) demonstrates fewer ribs projected above the

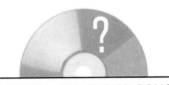

diaphragm. Because a smaller volume of air is contained within the lungs, the expiration radiograph requires an increase in exposure of approximately 6 to 8 kVp. A *lordotic* position projects the clavicles above the pulmonary apices. A *ventral decubitus* position may be used to demonstrate air–fluid levels and is made using a horizontal x-ray beam with the patient in the prone position. *(Ballinger & Frank, vol 1, p 516)*

112. **(B)** Each film passing through the processor solutions takes with it a certain amount of solution. Replenishment is also essential for maintaining each solution's level of concentration, to maintain solution activity and avoid chemical fog from exhausted solutions. One way to determine the quantity of replenisher solution to be added is by the *length of the film* entering the processor. A microswitch initiates and terminates replenishment as it senses the beginning and end of each film. Replenishment is also determined by the *number of films* (volume) processed. The greater the number of films processed, the lower the required replenishment rate. *(McKinney, p 106)*

113. **(B)** To demonstrate the intercondyloid fossa, the central ray must be directed perpendicular to the long axis of the tibia (Fig. 7–24). Because the knee is flexed so that the tibia forms a 40° angle with the IR, the central ray must be directed 40° caudad to place the central ray perpendicular to the long axis of the tibia.

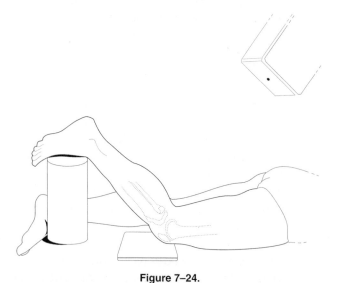

Figure 7–24.

Directing the central ray to the popliteal depression aligns the central ray parallel with the knee joint space. *(Bontrager, p 236)*

114. **(D)** In CPR for infants the rescuer places his index finger on the sternum just below the level of the intermammary line. The second and third fingers are used to compress the sternum 1/2 to 1 inch during compressions. The recommended rate is 100 compressions per minute. The volume of air delivered during ventilation should be just enough to make the infants chest rise and fall. *(Adler & Carlton, p 244)*

115. **(C)** The term *radiolucent* refers to a material through which x-rays will pass easily. Contrast agents such as barium and iodine are radioopaque; an example of a *radiolucent* contrast agent is *air*. Radioopaque contrast agents appear white on the finished image because many x-ray photons are absorbed by the dense agent. *Radiolucent* contrast agents appear *black* on the finished image because x-ray photons pass easily through. *(Shephard, pp 200–202)*

116. **(C)** The degree of anterior and posterior motion is occasionally diminished with a "whiplash"-type injury. Anterior (forward, *flexion*) and posterior (backward, *extension*) motion is evaluated in the lateral position with the patient assuming flexion and extension as best as he or she can. *Left and right bending* images of the thoracic and lumbar vertebrae are frequently obtained when evaluating scoliosis. The AP *open-mouth projection* is used to evaluate the first two cervical vertebrae. The *moving mandible* AP is used to demonstrate the entire cervical spine while blurring out the superimposed mandible. *(Ballinger & Frank, vol 1, p 398)*

117. **(D)** The processor's pumping mechanisms transport the solution through heating devices to maintain the proper *temperature*. The solution is then returned under pressure for recirculation. The added pressure functions to *agitate* the solution and keep it in *close contact* with the film emulsion. *(Bushong, p 212)*

118–119. **(118, C; 119, A)** An anterior view of the foot and ankle bones is illustrated. The ankle

joint is formed by the articulation of the tibia, fibula, and talus (7). The tibial (medial) malleolus is labeled 8; the fibular (lateral) malleolus is labeled 1. The talus articulates with the calcaneus (2) inferiorly and with the navicular (6) anteriorly. The cuboid (3) is seen anterior to the calcaneus, and the three cuneiforms (5) are anterior to the navicular. *(Saia, p 103)*

120. **(D)** When scheduling patient examinations, it is important to avoid the possibility of residual contrast medium covering areas of interest on later examinations. The IVP should be scheduled first, because the contrast medium used is excreted rapidly. The BE should be scheduled next. Finally, the upper GI is scheduled. Any barium remaining from the previous BE should not be enough to interfere with the stomach or duodenum (a preliminary scout image should be taken in each case). *(Torres et al, pp 233–234)*

121. **(D)** The *synchronous timer* is an older type of x-ray timer that does not permit very precise, short exposures. The *impulse timer* permits a shorter, more precise exposure, and the *electronic timer* may be used for exposures as short as 0.001 second. The *phototimer,* however, automatically terminates the exposure when the proper density has been recorded on the IR. The important advantage of the phototimer, then, is that it can accurately duplicate radiographic densities. It is therefore very useful for providing accurate comparison in follow-up examinations, and for decreasing patient dose by decreasing the number of "retakes" required because of improper exposure. Remember that proper functioning of the phototimer depends on accurate positioning (and centering) by the radiographer. *(Bushong, pp 115–117)*

122. **(B)** *Sterile* technique is required for administration of contrast media by the *intravenous* and *intrathecal* (intraspinal) methods. *Aseptic* technique is used for administration of contrast media by the oral and rectal routes, as well as through the nasogastric tube. *(Torres et al, pp 270–271)*

123. **(B)** As x-ray photons are produced at the tungsten target, they more readily diverge toward the cathode end of the x-ray tube. As they try to diverge toward the anode, they interact with and are absorbed by the anode "heel." Consequently, there is a greater intensity of x-ray photons at the cathode end of the x-ray beam. This phenomenon is known as the anode heel effect. Because shorter SIDs and larger IR sizes require greater divergence of the x-ray beam to provide coverage, the anode heel effect will be accentuated. *(Bushong, pp 138–140)*

124. **(C)** The infraorbitomeatal line (IOML) is an imaginary line extending from the infraorbital margin to the external auditory meatus and is represented by number 3. The IOML is used for most lateral skull projections, including lateral projections of facial bones. The skull is positioned so that the MSP is parallel to the cassette, the interpupillary line is perpendicular to the cassette, and the IOML is parallel to the long (transverse) axis of the cassette. Number 1 is the glabellomeatal line, 2 is the OML (orbitomeatal line), and 4 is the acanthomeatal line. These baselines are used to obtain accurate positioning in skull radiography. *(Ballinger & Frank, vol 2, p 252)*

125. **(B)** The patient is well positioned; the spinous processes and sternum are clearly seen without superimposition. Adequate penetration and long-scale contrast are present without excessive radiographic density. The patient had been properly shielded for the PA projection; however, the shield was not moved to the correct location prior to the lateral exposure. *(Ballinger & Frank, vol 3, p 162)*

126. **(D)** Follow-up studies have been done on individuals receiving accidental exposure to radiation (medical personnel, uranium miners, children irradiated in vivo). Pioneer radiation workers developed leukemia and other cancers, their vision was clouded by formation of cataracts, and their lives were shorter than those of their colleagues. With today's sophisticated equipment and knowledge of radiation protection, none of these situations should occur. *(Bushong, pp 537–540)*

127. **(A)** *Heparin* is produced by the body (especially in the liver) and functions to prevent

intravascular clotting. Heparin is also produced artificially and used to treat throm-
boembolic disorders. Lidocaine and Benadryl
are drugs that are usually available on crash
carts for emergency use. *Lidocaine* is used to
treat ventricular arrhythmias, and *Benadryl* is
used to treat allergic reactions and acute anaphylaxis. *(Torres et al, p 284)*

128. **(C)** Every radiographic image is composed of
a number of different densities. These densities may be measured and given a numeric
value with a device called a *densitometer.*
A *sensitometer* is another device used in quality control programs; it is used to give a precise exposure to a film emulsion. An *aluminum
step wedge* (penetrometer) may be used to
show the effect of kVp on contrast. A *spinning
top* is used to test the accuracy of the x-ray machine's timer or rectifiers. *(Bushong, p 275)*

129. (C) To change nongrid to grid exposure, or to
adjust exposure when changing from one grid
ratio to another, remember the factor for each
grid ratio:

No grid = 1 × original mAs
5:1 grid = 2 × original mAs
6:1 grid = 3 × original mAs
8:1 grid = 4 × original mAs
12:1 grid = 5 × original mAs
16:1 grid = 6 × original mAs

Therefore, to change from nongrid exposure
to an 8:1 grid, multiply the original mAs by a
factor of 4. A new mAs of 32 is required.
(Saia, p 324)

130. **(B)** The *midcoronal* plane (1) divides the body
into anterior and posterior halves. A *coronal*
plane is any plane parallel to the midcoronal
plane. The *midsagittal* plane (2) divides the
body into left and right halves. A *sagittal* plane
is any plane parallel to the midsagittal plane.
A *transverse* or *horizontal* plane (3) is perpendicular to the midsagittal plane and midcoronal
plane, dividing the body into superior and inferior portions. *(Saia, p 72)*

131. **(D)** Pulmonary vascular markings are often
prominent in the elderly and in smokers.

Quiet, shallow breathing may be used during
a long exposure (with a compensating low
mA) to blur them out. *Oblique sternum, AP
scapula*, and the *lateral thoracic spine* are examinations in which this technique is useful.
(Ballinger & Frank, vol 1, pp 202, 422, 474)

132. **(D)** Streptococcal pharyngitis (strep throat) is
caused by bacteria. To know this, you have to
remember that bacteria are classified according to their morphology (ie, size and shape).
The three classifications are spirals, rods
(bacilli), and spheres (cocci). Viruses, unlike
bacteria, cannot live outside of a human cell.
Viruses attach themselves to a host cell and
invade the cell with its genetic information.
Various fungal infections may grow on the
skin (cutaneously), or they may enter the skin.
Fungal infections that enter the circulatory or
lymphatic system can be deadly. Protozoa are
one-celled organisms classified by their motility. Ameboids move by locomotion, flagella
use their protein tail, cilia possess numerous
short protein tails, and sporozoans are actually
not mobile. *(Adler & Carlton, pp 196–199)*

133. **(C)** A lateral projection of the fourth finger is
best obtained if the finger is positioned so that
there is as little OID as possible. Therefore,
with only the fourth finger extended in the
lateral position, the arm is positioned on the
ulnar (medial) surface. This places the finger
closer to the IR than if it were positioned radial side down. Excessive magnification distortion is avoided, and better recorded detail
is obtained. *(Ballinger & Frank, vol 1, p 94)*

134. **(A)** The oblique axial projection is valuable
when the zygomatic arches cannot be demonstrated bilaterally with the submentovertical
projection, because they are not prominent
enough or because of a depressed fracture.
The patient may still be positioned as for an
SMV, but the head is obliqued 15° toward the
side being examined. This serves to move
the zygomatic arch away from superimposed
structures and provides a slightly oblique axial projection of the arch. *(Bontrager, p 401)*

135. **(A)** A PA axial Caldwell position is illustrated,
demonstrating the *frontal and ethmoidal* sinuses.

The Caldwell position requires an angle of 15° caudad, exiting the nasion. The petrous ridges should be projected in the lower third of the orbits. The illustrated radiograph demonstrates somewhat excessive angulation because the petrous pyramids are projected at the bottom of the orbits. The *maxillary* sinuses are demonstrated in the parietoacanthial projection (Waters position), and the *sphenoidal* sinuses are demonstrated through the open mouth in a modified Waters' position. The mastoid sinuses/air cells are part of the temporal bone and are radiographically unrelated to the paranasal sinuses. *(Bontrager, p 429)*

136. **(C)** A phototimer is one type of automatic exposure device. When it is installed in the x-ray unit, it is calibrated to produce radiographic densities as required by the radiologist. Once the part being radiographed has been exposed to produce the proper image density, the phototimer automatically terminates the exposure. *The manual timer should be used as a backup timer should the phototimer fail to terminate the exposure, thus protecting the patient from overexposure and the x-ray tube from excessive heat load. Circuit breakers and fuses are circuit devices used to* protect circuit elements from overload. In case of current surge, the circuit will be broken, thus preventing equipment damage. A *rheostat* is a type of variable resistor. *(Shephard, p 274)*

137. **(A)** It is occasionally necessary to view the lung apices free of superimposition with the clavicles. This objective can be achieved in the AP axial projection. The patient is positioned AP erect with the central ray directed 15° cephalad, entering the manubrium. An AP axial projection can also be obtained with the patient in the lordotic position. If sufficient lordosis can be assumed, the central ray is directed perpendicular to the IR. *(Ballinger & Frank, vol 1, p 544)*

138. **(C)** Contrast media may be administered in a variety of manners in cholangiography, including

1. an endoscope with a cannula placed in the hepatopancreatic ampulla (of Vater) for an ERCP.

2. a needle or small catheter placed directly in the common bile duct for an operative cholangiogram.
3. a very fine needle through the patient's side and into the liver for a percutaneous transhepatic cholangiogram.
4. via an indwelling T-tube for a postoperative or T-tube cholangiogram.

(Ballinger & Frank, vol 2, p 78)

139. **B.** Radiographic technique charts are highly recommended for use with every x-ray unit. A technique chart identifies the standardized factors that should be used with that particular x-ray unit, for various examinations/positions, of anatomic parts of different sizes. To be used effectively, these technique charts require that the anatomic part in question be measured correctly with a *caliper*.

A *fulcrum* is of importance in tomography, a *densitometer* is used in sensitometry and QA. *(Ballinger & Frank, vol 3, p 237)*

140. **(C)** Radiographic rating charts enable the operator to determine the maximum safe milliamperage, exposure time, and kVp for a particular exposure using a particular x-ray tube. An exposure that can be made using the large focal spot may not be safe when the small focal spot of the same x-ray tube is used. The total number of HU an exposure generates also influences the amount of stress (in the form of heat) imparted to the anode. *Single-phase HU* are determined by the product of mAs and kVp. *Three-phase, six-pulse HU* are determined from the product of mA × time × kVp × 1.35. *three-phase, 12-pulse HU* are determined from the product of mA × time × kVp × 1.41. In the examples given, then, group A produces 6091 HU, group B produces 14,805 HU, group C produces 1997 HU, and group D produces 7106 HU. Therefore, group *A* exposure factors will deliver the *least amount of heat* to the anode. *(Fauber, pp 36–37)*

141. **(D)** Converting from nongrid to an 8:1 grid requires about a fourfold increase in mAs. Increasing the kVp by 15% and cutting the mAs in half would reduce patient dose. When

changing from general radiographic technical factors to tomographic factors, it is generally recommended that the kVp remain the same and that mAs be increased by 50%. Changing from a 400 speed system to a 200 speed system will require the mAs to be doubled. Therefore, the largest increase would be required by the addition of a grid. *(Bushong, p 252)*

142. **(B)** Rotation of the chest is evidenced in the following ways: The distance between the medial aspect of the clavicles and the lateral portion of the vertebral column is asymmetrical, the air-filled trachea is off midline, and the scapulae and air-filled lungs are asymmetric. The exposure was made during reasonably good inspiration as evidenced by visualization of eight ribs above the diaphragm. The upper and lateral aspects of the lungs, including the pulmonary apices and costophrenic angles, are demonstrated. Even minimal rotation of the chest introduces significant distortion of the heart. *(Ballinger & Frank, vol 1, p 514)*

143. **(C)** To place the right posterior axillary ribs parallel to the IR, an *RPO* position is required. The *LAO* will also demonstrate the right axillary ribs, but primarily the anterior portion. The *RAO* position will demonstrate the left anterior axillary ribs, and the *LPO* will demonstrate the left posterior axillary ribs. *(Ballinger & Frank, vol 1, pp 490, 498)*

144. **(D)** Generally, contrast medium is injected into the subarachnoid space between the third and fourth lumbar vertebrae. Because the spinal cord ends at the level of the first or second lumbar vertebra, this is considered to be a relatively safe injection site. The cisterna magna can be used, but the risk of contrast entering the ventricles and causing side effects increases. Diskography requires injection of contrast medium into the individual intervertebral disks. *(Saia, p 200)*

145. **(D)** Improper support of a patient's fractured lower leg (tibia/fibula) while performing radiography could result in movement of the fracture fragments, which can cause tearing of the soft tissue, nerves, and blood vessels. In

addition, lack of support may cause muscle spasm, which can make closed reduction of some fractures difficult. *(Bontrager, p 295)*

146. **(B)** Intervertebral joints are well visualized in the lateral projection of all the vertebral groups. Cervical articular facets (forming apophyseal joints) are 90° to the MSP and therefore are well demonstrated in the lateral projection. The cervical intervertebral foramina lie 45° to the MSP (and 15° to 20° to a transverse plane), and are therefore demonstrated in the oblique position. *(Bontrager, p 295)*

147. **(D)** Postoperative, or T-tube, cholangiography is frequently performed to evaluate the patency of the biliary ducts and to identify any previously undetected stones. Following surgery, a T-tube is left in place within the common bile duct, with the vertical portion of the *T* extending outside the body. Water-soluble iodinated medium is injected, and fluoroscopic examination is carried out. *(Ballinger & Frank, vol 2, p 78)*

148. **(C)** During radiography and fluoroscopy, radiation scatters from the patient in all directions. In fact, the patient is the single most important scattering object in both radiographic and fluoroscopic procedures. The approximate intensity (quantity) of scattered radiation at 1 m from the patient is *0.1% of the entrance dose.* Therefore, if the entrance dose for this image is 320 mR, the intensity of radiation at 1 m from the patient is 0.1% of that, or 0.32 mR (0.001 × 320 = 0.32). *(Bushong, p 572)*

149. **(A)** Because patient dose is regulated by the quantity of x-ray photons delivered to the patient, mAs regulates patient dose. Highly energetic x-ray photons (high kVp) are more likely to penetrate the patient, rather than be absorbed by biologic tissue. Consequently, the use of high-kVp and low-mAs exposure factors is preferred in an effort to reduce patient dose. The use of high-speed screens can assist in the reduction of exposure factors. *(Bushong, p 162)*

150. **(B)** The most hazardous time for abdominal irradiation is in the earliest stages of pregnancy,

when many women are unaware that they are pregnant. For this reason, *it is recommended that elective radiologic procedures be performed within the first 10 days following the onset of the menses.* It is during this time that the danger of irradiating a recently fertilized ovum is most unlikely. About 14 days before the onset of menses is when the ovarian follicle ruptures and liberates an ovum. *(Bushong, pp 563–564)*

151–152. (151, C; 152, D) A parietoacanthial projection (Waters' position) of the skull is pictured. The chin is elevated sufficiently to project the petrous ridges below the *maxillary sinuses* (number 4). Note that the foramen rotundum is seen near the upper margin of the maxillary sinuses. Other paranasal sinus groups are not well visualized in this position, although a modification with the mouth open may be taken to demonstrate the *sphenoidal* sinuses. This is also the single best projection to demonstrate the *facial bones*. The *zygomatic arch* (number 2) is well demonstrated; the mandible, its *angle* (number 1), and the *coronoid process* (number 3) are also well demonstrated. The odontoid process is seen projected through the foramen magnum. The *mastoid* air cells are seen adjacent to the mandibular angle as multiple small, air-filled, bony spaces. *(Ballinger & Frank, vol 2, pp 333, 369)*

153. (B) Esophageal varices are best demonstrated when there is increased venous pressure and when blood is flowing against gravity. Therefore, to demonstrate the twisted, dilated condition of venous varicosities, esophagograms must be performed in the *recumbent* position. In the *erect* position, the veins appear more smooth and normal. *Fowler's* position describes a position in which the patient's head is higher than the feet, and *Sims'* position is preferred for insertion of the enema tip. *(Ballinger & Frank, vol 2, p 100)*

154. (B) In the *low-kilovoltage* ranges, a difference of just a few kVp makes a very noticeable radiographic difference, that is, there is little latitude. *High kVp* techniques offer a much greater margin for error, as do *slower film–screen* combinations. Grid ratio is unrelated to *exposure*

latitude, but higher ratio grids offer *less tube centering latitude* (leeway, margin for error) than low-ratio grids. *(Carlton & Adler, p 185)*

155. (A) As SID increases, so does recorded detail, because magnification is decreased. Therefore, SID is *directly* related to recorded detail. As focal spot size *increases*, recorded detail *decreases* because more penumbra is produced. Focal spot size is thus *inversely* related to radiographic sharpness or recorded detail. Tube current affects radiographic density and is unrelated to recorded detail. *(Fauber, pp 79, 81)*

156. (A) The sacroiliac joints angle posteriorly and medially 25° to the MSP. Therefore, to demonstrate them with an AP oblique projection, the *affected side* must be elevated 25°. This places the joint space perpendicular to the IR and parallel to the central ray. When the PA oblique projection is used, the *unaffected side* will be elevated 25°. *(Ballinger & Frank, vol 1, pp 442–443)*

157. (B) A double-focus tube has two *focal spot* sizes available. These focal spots are actually two available paths on the focal track. There are also two *filaments*. When the small focal spot is selected, the small filament is heated, and electrons are driven across to the smaller portion of the focal track. When the large focal spot is selected, the large filament is heated, and electrons are driven across to the larger portion of the focal track. *(Bushong, pp 132–134)*

158–159. (158, C; 159, B) An LPO of the lumbar spine is pictured. The patient is positioned so that the lumbar spine forms a 45° angle with the IR. The apophyseal joints (those closest to the IR) are well demonstrated in this position. The typical "scotty dog" image is depicted. The "ear" of the scotty is the superior articular process (number 1) and the front foot is the inferior articular process (4). The scotty's eye is the pedicle its "body" is the lamina (3), and its nose is the transverse process (2). *(Bontrager, p 312)*

160. (C) With the patient in the lateral position, the MSP is parallel to the x-ray tabletop. Because the *inter*vertebral foramina, which are formed by the *pedicles*, are 90° to the MSP, they

are well demonstrated in the lateral projection. The intervertebral joints (disk spaces) are also well demonstrated. The spinal cord passes through the *vertebral foramina,* which would not be visualized in conventional radiography of the lumbar spine. *(Saia, p 132)*

161. **(A)** Since 4500 mrad is equal to 4.5 rad, if 4.5 rad were delivered in 6 minutes, then the dose rate must be 0.75 rad/min:

$$\frac{4.5 \text{ rad}}{6 \text{ min}} = \frac{x \text{ rad}}{1 \text{ min}}$$
$$6x = 4.5$$
$$x = 0.75 \text{ rad/min}$$

(Selman, p 528)

162. **(D)** Breast tissue has very low subject contrast, but it is imperative to visualize microcalcifications and subtle density differences. Fine detail is necessary to visualize any microcalcifications; therefore, a small focal spot tube is essential. High contrast (and therefore low kilovoltage) is needed to accentuate any differences in tissue density. A compression device serves to even out differences in tissue thickness (thicker at chest wall, thinner at nipple) and decrease object–image recorder distance, and helps decrease the production of scattered radiation. *(Peart, pp 49–50)*

163. **(A)** It is our ethical responsibility to minimize radiation dose to patients. X-rays produced at the target make up a heterogeneous primary beam. There are many "soft" (low-energy) photons that, if not removed, would contribute only to greater patient dose. They are too weak to penetrate the patient and expose the IR. These soft x-rays penetrate only a small thickness of tissue before being absorbed. *(Fauber, pp 32–33)*

164–165. (164,B; 165, D) An anterior view of the forearm is pictured. The proximal anterior surface of the ulna (number 8) presents a rather large pointed process at the anterior margin of the semilunar (trochlear) notch (5) called the *coronoid process* (6). The olecranon process is identified as number 4, and the radial notch of the ulna is number 7. Distally, the ulnar head is number 9, and the styloid process is labeled

10. The radius (number 12) is the lateral bone of the forearm. The radial head is number 3, the radial neck is number 2, and the radial tuberosity is number 1. Distally, the radial *styloid* process is labeled 11. *(Saia, p 90)*

166. **(D)** The PA axial (Caldwell) projection of the paranasal sinuses is used to demonstrate the frontal and ethmoidal sinuses. The central ray is angled caudally 15° to the OML. This projects the petrous pyramids into the lower one-third of the orbits, thus permitting optimal visualization of the frontal and ethmoidal sinuses. *(Bontrager, p 429)*

167. **(B)** In mutual induction, two coils are in close proximity, and a current is supplied to one of the coils. As the magnetic field associated with every electric current expands and "grows up" around the first coil, it interacts with and "cuts" the turns of the second coil. This interaction, *motion* between magnetic field and coil (conductor), *induces* an emf in the second coil. This is mutual induction, the production of a current in a neighboring circuit. *Transformers* such as the high-voltage transformer and the filament (step-down) transformer operate on the principle of mutual induction. The *autotransformer* operates on the principle of self-induction. Both the transformer and the autotransformer require the use of alternating current. *(Bushong, p 99)*

168. **(A)** The line focus principle illustrates that as the target angle decreases, the effective focal spot decreases (providing improved recorded detail), but the actual area of electron interaction remains much larger (allowing for greater heat capacity). *It must be remembered, however, that a steep (small) target angle increases the heel effect, and part coverage may be compromised. (Saia, p 427)*

169. **(D)** Because the toes curve naturally downward, the interphalangeal joints are not well demonstrated in the AP (dorsoplantar) projection. To "open" the interphalangeal joints, the central ray should be directed 15° cephalad. Another method is to place a 15° foam sponge wedge under the foot, elevating the toes 15° from the IR; the central ray would then be directed perpendicularly. *(Bushong, p 137)*

170. **(B)** The most commonly used method of low-flow oxygen delivery is the *nasal cannula*. It can be used to deliver oxygen at rates from 1 to 4 mL/min at concentrations of 24% to 36%. The nasal cannula also provides increased patient freedom to eat and talk, which a mask does not. *Masks* are used for higher flow concentrations of oxygen, over 5 mL/min; depending on the type of mask, they can deliver anywhere from 35% to 60% oxygen. *Respirators* or *ventilators* are high-flow delivery mechanisms that are used for patients who are in severe respiratory distress or are unable to breathe on their own. *Oxyhoods* or tents are generally used for pediatric patients who may not tolerate a mask or cannula. The amount of oxygen delivered is somewhat unpredictable, especially if the opening is frequently accessed. Oxygen delivery may be between 20% and 100%. (*Adler & Carlton, pp 188–190*)

171. **(D)** A thin chest would require a *greater degree of obliquity* to separate the vertebrae and sternum from superimposition than would a thick chest. With the patient in the RAO position, the sternum is projected to the left of the vertebral column and superimposed on the heart. This superimposition promotes more uniform tissue density and therefore more uniform radiographic density. Prominent pulmonary vascular markings may be obliterated by allowing the patient to breathe (shallow breaths only) during a long exposure (with a very low mA). (*Saia, p 135*)

172. **(C)** A signed consent form (informed consent) is not necessary prior to performing an *upper GI* series. Informed consent is necessary before performing any procedure that is considered invasive or that carries considerable risk. A *myelogram*, a *cardiac catheterization*, and an *interventional vascular procedure* are all invasive procedures, and all carry some degree of risk. A physician should explain to the patient what those risks are, as well as the risk of not having the procedure. In addition, the patient should be made aware of alternative procedures and the risks associated with the alternatives. Only after the patient has been made aware and all questions have been answered appropriately should the informed consent be signed. A radiographer is not responsible for obtaining informed consent. However, in some institutions, it may be departmental procedure for the radiographer to check the chart and see if there is a signed consent form in place. (*Adler & Carlton, p 350*)

173. **(C)** Interviewing skills, the collection of valuable objective and subjective patient data (clinical history), are an important function of the health-care professional. Objective data are those that are discernible to the senses of the *interviewer: objective signs* that can be heard, seen, or felt. Subjective data are those that can be discerned only by the *patient:* pain, emotions, etc. *Chief complaint* is the principal medical problem as stated by the patient. (*Adler & Carlton, p 136*)

174. **(A)** The *control badge* is an important part of the monitoring system. It should be stored somewhere *away from radiation sources*. At the end of the monitoring period, when the badges are returned to the dosimetry service, the exposure to the control badge (which should be zero) is compared to the exposure received by the rest of the personnel monitors. If the control badge is stored near radiation or used to replace someone's lost badge, there is no standard for comparison for the rest of the group of monitors. (*Bushong, p 596*)

175. **(B)** The American Hospital Association identifies 12 important areas in its "Patients' Bill of Rights." These include the right to refuse treatment (to the extent allowed by law), the right to confidentiality of records and communication, and the right to continuing care. Other patient rights identified are the right to informed consent, privacy, respectful care, access to records, refuse to participate in research projects, and an explanation of the hospital bill. (*Torres et al, p 12*)

176. **(C)** Fidelity, veracity, nonmalficence, and beneficence are all ethical principles. *Nonmalficence* is the principle that refers to the prevention of harm. *Beneficence* is the ethical principle that refers to bringing about good or benefiting others. *Fidelity* refers to faithfulness and *veracity* refers to truthfulness. (*Adler & Carlton, p 308*)

177. **(C)** A radiographer who fails to wear a lead apron when performing portable radiography is in direct violation of the ARRT Code of Ethics for the Profession of Radiologic Technology. Although this may seem to some to be a personal decision, the fact is that our profession demands that we protect not only others, but ourselves as well from unnecessary radiation exposure. Participating in continuing education is every radiographer's duty, and not only is in keeping with the ARRT Code of Ethics, but now is also mandatory for renewal of ARRT certification. Under normal circumstances, patient confidentiality is of the utmost importance, and radiographers must always respect a patient's right to privacy. There are special circumstances, however, where a radiographer is negligent if he or she does not communicate confidential information to the proper individuals. These cases include suspected cases of child abuse and any instance where the welfare of an individual or community is at risk. The professional radiographer is encouraged to investigate new and innovative techniques. As technology continues to grow, we must grow with it. There are often new and better ways to perform procedures, especially as equipment changes occur. *(Torres et al, pp 8–9)*

178. **(C)** Hospital Information Systems must ensure confidentiality in compliance with Health Insurance Portability and Accountability Act of 1996 (HIPAA) regulations. Most institutions now have computerized, paperless systems that accomplish the same information transmittal; these systems must ensure confidentiality in compliance with HIPAA regulations. The health-care professional generally has access to the computerized system only via personal password, thus helping to ensure confidentiality of patient information. All medical records and other individually identifiable health information, whether electronic, on paper, or oral, are covered by HIPAA legislation and by subsequent Department of Health and Human Services (HHS) rules that took effect in April of 2001. *(Torres et al, p 20)*

179. **(A)** Evaluation of the acromioclavicular joints requires bilateral AP or PA erect projections with and without the use of weights. Weights are used to emphasize the minute changes within a joint caused by separation or dislocation. The use of weights should be avoided if a fracture of the affected area is suspected. *(Ballinger & Frank, vol 1, p 90)*

180. **(D)** Fidelity, veracity, nonmalficence, and beneficence are all ethical principles. *Nonmalficence* is the principle that refers to the prevention of harm. *Beneficence* is the ethical principle that refers to bringing about good, or benefiting others. *Fidelity* refers to faithfulness and *veracity* refers to truthfulness. *(Adler & Carlton, p 308)*

181. **(C)** There is no preparation required for an abdominal survey. For an upper gastrointestinal (upper GI) series and a lower GI series (BE), the patient should be npo, or have nothing by mouth, for 8 to 10 hours prior to the examination. In addition, a low-residue diet may be imposed, fluid intake may be increased, and cleansing enemas and laxatives may be prescribed to rid the colon of fecal matter. *(Adler & Carlton, p 307)*

182. **(B)** The pregnant radiographer poses a special radiation protection consideration, as the safety of the unborn individual must be considered. It must be remembered that the developing fetus is particularly sensitive to radiation exposure. Established guidelines state that the occupational radiation exposure to the fetus must not exceed 0.5 rem (500 mrem, or 5 mSv) during the entire gestation period. *(Bushong, p 557)*

183. **(D)** Epidemiologic studies indicate that AIDS can be transmitted only by intimate contact with body fluids of an infected individual. This can occur through the sharing of contaminated needles, through sexual contact, and from mother to baby at childbirth (perinatal). AIDS can also be transmitted by transfusion of contaminated blood. *(Torres et al, p 116)*

184. **(D)** Sterilization is the complete elimination of all living microorganisms, and it can be accomplished by several methods. *Pressurized steam*, in an *autoclave*, is probably the most familiar means of sterilization; the pressure allows higher temperatures to be achieved. *Gas*

or *chemical* sterilization is used for items that are unable to withstand moisture and/or high temperatures. Other methods of sterilization include *dry heat*, ionizing *radiation*, and microwaves (*nonionizing radiation*). *(Torres et al, p 116)*

185. **(A)** Mature white blood cells (*lymphocytes*) are considered the most radiosensitive cells. *Ova* (female germ cells) are very radiosensitive, but not to the same degree as lymphocytes. *Myocytes* (muscle cells) and especially *neurons* (nerve cells) are actually radioresistant. *(Gurley & Callaway, p 246)*

186. **(A)** Proper body mechanics includes a wide base of support. The *base of support* is the portion of the body that is in contact with the floor or some other horizontal plane. The *center of gravity* is the midpoint of the pelvis or lower abdomen, depending on body build. The *line of gravity* is the abstract line passing vertically through the center of gravity. Proper body mechanics can help prevent painful back injuries by making proficient use of the muscles in the arms and legs. *(Torres et al, pp 82–83)*

187. **(B)** Rare earth phosphors have a greater conversion efficiency than do other phosphors. Lanthanum oxybromide is a blue-emitting phosphor, and gadolinium oxysulfide is a green-emitting phosphor. Cesium iodide is the phosphor used on the input screen of image intensifiers; it is not a rare earth phosphor. *(Shephard, p 66)*

188. **(D)** Double-contrast studies of the stomach or large intestine involve coating the organ with a thin layer of barium sulfate and then introducing air. This permits seeing through the organ to the structures behind it, and most especially allows visualization of the mucosal lining of the organ. A barium-filled stomach or large bowel demonstrates the position, size, and shape of the organ and any lesion that projects out from its walls, such as diverticula. Polypoid lesions, which project inward from the wall of an organ, may go unnoticed unless a double-contrast examination is performed. *(Turley & Calloway, p 126)*

189. **(D)** A patient who has been recumbent for some period of time and gets up quickly may suffer from lightheadedness or feel faint. This is referred to as *orthostatic hypertension*. It is best to have patients sit up and dangle their feet from the table for a moment while being supported, and then assist them off the table. Patients will also feel better emotionally if they are not rushed or treated like they are on an assembly line. Always assist patients on and off of the radiographic table. Even healthy, young outpatients can injure themselves. Patients with *dyspnea* or *orthopnea* are unable to lie supine. Dyspnea and orthopnea refer to difficulty breathing; this may be due to a heart condition, asthma, strenuous exercise, or excessive anxiety. *Hypertension* refers to the condition of elevated blood pressure. *(Adler & Carlton, pp 148–149)*

190. **(D)** Most needle sticks occur while attempting to recap a needle. Several diseases, including hepatitis and HIV, can be transmitted via a needle stick. Therefore, do not attempt to recap a needle, but rather dispose of the entire syringe with needle attached in the special container that is available. *(Torres et al, pp 63–66)*

191. **(C)** Angina pectoris is a spasmodic chest pain that is frequently due to oxygen deficiency in the myocardium. The pain often radiates down the left arm and up to the left jaw. Angina pectoris attacks are frequently associated with exertion or emotional stress in individuals with coronary artery disease. Pain may be relieved with a vasodilator such as *nitroglycerin* given sublingually or transdermally. *Digitalis* is used to treat congestive heart failure. *Dilantin* is used in the control of seizure disorders, and *cimetidine (Tagamet)* is used to treat duodenal ulcers. *(Torres et al, p 282)*

192. **(A)** This is the definition of *fog*. Anything other than intensifying screen light or primary x-radiation is undesirable in terms of image exposure. *Log relative exposure* is the amount of exposure required to produce a given density as measured on the sensitometric graph. *Optical density* is normal radiographic density. An *artifact* is anything foreign

to the image; the term could include fog, but it also covers many physical interferences. (*Selman, pp 196–197*)

193. **(C)** The occupational dose limit is valid for *beta, x-,* and *gamma* radiations. Because alpha radiation is so rapidly ionizing, traditional personnel monitors will not record alpha radiation. Because alpha particles are capable of penetrating only a few centimeters of air, they are practically harmless as an external source. (*Selman, p 395*)

194. **(A)** With three-phase equipment, the voltage never drops to zero and x-ray intensity is significantly greater. When changing *from single-phase to three-phase, six-pulse equipment, two thirds of the original mAs are required* to produce a radiograph with similar density. (When going from three-phase, six-pulse to single-phase, add one-third more mAs.) When changing *from single-phase to 3-phase, 12-pulse equipment, only one half of the original mAs is required.* (Going from three-phase, 12-pulse to single-phase requires twice the mAs.) In this instance, we are changing from single-phase to three-phase, 12-pulse equipment; therefore the new mAs should be half the original 50 mAs, or *25 mAs.* The only selection that will provide 25 mAs is A, 200 mA. B will produce 75 mAs (600 mA × 1/8 s = 75 mAs); C will produce 50 mAs (400 mA × 0.125 s = 50 mAs); D will produce 100 mAs (400 × 0.25 = 100 mAs). (*Carlton & Adler, p 98*)

Comparison of Technical Factors Required

Single-Phase	Three-Phase, 6-Pulse	Three-Phase, 12-Pulse
x mAs	*2/3x* mAs	*1/2x* mAs

195. **(B)** In the parietoorbital projection (Rhese method), the patient is prone with the acanthomeatal line perpendicular to the IR. The head rests on the forehead, nose, and chin, and the MSP should form 53° with the IR (37° with the central ray). Radiographically, the optic canal should appear in the *lower outer quadrant* of the orbit. Incorrect *rotation* of the MSP results in *lateral displacement,* and incorrect positioning of the *baseline* results in *longi-*

tudinal displacement of the optic canal. (*Ballinger & Frank, vol 2, pp 290–293*)

196. **(C)** Although the *inferosuperior axial* projection can be used to evaluate the glenohumeral joint, the required abduction of the arm would be contraindicated when evaluating a shoulder for possible dislocation. The *transthoracic lateral* projection is used to evaluate the glenohumeral joint and upper humerus when the patient is unable to abduct the arm (as in dislocation). The *scapular Y* projection is an oblique projection of the shoulder and is used in demonstrating anterior or posterior dislocation. (*Ballinger & Frank, vol 1, pp 166, 179*)

197. **(B)** Standard blood and body fluid precautions serve to protect health-care workers and patients from the spread of diseases such as AIDS and AIDS-related complex. Although the precautions are indicated for *all* patients, special care must be emphasized when working with patients whose infectious status is unknown (eg, the emergency trauma patient). Gloves must be worn if the radiographer may come in contact with blood or body fluids. A gown should be worn if the clothing may become contaminated. Blood spills should be cleaned with a solution of 1 part bleach to 10 parts water. (*Torres et al, pp 62–65*)

198. **(C)** X-ray tube life may be extended by using exposure factors that produce a minimum of heat (a *lower mAs and higher kVp* combination) whenever possible. When the rotor is activated, the filament current is increased to produce the required electron source (thermionic emission). *Prolonged rotor time,* then, can lead to shortened filament life due to early vaporization. Large *exposures to a cold anode* will heat the anode surface, and the temperature difference between surface and interior can cause cracking of the anode. This can be avoided by proper warming of the anode prior to use, thereby allowing sufficient dispersion of heat through the anode. (*Selman, pp 147–148*)

199. **(D)** The thoriated tungsten filament of the cathode assembly is heated by its own filament circuit. This circuit provides current and voltage to *heat the filament* to incandescence, at

which time it undergoes thermionic emission (the liberation of valence electrons from filament atoms). The greater the *number of electrons* flowing between the cathode and the anode, the greater the *tube current (mA)*. *Rectification* (single- or three-phase) is the process of changing alternating current to unidirectional current. A greater number of secondary *transformer* turns functions to increase voltage and decrease current. *(Bushong, pp 132–133)*

200.   **(D)** Technique charts are exposure factor *guides* that help technologists produce radiographs with consistent density and contrast. They suggest a group of exposure factors to be used at a particular SID with a particular grid ratio, screen–film combination, focal spot size, and central ray angulation. *Technique charts do not take into account the nature of the part* (disease, atrophy, etc). *(Shephard, p 298)*

Subspecialty List

67. Radiation protection
68. Image production and evaluation
69. Radiation protection
70. Image production and evaluation
71. Radiation protection
72. Radiographic procedures
73. Equipment operation and quality control
74. Image production and evaluation
75. Radiographic procedures
76. Image production and evaluation
77. Image production and evaluation
78. Radiation protection
79. Image production and evaluation
80. Image production and evaluation
81. Radiation protection
82. Image production and evaluation
83. Image production and evaluation
84. Radiation protection
85. Patient care and education
86. Image production and evaluation
87. Image production and evaluation
88. Radiation protection
89. Radiation protection
90. Radiation protection
91. Image production and evaluation
92. Patient care and education
93. Radiation protection
94. Image production and evaluation
95. Image production and evaluation
96. Radiation protection
97. Equipment operation and quality control
98. Equipment operation and quality control
99. Image production and evaluation
100. Image production and evaluation
101. Radiation protection
102. Image production and evaluation
103. Image production and evaluation
104. Equipment operation and quality control
105. Radiographic procedures
106. Image production and evaluation
107. Equipment operation and quality control
108. Equipment operation and quality control
109. Image production and evaluation
110. Image production and evaluation
111. Radiographic procedures
112. Image Production and Evaluation
113. Radiographic Procedures
114. Patient Care and Education
115. Equipment operation and maintenance
116. Radiographic procedures
117. Image production and evaluation
118. Radiographic procedures
119. Radiographic procedures
120. Radiographic procedures
121. Equipment operation and quality control
122. Patient care and education
123. Image production and evaluation
124. Radiographic procedures
125. Radiographic procedures
126. Radiation protection
127. Patient care and education
128. Equipment operation and quality control
129. Image production and evaluation
130. Radiographic procedures
131. Radiographic procedures
132. Patient care and education
133. Radiographic procedures
134. Radiographic procedures
135. Radiographic procedures
136. Radiation protection
137. Radiographic procedures
138. Radiographic procedures
139. Radiation protection
140. Equipment operation and quality control
141. Radiation protection
142. Radiographic procedures
143. Radiographic procedures
144. Radiographic procedures
145. Radiographic procedures
146. Radiographic procedures
147. Radiographic procedures
148. Radiation protection
149. Radiation protection
150. Radiation protection
151. Radiographic procedures
152. Radiographic procedures
153. Radiographic procedures
154. Image production and evaluation
155. Image production and evaluation
156. Radiographic procedures
157. Equipment operation and quality control
158. Radiographic procedures
159. Radiographic procedures
160. Radiographic procedures
161. Radiation protection
162. Equipment operation and quality control
163. Radiation protection
164. Radiographic procedures
165. Radiographic procedures
166. Radiographic procedures
167. Equipment operation and quality control
168. Image production and evaluation

169. Radiographic procedures
170. Patient care and education
171. Radiographic procedures
172. Radiographic procedures
173. Patient care and education
174. Radiation protection
175. Patient care and education
176. Patient care and education
177. Patient care and education
178. Patient care and education
179. Radiographic procedures
180. Patient care and education
181. Radiographic procedures
182. Radiation protection
183. Patient care and education
184. Patient care and education

185. Radiation protection
186. Patient care and education
187. Image production and evaluation
188. Radiographic procedures
189. Patient care and education
190. Patient care and education
191. Patient care and education
192. Image production and evaluation
193. Radiation protection
194. Image production and evaluation
195. Radiographic procedures
196. Radiographic procedures
197. Patient care and education
198. Equipment operation and quality control
199. Image production and evaluation
200. Image production and evaluation